FDA'S ROLE IN PROTECTING THE PUBLIC HEALTH: EXAMINING FDA'S REVIEW OF SAFETY AND EFFICACY CONCERNS IN ANTI-DEPRESSANT USE BY CHILDREN

HEARING

BEFORE THE

SUBCOMMITTEE ON
OVERSIGHT AND INVESTIGATIONS

OF THE

COMMITTEE ON ENERGY AND COMMERCE
HOUSE OF REPRESENTATIVES

ONE HUNDRED EIGHTH CONGRESS

SECOND SESSION

SEPTEMBER 23, 2004

Serial No. 108–125

Printed for the use of the Committee on Energy and Commerce

Available via the World Wide Web: http://www.access.gpo.gov/congress/house

U.S. GOVERNMENT PRINTING OFFICE

96–099PDF WASHINGTON : 2005

For sale by the Superintendent of Documents, U.S. Government Printing Office
Internet: bookstore.gpo.gov Phone: toll free (866) 512–1800; DC area (202) 512–1800
Fax: (202) 512–2250 Mail: Stop SSOP, Washington, DC 20402–0001

COMMITTEE ON ENERGY AND COMMERCE

JOE BARTON, Texas, *Chairman*

W.J. "BILLY" TAUZIN, Louisiana
RALPH M. HALL, Texas
MICHAEL BILIRAKIS, Florida
FRED UPTON, Michigan
CLIFF STEARNS, Florida
PAUL E. GILLMOR, Ohio
JAMES C. GREENWOOD, Pennsylvania
CHRISTOPHER COX, California
NATHAN DEAL, Georgia
RICHARD BURR, North Carolina
ED WHITFIELD, Kentucky
CHARLIE NORWOOD, Georgia
BARBARA CUBIN, Wyoming
JOHN SHIMKUS, Illinois
HEATHER WILSON, New Mexico
JOHN B. SHADEGG, Arizona
CHARLES W. "CHIP" PICKERING, Mississippi, *Vice Chairman*
VITO FOSSELLA, New York
STEVE BUYER, Indiana
GEORGE RADANOVICH, California
CHARLES F. BASS, New Hampshire
JOSEPH R. PITTS, Pennsylvania
MARY BONO, California
GREG WALDEN, Oregon
LEE TERRY, Nebraska
MIKE FERGUSON, New Jersey
MIKE ROGERS, Michigan
DARRELL E. ISSA, California
C.L. "BUTCH" OTTER, Idaho
JOHN SULLIVAN, Oklahoma

JOHN D. DINGELL, Michigan *Ranking Member*
HENRY A. WAXMAN, California
EDWARD J. MARKEY, Massachusetts
RICK BOUCHER, Virginia
EDOLPHUS TOWNS, New York
FRANK PALLONE, Jr., New Jersey
SHERROD BROWN, Ohio
BART GORDON, Tennessee
PETER DEUTSCH, Florida
BOBBY L. RUSH, Illinois
ANNA G. ESHOO, California
BART STUPAK, Michigan
ELIOT L. ENGEL, New York
ALBERT R. WYNN, Maryland
GENE GREEN, Texas
KAREN McCARTHY, Missouri
TED STRICKLAND, Ohio
DIANA DEGETTE, Colorado
LOIS CAPPS, California
MICHAEL F. DOYLE, Pennsylvania
CHRISTOPHER JOHN, Louisiana
TOM ALLEN, Maine
JIM DAVIS, Florida
JANICE D. SCHAKOWSKY, Illinois
HILDA L. SOLIS, California
CHARLES A. GONZALEZ, Texas

BUD ALBRIGHT, *Staff Director*
JAMES D. BARNETTE, *General Counsel*
REID P.F. STUNTZ, *Minority Staff Director and Chief Counsel*

SUBCOMMITTEE ON OVERSIGHT AND INVESTIGATIONS

JAMES C. GREENWOOD, Pennsylvania, *Chairman*

MICHAEL BILIRAKIS, Florida
CLIFF STEARNS, Florida
RICHARD BURR, North Carolina
CHARLES F. BASS, New Hampshire
GREG WALDEN, Oregon *Vice Chairman*
MIKE FERGUSON, New Jersey
MIKE ROGERS, Michigan
JOE BARTON, Texas, (Ex Officio)

PETER DEUTSCH, Florida *Ranking Member*
DIANA DEGETTE, Colorado
TOM ALLEN, Maine
JANICE D. SCHAKOWSKY, Illinois
HENRY A. WAXMAN, California
EDWARD J. MARKEY, Massachusetts
JOHN D. DINGELL, Michigan, (Ex Officio)

CONTENTS

FDA'S ROLE IN PROTECTING THE PUBLIC HEALTH: EXAMINING FDA'S REVIEW OF SAFETY AND EFFICACY CONCERNS IN ANTI-DEPRESSANT USE BY CHILDREN

THURSDAY, SEPTEMBER 23, 2004

HOUSE OF REPRESENTATIVES,
SUBCOMMITTEE ON OVERSIGHT AND INVESTIGATIONS,
COMMITTEE ON ENERGY AND COMMERCE,
Washington, DC.

The subcommittee met, pursuant to notice, at 11:05 a.m., in room 2123, Rayburn House Office Building, Hon. Joe Barton (chairman) presiding.

Members present: Representatives Bilirakis, Stearns, Bass, Walden, Ferguson, Rogers, Barton (ex officio), Deutsch, DeGette, Allen, Schakowsky, and Waxman

Also present: Representative Stupak.

Staff present: Mark Paoletta, majority counsel; Alan Slobodin, majority counsel; Kelli Andrews, majority counsel; Joby Fortson, majority counsel; Billy Harvard, majority staff assistant; David Nelson, minority investigator; and Jessica McNiece, minority research assistant.

Chairman BARTON. Today we are continuing a series of hearings on FDA's role in protecting the public health, examining the FDA's review of safety and efficacy concerns in anti-depressant use in children.

As part of this committee's jurisdiction over public health, the subcommittee today will examine the FDA's process in determining the safety and public health concerns of anti-depressants in children.

The controversy over the use of anti-depressants in children is of great public interest. Over 10 million children a year are prescribed anti-depressants in the United States. The committee's interest in this issue began in January of this year in response to media reports about the concerns over the safety and efficacy of anti-depressants used by children.

One month earlier, in December 2003, British regulators contra-indicted all anti-depressants for children except Prozac due to the risk-benefit analysis of safety concerns related to suicidal behavior coupled with a weak showing of efficacy. Despite the action taken by British regulators in December 2003, at that time in the United States there appeared to still be substantial support in the medical community for the use of anti-depressants in children and for the belief that these drugs saved children's lives.

The U.S. psychiatric establishment had repeatedly assured the public that the drugs are very safe. At around the same time that the British regulators announced their decision, an internal FDA analysis of the pediatric clinical trials of these drugs did show an increased risk of suicide related events, and seemed to be at odds with these assurances of safety.

This analysis was prepared by a medical review officer specializing in pediatric anti-depressants named Dr. Andrew Mosholder. Dr. Mosholder was first requested in June 2003 by the Neuropharm Division of FDA to perform this consult after GlaxoSmithKline provided the FDA and other regulatory agencies with an internal analysis showing an increase in suicidality during their pediatric clinical trials of the anti-depressant Paxil.

The Neuropharm Division requested that Dr. Mosholder review the Paxil data as well as the data from other pediatric clinical trials to determine whether the signal was limited to Paxil or whether other anti-depressants showed a similar association.

In September of this year—excuse me, in September 2003 Dr. Mosholder informed the agency at an internal briefing of his preliminary conclusions. He concluded that the pediatric clinical data showed an association between children taking the drug and suicide related behavior.

Dr. Mosholder completed a second consult in December 2003 which confirmed his preliminary findings reported in September. Although initially scheduled to present his findings at a February 2004 Advisory Committee meeting, the purpose of which was to publicly discuss how the agency should handle the safety issues raised in pediatric anti-depressant trials, Dr. Mosholder was informed in early January of this year he would not be presenting at the Advisory Committee.

It is my understanding that the individuals within the Neuropharm Division, who incidentally were in charge of this February meeting, told Dr. Mosholder that they had, "reached a different conclusion" about the data. As a result of this disagreement, he was prevented from presenting his analysis before the FDA Advisory Committee.

The first question that this raises is quite simple: Why? Isn't an Advisory Committee a panel of experts? Aren't those people capable of hearing different points of view and making decisions? What was the harm in allowing Dr. Mosholder an opportunity to present his data, his analysis, and his opinion to a group of experts?

I am looking forward to hearing from Dr. Mosholder and some of the other FDA witnesses about these issues to get to the very heart of this matter.

On September 13, 2004, which was just several weeks ago, the FDA convened another meeting of the Advisory Committee to consider the question again, whether there was an increased risk of suicide related behavior in children taking anti-depressants. This time at this meeting, Dr. Mosholder did present his data.

As I understand it, the FDA also presented another analysis recently completed by Dr. Hammad. Both Dr. Hammad's analysis and Dr. Mosholder's December 2003 analysis essentially reached the same conclusions. There is an increase in suicide related behavior with children taking anti-depressants.

Let me repeat that. Their two analyses essentially reached the same conclusions. There is an increase in suicide related behavior with children taking anti-depressants. The agency now acknowledges this association.

Where do we go from here? The FDA has now looked at the issue in depth and has indicated that they are just about ready to announce a final course of action. What that course of action is and when it will be implemented are two questions this committee is very interested in knowing.

Will we have a black box on these drugs? Will we have a new and stronger warning label? Will we have a pamphlet, known as a Med Guide, attached to the drug? Will we contra-indict the drug like they did in Britain when they banned it from pediatric populations? Will we have an informed consent form signed by the patient, parent and physician? These are all questions that need to be addressed at today's hearing.

We look forward to getting answers to these questions and a better sense of direction about where the FDA is going.

One final issue that I want an answer today from the FDA: When the FDA first become aware of the potential link between anti-depressants and suicidality in children, and what did they do to get to the bottom of it?

Throughout our investigation, we have learned that as far back as 1996, 8 years ago, a medical review at FDA, Dr. James Knudsen, raised the question of an increase in suicidality in pediatric clinical trials of a drug called Zoloft. There was also an analysis in 1997 of Luvox, another anti-depressant, where the review, the same Dr. Mosholder, noted that there was an increase in hostility in children versus adults. The issue is noted in the Luvox labeling as a result.

The fact that children taking anti-depressants were experiencing psychiatric adverse events at greater rates than adults was known at the agency as far back as 1996 and 1997. This committee wants to know what did the agency do to respond to these concerns? Did they require that pediatric clinical trials conducted pursuant to the Best Pharmaceuticals for Children Act be designed to capture these types of safety issues? If not, why not? Did the agency alert their medical reviewers to this potential issue, tell them to look closely at that type of data that the companies were submitting in their pediatric trials? If not, why not?

I hope that today we will be able to view the whole picture concerning anti-depressants and their effect on children as well as the FDA approval process as a whole. The FDA's task is quite commendable. It is not easy. They are entrusted with being the guardians of our safety. That is a very difficult trust to maintain.

As Members of Congress, it is our duty to ensure through the oversight process that the FDA undertake this task in an earnest and diligent and, I might also say, an open and transparent fashion. We must ensure that the FDA fulfills its public health role and its public trust.

The FDA serves the American people. We are the client. The mission of the FDA is not to protect the FDA's internal workings, but to promote and protect the public health by helping safe and effective products reach the market by monitoring for safety, by disclosing the accurate, science based information, and for providing this in a clear and concise and timely fashion to the American people.

Is the FDA accomplishing its mission with anti-depressants used by children? I would have to say the record is open on that, and I would say that, unless we get some very straight answers at today's hearing, it is probably going to be answered that the FDA is not fulfilling its mission in this particular issue.

At the September 9 hearing concerning the publication of anti-depressant clinical trial data, I was upset with the FDA's lack of full cooperation with the documentation production process pursuant to this committee's request. Since that hearing, I have met with the Acting FDA Commissioner, Dr. Lester Crawford, about the issue of FDA's cooperation in this matter.

I would like to take note that, since that meeting, there has been improvement in the FDA's cooperation in document production, and for that I want to thank Dr. Crawford publicly. I also want to thank Dr. Crawford for his assistance with securing the appearances of some of the witnesses that will be speaking today.

Finally, I would like to thank the FDA in their diligence to responding to several member questions that were raised at the September 9 hearing.

Having said that, I must say that we continue to be somewhat surprised when we questioning them about their policy of document retention at the FDA. The answer we got back was, in writing, that they had none—that they have no policy for document retention, which is something that we still need to address with them.

I must say, though, that since the last hearing the FDA is cooperating much more cooperatively with this committee, and again for that I want to thank all of our FDA representatives.

[The prepared statement of Hon. Joe Barton follows:]

PREPARED STATEMENT OF HON. JOE BARTON, CHAIRMAN, COMMITTEE ON ENERGY AND COMMERCE

As part of the Committee's jurisdiction over public health, the Subcommittee today will examine the Food and Drug Administration's (FDA's) process in determining the safety and public health concerns of anti-depressants in children.

The controversy over the use of anti-depressants in children is of great public interest. Over 10 million children a year are prescribed anti-depressants in the United States. The Committee's interest in this issue began in January of this year in response to media reports about the concerns over the safety and efficacy of anti-depressants used by children. One month earlier, in December 2003, British regulators contraindicated all anti-depressants for children, except Prozac, due to the risk-benefit analysis of safety concerns related to suicidal behavior coupled with a weak showing of efficacy.

Despite the action taken by British regulators in December of 2003, at that time, in the United States there appeared to still be substantial support in the medical community for the use of antidepressants in children, and for the belief that these drugs save children's lives. The U.S. psychiatric establishment had repeatedly assured the public that the drugs are very safe. At around the same time that the British regulators announced their decision, an internal FDA analysis of the pediatric clinical trials of these drugs showed an increased risk of suicide-related events and seemed to be at odds with these assurances of safety. This analysis was prepared by a medical review officer specializing in pediatric anti-depressants named Dr. Andrew Mosholder. Dr. Mosholder was first requested in June 2003, by the Neuropharm division of FDA to perform this consult, after GlaxoSmithKline provided the FDA and other regulatory agencies, with an internal analysis showing an increase in suicidality during their pediatric clinical trials of the anti-depressant

Paxil. The Neuropharm division requested that Dr. Mosholder review the Paxil data, as well as the data from the other pediatric clinical trials, to determine whether the signal was limited to Paxil or whether other anti-depressants showed a similar association. In September 2003, Dr. Mosholder informed the agency at an internal briefing of his preliminary conclusions: the pediatric clinical data showed an association between children taking the drug and suicide-related behavior. Dr. Mosholder completed a second consult in December 2003, which confirmed his preliminary findings reported in September. Although initially scheduled to present his findings at a February 2004 Advisory Committee meeting-the purpose of which was to publicly discuss how the agency should handle the safety issues raised in pediatric anti-depressant trials-Dr. Mosholder was informed in early January 2004, he would not be presenting at the Advisory Committee meeting. It is my understanding that individuals within the Neuropharm Division, who incidentally were in charge of this February meeting, told Dr. Mosholder-they had "reached a different conclusion" about the data. As a result of this disagreement, he was prevented from presenting his analysis before the FDA Advisory Committee.

The first question this raises is simply: why? Isn't an Advisory Committee a panel of experts? Aren't those people capable of hearing differing points of view and making decisions? What was the harm in allowing Dr. Mosholder an opportunity to present his data, his analysis and his opinion to this group of experts? I am looking forward to hearing from Dr. Mosholder and some of the other FDA witnesses about these issues, to get to heart of this matter.

On September 13, 2004, the FDA convened another meeting of the Advisory Committee to consider the question again: whether there was an increased risk of suicide-related behavior in children taking anti-depressants. This time, at this September meeting, Dr. Mosholder did present his data. As I understand it, the FDA also presented another analysis, recently completed by Dr. Hammad. Both Dr. Hammad's analysis and Dr. Mosholder's December 2003 analysis essentially reached the same conclusions-there is an increase in suicide-related behavior with children taking anti-depressants. The agency now acknowledges this association.

Where do we go from here? The FDA has now looked at the issue in depth and has indicated that they are just about ready to announce a final course of action. What that course of action is, and when will it be implemented-are two questions I am very interested to know. Will we have a "black-box" on the drugs? Will we have a new and stronger warning label? Will we have a pamphlet, known as a "Med Guide," attached to the drug? Will we contraindicate the drug like they did in Britain when they banned it from the pediatric population? Will we have an informed consent form signed by patient, parent and physician? I look forward to getting feedback on these questions and a better sense of that direction today.

One final issue that I want an answer from FDA today: When did the FDA first become aware of a potential link between anti-depressants and suicidality in children and what did they do to get to the bottom of it? Through our investigation, we have learned that as far back as 1996, a medical reviewer at FDA-a Dr. James Knudsen—raised the question of an increase in suicidality in pediatric clinical trials of Zoloft. There was also an analysis in 1997 of Luvox-another anti-depressant-where the reviewer, the same Dr. Mosholder, noted that there was an increase in hostility in children versus adults. This issue was noted in the Luvox labeling as a result.

The fact that children taking anti-depressants were experiencing psychiatric adverse events-at greater rates than adults-was known at the agency as far back as 1996 and 1997. I want to know: What did the agency do to respond to these concerns? Did they require that pediatric clinical trials conducted pursuant to the Best Pharmaceuticals for Children Act be designed to capture these types of safety issues? If not-why not? Did the agency alert their medical reviewers to this potential issue and tell them to look closely at that type of data the companies submitted in pediatric trials? If not-why not?

I hope that after today we will be able to view the whole picture concerning antidepressants and their effect on children, as well as the FDA approval process as a whole.

The FDA's task is quite commendable and not easy. They are entrusted with being guardians of our safety. As Members of Congress, it is our duty is to ensure through the oversight process that this vital agency undertake this task in an earnest and diligent manner. We must ensure that FDA fulfills its public health role. The FDA serves the American people. We are the client. The mission of the FDA is not to protect the FDA, but to promote and protect the public health by helping safe and effective products reach the market, by monitoring for safety, and by disclosing accurate, science-based information. Is FDA accomplishing its mission with anti-depressants used by children?

At the September 9th hearing concerning the publication of anti-depressant clinical trial data, I was upset with the FDA's lack of full cooperation with the document production process pursuant to the Committee's request. Since that hearing, I have met with Acting FDA Commissioner Dr. Lester Crawford about the issue of FDA's cooperation in this matter, and I would like to note that since that meeting, there has been some improvement, in FDA's cooperation and document production. I also want to thank Dr. Crawford for his assistance with securing the appearances of some of witnesses that will be speaking today. Finally, I would like to thank the FDA in their diligence in responding to several member questions that were raised at the September 9th hearing.

However, if FDA does not continue this cooperation, I will be forced to address this issue again just as I did at the September 9th hearing. Nevertheless, I am hopeful that we can continue to move forward on improved document production from the agency.

Once again, I would like to thank the witnesses for appearing today and the other members present today, and I look forward to this hearing.

Chairman BARTON. I would now like to turn to our ranking member, Mr. Deutsch for any opening statement that he wishes to make.

Mr. DEUTSCH. Thank you, Mr. Chairman, for holding this hearing and its counterpart earlier this month.

The September 9 hearing dealt with the fact that the FDA and drug companies withheld from the public the important information that all but one of the pediatric trials of anti-depressants failed to show efficacy in adolescents. Sadly, we got no good answers from the FDA witness at that time, Dr. Woodcock.

Today we deal with the critical question of the safety of these potent medications in children. Specifically, we need to understand if the risk of suicidal behavior of teens taking SSRIs is greater than the suicide risk associated with a failure to take these anti-depressants.

That is exactly the kind of straightforward, scientific question that the Congress expects FDA to answer for the American people. Unfortunately, the FDA has handled the decisions involving both the safety and efficacy of these drugs in adolescents in such an unscrupulous manner that it is very hard for anyone to accept that objective science is the basis of the agency's conclusions.

Consider that the FDA extended the monopoly status of these drugs for 6 months, costing American taxpayers and consumers over $4 billion, and then decided that the public didn't even need to know that all but one of these drugs could not demonstrate efficacy.

The only labeling change was for Prozac, the only SSRI shown to work at all in kids. Shockingly, the FDA made a deliberate decision to withhold information on the clinical failures from parents as well as pediatricians and other prescribers. But it gets even worse.

When Wyeth found evidence of elevated risk of suicidal ideation and hostility among adolescents taking its drug and tried to change its label to warn parents and providers about this increased danger, the FDA said no label change to reflect those warnings is permissible.

It is incredible that this agency charged with protecting the public health would stop a company from warning the public about risks associated with the use of its products by children. But the FDA was far from finished with its cover-up at that point.

As information flooded in from the industry and the British authorities who had banned the use of these drugs in kids, the FDA began a review of the 15 studies that had been done on pediatric use of SSRIs. They turned the project over to a scientist, Dr. Andrew Mosholder, a medical doctor, psychiatrist and epidemiologist in the Office of Drug Safety.

Dr. Mosholder's analysis of multiple studies concluded that there was indeed an elevated risk of suicidal behavior discernible from the pediatric studies. Dr. Mosholder was scheduled to present his findings before the Advisory Committee charged with recommending action to the FDA on anti-depressant drugs in February.

Someone within the FDA did not want those conclusions to be public and ripped his presentation from the program. Perhaps it was the same people who thought Wyeth shouldn't warn the public either. The FDA excuse was that the underlying data needed to be examined more critically before such a sensational conclusion could be broached publicly.

When the San Francisco Chronicle got wind of the story that the FDA had squelched its own investigator's report, the real cover-up began. Both this subcommittee and the Senate Finance Committee chaired by Senator Grassley began inquiries, but even as Congress was gearing up, senior officials within the FDA decided to conduct a witch hunt.

They sent criminal investigators to probe the source of the leak. It is readily apparent that the probe was not about information but, rather, about intimidation. It was a warning to Dr. Mosholder and other dedicated epidemiologists at the Office of Drug Safety, and the ostensible initiating officer was the Director of the Office of Drug Safety.

When we authorized the Prescription Drug User Fee Act in the last Congress, the clear tradeoff for the continuing rapid review and approval of new drug applications was that the FDA would place a renewed emphasis on post-marketing surveillance to detect safety problems with drugs just as soon as they emerged.

The Mosholder investigation is a substantive demonstration that drug safety remains a stepchild in the FDA-drug company partnership at the Center for Drug Evaluation and Research. But it gets even worse.

To be clear, the events I am about to describe involve response to requests from Senator Grassley, although I have no doubt that, had this ploy succeeded, false documents would have been supplied to this committee as well.

Andy Mosholder was forced to supply a statement to the Office of Internal Affairs regarding the events surrounding the decision to remove his analysis from the Advisory Committee's agenda and the leaking of that story to the Chronicle. This document was apparently in response to a request from Senator Grassley.

Apparently, officials in the FDA Office of Legislative Affairs and the Office of Chief Counsel met to decide how to respond. They decided that not only should the Mosholder affidavit be redacted, but that a new document needed to be created to hide the fact that an investigation had even taken place.

Ultimately, Dr. Mosholder on advice of his personal counsel declined to sign the phony document suggested and drafted by an

FDA lawyer. Had Dr. Mosholder not acted to thwart the submission of an altered document to a bona fide Congressional investigation, a criminal act of obstruction of justice would have occurred. As it was, the FDA and its lawyers are only guilty of attempting to obstruct justice.

As you are well aware, Mr. Chairman, the FDA has stonewalled lawful requests from this committee regarding documents in the past. It has also slow-rolled and stonewalled our requests for interviews.

I applaud the determination that you have shown to get to the bottom of this, despite the obstruction that has been employed by FDA and its attorneys. As a result of this committee's efforts, the Advisory Committee did receive the Mosholder analysis last week, as well as subsequent analysis done by Dr. Tarek Hammad. That reached the same conclusion.

As we are all well aware, the Advisory Committee recommended that a black box warning of increased suicide risk in children be attached to the labels of these drugs, and that patients be informed of the increased risk when each prescription is dispensed. They also recommended that each drug that has failed its efficacy test be so labeled.

I expect that the FDA will tell us at this hearing that it will adopt the recommendations of its Advisory Committee. if so, this may be an appropriate result. But for the investigations by Congress, specifically this committee, and the media, I doubt that we would have reached the level of public knowledge and concern that has prompted this result.

Mr. Chairman, I congratulate you on the witness panel you have assembled before us today. I hope that the Secretary will provide us with an accurate account of events that were exposed today.

There is something terribly rotten at the FDA. No agency charged with protecting the public health should behave with such indifference to the public safety as is evidenced in this case, and no agency should ever treat Congress with the disrespect shown by the FDA during the course of this investigation.

Again, Mr. Chairman, you are to be applauded for your determination and commitment to the public interest in pursuing this difficult inquiry.

Chairman BARTON. Thank you, Mr. Deutsch, and let me say before I recognize our vice chairman: This has been a bipartisan effort. Mr. Deutsch has been applauding me, but it is actually the entire subcommittee and the staffs on both sides. We have worked together on this, and we are finally beginning to get the truth out to the American people.

With that, I would like to recognize the distinguished vice chairman of the committee, Mr. Walden, Mr. Greg Walden, for an opening statement.

Mr. WALDEN. Thank you, Mr. Chairman. I thank you for holding this second hearing on the safety and efficacy concerns of anti-depressants in children.

Giving parents and doctors as much information about the benefits or lack thereof and the risks associated with drugs that are being prescribed for millions, tens of millions, of our Nation's children should be at the forefront of FDA's mission. I am troubled by issues raised at the last hearing about what information is on the label of these drugs and what information was publicly presented to doctors and parents about these pediatric anti-depressant trials.

Testimony from certain pharmaceutical companies at the last hearing raised two issues that I would like the agency to fully discuss today. The first question is about stronger warnings.

As I understand it, in August 2003, Wyeth Pharmaceuticals issued a "Dear Health Care Provider" letter to more than 450,000 health care practitioners warning them of increased hostility in children taking Efexir and recommending that it not be prescribed to anyone under 18 years of age. Wyeth also added a stronger warning to their label reflecting this safety issue.

Approximately 8 months later when the FDA finally decided to change the warnings on all the labels of all anti-depressants, they required Wyeth to remove—to remove this stronger labeling. What this tells me is the regulatory agency charged with protecting the public health is preventing a company from disseminating important safety information to parents, the public and physicians.

I want answers from the folks at the Neuropharm Division at FDA that made this decision to explain their rationale for it.

The second question concerns efficacy. In testimony from various pharmaceutical companies at the last hearing, it became clear that many companies—in fact, most except Eli Lilly—conducted anti-depressant clinical trials in kids that showed no efficacy. That is why none of the anti-depressants except Prozac is approved by the FDA for use in treating depressed kids.

Yet the FDA also decided not to allow the companies' product labeling to state that clinical trials conducted in kids did not demonstrate efficacy. The question is why? Why wouldn't you put that on the label? Why shouldn't the label reflect that information?

I note that the Advisory Committee just recommended that this labeling change take place, but the point is that the FDA knew about the lack of efficacy in these trials several years ago, and nothing has been done to change the label to inform doctors, patients and parents of this finding.

I am also interested to learn more about the FDA Advisory Committee process and the recommendations that the Advisory Committee made last week concerning how to notify the public that clinical trial data indicate that there is an increased risk of suicide related behavior in children that take anti-depressants.

I was struck by the press release that the FDA sent out on September 16, just a few days after their Advisory Committee meeting. Now in that release, the FDA states, "that it generally supports"—generally supports—"the recommendations of the Advisory Committee." Generally supports? To me, that sounds like the FDA has some doubts about the Advisory Committee's recommendations.

So I would like to know if the FDA has reservations about these recommendations; if so, what they are, and why. I would also like to know more about FDA's characterization of the Advisory Committee's 15 to 8 vote as, "a split decision" on whether a black box warning label should be on the labels of SSRIs.

Now it is my understanding that a black box warning will alert doctors, patients and parents about the risks of taking these drugs without preventing these drugs from being prescribed to depressed children. Now here in the House, if you get a 15 to 8 vote, a 2 to 1 margin, that is a pretty significant vote, not generally described as a split decision.

So it is my question as to how that is being described and why in the FDA's press release. Is the FDA going to follow the clear majority recommendation and implement this labeling change and, if not, why? It is my understanding that Dr. Temple and Dr. Laughren will be able to address these questions.

Finally, I hope to get some answers from the agency about the timeline of events in terms of what they told the public about safety concerns raised within the agency about children taking these drugs, and then when they told the public.

As we know, the British drug regulatory agency seemed to act much swifter on this than the FDA with the same data. So I think it is a fair question to ask this agency: Was the public health served by a longer deliberative process in this case?

I also would like to know why the agency made the decision, as you have heard from my colleagues, to prevent Dr. Mosholder from presenting the findings from his extensive 6-month analysis of data on SSRI clinical trials at the February 2004 Advisory Committee meeting.

So I will be interested in hearing Dr. Mosholder's perspective on his consult, why he believed the safety signals were robust even in December 2003, and how he believes his consult would have contributed to the February Advisory Committee's deliberative process.

We have many witnesses from the FDA today, and I am hopeful they will provide a more complete picture of this process and answer these questions that are on our minds and those of the people we represent. I thank them for being here, and I thank you, Mr. Chairman.

Chairman BARTON. We thank you, Congressman.

Now I will recognize the distinguished member from Colorado, Congresswoman DeGette, for an opening statement.

Ms. DEGETTE. Thank you, Mr. Chairman. I would ask unanimous consent to put my full statement in the record.

Chairman BARTON. Without objection, so ordered.

Ms. DEGETTE. Thank you. I would just like to make a couple of observations.

When I walked into our last hearing on September 9, I didn't know anything about this rampant off-label prescription of anti-depressants for kids, and I didn't know about the risks about it, and I don't think most Americans did know about it.

Sometimes when I go out in my district, as I have the last few weeks, my constituents say how can you stand doing the job that you do; how can you stand it back there? What I have been saying the last couple of weeks is, well, let me tell you a little story about this hearing we had in Congress where we found out that anti-depressants, which have been approved by the FDA for adults, are being prescribed for kids in rampant off-label use and, furthermore, there was data that showed that, at best, those drugs did not work, at worse and quite possibly, some of those drugs increase the risk of suicide for kids.

So after we had that hearing, and with all the press associated with that hearing and the witnesses, well, lo and behold, the FDA's Advisory Committee decided there was an increased risk of suicidality, and they recommended a black box label.

So, Mr. Chairman, I guess every so often we do do some good in Washington, but I think it is a damn shame that we have to have Congressional hearings to make that happen.

Frankly, the public is desperate. Teen depression, in particular, is on the rise. We only have one drug that has been approved by the FDA for use in kids, and parents are desperate to find some way to treat their kids. But they were unaware how the off-label use of anti-depressants could really not only not help their kids but could actually kill their kids.

Now I think that the FDA has to answer a lot of questions. They need to answer questions about, for example, why there were delays of presentation of data between the links of suicide and anti-depressants. The FDA needs to answer what steps will be taken to ensure that scientists at FDA are able to present their findings to advisory committees. They have to answer as to what future actions the FDA is taking for pediatric and adult use of anti-depressants.

The American public and the U.S. Congress rely on the FDA to ensure that all approved pharmaceuticals are safe. This is the responsibility that is at the very core of the FDA's mission, and to fulfill that mission the FDA must conduct objective studies with rigorous scientific inquiry, and then they must present the results to the public. They can't simply just sweep this under the carpet or put it in the back room because they are concerned about the rise of teen depression and the lack of medications to deal with this.

So I think—I am really glad we are having this series of hearings, but I think the FDA has a lot to answer for. I would also like to add that at the last hearing, Mr. Chairman, you chastised the FDA for its lack of cooperation with this committee, and rightly so. But we are still having difficulty getting information from the FDA.

Some of the documents that we requested were not produced until 36 hours before this hearing. The questions posed by the Democrats at and after the last hearing, including myself, have still not been answered, and the FDA did finally, I heard, respond to some questions that Mr. Walden had last night.

We didn't get Doctors Temple and Mosholder's testimony until after 7 o'clock last night, and I don't know if Dr. Temple testimony required OMB review, which is why the FDA usually says the testimony is tardy, but the delay is certainly a burden on the committee and our hard working staff. Some of us on this subcommittee were here until after 6 o'clock in a different hearing last night, and it makes it very difficult to prepare for these hearings.

So in sum, Mr. Chairman—and I have an extension of remarks I will put in the record—we have got to have cooperation in this hearing by the FDA and by all the other Federal agencies. We are elected as representatives of the American people to find the truth, and I know. one of the things I love about this subcommittee, we work on a bipartisan basis, as the chairman said.

We intend to get to the bottom of this, and I really want to thank the chairman for not relenting, and I would hope these agencies would realize they have got to cooperate.

I yield back the balance of my time.

Chairman BARTON. I thank the distinguished Congresswoman from Colorado. You statement is the first I had heard that we hadn't had those questions answered. I wish I had known that yesterday, because I had a phone conversation with Dr. Crawford. But what we might do is do another—maybe another meeting and get you and Mr. Dingell and Mr. Deutsch involved, and we will get your answers.

Ms. DEGETTE. Thank you, Mr. Chairman.

[The prepared statement of Hon. Diana Degette follows:]

PREPARED STATEMENT OF HON. DIANA DEGETTE, A REPRESENTATIVE IN CONGRESS FROM THE STATE OF COLORADO

Today's hearing is the second of this series on antidepressant use in pediatric populations. Parents, children and physicians seeking improved mental health carefully weigh the risks and benefits of taking antidepressants. The Committee's investigation has uncovered that the risks of taking antidepressants had not been fully shared.

This hearing is more broadly about the Food and Drug Agency's ability and efforts to ensure that all approved pharmaceuticals are safe. This responsibility is at the very core of the FDA's mission. To fulfill that mission, FDA must conduct objective studies with rigorous scientific inquiry. When risks are identified, it is essential that they be communicated to the public.

The FDA staff here with us today must answer to this Committee and to the American public. Why were there delays in the presentation of data on the link between suicides and antidepressants? What steps will be taken to ensure that scientists at FDA are able to present their findings to Advisory Committees? What future actions is FDA taking for pediatric and adult use of antidepressants?

This investigation on antidepressant use in pediatric populations has revealed that transparency and availability of information may have been compromised. I would once again like to remind the FDA of the importance of their role. It greatly concerns me that the United Kingdom's equivalent to FDA (the MHRA), contraindicated all anti-depressants for individuals less than 18 years of age in December 2003. That was almost one year ago. Why has the FDA not taken similar steps?

The FDA's recent Advisory Committee meeting has determined that there is an increased risk of suicidality in pediatric patients taking antidepressants. They have recommended warning labels, but not contraindication. But the data has shown that a risk of suicide does exist for two antidepressants (Effexor and Paxil). How can we not provide that information to physicians and parents?

I, like many of my colleagues believe that we must balance safety concerns with access to medication. I do not believe that this balance can exist when the risks are hidden.

In addition to considerations about analysis of the data, this investigation has revealed that post-market surveillance of pharmaceuticals has not perhaps been as strict as this Committee would like. I hope that the witnesses from the FDA will provide some insight on how this monitoring process may be limited and what Congress can do to improve it.

I continue to be concerned about the inadequacy of our mental health research and treatment system. While antidepressants have greatly improved treatment options, much more must be done. In addition to examining the FDA's actions, this hearing highlights the areas of improvement needed. While safety of medications is of immediate importance, this Committee should not turn a blind eye to the more significant shortcomings in our health system.

Chairman BARTON. The Chair would recognize Mr. Rogers for an opening statement.

Mr. ROGERS. I will yield.

Chairman BARTON. Would Mr. Bilirakis like to make an opening statement, distinguished subcommittee chairman?

Mr. BILIRAKIS. Well, thank you, Mr. Chairman, just very briefly. Obviously, the recent reports of anti-depressant drugs possibly increasing the risk of suicidal thoughts and actions in children taking these drugs are certainly extremely disturbing. While there are, as I understand it, no actual suicides, it is important to recognize any possible adverse effects that these drugs may have on adolescents and children.

Mr. Chairman, I don't disagree with any of the comments made by you or any of the other members of the committee up here and the fault on the part of the FDA and that sort of thing, but I guess, as I understand it also, there have been some positive things that have taken place.

I think we all can agree that the new FDA labeling requirements are a step in the right direction. The FDA has been closely reviewing the results of anti-depressant studies in children since June 2003, and asked that the matter be investigated by the Psychopharmacologic Drugs Advisory Committee, PDAC, and the Pediatric Subcommittee of the Anti-Infective Drugs Advisory.

The Advisory Committee did recommend to the FDA that the labeling of these drugs be revised to advise the need to monitor patients closely when the anti-depressive therapy started and, based on this recommendation, FDA did require changes to the labels for anti-depressant drugs used for adolescents to include stronger cautions and warnings about the need to monitor patients for worsening of depression and the emergence of suicidality.

I don't know that this will solve the problem, Mr. Chairman, and certainly things like delays and not being apparently cooperative and all that are concerns, but I suppose that this is a step in the right direction. And thanks to you and Mr. Walden, the ranking members in the committee, hopefully, this brings it out to the fore, and these matters will be solved on an adequate basis, and I look forward to hearing from all the witnesses.

Thank you, Mr. Chairman.

Chairman BARTON. Thank the distinguished subcommittee chairman. We now recognize Mr. Allen for an opening statement—Congressman Allen, I mean.

Mr. ALLEN. Thank you, Mr. Chairman, and thank you for calling this second hearing to examine concerns surrounding the safety and efficacy of anti-depressant use by children.

This committee must closely examine the FDA's role in reviewing clinical trial data indicating serious side effects associated with certain prescription drugs. The FDA's mission is to protect public health and, therefore, it has the responsibility to alert physicians and the public to safety and efficacy concerns associated with various medical treatments.

I do find it very troubling that FDA officials appear to have attempted to suppress information indicating that SSRI anti-depressants may increase the risk of certain suicide related thoughts and/or behaviors in children. I am disturbed that Dr. Mosholder's full report on this issue conducted at the behest of the FDA was not allowed to be presented at FDA's February Advisory Committee meeting on this issue.

I look forward to hearing from Dr. Mosholder about the directive under which he conducted his review on clinical trial data of SSRIs and the conclusions of his report.

Clearly, there is debate among the scientific community about whether episodes of attempted suicide while taking SSRIs are attributed to the underlying depression of an individual patient or to the taking of SSRIs. However, disagreement about clinical trial data does not mean that the studies and conclusions of specific researchers should be dismissed or suppressed. Rather, vigorous debate in the scientific community should be encouraged and conclusions challenged in order to arrive at the best determination of what information should be disseminated to physicians and their patients.

The increasing rate of clinical depression in children is a serious public health issue. Children diagnosed with depression are clearly at an increased risk for suicidal thoughts and behaviors. Each year, more than 500,000 children and adolescents attempt suicide, and approximately 2,000 young people die as a result of suicide.

I had the opportunity to discuss the link between SSRI use and the possible increase in suicidal thoughts and behavior with a pediatric physiatrist in Maine. He said that there is a solid agreement among physicians that they need better clinical data on the side effects of anti-depressants and not just studies financed by the drug manufacturers.

He also stressed that physicians need to have a variety of drugs available to them in order to make the best choice for their patients. Research indicates that between 30 and 40 percent of children and adolescents with depression will not respond to the first medication. The debate surrounding this issue clearly indicates a need for greater post-marketing studies on prescription drugs.

I am interested in learning from Dr. Temple about the recent recommendations of the Psychopharmacologic Drugs and Pediatric Advisory Committee, including the suggestion of requiring the black box warning on all anti-depressant drugs, indicating an increased risk for suicidality in pediatric patients.

Certain drugs prescribed to children can be ineffective or dangerous. It is FDA's responsibility to investigate the risks associated with prescription drug use in order to protect the safety of our Nation's children. FDA has a critical role in ensuring that doctors and consumers receive balanced information.

I look forward to hearing the testimony of all of you on this very important topic. Mr. Chairman, I yield back the balance of my time.

Chairman BARTON. Thank the distinguished member for that statement.

Does the gentleman from New Hampshire wish to—Okay. Does the gentleman from California, Congressman Waxman, wish to make an opening statement? Mr. Stupak is not a member of the subcommittee.

Mr. WAXMAN. Thank you very much, Mr. Chairman. I want to commend you for holding this hearing. I am pleased with the bipartisan way the committee has operated, and this is an important issue, the question of anti-depressant use in children.

The issue has a lot of different implications. Certainly, we ought to learn how FDA oversees the safety and effectiveness of drugs, both in the approval process and after the approval process when drugs are used for an off-label use, and especially when we are talking about children.

The issue also has implications for how the pharmaceutical industry shares data on its products with the public, and especially the medical community.

The subcommittee's investigations have revealed that all too often the drug industry has concealed data from physicians and patients. In the case of anti-depressants, the data that was concealed would have shown that the drugs failed to work in children.

Concealing these negative results had very serious consequences. It now appears that many children taking these potentially ineffective drugs were put at an unnecessary risk, because the drugs they were given may have actually increased the likelihood that they might commit suicide.

Today the FDA is going to respond to allegations that the agency failed to act quickly enough when the risk of suicide as first brought to light. I am very interested in hearing what they have to say, and hearing their responses.

In the weeks and months to come, I hope that the subcommittee will continue to examine the broader issue of how information about pharmaceuticals is made in general, so that we can better protect patients from serious drug risks in the future. I think FDA has a lot to answer to today, and I am pleased that we have them here and under oath, so that the questions may be asked of them and that we can pursue the matter fully.

I am disturbed to hear that perhaps they had not given the committee all the information that has been requested. I have very little patience, and I know the chairman feels this way as well, that when we request information from any government agency in order to do our job of oversight—and it is an important constitutional function to do that job—we need to given all the information that is requested so that we can make a better evaluation of the matter before us.

So I commend you, Mr. Chairman, again for holding these hearings, and I look forward to the testimony today and working with the members of this committee to figure out what actions we need to take thereafter.

[The prepared statement of Hon. Henry Waxman follows:]

PREPARED STATEMENT OF HON. HENRY A. WAXMAN, A REPRESENTATIVE IN CONGRESS FROM THE STATE OF CALIFORNIA

I'd like to thank the Subcommittee for holding this series of hearings on anti-depressant use in children. This is an extremely important issue, which has implications for how the FDA oversees the safety and effectiveness of drugs. The issue also has implications for how the pharmaceutical industry shares data on its products with the public.

The Subcommittee's investigations have revealed that all too often the drug industry has concealed data from physicians and patients. In the case of anti-depressants, the data that was concealed would have shown that the drugs failed to work in children. Concealing these negative results had very serious consequences. It now appears that many children taking these potentially ineffective drugs were put at unnecessary risk, because the drugs that they were given may have actually increased the likelihood that they might commit suicide.

Today, the FDA will respond to allegations that the agency failed to act quickly enough when the risk of suicide was first brought to light.

I am very interested in learning the response of the FDA to these allegations.

In the weeks and months to come, I hope that the Subcommittee will continue to examine the broader issue of how information about pharmaceuticals is made public in general, so that we can better protect patients from serious drug risks in the future.

Chairman BARTON. We thank the gentleman from California.

The gentleman from New Jersey, Congressman Ferguson, is recognized for an opening statement.

Mr. FERGUSON. Thank you, Mr. Chairman. I thank you for holding this important hearing, continuing the committee's investigation of adverse effects of anti-depressants in children.

Two weeks ago, we discussed how vital it is that doctors receive all the latest relevant study data and results so they can make the most informed decisions possible on the safety of the drugs that they are prescribing. The drug makers discussed steps that they are taking to make their trials available to doctors so they can have all the information they need to confidently prescribe medicines to patients.

I commend the work of the committee and, most importantly, the parents of children who have suffered unspeakable pain because of the adverse reactions to some of these anti-depressants.

In the last hearing 2 weeks ago, I spoke about a constituent and friend of mine, Lisa Van Sickel. Lisa is here with us again today. I spoke about Lisa and her daughter, Michelle, as well as other constituents of mine who have suffered in this way. Lisa, as I say, is with us again here today.

I am told that Michelle, who is away at college, will be watching via the committee's webcast today. If that is the case, hello, Michelle.

Since our last hearing, there have been developments from the FDA regarding their recommendations for doctors prescribing anti-depressants to children. Last week the FDA's Psychopharmacological Drugs and Pediatric Advisory Committees met and made their recommendations on the prescribing of anti-depressants to children.

I am interested to hear today what the panel has to say about the recommendations and whether or not the FDA plans on fully implementing the Advisory Committee's recommendations, but also of particular interest is the path that the FDA took to come to the conclusions that they have decided upon.

I look forward to hearing the testimony of Dr. Mosholder today, and then the testimony of the second panel about how we have arrived at the point that we are at now.

Question: Why was Dr. Mosholder's work not presented to the FDA's February 2004 advisory committee, and when did the Neuropharm Division first become aware of an increase in psychiatric adverse events occurring in pediatric randomized controlled trials of anti-depressants as compared with the adult population?

My constituents and I and members of this panel are looking forward to hearing the answers to these and a number of other questions from today's panels of witnesses.

Thank you again, Mr. Chairman, for holding this hearing, and I yield back.

Chairman BARTON. Thank the gentleman from New Jersey. The gentlelady from Illinois, Ms. Schakowsky, is recognized for an opening statement.

Ms. SCHAKOWSKY. Thank you, Chairman Barton, for recognizing me for the purpose of making an opening statement and for agreeing to hear the opening statement of a Member of Congress not on this subcommittee, Mr. Stupak. I hope that the tradition of opening statements will continue going forward.

I look forward to hearing the testimony of the members of the panel who took part in reviewing the safety of anti-depressants in children over the past 1½ years. We need to get some straightforward answers as to why specific concerns regarding the safety of those medications were kept not just from the public and from the medical community, but from the Advisory Committee whose job it is to advise the FDA on these issues.

The process of reviewing the safety and efficacy of medications is complex. What is not complex is that the findings of someone who is charged at taxpayers' expense with the review should not be hidden from sight. This is a particular concern when we talk about the health and safety of our children.

I would like to hear an explanation today as to why, after spending months examining the connection between anti-depressant use in children and increased suicidal ideation at the request of his superiors, an FDA medical examiner would be prevented by those same superiors from presenting his conclusions to the FDA's Advisory Committee.

I find this apparent suppression of information appalling, particularly when it serves to hide information that could have a significant impact on how medications are used by children.

In order for an advisory committee to come up with well-informed and accurate recommendations, it is absolutely crucial that they are provided with the most comprehensive, up-to-date and accurate information available. When this does not happen and the committee is prevented from hearing the conclusions of those who actually conducted the reviews, the recommendations of the committee inevitably will fail to reflect the best interests of children and their families. This not only leads to continued misuse of medications by misinformed parents and physicians, it results in a serious breach of trust of the FDA in its role of protecting the public from unsafe foods and medications.

There already exists a great deal of misunderstanding and mistrust within our society regarding the diagnosis and treatment of mental health disorders. Incidents such as these only serve to add fuel to the fire and increase the anger and frustration on all sides.

Over the past weeks, we have heard from many mental health professionals and parents who are convinced that these medications can be effective in the treatment of major depression in their children if they are used in an appropriate manner and under the right circumstances. Many parents are also very concerned about the possible negative impact of these drugs on their children. All of them, however, deserve to know that the decisions about these drugs are based on a full, fair and independent analysis, and that critical information has not been denied them. Thank you.

Chairman BARTON. The Chair would now recognize the distinguished member of the full committee, Congressman Stupak of Michigan, for an opening statement.

Mr. STUPAK. Thank you, Mr. Chairman, and thank you once again for allowing me to take part in this series of hearings concerning the safety and effectiveness of anti-depressants used by children.

Two weeks ago, this committee heard the FDA repeatedly claim the jury was still out about the safety of anti-depressants. Just 4 days later before an advisory committee in Bethesda, the FDA finally admitted what they had known for a year: There is an increased risk of suicidal thoughts and behavior in children who take anti-depressants.

I am appalled but, frankly, not surprised by the systematic efforts of the FDA to suppress information that could have prevented the senseless deaths of too many children.

I believe these anti-depressants should be banned until the jury comes back with proof that they are safe and that they work. They are not effective to treat depression. Increased risk, no matter how large or small, is still an increased risk for suicidal behavior.

The American people have a right to demand the FDA to look out for their interests and not the interests of the drug companies. When safety is questioned, FDA should err on the side of caution.

The tragedies experienced by the families in the audience today may have been prevented. The jury is no longer out. Congress at a minimum should demand that the FDA to immediately and completely implement all the Advisory Committee recommendations made last week. Those recommendations included warnings on all anti-depressants, black box labeling, and easy to understand warnings on the packaging where parents and patients can see it.

What many here may not realize is the FDA is under no obligation to implement those recommendations. There are many instances when the FDA has ignored or scaled back Advisory Committee recommendations, caving to drug company pressure.

I know from my own experience that the FDA has repeatedly ignored for the past 4 years advisory committee recommendations concerning the acne drug, Accutane. I am particularly concerned the FDA might back away from the recommendation of package labeling that parents and patients can see and understand. The FDA should require that information about the safety and efficacy of these drugs be dispensed with every prescription and on the package labeling.

The FDA should also require parents to sign an informed consent before treatment can begin. The FDA cannot ignore these recommendations like they ignored Dr. Mosholder's analysis. They can't drag their feet on implementing the recommendations as they dragged their feet on posting these studies on their website.

Congress and the American people have had enough of the stonewalling and excuse making. It is time to take action. Let's be clear. Package labeling is the least the drug companies can do.

In 1997 Congress passed a law beginning a system where the drug companies get patent extensions worth billions of dollars to study these drugs in children. Children, the most vulnerable members of our society, are the only group that we grant patent extensions to drug companies in exchange for studies.

We don't grant patent extensions to drug companies to study the effect of drugs in women. We just demand it, and the drug companies do it. We don't grant patent extensions worth billions of dollars to drug companies to study drugs in minorities. We just demand it, and drug companies do it.

Patents are extended once pediatric studies are turned in to the FDA. There is no requirement that the studies were actually well done or actually show whether the drug worked or was safe, and there is no requirement that the packaging label on these drugs are actually changed before the patent extension is granted.

At the very least, parents should get the facts in exchange for these billions in profits. It is clear today that they are not.

Mr. Chairman, thank you again for calling these hearings and for your leadership on this issue. This hearing illustrates a larger problem at the FDA where too often drug companies trump parents where medical evidence is suppressed and where expert opinion is silenced, and it illustrates that our system to study the effects of drugs on children is broken.

It is a system that gives billions of dollars to drug companies and asks little in return. The FDA is failing to live up to its responsibility to the American people.

I yield back the balance of my time.

Chairman BARTON. We thank the distinguished gentleman from Michigan.

The Chair would now recognize the gentleman from Florida for an opening statement, Mr. Stearns.

Mr. STEARNS. And good morning and thank you, Mr. Chairman, for holding this hearing.

I think, as Mr. Stupak and others who are parents of children are very much interested in this, 2 weeks ago we explored the measures to make the results of clinical drug trials more accessible to doctors and parents, and I think that goes without saying.

You know, in our society today there seems to be a pill for everything that ails you and, of course, this is especially true for depression where millions of American children are being prescribed anti-depressants. It is probably unquestionable that anti-depressants have improved the quality of life for many children and their families, and may have even saved some lives. But for years now, we have heard anecdotal evidence that some of these same anti-depressants increase suicidal behavior in some children.

Lately, the evidence has become less anecdotal and more and more compelling. In March 2004 the FDA issued a warning that 10 popular anti-depressants can cause deeper depression, agitation, and other forms of violent behavior, including suicide.

A month later, it was reported that the number of American children being treated with anti-depressants has soared over the past decades—it has been in all the press—even though the vast majority of clinical trials have failed to prove that the medicines even help—even help children at all.

Now we have also heard that the agency's own drug safety analyst found a link between some anti-depressants and suicidal behavior in children. Yet, my colleagues, these findings were suppressed, and his analysis deemed unreliable.

Finally, a recent FDA commission study by Columbia University researchers have confirmed the adverse results, and we are forced to admit finally the truth that there is indeed an increase in suicide and suicidal thoughts and behavior for some children who are prescribed certain anti-depressants.

Mr. Chairman, the FDA is responsible for protecting the public health by assuring the safety and efficacy of these prescription drugs. We all know that. The widespread use of these anti-depressants should provide even more incentive for this FDA to fulfill its stated mission. At the very least, the drugs in question should contain strong warning labels to help physicians and parents evaluate the risks.

So truly, all of us here hope that this hearing will help us get to the bottom of these disturbing findings and that we will have a chance to fully explore the findings with the panel.

So I look forward to this hearing and to learning more about the FDA's role in making sure anti-depressants used by children are safe and do what they are supposed to do.

Thank you, Mr. Chairman.

Chairman BARTON. We thank the distinguished gentleman from Florida for his opening statement. Seeing no other members of the subcommittee on either side of the aisle present, the Chair would ask unanimous consent that all members of the subcommittee not present have the requisite number of days to put their formal opening statement in the record. hearing no objection, so ordered.

[Additional statement submitted for the record follows:]

PREPARED STATEMENT OF HON. EDWARD J. MARKEY, A REPRESENTATIVE IN CONGRESS FROM THE STATE OF MASSACHUSETTS

Thank you Mr. Chairman for calling this important hearing.

As we continue the Subcommittee's examination of how the FDA and the pharmaceutical industry evaluated, reported, and responded to data linking certain anti-depressants to an increased risk of suicide in children and adolescents, I think it is important to recognize that these drugs have played a very positive role in expanding the treatment options for so many people around the country who have been struggling with depression. For them and their families, anti-depressant medications have been a real life line.

However, we have learned that until very recently we did not have the whole truth about the impact of these drugs on our children. Today's hearing will help the Subcommittee understand how this could have occurred.

Based on what I have heard and read so far, it seems to me that our current system for informing the public about potential risks associated may be broken. It failed to inform the public about potential risks of anti-depressants at two points. The first failure was when the pharmaceutical companies did not disclose the negative results of their clinical trials. Congressman Waxman and I will soon introduce legislation to address this issue. We are proposing the creation of a federal registry of clinical trials. This will ensure that companies cannot pick and choose what information they want to share with the public.

The second failure was when the pharmaceutical companies told the FDA about negative trials, the FDA did not move quickly and aggressively to fulfill its role as the watchdog for public health. After conducting their own study and confirming the risk, the Agency hesitated, suppressed their own data and left the public in the dark for months. Meanwhile, regulators in Great Britain were already taking action to protect their citizens from the same risks revealed by the data.

The public absolutely needs to know about the risks associated with the drugs that they are taking. Even if Dr. Mosholder's conclusions were wrong (which does not appear to be the case) it was completely inappropriate for the FDA to suppress his findings. Instead, the he should have been allowed presented his findings and conclusions to the FDA's Advisory Committee and allowed the experts to evaluate the data, question the study and have a complete discussion of the available information. Instead the FDA hid the data, got embarrassed when the public found out about their actions from the press, and initiated an internal criminal investigation that appears aimed at scaring its own employees into silence.

Today we are going to examine the nature of the FDA's failure. The FDA plays a critical role in protecting the public health so I am very concerned about the maintaining the integrity of the FDA process. It is my hope that in the future the FDA will provide a fair, thorough evaluation of the risks associated with drugs and promptly inform the public of those conclusions in a timely fashion. I am looking forward to hearing what steps the FDA is taking to restore the public's trust. I look forward to hearing the testimony of today's witnesses.

Chairman BARTON. The Chair would now call forward our first witness, the distinguished representative from the Food and Drug Administration, Dr. Andrew Mosholder. Would you please come forward and be seated.

Welcome, Dr. Mosholder. You are aware that the committee has the tradition of taking all testimony under oath. Do you object to testifying under oath?

Mr. MOSHOLDER. Thank you. As a member of the Religious Society of Friends or Quakers, I would prefer to affirm rather than swear.

Chairman BARTON. We have the oath so that you can affirm rather than swear. But you don't oppose to affirming under oath?

Mr. MOSHOLDER. That is correct.

Chairman BARTON. Thank you. You also have the right as a citizen of the United States of America under the Constitution of our great Nation to be advised by counsel during your testimony. Do you wish to be so advised during your testimony?

Mr. MOSHOLDER. No, I do not.

Chairman BARTON. Would you please stand and raise your right hand.

[Witness sworn.]

Chairman BARTON. Be seated. Dr. Mosholder, we welcome you to the subcommittee. Your testimony in its entirety is in the record. We would recognize you for 7 minutes to elaborate on that formal testimony.

TESTIMONY OF ANDREW D. MOSHOLDER, FOOD AND DRUG ADMINISTRATION

Mr. MOSHOLDER. Thank you. I have a brief oral statement which I can read now.

Mr. Chairman and members of the subcommittee, I am Dr. Andrew Mosholder, a medical officer in the Office of Drug Safety at FDA's Center for Drug Evaluation and Research. My statement will briefly summarize my role in FDA's review of suicidality in pediatric anti-depressant drug trials.

Before joining the Office of Drug Safety, or ODS, I was medical officer in the Division of Neuropharmacological Drug Products, DNDP, where I reviewed a number of submissions of pediatric data for anti-depressant drugs, including Paxil. In my review of the Paxil pediatric data, I noted that some of the clinical trial adverse events classified as emotional ability involved suicidal behavior or ideation.

So DNDP requested clarification from the manufacturer, GlaxoSmithKline. In May 2003, GlaxoSmithKline provided new analyses showing an increase in suicidal thoughts and behaviors with paroxetine compared to placebo. Dr. Russell Katz, the Director of DNDP, requested my assistance in the evaluation of these data, and my managers in ODS agreed.

In July, DNDP asked the sponsors of other anti-depressant drugs to reproduce GlaxoSmithKline's analysis of suicidal events for Paxil by applying the same method to their own pediatric trial data bases.

By September 2003, I had completed an analysis of the paroxetine data and a preliminary analysis of pediatric data on seven other anti-depressant drugs. I presented these analyses at a briefing for CDER management September 16, 2003.

DNDP forward responses from the other manufacturers to me for review. I completed the first written draft of my report in December 2003. DNDP apparently was reaching a conclusion that these data were not adequate for definitive analysis. DNDP requested additional data from each sponsor, and also arranged for the possible suicidal events in these trials to be reclassified by outside experts.

On December 18, 2003, at a planning session for the February 2 Advisory Committee meeting on this issue, I shared a proposed outline of my Advisory Committee presentation. I noted that suicidal events designated as serious in pediatric clinical trials for major depressive disorder were 1.9 times more frequent with anti-depressant drug treatment than with placebo, and that this was statistically significant. There was some discussion of the pros and cons of my analysis.

On January 6, Dr. Katz informed me by telephone that someone else would present the clinical trial data at the February 2 meeting, since I had a different view of the data from that of DNDP.

News of my analysis and the fact that it would not be presented at the February 2 AC meeting reached Mr. Rob Waters, a reporter for the San Francisco Chronicle. The Chronicle ran the story on February 1, 1 day prior to the AC meeting.

On February 18, I completed my written report. In it I recommended discouraging off-label pediatric use of the anti-depressant drugs. When my report received supervisory signoff March 19, Dr. Mary Willy concurred, and Doctors Anne Trontell and Mark Avigan attached cover memoranda indicating their areas of disagreement.

On March 3, 2004, two special agents from the FDA Office of Internal Affairs interviewed me regarding the disclosure of my findings in the February 1 San Francisco Chronicle article. I later provided the Office of Internal Affairs with a written statement about the matter. I indicated that I was not the source of the disclosure.

On March 22, FDA issued a public health advisory stating in part, “health care providers should carefully monitor patients receiving anti-depressants for possible worsening of depression or suicidality.”

In mid-July Dr. Tarek Hammad of DNDP shared the results of his analysis of the clinical trial events as reclassified by a panel of suicide experts convened by Columbia University. The new analysis confirmed the previous finding: Definitive suicidal behaviors and ideation in short term pediatric trials were 1.8 times more frequent with anti-depressant drug treatment compared to placebo, and this was statistically significant.

Shortly thereafter, data from a new study of paroxetine, the treatment of adolescent depression study or TADS, became available. The TADS data indicated a therapeutic effect of fluoxetine, but also showed an excess of suicidal events among those receiving fluoxetine compared to patients who received placebo, which was a new finding for fluoxetine.

On September 13 and 14, FDA held an AC meeting to consider this issue. I was among the presenters, and I provided a comparison of my analysis to the current analysis. The Advisory Committee members voted 15 to 8 in favor of a boxed warning to the labeling of anti-depressant drugs.

Thank you.

[The prepared statement of Andrew D. Mosholder follows:]

PREPARED STATEMENT OF ANDREW D. MOSHOLDER, MEDICAL OFFICER, OFFICE OF DRUG SAFETY, U.S. FOOD AND DRUG ADMINISTRATION

Mr. Chairman and Members of the Subcommittee: I, Andrew D. Mosholder, am a licensed physician and board certified in child and adolescent psychiatry. I obtained my medical degree from the University of Virginia. I also have a Master of Public Health degree from Johns Hopkins University.

I am currently employed by the U.S. Food and Drug Administration and have been so employed since 1992. During my employment, I have been a medical officer with the Center for Drug Evaluation and Research (CDER) for twelve years. For about the past 20 months, I have worked as an epidemiologist in the Division of Drug Risk Evaluation, Office of Drug Safety (ODS). Prior to that, I was a medical officer in CDER's Division of Neuropharmacological Drug Products (DNDP) for over 10 years.

In this statement, I will briefly summarize my role in FDA's review of pediatric use of antidepressant drugs, with particular attention to recent concerns about the effects of these drugs on suicidal thoughts and behaviors in children and adolescents.

As a medical officer in DNDP, I reviewed a number of submissions of pediatric data for antidepressant drugs, including pediatric data submitted for Paxil (paroxetine), manufactured by GlaxoSmithKline. In my review of the Paxil pediatric supplement, I noted that a number of clinical trial adverse events designated as "emotional lability" involved suicidal behavior or ideation. Accordingly, DNDP requested clarification regarding such behavioral adverse events from GlaxoSmithKline. In May of 2003, after I had transferred to ODS, DNDP received new data analyses from the manufacturer, indicating an increase in suicidal thoughts and behaviors with paroxetine compared to placebo in pediatric clinical trials. A consultation request from DNDP to ODS signed June 6, 2003 by Dr. Russell Katz stated: "Since the original review of the Paxil supplement, as well as the reviews of most other pediatric supplements for SSRIs, was done by Andrew Mosholder, M.D, . . . we ask that this consult be assigned to him. We seek his advice on further analysis and interpretation of the Paxil results, as well as more general advice on what might be done to re-evaluate the risk of suicidality in the pediatric databases for other SSRIs . . ."

My managers in ODS agreed to Dr. Katz's request and assigned me to this consultation on June 9, 2003. To determine whether the apparent increase in suicidal events applies to pediatric use of other antidepressant drugs as well, I started to review FDA's pediatric data for other antidepressant drugs. DNDP ultimately decided that the best way to proceed would be to ask the sponsors of other antidepressant drugs to reproduce GlaxoSmithKline's analysis of suicidal events for Paxil, with each sponsor applying the same method to their own pediatric trial databases. In July of 2003, DNDP sent requests for such analyses to other antidepressant drug sponsors.

By September of 2003, I had completed an analysis of the paroxetine data and a preliminary analysis of pediatric data on seven other antidepressant drugs. At the request of management, I presented these analyses at a CDER Regulatory Briefing for upper level management on September 16, 2003. During the briefing, I presented the paroxetine pediatric data, along with preliminary findings for other antidepressant drugs. As noted in the briefing minutes, there was discussion about the clinical significance of some of the events in the analysis: "We need to get a better sense of what the events from these studies really are, i.e., are they legitimate, suicide-associated thoughts/actions or self-mutilation acts that are becoming increasingly common in the adolescent population today and are not generally associated with a sincere intent to die."

The Federal Register on October 31, 2003 contained this announcement to the public regarding an Advisory Committee meeting scheduled for February 2, 2004: "The Psychopharmacologic Drugs Advisory Committee and the Pediatric Subcommittee of the Anti-Infective Drugs Advisory Committee will discuss reports of the occurrence of suicidality (both suicidal ideation and suicide attempts) in clinical trials for various antidepressant drugs in pediatric patients with major depressive disorder (MDD). The committee will consider optimal approaches to the analysis of data from these trials, and the results of analyses conducted to date, with regard to the question of what regulatory action may be needed pertinent to the clinical use of these products in pediatric patients. The committee will also consider further research needs to address questions on this topic."

As DNDP received responses from the other manufacturers to the July information requests, those responses were forwarded to me for review. I then worked on my analysis of these responses over the next couple of months and completed the first written draft of my results in December of 2003.

DNDP apparently was reaching a conclusion that the responses from the sponsors to the July requests were not going to be adequate for a definitive analysis. In October of 2003, DNDP sent requests to the manufacturers asking for patient level data sets, to permit a more sophisticated statistical analysis than what I could accomplish using only the responses to the July requests. DNDP also decided that all of the possible suicidal events in these trials should be reclassified by outside experts in suicidology.

On December 10, 2003, the U.K.'s Medicines and Healthcare products Regulatory Agency issued their statement, "Use of Selective Serotonin Reuptake Inhibitors (SSRIs) in children and adolescents with major depressive disorder (MDD)—only fluoxetine (Prozac) shown to have a favourable balance of risks and benefits for the treatment of MDD in the under 18s."

On December 18, 2003, we held one of our planning meetings for the February 2 Advisory Committee (AC) meeting. A draft agenda distributed for the December 18 planning meeting included a 45-minute presentation by me entitled, "Limited Overview of Paxil Controlled Trials and Controlled Trials of Other Antidepressants." At that meeting, I shared a proposed outline of my presentation, which included my finding that suicidal events designated as "serious" in pediatric clinical trials for major depressive disorder were 1.9 times more frequent with antidepressant drug treatment than with placebo, and that this was statistically significant. I recall some discussion of the pros and cons of my analysis.

On January 6, 2004, Dr. Katz sent me an email asking to speak with me by phone regarding my presentation at the February 2 AC meeting. In our subsequent telephone conversation on that date, he told me that someone else would present the clinical trial data at the February 2 AC meeting since I had reached a different view of the clinical trial data from that of DNDP. On January 7, 2004, I sent an email to the team members planning the February 2 meeting, confirming that I would not be giving the presentation as originally planned and attaching a draft of my slides for their use and interest.

On January 12, 2004, the Agency issued a Federal Register notice with a revised agenda for the February 2 meeting. The notice stated, "The committee will not be considering options for definitive regulatory action at this meeting because definitive analyses of the data have not been completed. This topic will be covered in a second meeting to be scheduled by summer 2004."

News of my analysis, and the fact that the findings would not be presented at the February 2 AC meeting, reached Mr. Rob Waters, a reporter for the San Francisco Chronicle. I was not the source of this information, however, and in the course of a number of contacts from Mr. Waters I did not disclose to him any confidential information. Nonetheless, his story about this matter ran on February 1, 2004 in the San Francisco Chronicle, one day prior to the AC meeting.

At the February 2, 2004 AC meeting, I delivered a presentation entitled, "Office of Drug Safety Data Resources for the Study of Suicidal Events Associated with Pediatric Use of Antidepressants." This presentation emphasized postmarketing surveillance (MedWatch) data regarding suicidal events with pediatric use of antidepressants, but it did not include findings from my analysis of the pediatric clinical trial data. Dr. Anne Trontell, the Deputy Director of ODS, instructed me to prepare brief remarks regarding my analysis of the pediatric clinical trial data, to be used if any members of the Advisory Committee inquired about it. No AC members asked any questions about this, however, and so I did not deliver the brief remarks that I had prepared.

Subsequent to the February 2 AC meeting, I completed my written consultation memorandum regarding suicidality in pediatric clinical trials of antidepressants, dated February 18, 2004. In it, I recommended discouraging off-label pediatric use of antidepressant drugs, chiefly because the one drug that appeared to have the least risk of suicidal adverse events from the data available at that time was also the only drug to have won approval for pediatric depression, i.e., fluoxetine. I had extensive discussions with my management in ODS regarding my findings and their interpretation, and when my report received final supervisory sign-off on March 19, Dr. Mary Willy concurred, while Drs. Anne Trontell and Mark Avigan wrote separate cover memoranda indicating their areas of disagreement. That essentially ended my involvement with this project until mid-July when the results of the Columbia University reclassification analysis became available.

On March 3, 2004, two Special Agents from the FDA Office of Internal Affairs interviewed me regarding the disclosure of my findings in the February 1 San Francisco Chronicle article. I was also asked to produce a written statement regarding this matter for the Office of Internal Affairs, and in that statement I indicated that I was not the source of the disclosure.

On March 22, 2004, FDA issued a public health advisory which included the following statement: "Health care providers should carefully monitor patients receiving antidepressants for possible worsening of depression or suicidality, especially at the beginning of therapy or when the dose either increases or decreases. Although FDA has not concluded that these drugs cause worsening depression or suicidality, health care providers should be aware that worsening of symptoms could be due to the underlying disease or might be a result of drug therapy."

During the spring and summer of this year, I had several meetings with investigative staff of this Committee and of the Senate Finance Committee, as part of each committee's examination of this issue. FDA's written response to this Committee, dated April 14, 2004, summarized the rationale for withholding the results of my analysis at the February 2 AC meeting as follows: ". . . given the Agency's concerns regarding the limitations of the data and the plans to pursue case reclassification and more in-depth analyses, CDER decided that having Dr. Mosholder present his conclusion to the Advisory Committee, with the appearance that it was an Agency determination, would be potentially harmful to the public health as it might lead patients who were actually benefiting from the use of these drugs to inappropriately discontinue therapy."

My next involvement with the analysis of the clinical trial data came in mid-July, when Dr. Tarek Hammad was completing the DNDP analyses of suicidal adverse events as reclassified by a panel of suicide experts convened by Columbia University. The reclassification of potential suicidal events by the panel of experts had apparently confirmed the finding; definitive suicidal behaviors and ideation in short-term pediatric trials were 1.8 times more frequent with antidepressant drug treatment compared to placebo, and this was statistically significant. I was asked by my management to work with Dr. Hammad to prepare a comparison of his analysis to my previous analysis. We both participated in an August 9 briefing for CDER management on this issue, during which I presented such a comparison.

Subsequently I prepared a memorandum summarizing this comparison, along with some additional supplemental topics, and this memorandum received supervisory sign-off August 16.

Shortly after this, Dr. Hammad obtained data from a new study of fluoxetine (Prozac), called the Treatment of Adolescent Depression Study (TADS). The TADS data indicated a therapeutic effect of fluoxetine, as seen in the previous fluoxetine pediatric depression trials, but TADS also showed an excess of suicidal events among those receiving fluoxetine compared to patients who received placebo. The latter was a new finding, since there did not appear to be such an excess in previous fluoxetine trials.

On September 13 and 14, FDA held an AC meeting to consider this issue. The consult document signed March 19 and the follow-up memorandum dated August 16 were both included in the briefing materials for the AC meeting, and in fact FDA posted these documents on its web site several weeks in advance of the meeting. At the first day of the AC meeting, I was among the presenters and provided a comparison of my previous analysis to the current analysis, this time including the new findings from the TADS data, which were not included in the August 16 memorandum. The following day, the AC members voted 15-8 in favor of a boxed warning for the labeling of antidepressant drugs, to note the observed increase in suicidal behavior and ideation among pediatric patients treated with antidepressant drugs in clinical trials.

Chairman BARTON. Thank you, Dr. Mosholder.

The Chair would recognize himself for the first series of questions, and we will set the clock at 10 minutes.

Before I ask questions, I want to commend you for your work on behalf of the American people. I want to thank you for your perseverance. I want to applaud you for insisting on honesty and integrity in the review process. My guess is it has not been easy. So on behalf of at least this subcommittee and the full committee, and I would think I can say on behalf of the American people, just let me say thank you. We appreciate you being here today.

Mr. MOSHOLDER. Thank you very much.

Chairman BARTON. My first question to you is: Do you feel that you have been pressured in any way at the FDA to suppress or change your conclusions regarding your consult or consults—I think there were two of them—with regard to the efficacy of antidepressant drugs being prescribed off-label for children in this country?

Mr. MOSHOLDER. With regard to efficacy, not per se, but as far as the suicidality issue, at the time of finalizing the March consult document I had considerable discussion with my managers in the Office of Drug Safety about my interpretation of the data and the recommendation, and at one point alternative conclusions were offered to me which I declined to incorporate into my written document. Accordingly, we had the document finalized with cover memoranda which in our system indicated disagreement between the manager signing the document and the original author of the document.

Chairman BARTON. Okay. What are your thoughts on why you were refused to participate in the February 2004 Advisory meeting?

Mr. MOSHOLDER. Well, I would describe that as lack of confidence in the data and the meaning of the data on the part of those who made the decision to remove my presentation from the agenda. My understanding is that that lack of confidence centered around concern about whether the cases that I had counted in my analysis were really bona fide suicidal events or were perhaps events that were more clinically trivial or not meaningful.

Chairman BARTON. My understanding is that you are a medical doctor, an M.D. Is that correct?

Mr. MOSHOLDER. Yes, that is correct.

Chairman BARTON. And it is pediatric psychiatry. Is that correct?

Mr. MOSHOLDER. Child and adolescent psychiatry. Yes.

Chairman BARTON. Okay. So you feel that you are qualified—because of your medical training and your background, you are professionally qualified in the medical field to make some of the judgments and decisions that you had to make in the analysis of this data. Nobody has questioned your credentials. Is that correct?

Mr. MOSHOLDER. Not as far as my clinical background, no.

Chairman BARTON. So there was no—It is not one of the reasons you were not allowed to participate in the February Advisory, because somebody questioned your credentials or anything like that?

Mr. MOSHOLDER. Not to my knowledge.

Chairman BARTON. Okay. Do you agree with the British decision to prohibit the use of these anti-depressant drugs in children?

Mr. MOSHOLDER. Well, my comment there is—well, of course, in the sequence of events, that came shortly before I was completing my own report, and I am sure it had some influence on my thinking.

A close reading of the British contraindication actually would suggest that, under certain circumstances, physicians might choose to use the drugs for children. So that the term contraindication means something a bit different on either side of the Atlantic perhaps.

In the U.S. a contraindication basically means never, that the risk is never justified. So that I did support the British action with the understanding that their term contraindication is not an absolute and recognizing the fact that there might be selected circumstances where a clinician and patient might choose to use the drug.

Chairman BARTON. This is a personal question. You don't have to answer it if you don't want to. Do you have children?

Mr. MOSHOLDER. I have one step-son who is married, grown and married.

Chairman BARTON. If you did have young children, would you prescribe these anti-depressant drugs for them if they exhibited some of the symptoms of depression and suicidality?

Mr. MOSHOLDER. Well, my own opinion would be that, based on the evidence we have, the so called evidence based approach to clinical practice would be that fluoxetine appears to have the best data for depression as far as its efficacy.

We now have data that indicate, even with fluoxetine, there could be an increase in the suicidal events. So that that would have to be weighed, the risk and the benefit. So I would think that fluoxetine would sort of emerge as the default choice among the drugs for depression. But even there, it would have to be with careful attention to the potential risks.

Chairman BARTON. So I take that, if you personally had a child, what I heard you say is the best of a bad choice is this fluoxetine, but you really didn't say whether you would recommend that it be prescribed or not.

Mr. MOSHOLDER. Well, in certain circumstances—I think my view of the data that we have now is that we should think more carefully about the place of medication in the broader treatment of juvenile depression. And just again on a personal note, I trained long enough ago in psychiatry where we did not have Prozac or any of the other SSRIs, and in those days using medication was something that was not necessarily the first choice.

So I would say I would not never use it if it was my child or my patient, for that matter, but I would do it with careful attention to all the risks and benefits.

Chairman BARTON. Why do you think that the FDA, in spite of all these studies and all the evidence and all of the analysis that you have done, has been so reluctant to withdraw or more firmly encourage the medical community to stop prescribing these drugs off-label? Why wouldn't our FDA, which is viewed as the gold standard of the world, given the studies that have been done and your work—why do you think they haven't followed the lead of the British? Why have they continued to, even after last week—you know, this 51 to 8 decision which has just put a black box warning—It just seems to me that the cautious, prudent, conservative approach would be to strongly indicate to the medical prescribing community that these drugs shouldn't be used in children.

What has caused this reluctance at the FDA which, in my view, is quite contrary to their normal procedure, which is to be totally cautious?

Mr. MOSHOLDER. Well, I'm not sure I can give a complete explanation, but I think, on the other hand, there is some concern with abandoning the utility of these drugs perhaps to quickly—there's concerns about whether the studies which failed to show efficacy, whether that is due to the drug not being effective or whether the trial was not done properly, and it is often difficult to tell.

Another limitation is that we don't have good data on long term effects of these drugs. All of the studies that I looked at and that Dr. Hammad looked at were just a matter of several weeks. So there is also the possibility there could be long term benefits but short term risks. We just don't know.

So I think those are the caveats that perhaps the other people in the agency are looking at.

Chairman BARTON. Well, my time has expired. The Chair recognize the distinguished gentlelady from Colorado, Ms. DeGette, for 10 minutes.

Ms. DEGETTE. Thank you, Mr. Chairman. Dr. Mosholder, you told the chairman that after you presented your initial findings, alternative conclusions were offered to you. I wonder if you could tell us what those alternative conclusions were.

Mr. MOSHOLDER. Well, this was, as I recall, an e-mail from Dr. Trontell, one of my supervisors who wrote a cover memorandum to the report. As I recall, the difference was whether to take the step of channeling patients toward fluoxetine, as I said, as sort of a default choice or——

Ms. DEGETTE. That is Prozac, which has been approved for pediatric use.

Mr. MOSHOLDER. Yes, for both depression and obsessive compulsive disorder—whether to sort of actively advise people that that looks like the best choice or to be more cautious and just say sort of to use the drugs with caution.

Ms. DEGETTE. And they were recommending that you change it to say just use the drugs with caution?

Mr. MOSHOLDER. That is my recollection, yes.

Ms. DEGETTE. And you said you rejected that. Right?

Mr. MOSHOLDER. Yes, and the reason was I thought we had some good reasons to sort of point toward fluoxetine as perhaps——

Ms. DEGETTE. To take the stronger position, saying this is the drug that's been approved for pediatric use, this is what you should be prescribing. Right?

Mr. MOSHOLDER. Yes.

Ms. DEGETTE. Okay. I want to ask you, Doctor, in layman's terms what did you consult reveal about the link between suicidality and anti-depressants?

Mr. MOSHOLDER. Well, to put it simply, in the short term studies events which involved suicidal thoughts or behaviors were almost twice as frequent among the children and adolescents who received drug compared to the placebo or sugar pill control.

Ms. DEGETTE. So, basically, what your research showed: Kids are twice as likely to commit suicide on anti-depressants, at least in the short term, than on placebo?

Mr. MOSHOLDER. Well, I don't think I would say suicide, because, of course, there were no actual suicides. So suicidal thoughts and behavior.

Ms. DEGETTE. Okay. Thanks. Now did these conclusions apply to all anti-depressant drugs?

Mr. MOSHOLDER. That is a very good question. That is the conclusion from putting all of the studies together. When you break that apart by individual drug, the numbers become much smaller, and it is harder to have the same level of confidence that you have when you combined all the studies, as I did to get that figure.

So—But it is certainly true that in almost all of the drugs that have been looked at individually, there is at least an excess of such events with the drug versus the placebo.

Ms. DEGETTE. It would probably be helpful to have additional research, wouldn't it? More data?

Mr. MOSHOLDER. There is no question about that. Yes.

Ms. DEGETTE. That is what I think, too. Were any of your conclusions or findings about increased risk of suicidality ever disproved by the FDA, by the Columbia data review, or by Dr. Hammad's reanalysis?

Mr. MOSHOLDER. In general, I think Dr. Hammad's analysis and mine were consistent.

Ms. DEGETTE. Did anybody else disprove your findings?

Mr. MOSHOLDER. Not that I am aware of.

Ms. DEGETTE. Okay. Now I am curious about the February 2 Advisory Committee meeting that you testified about. I am wondering, if you know, why they decided not to let you present your findings at that meeting?

Mr. MOSHOLDER. Well, it was explained to me by Dr. Katz that I had reached a different point of view about the data from the Neuropharm Division, and by that I understood that I felt the data were of sufficient quality to perform an analysis, which I did, while the Neuropharm Division felt that any analysis should await the Columbia University reclassification project.

Ms. DEGETTE. So they felt like your data was not as conclusive as you thought it was? Would that be a fair characterization?

Mr. MOSHOLDER. Yes, you could characterize it that way.

Ms. DEGETTE. Okay. Let me ask you this. The chairman was asking you about some of your background, and you have been at the FDA quite sometime. Is that right?

Mr. MOSHOLDER. Twelve years.

Ms. DEGETTE. And how long have you been in your current position?

Mr. MOSHOLDER. Just over 1½ years.

Ms. DEGETTE. And before that, what did you do at the FDA?

Mr. MOSHOLDER. I was a medical officer in the Neuropharm Division.

Ms. DeGette. And part of your job, as I understand, is you were a reviewer of adult anti-depressants in that job. Correct?

Mr. Mosholder. Yes, that was part of my assignments. Yes.

Ms. DeGette. In your 12 years at the FDA, I am wondering if you have ever been in a situation like this before where you were asked to do a medical consult, where you completed the consult, where you presented the findings to your supervisors and got approval, and then where ultimately the FDA said, well, don't worry about it, just keep your conclusions to yourself?

Mr. Mosholder. Well, certainly, disagreements are not an uncommon event. Personally, I had never had the experience of having my presentation removed from an Advisory Committee meeting agenda.

Ms. DeGette. Have you ever known that to happen at the FDA?

Mr. Mosholder. Not by direct knowledge, but I have heard reports of other types of events like that.

Ms. DeGette. Is it your impression that it is a rare or a common occurrence at the FDA?

Mr. Mosholder. Well, it is hard to give an exact frequency, I guess, but I would say I have heard of several such circumstances, just incidentally.

Ms. DeGette. And how often is it that people are asked to do consults like this and make presentations as to their finding? I mean, you said you have heard of people being told they can't do their presentations a couple of times. I am wondering how often that happens, how often we have these types of presentations at the FDA.

Mr. Mosholder. Advisory Committee meetings, I think, are fairly frequent, probably on a monthly basis. There's probably other people who can give you real figures.

Ms. DeGette. So the Advisory Committee meetings happen fairly often. How many cases do they review at the meetings?

Mr. Mosholder. Typically, one issue or one drug per meeting.

Ms. DeGette. Okay. So your view would be it has been infrequent that people have been told that they can't—and again it is anecdotal, I know, because this only happened to you this one time.

Mr. Mosholder. That is correct.

Ms. DeGette. Okay. Now is it—I think that you—now you did present at the February 2 meeting, but you didn't present on your findings from the analysis of the pediatric clinical trial data. Is that right?

Mr. Mosholder. That is correct.

Ms. DeGette. What did you testify about?

Mr. Mosholder. I did a presentation which looked at the Office of Drug Safety's resources to evaluate this issue, the chief resource being, of course, the post-marketing reports, as we call them, or reports obtained through the MedWatch program from patients and doctors about adverse experiences with drugs—that is outside of clinical studies—along with examining some other potential sources of information, the conclusion being that the best source of information was the actual clinical studies.

Ms. DeGette. But you didn't testify about your latest consult?

Mr. Mosholder. No, that is correct.

Ms. DEGETTE. Mr. Chairman, I have more questions. I will ask them during the next round. Thank you.

Mr. WALDEN [presiding]. I assume we will have one. Dr. Mosholder, thank you for being here. Thank you for your good work on all these issues.

I would like you to turn to Tab 1 in that giant notebook in front of you there, and I would ask unanimous consent to be able to put the binder with all the data in our official record. Without objection, so ordered.

This is an e-mail, and I will read it or parts of it at least, to you and then your response to Dr. Katz. It is an e-mail from Rusty Katz to you, and then your response. Can you tell us—Well, let me read part of it, and then maybe you can respond to it, sir. This is dated June 2, 2003, and Dr. Katz says:

"We have recently become aware of a presumed association between Paxil and suicidality in pediatric patients. We received a call from the EMEA a little over a week ago. Dr. Raines told us the company, GSK, had submitted data that demonstrated that use of Paxil in kids was associated with increased suicidality compared to placebo and that the company proposed labeling changes. I believe she also said that it was in the news, and it was a big issue. Tom and I told her that the company had not informed us of any of this, and we agreed to look into it."

Then it goes on to talk about some things, and it says: "The sponsor has not proposed labeling changes and makes a feeble attempt to dismiss the finding. We are also awaiting the submission of what the sponsor submitted to UK. We want to move quickly to evaluate this signal. We are planning to look at the NDAs for other SSRIs to see whether or not similar events are being hidden by various inappropriate coating maneuvers."

Then they want to compare other things. Then they go on to say to you: "Given your history with this application and this general issue, we think you would be the right person to help us think about the best approach to the data in the other NDAs and their sponsors, as well as to provide ideas for further sources of potential relevant data and possible approaches to better evaluate this signal study."

They go on to say, you know, we want to know if you want to do this, basically, and want to move soon.

Can you tell us, basically, what you were tasked to do as a result of this?

Mr. MOSHOLDER. Well, I approached my own management, and they agreed to assign me to this issue, and it involved, initially last summer, a review of the Paxil submission that was referred to, and then a preliminary search of submissions for the other drugs, looking for any kind of similar pattern with these events.

Mr. WALDEN. So you looked at all the drugs, similar drugs being prescribed to kids for anti-depression?

Mr. MOSHOLDER. All the ones that we had the pediatric supplement NDA applications for.

Mr. WALDEN. And you were specifically looking at suicidality among adolescents? Wasn't that——

Mr. MOSHOLDER. That is correct. Children and adolescents, yes.

Mr. WALDEN. When did you first report the results of your consult to your superiors?

Mr. MOSHOLDER. As I recall, I completed a written consult in early September 2003, and then there was a briefing for CDER management also in September.

Mr. WALDEN. I believe it was September 16, our records would indicate, of 2003, that the regulatory briefing took place.

Did you attend an internal regulatory briefing then in September 2003, and at that briefing did you present the results of your first consult to FDA's Neuropharm Division?

Mr. MOSHOLDER. Yes, I did.

Mr. WALDEN. And was Robert Temple and Tom Laughren and Russell Katz among those who attended the briefing?

Mr. MOSHOLDER. As I recall, they were.

Mr. WALDEN. What were your general conclusions about the pediatric suicidality data you reviewed and your September 2003 consult in Tab 3, if you need to refer to it—or excuse me, Tab 8, if you need to look at that? What were your general conclusions about suicidality?

Mr. MOSHOLDER. Well, I need to refer to my summary here.

Mr. WALDEN. Sure. Absolutely.

Mr. MOSHOLDER. Well, basically this had two components. One was a thorough look at the Paxil data, and then a preliminary look at the data for the other drugs. Basically, I was saying that there did seem to be a risk with Paxil based on the data the company had submitted and that a first look at the other drugs showed that it was not limited necessarily to Paxil. That was the question at the time, and it might be what we call a class effect, which means that it applies to all of the drugs in a particular type of drug.

Mr. WALDEN. So am I correct then in understanding that what you were saying in that document is that Paxil definitely showed potential suicidality increase in adolescents, and that the others may also show that in a whole class?

Mr. MOSHOLDER. Yes, and I recommended looking further at the other drugs, which was already underway at that time.

Mr. WALDEN. And that was September 16, 2003?

Mr. MOSHOLDER. Yes. The briefing presentation basically mirrored the written document.

Mr. WALDEN. When this consult was first given to you and you had experience previously in looking at some of these pediatric anti-depressant trials, did you have any sense of what the conclusion would likely be?

Mr. MOSHOLDER. No, I did not.

Mr. WALDEN. What type of data did you review from the other SSRIs to come to the conclusion you did come to?

Mr. MOSHOLDER. For this work, it involved a manual review of the reports from those pediatric trials.

Mr. WALDEN. That would be the adverse event reports?

Mr. MOSHOLDER. Right, as written up in the clinical trial reports for those drugs.

Mr. WALDEN. And at that time, were you waiting to receive more data from the pharmaceutical companies. So, therefore, this was a preliminary consult?

Mr. MOSHOLDER. Yes, and I think, as I mentioned earlier, what GlaxoSmithKline did was they had an electronic search of their clinical trial data base, looking for certain key words that had been used to describe adverse events, and that is how they produced the data which yielded the signal for Paxil.

So what DNDP had done in July was ask all the other sponsors to reproduce that, using the same methods that GSK had used for Paxil, so that we had, you know, a reasonable comparison between the drugs. Then that was still being awaited at the time—I think those data were just arriving at the time I was finishing this September report.

Mr. WALDEN. And were you the one who was going to review those data?

Mr. MOSHOLDER. Yes.

Mr. WALDEN. Okay. And did anyone at that meeting express to you that your work was done and not to continue with it?

Mr. MOSHOLDER. No, although there was considerable discussion about how to pursue it and how to classify the events, but nobody thought it was finished, although there wasn't—there was a lot of discussion about what the next steps should be.

Mr. WALDEN. Incidentally, who signed off on this consult, because I see that the last page of it only has signature blocks for you and Dr. Willy. Did you need to get anyone else's approval to finalize the September consult?

Mr. MOSHOLDER. Let's see. In my copy, if you turn to another couple of pages, you will see that Dr. Avigan, who is my Division Director, signed it electronically, which is our system for sign-off.

Mr. WALDEN. All right. But not Anne Trontell?

Mr. MOSHOLDER. No. Dr. Trontell did not.

Mr. WALDEN. Okay. So it was finalized shortly after you completed it, and there was not a significant lag time between you completing it and getting it signed off?

Mr. MOSHOLDER. Well, let's see. The date I have is September 4, and then it looks like it was signed off September 5.

Mr. WALDEN. Okay. If you would turn to Tab 10 then, this is an e-mail from Russell Katz to you dated September 17, 2003 in which he stated you had done a superb job. Is this in reference to the presentation you made about the signal of suicidality in children taking anti-depressants?

Mr. MOSHOLDER. This was in reference to that September briefing.

Mr. WALDEN. Okay. But on that issue. Right?

Mr. MOSHOLDER. On this issue. Correct.

Mr. WALDEN. Did he or any other person in an advisory role express any concerns with your conclusion at this time? That is, did anyone take the position that your analysis was wrong?

Mr. MOSHOLDER. Not wrong per se, but there was a lot of discussion about whether the events could be more appropriately classified and whether—which—that is the concern that led ultimately to the Columbia reclassification project.

Mr. WALDEN. But one more question. Then I will yield to my colleagues. Were there any concerns expressed by anyone within Neuropharm or the agency at that time that the method in which you approached the data and your analysis was incorrect or problematic?

Mr. MOSHOLDER. As I recall, there was—I had some suggestions from the statisticians about how to improve the methodology from that standpoint.

Mr. WALDEN. But did you ever think that—I mean, yes, how confident were you in that consult in your methodology? Was it any different than what Columbia ended up when they reclassified the data?

Mr. MOSHOLDER. Well, I mean, I would say I was reasonably confident. People may have different opinions about that, you know. The Columbia project was—their involvement was to classify the events into whether they were definitive suicidal behaviors or not, basically, and they had a more refined methodology than what I had used.

Then the other part of that is that Dr. Hammad's analysis from a statistical standpoint is more sophisticated than what I did. So——

Mr. WALDEN. But the outcome was the same, wasn't it?

Mr. MOSHOLDER. The results were very similar.

Mr. WALDEN. Thank you. I now recognize the gentleman from Michigan, Mr. Stupak, for questions.

Mr. STUPAK. Thank you, Mr. Chairman. Doctor, Ms. DeGette asked a question about not being allowed to testify at the Advisory Committee. Is it your understanding that Dr. Graham has not been allowed to testify at the Accutane Advisory Committees?

Mr. MOSHOLDER. I am not—I don't have direct knowledge of the Accutane Advisory Committees.

Mr. STUPAK. Okay. When we talk about these anti-depressants, Paxil, Zoloft, Prozac, etcetera, we are talking about SSRIs, which is selective serotonin reuptake inhibitors. Correct?

Mr. MOSHOLDER. Correct. There are also—in the group of drugs that were looked at, there are some so called atypical anti-depressants which are not SSRIs.

Mr. STUPAK. Sure. Let me show you a document. We will give the doctor one and the rest of the committee members a copy of this document. I am going to show you three of them, but the first one is a September 19, 2001, FDA pharmacology/toxicology consultation.

In there, they are reviewing three previously unreported Accutane studies, and a pharmacologist reported—and I am on page 3, the last paragraph, sort of the conclusions. It is a seven or nine-page document there, but on page 3 there are conclusions, and I am quoting now. I think it is the second to last line. "Although possible psychiatric correlates of excessive serotonagenic function cannot be ruled out, it should be noted that increased serotonagenic function is presumed to be the mechanism of action of a major class of anti-depressants, the SSRIs, i.e., selective serotonin reuptake inhibitors."

Since the excessive serotonic function discovered with Accutane use mimics the SSRIs of these anti-depressants, I as you then: Do you believe that this relationship between Accutane and the SSRIs warrant the same type of notification to patients, to the parents, consisting of an informed consent, a clear and concise package warning, a Med Guide, and a certification of the physician and the registry of all patients, as is recommended for Accutane? Do you think we should have that same kind of notice, if we are talking about SSRIs which somehow, some are similar to function we find in Accutane?

Mr. MOSHOLDER. That is a good question. As I understand it, you are suggesting that a risk management program——

Mr. STUPAK. That has been recommended for Accutane, which Accutane, according to this consult 3 years ago, talks about SSRIs and the mechanism which is similar—it is the same thing we are talking about right here with Paxil and Zoloft and Prozac.

So if we are going to have that kind of a recommended warning for Accutane, shouldn't we have that kind of notification or warning to patients who are using these anti-depressants that again have the SSRI function in them?

Mr. MOSHOLDER. That is something I haven't really thought about. I guess that would be going beyond the boxed warning and more——

Mr. STUPAK. Sure, it is.

Mr. MOSHOLDER. The real issue being how can we be sure that patients——

Mr. STUPAK. Have the full information before they make this decision. Right? As you said earlier talking to Mr. Chairman, the benefits and the risks have to be known before you can have had the whole thing—before a parent should make that decision. Correct?

Take a look at the second document I showed you there. This document, if you look, is a PET scan of the orbital frontal cortex in the area of the brain that mediates depression. The PET scan is of a 17-year-old, and the brain starts—17-year-old brain. It starts with baseline of the orbital frontal cortex, and then it shows this area of the brain after 4 months on Accutane. Please note the changes. As demonstrated in color, the brain after 4 months on Accutane, there's some clear differences.

The PET scan clearly shows changes in the brain after 4 months. The researcher took PET scans of Accutane patients and patients who received a different oral antibiotic. The researcher took a baseline PET scan of all the patients' brains and then again at the 4 month stage of their Accutane or oral antibiotic treatment.

Some of the Accutane patients showed a pronounced difference in the brain's metabolism in the area that we recognize causing depression.

Since the FDA in their previous memo has equated Accutane with SSRIs, and we know from this research that, while metabolic changes are occurring in the brain of Accutane user, then my question is this. Is the FDA, by allowing anti-depressants be used in young people, creating another situation like we have in Accutane where these drugs are destroying part of the brain, destroying young people, but the evidence is ignored as not being scientifically established and, therefore, the drug manufacturer continues to market their products, despite the research which suggests that the drugs are actually destroying a person's brain, causing depression, and is doing more harm than good? Based on the PET scan, research of this metabolism that is going on in the brain may or may not be reversible. Can the brain regenerate itself to repair the damage done by the SSRIs? What are we telling parents whose children have not improved after taking the anti-depressants? That the drug their children are taking may have actually destroyed part of the brain?

You and I don't have the answers to this, but in summation: Since there appears to be an established link, at least in one research project, by giving our children Accutane and these SSRIs, Prozac, Zoloft and Paxil, we may actually be causing more harm than good in the brains of young people.

Should the FDA—and here is my question. Should the FDA prevent the use of these drugs in children until these very serious questions are answered? I think it is the same question—maybe we have a little bit of evidence here that Mr. Barton didn't have—that Mr. Barton asked you about the risk versus benefits, and I think in response you said to him, risk is never justified in dealing with suicidal behavior.

So if we have some evidence here showing changes in the brain in Accutane, which is equated to the previous documents SSRIs, should we not be very cautious on continuing to prescribe these SSRIs to young people under the age of 18 until we answer these questions?

Mr. MOSHOLDER. Well, I would say that the findings from—actually from the clinical trial data—you know, without turning to even neuroimaging, one can look at the clinical trial data, and that would certainly give one pause about the usefulness of these drugs for children and adolescents for depression.

It is also true that we don't know nearly enough about the long term effects of these anti-depressant drugs or other drugs on children and adolescents who are growing and developing.

Mr. STUPAK. Well, as you said, we don't know enough about it. So as I said in my opening statement, shouldn't we really err on the side on caution? You know, suicide is final, and we have had a number of suicides related to these SSRIs and, say, with Accutane. I mean, if there is a question here as to the safety, and to date this is probably the only evidence we have showing a change in the brain in some of these Accutane patients which equate to your SSRIs—if we have brain changes, until we answer these questions, if it is reversible, can the brain rehabilitate itself, grow new cells, shouldn't we really be very, very cautious in how we use these drugs, and should we not even consider not prescribing to young people under age 18?

I asked that same question of the drug manufacturers 2 weeks ago, and they really wouldn't give me an answer. They thought it was still okay to prescribe drugs to people under 18, even though the jury is still out, as they wanted to say. Shouldn't we err on the side of caution here?

Mr. MOSHOLDER. Well, my own opinion is, as I said before, that we should be mindful of the fact that the best data, the best evidence for benefit is limited to the single drug, Prozac, at least in terms of depression. Obsessive compulsive disorder is a different story, but for depression.

So that faced with the question of possible harm, on the one hand, and then lack of evidence of benefit, on the other, that should certainly be part of the evaluation of whether or not to use the drugs.

I am not prepared to say that the drugs shouldn't be used in children.

Mr. STUPAK. I believe you got one more document there. My time has almost run out. Let's go to that. In dealing with pediatric studies, and again we are still in question here, dosage is usually a question as to the proper amount that should be given, of the amount, the percentage, things like that.

For example, in Accutane we know that the dosage is way too high, and in one FDA source—in fact, it is there with you—it states that the Accutane formula dose may be 240 times more than necessary for safe treatment, and that was followed up with discussions to have Hoffman La Roche do a dosage study and, as far as I know, it was never done.

So my question is: Since these anti-depressants and Accutane have sort of been linked here today, has there been shown to be—has the FDA given any thought to determine whether proper dosage is given to children and adolescents with these anti-depressants, because they were developed for adults. So are we dealing with the proper dosage when we are dealing with young people and adolescents?

Mr. MOSHOLDER. Well, that is a very good question, and unfortunately, to the best of my recollection, the clinical trials that we have for the anti-depressants in children were done with what we call flexible dosing where it is left up to the clinician/investigator to determine the dose within a certain range.

So there might have been one or two exceptions to that, but what is really needed is a study in which patients are assigned to a specific dose, and then both the benefits and the side effects can be compared to get a judgment of what the best dose is.

So there is clearly—apart from even figuring out if the drugs are effective in children, there is clearly more need for data on the proper dosage.

Mr. WALDEN. I want to thank the gentleman.

Mr. STUPAK. Thank you. Mr. Chairman, I ask that those three documents referred to by Dr. Mosholder and given to the committee be made part of the record.

Mr. WALDEN. Without objection.

[The documents referred to follow:]

PHARMACOLOGY/TOXICOLOGY CONSULTATION

From: Division of Dermatologic and Dental Drug Products, HFD-540.
Date of request: 9/19/01.
Desired date of completion: 10/30/01.
Requested by: Indira Hills, PM; A. Nostrandt, P/T.

NDA 18-662
Type of document: Articles dated 9/5/01, consisting of 3 study reports (see listing below).
Name of drug: Isotretinoin Oral Capsules (Accutane).
Drug classification: Retinoid; indication, acne.
Name of firm: Hoffman-La Roche/Basilea.

Reviewer name: Linda H. Fossom.
Division name: Neuropharmacological Drug Product
HFD #: 120.
Review completion date: 10/31/01.

Reason for request: To determine whether there is any preclinical basis for concern regarding possible clinical psychiatric events, e.g. suicide, evident in the submitted studies on 13-cis-retinoic acid (isotretinoin; Accutane) and 9-cis-retinoic acid (alitretinoin, an isomer that is an active metabolite of isotretinoin and directly binds the physiologic retinoic acid receptor).

Studies submitted: [These are old preclinical studies that were recently submitted by Basilea, a Roche-related company, related to a pre-IND for a different systemic retinoid, at the request of HFD-540.]

- General pharmacological and drug interaction studies with Ro 04-3780 (13-cis retinoic acid) [isotretinoin] administered orally; Report no. W-5615; dated 1/13/82.
- Preliminary acute toxicity of Ro 04-4079/001 [alitretinoin, isomer and active metabolite of isotretinoin] after oral administration in rats and behavioral observation of rats during subchronic (p.o. and i.v.) treatment with Ro 04-4079; Research Report B-159'819; 12/20/93.
- A 26-week oral (gavage) administration study in the rat with Ro 04-4079/001 (9-cis-RA[alitretinoin, an isomer and active metabolite of isotretinoin]); Research Report B-157'294; 11/9/95.

Specifically, I reviewed these studies focusing on behavioral effects of the 2 retinoids (see the Appendix to this consultation for more details).

SUMMARY: Three study reports were submitted with this request for consultation, however, the data in these reports was very limited in terms of the behavioral effects of isotretinoin (Accutane), with somewhat more information on the behavioral effects of alitretinoin, an isomer and active metabolite of isotretinoin.

Isotretinoin was tested at a single dose (30 mg/kg po) administered daily for 10 days to male mice. Behaviors noted were not unusual and included: increased touch response, increased irritability, and hyperactivity in some mice (i.e., 1 to 3 out of 6) at 1 hr after dosing (the only time noted) throughout the 10 days of dosing. Several instances of reduced abdominal tone were noted in 1 mouse (out of 6). There was a tendency for average rectal body temperature to be slightly increased in drug-treated mice. (up to 1.5 degrees C higher than controls, measured 1 hr after dosing). Additionally, anticonvulsant activity was investigated in mice using the same dosing schedule (i.e., 30 mg/kg/d po for 10 days) with the last dose 1 hr before precipitation of convulsions with either electroshock or iv injection of leptazol; isotretinoin was not anticonvulsant in either of these models, however, only a single dose was tested. It should be further noted that the design of these studies was probably not adequate to determine whether isotretinoin could potentiate seizures.

Alitretinoin was tested acutely at high doses and subchronically at lower doses in rats. Acute oral (gavage) administration of high doses (from 375 to 3000 mg/kg) of alitretinoin did not alter the appearance/behavior of rats for 2 days after dosing. However, from day 3 through day 10 (the last time monitored) after dosing, notable behaviors, including forepaw treading, high stepping gait, hindlimb abduction, and salivation, emerged and disappeared in a dose-related manner. One rat died 7 days after administration of the highest dose, however, the cause of death was not clear. In a repeated dose study of 6 mg/kg/d po to 2 strains of rats, notable behaviors also developed, including increased locomotion, rearing and sniffing, reciprocal forepaw treading, chewing, and rare salivation. Forepaw treading was evident in the home cage by day 7 of dosing, while the other behaviors were noted at day 23 (apparently the first time they were monitored). The treading behavior, evident immediately after dosing, was completely blocked by 30 min pretreatment with methiothepin, a non-selective serotonin receptor antagonist, before the 52nd day of dosing. This treading or paddling behavior also developed when alitretinoin was administered by the intravenous route (at a dose of 0.4 mg/kg/d, which the sponsor claims is equivalent to the 6 mg/kg/d po dose); the treading was not noted after the first dose, but apparent in some rats after 17 daily doses. In another repeated-dose study of oral (gavage) alitretinoin at doses from 0.67 to 6 mg/kg/d, these same behaviors, including paddling, high stepping gait and salivation, again developed with incidences and latencies that were dose-related. In this study, vehicle was substituted for drug on one day of week 7 in the high-dose group and paddling behavior was seen immediately after dosing, suggesting a conditioning effect on this behavior.

CONCLUSIONS: The behavioral effects of the retinoids, isotretinoin (in mice) and alitretinoin (in rats), in the studies submitted for review here were limited to clinical signs observed during the course of a few pharmacology and/or toxicology studies in mice and rats.

Given this understanding of the limitations of these studies, there were some behaviors exhibited by both rats and mice that are consistent with serotonergic receptor stimulation. Following the clinical availability of MAO inhibitors and tricyclic antidepressants in the 1950's, a behavioral reaction characterized by hyperactivity was described in both humans and animals given combinations of these agents, such as imipramine with an MAOI. A constellation of behaviors called the "serotonin syndrome" has been characterized in rodents under conditions of excessive stimulation of serotonin receptors, e.g., by administration of 5-HTP (the precursor of serotonin) in combination with an MAO inhibitor (e.g., pargyline) and includes, but is not limited to, increased locomotor activity, forepaw treading, tremors, hyperexcitability, salivation, lateral head weaving, hindlimb abduction, arched (Straub) tail, pyrexia, and seizures. Several of these behaviors were exhibited by the animals in the studies reviewed here, especially in the rat studies. Mice treated with isotretinoin developed increased irritability, hyperactivity and reduced abdominal tone. Rats treated with alitretinoin (po or iv) developed several of the more unusual behaviors, including forepaw paddling/treading, high stepping gait, hindlimb abduction, and salivation.

These behaviors, especially those seen in rats after alitretinoin administration, are characteristic of excessive serotonergic stimulation; in fact, the forepaw treading behavior was shown to be blocked by a (non-selective) serotonin receptor antagonist in a study reviewed here. An unusual feature of these behaviors in this case is the long latencies: at least 48 hr after a high acute oral dose and after several days of oral or intravenous administration of lower doses. This long latency to development of these behaviors is consistent with either an adaptive change or accumulation of drug and/or a metabolite. It might be helpful to know the temporal relationship between systemic exposures to alitretinoin and/or metabolites and the expression of these behaviors to clarify the underlying mechanism. Additionally, it seems likely that the expression of some (e.g., forepaw treading) if not all of these behaviors may be enhanced by conditioning in the repeated dosing studies; probably conditioning related to the oral dosing procedure, but also possibly conditioning to other aspects of the administration and testing procedure.

In conclusion, the only remarkable behavioral responses reported in the studies reviewed here apparently indicate an excessive serotonergic response that seems to develop in response to alitretinoin administration (to rats) and possibly in response to isotretinoin administration (to mice). However, the interpretation of this response in rodents for humans taking isotretinoin is difficult. Because of the long latency to the response in rodents seen here, it is not clear that this response is analogous to the clinical "serotonin syndrome," a potentially fatal neurological syndrome. Additionally, although possible psychiatric correlates of excessive serotonergic function cannot be ruled out, it should be noted that increased serotonergic function is presumed to be the mechanism of action of a major class of antidepressants, the SSRIs (i.e., selective serotonin reuptake inhibitors). Generalization from (apparently) excessive serotonergic function in rodents to any psychiatric problems in humans seems unwarranted at this time.

Linda H. Fossom, Ph.D., Pharmacologist, HFD-120
Barry Rosloff, Ph.D., Supervisor

cc: [in DFS]
HFD-540: /KHills/MJKozma-Fornaro/KO'Connell/ANostrandt
HFD-120: /AMosholder/TLaughren

Appendix: Brief reviews of relevant behavioral effects from 3 submitted studies:

- General pharmacological and drug interaction studies with Ro 04-3780 (13-cis retinoic acid) [Accutane] administered orally; Report no. W-5615; dated 1/13/82.
- Preliminary acute toxicity of Ro 04-4079/001 after oral administration in rats and behavioral observation of rats during subchronic (p.o. and i.v.) treatment with Ro 04-4079; Research Report B-159'819; 12/20/93.
- A 26-week oral (gavage) administration study in the rat with Ro 04-4079/001 (9-cis-RA); Research Report B-157'294; 11/9/95.

Cardiovascular, respiratory, and autonomic systems:
Antiarrhythmic potential in female mice: same 10-day, 0 or 30 mg/kg/d, treatments as above, but challenge with ouabain (300 ug/min iv, tail vein): mean survival times were 95 sec for vehicle controls and 99 sec for Ro group.
Vital signs (BP, HR and RR) in unanesthetized cats: 0 or 80 mg/kg/d po for 10 days, 2/sex/dose, then crossover after 10 treatment-free days; vital signs before and 1 hr after each day of dosing, plus next 2 treatment-free days; no notable effects.
Vital signs [basal and pharmacologically stimulated EKG, BP, HR, RR, and nerve-stimulated contraction of nictitating membrane] in [chloralose/pentobarb-] anesthetized cats: 30 mg/kg intraduodenal, 2/sex: small increases in arterial BP and HR in ¾cats noted by Sponsor; the Sponsor also notes that, based upon interactions with NE, ISO, HIST and 5-HT on HR, Ro was a weak inhibitor of tachycardia and increased bradycardia; this was associated with a possible increased hypotensive response to HIST and 5-HT; overall, without significant effects.

GI: motility in mouse: no effect reported, not reviewed.

Renal: diuresis in rat: no effect reported, not reviewed.

Immune: mouse: sheep red cell antibody test: reported negative, not reviewed; methylated BSA test: reduced the delayed hypersensitivity reaction, i.e., apparent immunosuppression, in contrast to cited literature reports of retinoid induced immunostimulation in vivo and in vitro; difference attributed to possible dose-effect, immuno stimulation at low doses, suppression at higher doses.

Drug interaction studies:

CNS: mouse: vs diazepam-attenuated leptazol-induced seizures; vs phenobarbitone- or phenytoin-attenuated electroshock-induced seizures; vs ethanol-induced sedation (loss of righting reflex); vs aspirin- or dextropropoxyphene-induced analgesia (acetylcholine iodide-induced writhing); no apparent interactions, but experimental designs were limited.
Immune and inflammatory: rat vs dexamethasone (developing adjuvant arthritis test); Ro had **no intrinsic anti-inflammatory activity** and did not alter dexamethasone's activity; Ro **reduced the secondary response (esp, non-injected paw swelling, lesion score, and joint mobility) similar to dexamethasone, but with lower potency and no interaction.**

Figure 2. Chemical structure of alitretinoin (9-cis retinoic acid; Ro 04-4079/001; active metabolite of isotretinoin).

Structural formulae and/or NAMES of Ro 04-4079/000

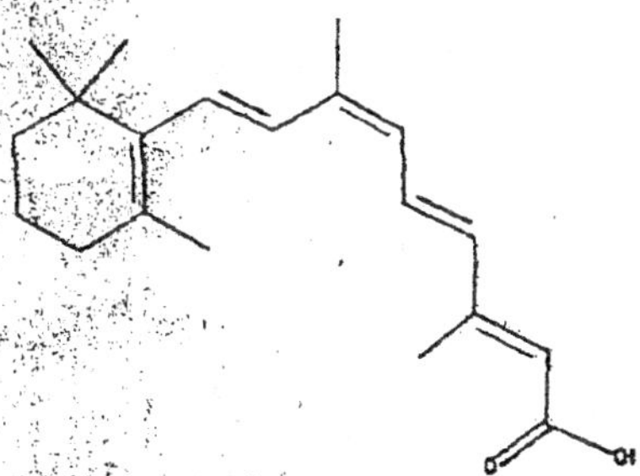

Systematic_NAME

(2E,4E,6Z,8E)-3,7-Dimethyl-9-(2,6,6-trimethyl-1-cyclohexen-1-yl)-2,4,6,8-nonatetraenoic acid

(9Z)-Retinoic acid

Preliminary acute toxicity of Ro 04-4079/001[isomer and active metabolite of Accutane] after oral administration in rats and behavioral observation of rats during subchronic (p.o. and i.v.) treatment with Ro 04-4079; Research Report B-159'819; 12/20/93.

Acute toxicity: 375, 750, 1500, and 3000 mg/kg po (in rapeseed oil, 10 ml/kg) to female rats (Ibm:RORO, ~100 g), 2/dose, observed in pairs daily; normal appearance for days 1 and 2, from days 3 through 10 after dosing, **behaviors consistent with "serotonin syndrome" emerged that were dose-dependent (the higher the dose, the more behaviors that were exhibited, e.g., only forepaw treading and high stepping gait at LD, expanding to include abduced hind legs and salivation at higher doses.** These signs persisted in a dose-related manner also, with signs subsiding by day 5 at LD, but reciprocal forepaw treading continuing through day 10 (but normal at days 11 and 12) at HD. Other behaviors, not clearly related to SS, were also noted with similar dose-relatedness, including chewing, loss of righting reflex, vocalization, ataxia, decrease in muscle tone, loss of body weight. No mention was made of other classic SS signs, such as hyperexcitability, lateral head weaving, Straub tail, myoclonous or seizures. One out of 2 (1/2) HD rats died on day 7.

NB It's unclear why these behaviors took so long to develop after acute dosing. This long latency suggests that some adaptive change(s) in response to drug administration or some metabolite with delayed synthesis/accumulation is responsible for the serotonin syndrome-like behaviors, rather than a more direct activation of serotonin receptors.

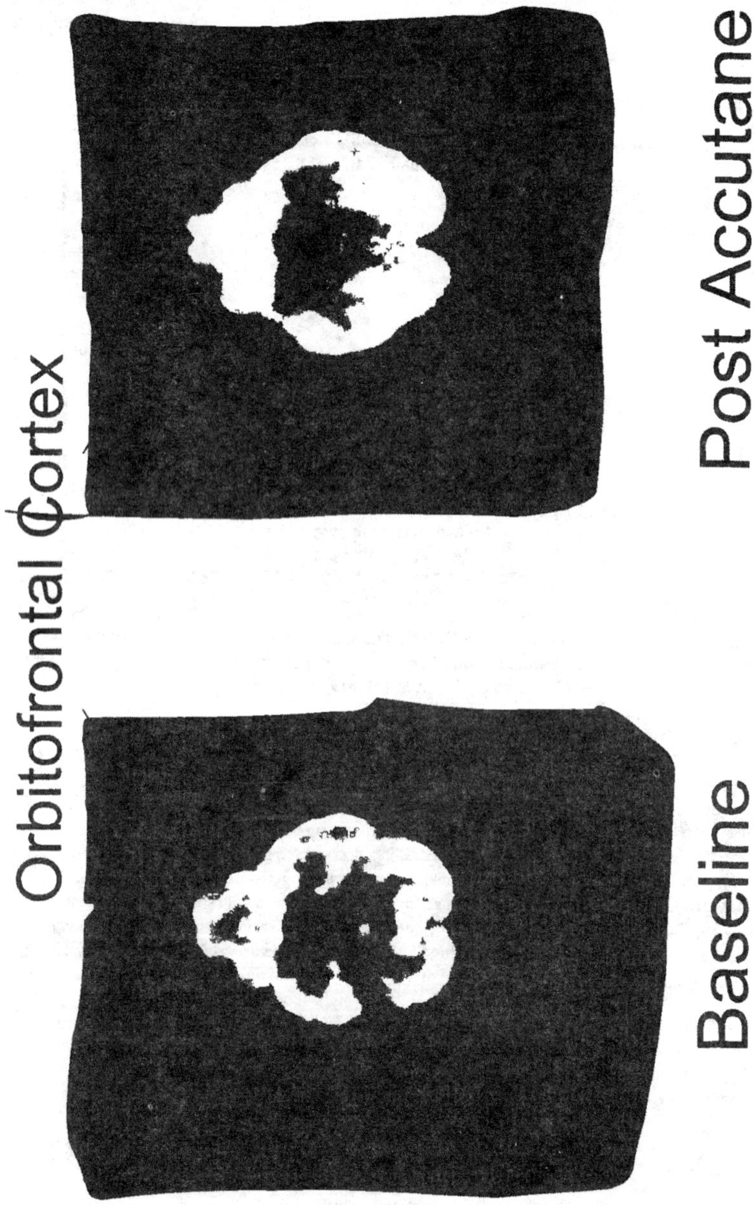
Orbitofrontal Cortex
Post Accutane
Baseline

Abstract View

FUNCTIONAL BRAIN IMAGING ALTERATIONS IN ACNE PATIENTS TREATED WITH ISOTRETINOIN

J.D.Bremner[1*]; N.Fani[2]; N.Ashraf[2]; J.Votaw[1]; M.Brummer[2]; V.Vaccarino[2]; M.Goodman[1]; L.Reed[2]; C.B.Nemeroff[2]

1. Emory Ctr for Positron Emission Tomography, 2. Psychiatry, 3. Radiology, Emory Univ Hosp, Atlanta, GA, USA

Although there have been case reports suggesting a relationship between treatment with the acne medication isotretinoin (Accutane) and the development of depression and suicide, this topic remains controversial. In order for isotretinoin to cause depression it must have an effect on the brain; however no studies to date have examined the effects of isotretinoin on brain function in acne patients. The purpose of this study was to assess the effects of isotretinoin on brain function in acne patients. Brain function was measured with [F-18]-2-fluoro-2-deoxyglucose (FDG) positron emission tomography (PET) before and after four months of treatment with isotretinoin (N=13) and antibiotic (N=15). Isotretinoin (but not antibiotic) treatment was associated with decreased brain metabolism in the orbitofrontal cortex (-21% change versus a +2% change for antibiotic) ($p<0.05$), a brain area known to mediate symptoms of depression. There were no differences in severity of depressive symptoms between the isotretinoin and antibiotic treatment groups before or after treatment. This study suggests that isotretinoin treatment is associated with changes in brain function.

Citation:J.D. Bremner, N. Fani, N. Ashraf, J. Votaw, M. Brummer, V. Vaccarino, M. Goodman, L. Reed, C.B. Nemeroff. FUNCTIONAL BRAIN IMAGING ALTERATIONS IN ACNE PATIENTS TREATED WITH ISOTRETINOIN Program No. 114.2. *2004 Abstract Viewer/Itinerary Planner.* Washington, DC: Society for Neuroscience, 2004. Online.

Translator: A. Rix
October 22, 1971

Vol 2 IND 9648

Investigational Drug Brochure
RO 4-3780
13-cis- Retinoic Acid
A. Glick, MD

p. 14 Contraindications

"At this early state of clinical evaluation, it is also contraindicated in children"

p. 15 Precautions and Warnings

With oral retinoic acid, headaches, nausea, vomiting, vertigo and some of the skin and mucous membrane lesions seen with hypervitaminosis A have been reported. Because of the chemical and pharmacological similarities between RO 4-3780, retinoic acid and retinol, one should be on the look out for the above adverse reactions in patients taking RO 4-3780.

March 17, 1976

HLR submits an Addendum to schedule 6 [Vol 1 has the schedules]
Preclinical Study Report
The Distribution of 13-cis Retionoic Acid Studied By
Whole-Body Autoradiography in the Rat

Results
Nervous System

Only transient but considerable uptake of radioactivity was seen in the cerebellum and in the brain stem. The concentrations in these organs and in the spinal medulla decreased to zero between 5 and 24 hours after application. [page 3]

Discussion

The aim of the investigation was to demonstrate the distribution and retention of labeled 13-cis retinoic acid in the rat. During the first hour after the intravenous injection of the labeled compound a wide-spread distribution over the whole body was observed. After 5 hours most of the radioactivity was eliminated from the blood and then temporarily accumulated in some tissues. The 13-cis retinoic acid – like all-trans retinoic acid – was found to be absorbed for a short time by the brain at a considerably higher degree than is vitamin A. As far as whole-body autoradiographs can be quantifatively evaluated, it can be said that no differences seen to exist between absorption of 13-cis retinoic acid and all-trans retinoic acid by the rat brain.

Vol 3 IND 9648

Supplemental Pharmacology Review of IND 9648 and 13,669
Completed 5/3/78

Evaluation and Comment
5) If RO 3780 is effective as a dermatological agent local application of the drug should **be test to overcome** some of the potential systemic adverse effects. As **Hypervitaminosis A is damaging** to normal bone structure and development use in growing children by systemic route is questioned and could possibly be overcome by local application.

May 30, 1978
RO 4-3780 – One Year Dog Study

"The nature of the toxic signs which are observed are considered to be similar to symptoms of hypervitaminosis A which have been observed in man."

May 8, 1978
Medical Officer Review

Clinical Evaluation

J. Peck, MD at NIH has 81 patients entered in his study and reports that results are under analysis. He notes that 9 patients have been removed from the protocol because of adverse reactions such as Xerosis, cheilitis, pruritus, blurred vision and dizziness. The dose range is 10-600 mg/day or 0.4-7.4 mg/kg.

HLR
Investigational Drug Brochure
RO 4-3780
13-cis Retinoic Acid
February 1978

p.18 Pharmacokinetics
Discusses Whole-body Autoradiography .... But leave out the lines on 13-cis hitting the brain!

p. 38 Recommendations for Clinical Use
B. Contraindications

At this stage of clinical evaluation, its use in children should be restricted to severe conditions in which the possible benefits to be gained are expected to outweigh the risks involved.

Mr. STUPAK. Thank you.

Chairman BARTON. Thank you.

Mr. WALDEN. Dr. Mosholder, given the new TAD study on fluoxetine, do you believe that that raises any issues parents and physicians should be concerned about relative to suicidality?

Mr. MOSHOLDER. My opinion is that it does raise some concerns about that, and as I was saying earlier, when I did my initial—well, actually, the March consult document didn't have the TADS study, and it looked at sort of conveniently the one drug that had the best efficacy for depression, also didn't seem to have this risk of increasing suicidal events, which made a certain amount of sense. But I think now it is a little different picture that, although the TAD study again showed that Prozac is effective in ameliorating the symptoms of depression, it suggests there is a certain number of patients who have an increased risk of suicidal behaviors or thoughts at the same time.

So there is both a risk and a benefit, in other words.

Mr. WALDEN. Do you recall what the suicidality rate was in the TAD study and how that compares to the other studies?

Mr. MOSHOLDER. As I recall from Dr. Hammad's analysis, the relative risk, as we call, which is—or risk ratio is between 4 and 5. I can look that up.

Mr. WALDEN. And what does that mean to a layperson like me?

Mr. MOSHOLDER. Well, one way that we measure these risks is to do what we call a risk ratio, and that is—I guess the simplest way to explain would be with a brief example. A study with 100 patients on drug, 100 on placebo, if one had 10 suicidal events on drug and 5 on placebo, the ratio would be 10 out of 100 to 5 out of 100, or 2.

So we would say that that relative risk is 2, and that is—and as I recall, in the TAD study it's actually higher than that.

Mr. WALDEN. And is that a—is 4, if that was the number, is that one that should raise a flag? I mean, you do this work all the time.

Mr. MOSHOLDER. Well, I think it raises a flag, and it has to be judged against the benefit. so that there is a study in which in the same study, you can look at the benefits and the risks simultaneously.

Mr. WALDEN. All right. The question is: Does it suggest a point of underreporting in the other studies?

Mr. MOSHOLDER. No, I'm not sure that is the—I'm not sure the answer is as simple as that. There are some differences between the TAD study and the other studies that might or might not account for the different in the data. It is kind of hard to tell after the fact.

Mr. WALDEN. Could you turn to Tab 11 in our notebook there. This is an e-mail dated October 2, 2003. Mary Willy who is your direct supervisor—correct?—in the Office of Drug Safety at that time, suggests to the Neuropharm Division and others that you should present your Paxil suicidality conclusions that were first presented in September to a Pediatric Advisory Subcommittee meeting that was meeting in October.

Then Russell Katz writes back to her and states: "We recognize that some folks outside the Division have concluded there is enough of a signal already established to make some sort of a meaningful statement about the data, but we haven't, and we think that publicly presenting part of the data in its current state has the great potential to be misleading and uninformative."

Do you agree with Dr. Katz' statement that publicly presenting your data and conclusions you reached at that time has the great potential to be misleading and uninformative?

Mr. MOSHOLDER. Well, my opinion was—and that of Dr. Willy at the time was that we thought it could be done and might have been useful, which is why she proposed it. But as you see, there was a difference of opinion about that.

Mr. WALDEN. You know, it strikes me that when word came over from Europe that there may be a problem here, they went right to you quickly and said we have to act quickly.

I guess what is troubling to us is it appears there was a fairly long delay between the time you did your quick review, your consult, came back and said I see some problems here, if I am characterizing that correctly, and then when it finally gets presented up the chain. It seems like somebody put a brake on somewhere. Did you ever feel that way?

Mr. MOSHOLDER. You know, it is really hard to be specific and say that—I'm not sure I have much of an answer to that, really.

Mr. WALDEN. All right. Did you present at that October Pediatric Advisory Committee meeting?

Mr. MOSHOLDER. No.

Mr. WALDEN. Throughout the fall of 2003, did you continue to work on this consult and, if so, can you briefly describe what you were looking at?

Mr. MOSHOLDER. During that fall, what I was doing was an analysis of the responses from the other anti-depressant manufacturers. As you recall, in July they had been asked to reproduce GSK's methods that found the problem with Paxil. So we wanted to—for comparability purposes, we wanted to have that reproduced by each of the other manufacturers.

We received that information in the late spring/early fall of 2003, and that is what I was working on.

Mr. WALDEN. You were reviewing all those data?

Mr. MOSHOLDER. Yes.

Mr. WALDEN. Would those data have been ready for the October presentation? Were you ready?

Mr. MOSHOLDER. For the October presentation, it would not have been the—what we would have had at that point would have paralleled the regulatory briefing that I had given in September to CDER management.

Mr. WALDEN. Okay. So at the end of October, the FDA noticed a public Advisory Committee meeting for February 2 and 3, 2004. Was it your understanding that you were going to present at this meeting on the topic of your consult and what your findings were regarding suicidal behavior in these pediatric clinical trials?

Mr. MOSHOLDER. Yes, that was my understanding.

Mr. WALDEN. That's what you were going to go do. Did the fact that in October 2003 Neuropharm decided to involve Columbia University in reclassifying the events provided by the companies mean that you were to stop working on your consult?

Mr. MOSHOLDER. I remember wondering that and discussing it with Dr. Willy, my team leader, and we decided that at that point I had gone far enough and had devoted a lot of time to this project that it made most sense just to have me finish with my analysis, which was the one that I completed the draft in December.

Mr. WALDEN. So it was your understanding, both your consult and any work that Columbia did would be pursued simultaneously?

Mr. MOSHOLDER. Correct, although the timeline—it seemed obvious that the Columbia—it seemed obvious pretty early that the Columbia data would not be ready for analysis and presentation by February 2.

Mr. WALDEN. But it was important enough that you wanted to get answers sooner than that?

Mr. MOSHOLDER. Yes, which is not to say that it had to be either one or the other, but both efforts were continuing full speed, you know, as far as I was concerned.

Mr. WALDEN. Were you involved in the planning meetings for the February 2 Advisory Committee meeting?

Mr. MOSHOLDER. Yes, I was.

Mr. WALDEN. When did you complete your final meta analysis of all the data from the SSRI pediatric clinical trials?

Mr. MOSHOLDER. As I recall, my draft was turned in to my management around mid-December.

Mr. WALDEN. Of 2003?

Mr. MOSHOLDER. Of 2003. I made some refinements to it in the subsequent couple of months.

Mr. WALDEN. And basically—correct me if I am wrong, but didn't those data, or didn't your findings show a 1.9 or 1.89 times more likely serious suicide-related event on drug than placebo?

Mr. MOSHOLDER. Yes.

Mr. WALDEN. Across the trials. Right?

Mr. MOSHOLDER. That's correct, yes.

Mr. WALDEN. All right. And didn't you recommend interim measures?

Mr. MOSHOLDER. Yes. I recommended—I wasn't very specific, I realize, but I had in mind some kind of interim measures to announce that there could be a problem.

Mr. WALDEN. Did you feel a sense of urgency?

Mr. MOSHOLDER. Yes, I did.

Mr. WALDEN. To get this information and your findings out?

Mr. MOSHOLDER. Yes, I thought it was—and that was one of the points I made at the September regulatory briefing, that these drugs are widely used in this population, and so that it was an important public health issue.

Mr. WALDEN. Did you reclassify any of the events that the sponsor gave? That is, did you change the classification from serious to nonserious or discount it completely?

Mr. MOSHOLDER. What I did for my meta analysis, I took the events which had been identified by each sponsor, using GSK's method, and then the result that I emphasized was the subgroup of those events which also met a regulatory definition for seriousness. That is a definition that—it is in the Code of Federal Regulations. It is something that each sponsor designates when they report the studies to the FDA as to whether or not a particular adverse event is serious or not.

Mr. WALDEN. And didn't your consult focus on serious suicidal events?

Mr. MOSHOLDER. Yes, it did.

Mr. WALDEN. Including the famous girl slapping face?

Mr. MOSHOLDER. Well, that was not a serious event which was——

Mr. WALDEN. So that wasn't——

Mr. MOSHOLDER. Well, that was the rationale that, without being able to do anything as elaborate or sophisticated as the Columbia University project, as a first cut to eliminate some of the questionable cases, I took the subgroup that met the criteria for seriousness, which in this case is mostly either life threatening or resulting in hospitalization.

Mr. WALDEN. Okay. So the girl slapping face scenario was not even included in your data that resulted in a 1.9 times——

Mr. MOSHOLDER. No.

Mr. WALDEN. I mean, you were pushing the upper end here in terms of suicidality issues then. Is that right? My reading as a layperson.

Mr. MOSHOLDER. Well, it was an attempt to hone in on the events that were clinically meaningful.

Mr. WALDEN. But it also says there are other events below that, including the girl slapping face situation that—I guess my point is, that could be occurring out there in adolescents——

Mr. MOSHOLDER. Yes.

Mr. WALDEN. [continuing] are not even in your data. That is not a criticism. I am just trying to get the range here.

Mr. MOSHOLDER. Well, I did look at it with the broader category, too, but I thought the more important result was with the subgroup of the serious events.

Mr. WALDEN. Indeed. My time has long since expired. I turn to my colleague from Colorado.

Ms. DEGETTE. Thank you, Mr. Chairman. Dr. Mosholder, if you could turn to Tab 67 of the notebook in front of you, do you see that statement? It is entitled Written Statement.

Mr. MOSHOLDER. Yes.

Ms. DEGETTE. Was this statement prepared by you?

Mr. MOSHOLDER. Yes, it was.

Ms. DEGETTE. Can you tell me how you came to prepare that document?

Mr. MOSHOLDER. I was—well, this is a statement that I provided to the Office of Internal Affairs, and this was pursuant to an interview that I had with two Special Agents of the Office of Internal Affairs regarding the San Francisco Chronicle story about my analysis of the suicidal events.

Ms. DEGETTE. Did those agents ask you to prepare that?

Mr. MOSHOLDER. Yes, subsequent to the interview they asked me to provide a written statement.

Ms. DEGETTE. And that is how you came to prepare that?

Mr. MOSHOLDER. Yes.

Ms. DEGETTE. Okay. And that statement was under oath. Correct?

Mr. MOSHOLDER. It was given——

Ms. DEGETTE. It was an affidavit?

Mr. MOSHOLDER. Right. That's correct, yes.

Ms. DEGETTE. And what it was about was the circumstances surrounding the removal of your analysis of the incidence of pediatric suicidality in clinical studies of anti-depressants from the agenda of the Advisory Committee meeting that we talked about, and also the conversations that you had with the San Francisco Chronicle reporter about that analysis and the decision to omit it from consideration by the Advisory Committee. Is that right?

Mr. MOSHOLDER. That is correct.

Ms. DEGETTE. And so what this written statement was attempted to be was an accurate account of the events as you knew them about the presentation and the decision to cancel that presentation, and also about your contacts with the reporter. Right?

Mr. MOSHOLDER. That is correct, and importantly, to include the statement that I did not divulge the information to the reporter.

Ms. DEGETTE. Right, and you wanted to—so part of what you wanted to do was set out a chronicle of the events, including how and why and in what way you communicated with this reporter. Right?

Mr. MOSHOLDER. That is correct. And that was part of the request that they gave me to include in the statement.

Ms. DEGETTE. Okay. Now when did you provide that statement to the OIA?

Mr. MOSHOLDER. I believe it was—it was middle of March, I think maybe March 15.

Ms. DEGETTE. That is the information I've got as well. Did there come a time when the U.S. Senate Finance Committee made inquiries regarding the events described in your statement?

Mr. MOSHOLDER. Yes, that's correct.

Ms. DEGETTE. And when did you know about that? How did you find out about that?

Mr. MOSHOLDER. I believe I saw a news report in late March of this year.

Ms. DEGETTE. And then were you contacted by the Office of Legislative Affairs?

Mr. MOSHOLDER. Yes, I was, when the Senate Finance Committee investigators wanted to arrange an interview.

Ms. DEGETTE. So it was sometime after March 15?

Mr. MOSHOLDER. That's correct.

Ms. DEGETTE. Okay. Did you meet with folks from the Office of Legislative Affairs subsequent to the TV report that you saw or the media report?

Mr. MOSHOLDER. Yes. We had a couple of preparatory meetings, as I recall, to prepare me for the Senate Finance Committee interview.

Ms. DEGETTE. Okay. Was that with Patrick McGarry and Karen Meister?

Mr. MOSHOLDER. I believe they were some of them.

Ms. DEGETTE. And there were others as well as them?

Mr. MOSHOLDER. Yes. We had a series of meetings, and I am not entirely clear on who precisely was at which meeting, but there was a number of them.

Ms. DEGETTE. Okay. Doctor, take a look at Exhibit 64, which is an e-mail from Ms. Meister to you regarding a May 3, 2004, meeting in Mr. McGarry's office. Do you see that memo, Tab 64?

Mr. MOSHOLDER. Yes.

Ms. DEGETTE. There are some people who are copied on that e-mail: Ann Hennig, Donna Katz, and Kim Dettlebach. Do you see those names?

Mr. MOSHOLDER. Yes.

Ms. DEGETTE. Do you know those individuals?

Mr. MOSHOLDER. Yes, I do.

Ms. DEGETTE. Do you know who they are?

Mr. MOSHOLDER. Ms. Hennig works with the CDER Office of Executive Programs, as I believe it is called. Ms. Katz and Ms. Dettelbach are, as I understand, with the Office of Chief Counsel at FDA.

Ms. DEGETTE. Okay. Now can you tell me what the subject of that meeting was?

Mr. MOSHOLDER. As I recall, it was a preparatory meeting for my Senate Finance Committee interview.

Ms. DEGETTE. And after that meeting, were there exchanges of various revisions to the written statement that you talked about a little while ago that you had prepared earlier that was to be provided to the Senate Finance Committee?

Mr. MOSHOLDER. Yes. That became an issue, and I can explain it this way. Having given the statement under penalty of perjury, as we said, I had a legal interest, and my attorney confirmed this, in being consistent with that statement. So that——

Ms. DEGETTE. And telling the truth, because you were under oath.

Mr. MOSHOLDER. Yes. And also not even inadvertently contradicting a previous statement. So——

Ms. DEGETTE. A previous statement made by you?

Mr. MOSHOLDER. Right. So to ensure my own consistency and knowing that the Senate Finance Committee would be asking about the same sequence of events, it was to my advantage to make use of that statement for the Senate Finance Committee investigation as well.

So I wanted to provide them with a copy of the statement as sort of my official record.

Ms. DEGETTE. Right, your take on what happened, to the best of your recollection.

Mr. MOSHOLDER. The issue was that at that time the Internal Affairs investigation, as I understand it, was still an open investigation, and apparently FDA's policy or the executive branch policy is not to reveal the existence of such investigations. So that I was advised to redact the statement so that it didn't have any reference to the Internal Affairs investigation.

Ms. DEGETTE. And they also wanted you to take the names out?

Mr. MOSHOLDER. Right. The other issue was personal privacy of not revealing the names of other people who were subject of an Internal Affairs investigation. So although I was free to reveal my own involvement, but that it wouldn't be appropriate to divulge other people who were subject to that same investigation.

Ms. DEGETTE. And were you willing to make those redactions?

Mr. MOSHOLDER. I said that I was uncomfortable redacting the document in a way that it wasn't transparent that it had been redacted.

Ms. DEGETTE. So you didn't mind taking out the names or the reference to the internal investigation, but you wanted the document to reflect that it had been altered. Correct?

Mr. MOSHOLDER. That is correct.

Ms. DEGETTE. And they wanted to alter it so that there would be no record of the redactions. Correct?

Mr. MOSHOLDER. That is my understanding. That is how I understood it, yes.

Ms. DEGETTE. Now ultimately you decided not to sign the revised document that they had sent you. Correct?

Mr. MOSHOLDER. Well, I said that, when I went to the Finance Committee for my interview, that I preferred to use my version, which indicated that the document had come from a previous document, and in the—actually, what happened was in the interim the Internal Affairs investigation was closed. So that that made that issue moot. So I was able to ultimately provide the Finance Committee with my affidavit, only minus the names for personal privacy.

Ms. DEGETTE. Okay. Take a look at Exhibit 57. That is an e-mail from Donna Katz to you with copies to various people. Do you see that there?

Mr. MOSHOLDER. Yes.

Ms. DEGETTE. Now attached to that e-mail is a copy of the written statement, your written statement, with lines through a number of sentences, and a copy where the deletions had been made. Do you see that?

Mr. MOSHOLDER. I see the—I only have the copy with the deletions indicated.

Ms. DEGETTE. All right. We are going to hand it to you. Apparently, it is not attached in the notebook, but do you recall seeing a draft of a document that Ms. Katz wanted you to look at?

Mr. MOSHOLDER. Yes. That is actually the situation I just described.

Ms. DEGETTE. Right, and here it is.

Mr. MOSHOLDER. Thank you.

Ms. DEGETTE. Is that the document?

Mr. MOSHOLDER. Well, this is the document showing where the lines have been dropped. Yes.

Ms. DEGETTE. Right, where she wanted to redact it, and in fact, her e-mail to you says, "Andy, I have taken a look at your written statement and made some suggested edits. Given this will be a new document created to give to the Senate Finance Committee, albeit based on an earlier document, I think it is cleaner to make this a stand-alone document, i.e., to include everything in it that is current and you would like to include, and just delete out anything you would like to leave out. I don't think it is necessary to indicate that this document represents a version of the earlier one by noting that the things that have been omitted. This simply invites the Committee to ask further questions about what was omitted in the earlier document. Please let me know if you have any questions, etcetera. Thanks, Donna."

Is it your understanding that, had you signed the revised statement, it would have been submitted to Senator Grassley and probably also this committee without notation regarding its alteration?

Mr. MOSHOLDER. Well, it wasn't a matter of signing it, but the plan was that I would provide this to the Committee at the start of my interview with them. So——

Ms. DEGETTE. Right. So if you had gone alone with this, this redacted document without the—I mean the lines would have been taken out. It would have been cleaned up, and that is what would have been given to the Senate and also probably to us, without notation of the things that had been taken out. Right?

Mr. MOSHOLDER. That is my understanding of what was proposed.

Ms. DEGETTE. And that is what you objected to?

Mr. MOSHOLDER. Yes. I said I was not comfortable with that.

Ms. DEGETTE. Okay. Now take a look at Tab 58. What that is, your reply to Ms. Katz the same day, which says, attached is a version of the statement that you say you would have been comfortable with. Right?

Mr. MOSHOLDER. Yes, that's correct.

Ms. DEGETTE. And the e-mail reads: "Thanks very much, Donna. Your version is actually very similar to the one I came up on my own this a.m. See attached. Although it might be cleaner to do so, as you say, I am uncomfortable with concealing from the Committee the fact this is not a new document. Accordingly, I prefer to use the version I edited as in the attached e-mail which otherwise incorporates all the edits we have discussed. Thanks, Andy." Right?

Mr. MOSHOLDER. Yes.

Ms. DEGETTE. And it is clear that you chose against the wishes of Ms. Katz and, I assume, the other lawyers to revise that document in such a way as to put the interest of Congressional committees on notice the document had been altered. Right?

Mr. MOSHOLDER. Well, that was my intent.

Ms. DEGETTE. Right. Thank you very much, Mr. Chairman.

Mr. WALDEN. The Chair recognizes the gentleman from Michigan, Mr. Stupak, for 10 minutes.

Mr. STUPAK. Thank you. Did you incur legal expenses while you were doing all these interviews with your Internal Affairs and all this?

Mr. MOSHOLDER. I did obtain legal representation. In point of fact, I have a Federal employee liability policy which provided for that. So my only expense was the insurance premium.

Mr. STUPAK. I can see an internal investigation on something about some newspaper leak or something, but sounds like here, and I think Ms. DeGette was being much too polite, you were being squeezed here to change your testimony. Correct?

Mr. MOSHOLDER. I'm not sure I would——

Mr. STUPAK. I was police officer for 12 years. I would have squeezed you and got it, too, you know. I mean, look, let me ask you this. Go to Tab 89.

Mr. MOSHOLDER. I'm sorry. Eighty?

Mr. STUPAK. Eighty-nine, please. It is a June 16 letter from Representative—I guess it is Senator Grassley to the FDA, and on the fourth page the letter states—it is on Tab 89. It says on page 4: "Perhaps most troubling, however, was the fact that the OND attempted to have Dr. Mosholder present reporting rates of suicidal thoughts rather than the available clinical trials data on anti-depressants in children which form the foundation of his analysis."

Can you please clarify the difference between the reporting rates of suicidal thoughts and available clinical trials data? Which is more reliable and relevant?

Mr. MOSHOLDER. A reporting rate is a term we use when we have spontaneous reports obtained through the MedWatch program, and as the enumerator. Then that is divided by some measure of the number of prescriptions in the U.S.

The problem with reporting rates is that it is usually assumed we only have only a small fraction of the number of events that are actually occurring in the population.

Mr. STUPAK. Well, clinical trial data is far more reliable than reporting rates. Right?

Mr. MOSHOLDER. That is correct. When——

Mr. STUPAK. And isn't it true that you were asked to present the reporting rates instead of the clinical trial rates or clinical trial data?

Mr. MOSHOLDER. You could put it that way. That is true, yes.

Mr. STUPAK. Okay. Then why did you choose not to present the reporting rates instead of your clinical trials data?

Mr. MOSHOLDER. Well, this was an issue we had considerable internal discussions about in preparation for the February 2 meeting. Ultimately, we in the Office of Drug Safety felt that, given that suicidal behaviors are part of the reason why the patients would be receiving the drug in the first place, giving a rate of such events really is not very useful information, and that the better data is done from trials where there could be comparisons.

Mr. STUPAK. So the better data is from the clinical trials data, and they were requesting, pressuring you—whatever word you want to use—to use the reporting rates and not the clinical trials data. OND asked you to present reporting rates instead of the clinical trials data. They wanted you to soften your conclusions.

Mr. MOSHOLDER. Well, at that point I was not presenting the clinical trials data at all.

Mr. STUPAK. But it was in your paper, your affidavit, if you will. So you had it. Correct?

Mr. MOSHOLDER. In my presentation to the Advisory Committee February 2 I presented simply a number of reports, as I recall, without the reporting rates in the end.

Mr. STUPAK. Right, but you used clinical trials data, because it is more reliable.

Mr. MOSHOLDER. Yes. My opinion is that is better data. Yes.

Mr. STUPAK. And OND wanted you to use reporting rates instead of clinical trials data. Correct?

Mr. MOSHOLDER. That is correct that they asked for that.

Mr. STUPAK. Correct. And the reason for that is it softens your conclusions that you put down in this paper, the affidavit. Isn't that correct?

Mr. MOSHOLDER. I'm not——

Mr. STUPAK. Let me put it this way. The numbers look better if you use reporting rates as opposed to the more reliable clinical trials data. Isn't that correct?

Mr. MOSHOLDER. My own opinion—well, that was a concern of the Finance Committee investigator. My own opinion is that the reporting rates simply are not informative. You can interpret it as an attempt to—I wouldn't go——

Mr. STUPAK. I'm not trying to put words here, but look it, we established that the clinical trials data is more reliable than the reporting rates. You were asked to change your clinical trial data to reporting rates, which is not as reliable. The reason to do that is then your affidavit, your conclusions are not as firm and solid. It is a softening of your conclusions, is it not? Softening is my word, not yours.

Mr. MOSHOLDER. Well, I would say that the reporting rates are inconclusive. There are no conclusions that you can draw from reporting rates, in my opinion. So——

Mr. STUPAK. Then why would OND want you to use reporting rates, if they are not as solid, not as reliable?

Mr. MOSHOLDER. Well, again there was difference of opinion about that. My understanding was that it was for completeness, because ordinarily this had been done and——

Mr. STUPAK. How do you get completeness if you don't use the most reliable data?

Mr. MOSHOLDER. Well, that was——

Mr. STUPAK. Completeness is the conclusion that one wishes to draw from the report that you did, completeness in the eye of the beholder. Right?

Mr. MOSHOLDER. Well, my own preference would have been to present the clinical trial data. Yes.

Mr. STUPAK. Correct. Okay. Reporting rates—to your knowledge, how many other instances were reporting rates provided when more reliable data was available? Is this a common thing? You medical officers do your reports. You look at the most reliable evidence, which may be your clinical trials data, and then you are told, well, geez, don't use that, let's look at the reporting rates, and let's use reporting rates as opposed to clinical data? Does that occur fairly often at the FDA?

Mr. MOSHOLDER. Not that I can recall, for just those reasons, that situations where reporting rates are useful are for very rare events that wouldn't necessarily be part of the reason why the patient was receiving the drug. So that it——

Mr. STUPAK. Absolutely. I agree with 1000 percent. Clinical trial data is always better than reporting rates. My question is: In the past, to your knowledge, has the FDA pressured medical review officers who review the drugs and deal with the data all the time to change from clinical trial data to reporting rates?

Mr. MOSHOLDER. I am not aware of any comparable situations, personally.

Mr. STUPAK. Your statement you gave here today—did the FDA have to approve your statement you are giving here today before the committee, your written statement?

Mr. MOSHOLDER. No, they did not.

Mr. STUPAK. Okay. If we do this labeling, packaging labeling that was suggested in the Advisory Committee, will you be involved in that process?

Mr. MOSHOLDER. Not to my knowledge.

Mr. STUPAK. I think someone may have asked you this, but let me just clarify this.

What is your impressions of Dr. Hammad's study?

Mr. MOSHOLDER. Well, I think the important point is that it is very consistent with the findings I had in my analysis.

Mr. STUPAK. That was my second question.

Mr. MOSHOLDER. You know, it lends strength to the finding.

Mr. STUPAK. So you would—Dr. Hammad's study is good work, and you would agree with it?

Mr. MOSHOLDER. Yes, and in many respects it is more sophisticated than my first crack at the data.

Mr. STUPAK. And it confirmed what your initial findings were? Dr. Hammad's report confirmed what your initial preliminary report showed. Correct?

Mr. MOSHOLDER. That is my—my own biased opinion is that it did confirm it, yes.

Mr. STUPAK. Someone, I think, asked you this one, too, on Tab 15 in which Dr. Avigan writes on your consult, "Andy, great job." If Dr. Avigan thought you did a great job with your analysis, why did he later issue a dissenting memo to your consult? It is in Tab 15.

Mr. MOSHOLDER. Yes. I believe Dr. Avigan did not feel that the data were ready to make the—or was sufficiently conclusive to make the recommendations that I made in my consult.

Mr. STUPAK. So you went from great job to being inconclusive?

Mr. MOSHOLDER. Well, to be fair, he did say that—at the time of the first draft, I remember him telling me that we would have to think about the recommendations some, but in the end he felt that the data were not persuasive enough to endorse my recommendations.

Mr. STUPAK. Thank you, Mr. Chairman.

Mr. WALDEN. Thank you. Dr. Mosholder, I want to refer you to Tab 78, if you would, sir, and go to—this is a memo. You were the medical officer on review and evaluation of clinical data. It is dated 12/13/96, received 12/16/1996, to Sulvay Pharmaceuticals regarding Luvoxamine maleate.

Mr. MOSHOLDER. Maleate, yes.

Mr. WALDEN. Thank you.

Mr. MOSHOLDER. Or Luvox.

Mr. WALDEN. Thank you. That is even easier. I want to refer you, though, to the second page, and it says: "it's of interest that in the adult studies the incidence of agitation was 2 percent and 1 percent for fluoxomine and placebo, respectively, while the pediatric study, the corresponding incidences were 12 percent and 3 percent. That is, the risk ratio for adults was two and for children was four. It is possible this reflects a real difference in adverse reactions between adults and children. There is an emerging literature pointing to behavioral reactions to SSRI drugs in children." Then you make some references there or some references are made here. "It may be that this is a reaction to SSRIs that is more prominent in children than adults. Further data would help clarify this."

Now I think what is interesting about this, this is a December 1996 memo. The review was completed in February 1997. Was this a flag you were raising in 1997?

Mr. MOSHOLDER. Well, as I said, this was one of the very first pediatric clinical trials we had seen with this class of drugs, and although there had been some other reports, apparently—I don't recall that reference at this point, but it seemed to be raising the question of whether the behavioral adverse effects might be different for kids versus adults.

Mr. WALDEN. Right. And you also said this is also reflected in Pfizer's recently submitted study of Certraline in the treatment of juvenile OCD as well in that reference. I guess the reason I asked is it looks like from this documentation, perhaps others, that this was sort of coming up as an issue back in 1996-1997.

I wonder, as we go into these pediatric clinical trials, could they have been designed better to go look at this issue of suicidality in children and adolescents? Should we have picked up on that sooner?

Mr. MOSHOLDER. Well, that is a good question. Historically, these two, as I recall, were the first actual studies we had with this class of drugs in kids. So it suggests that a pattern was starting to emerge. We, of course, didn't get more data until several years later, but the——

Mr. WALDEN. But should the FDA have sought more data in the way they designed the clinical trials for children?

Mr. MOSHOLDER. Well, the question being, as we were writing the request for pediatric studies, part of the pediatric exclusivity, could we have done more to get at this issue. Well——

Mr. WALDEN. In retrospect.

Mr. MOSHOLDER. Yes, in retrospect, you know, perhaps more attention could have been given to that. On the other hand, these trials had done nothing special to look for this type of event, and it seemed to be turning up. So that would be on the side of saying routine adverse event monitoring was sufficient to turn up this possibility.

Mr. WALDEN. Were you aware that apparently Dr. Knudsen also had some warnings that go back to 1996?

Mr. MOSHOLDER. I recall the——

Mr. WALDEN. For Zoloft.

Mr. MOSHOLDER. [continuing] something about that at the time. Then, of course, in preparation for this hearing I've been reminded of that. Yes.

Mr. WALDEN. I guess that the question we keep going back to is: Should this signal have been spotted sooner?

Mr. MOSHOLDER. Well——

Mr. WALDEN. Because it raises the issue, are there other signals that are bouncing around out there on other drugs being prescribed off-label for people that we are not catching. How do we fix the system, I guess, is part of it. Should we have spotted this one sooner? Should FDA?

Mr. MOSHOLDER. Well, one always wants to spot a problem as soon as possible, of course. The issue here, I think, at least in my own mind, was that we were lacking clinical trials in children until the past few years, that the Luvox and Zoloft studies were really sort of on the forefront of that, and so it was more just a plain lack of data rather than lack of any specific attention to it.

Mr. WALDEN. Okay. And I guess—but if we designed trials right, you would have the data. You would have had the data. Right?

Mr. MOSHOLDER. And in fact, that is what we have currently.

Mr. WALDEN. And I guess what I also want to make sure of is that, when we do have the data and they are evaluated by people of your credibility, that those data then are applied appropriately and the results are put out there appropriately.

I am troubled by an article that appeared in the August 7, 2004, British Medical Journal, and it states that Dr. Thomas Laughren reported the relative risk ratios of all the anti-depressants evaluated at the Pediatric Drug Advisory Committee meeting, and that it was—"it was Dr. Mosholder's conclusions and not the data that were withheld."

Do you agree with Dr. Laughren's reported characterizations?

Mr. MOSHOLDER. Is this what was——

Mr. WALDEN. This is the article. He also says—you will see in the second graph on this particular page—I'm sorry, second column, the last paragraph on the page, both the raw data and Dr. Mosholder's interpretation "were imperfect," said Dr. Temple, adding that some of the behaviors labeled suicidal were highly suspect and could have been accidents, such as a child "who hit her head with her hand." FDA officials acknowledged, however, that some cases classified as accidental injury could be suicide related. Because of this, they have gone on then to Columbia University.

That is why I raise that issue about whether or not your study included the incident of the girl slapping her head, because it didn't include that, did it?

Mr. MOSHOLDER. I included it in one analysis but not the result that I——

Mr. WALDEN. But not in the results, not in your conclusions.

Mr. MOSHOLDER. Yes.

Mr. WALDEN. And so why would then Dr. Temple tell this, allegedly, I suppose—it is printed here—say that that may be part of the problem here, that it is imperfect. Did you think your conclusions were imperfect?

Mr. MOSHOLDER. Well, I'm not sure I can give an unbiased answer to that. I think there was——

Mr. WALDEN. Well, do you think—let me ask this. Do you think his characterization of your consult is correct?

Mr. MOSHOLDER. I think we have had some—perhaps some communications issues where I am not sure that it was—I perhaps could have done more to make it obvious that I was trying to get away from the question of the clinically trivial events, if you will, such as the slapping in the face.

Mr. WALDEN. And I know we are putting you in a tough spot here with some of these folks that are, you know, your superiors sitting right behind you. I mean, I don't envy that position. Trust me. But these are critically important issues we have to get to.

Was your data analysis fully and fairly presented at the February 2004 Advisory Committee meeting and, if not, what should have been presented? What was presented, first of all, since you didn't do the presentation?

Mr. MOSHOLDER. As far as the clinical trial data, Dr. Laughren gave the presentation of that.

Mr. WALDEN. Was it full and fair?

Mr. MOSHOLDER. It did not include all of the results or data that I had in my draft presentation.

Mr. WALDEN. I guess the point is did it include the most important recommendations?

Mr. MOSHOLDER. Well, it didn't include—well, apart from the recommendations, the data I think that I would have included—let me put it that way—would——

Mr. WALDEN. If you had been there presenting it, what would you have included that wasn't included?

Mr. MOSHOLDER. I would have included the analysis of the serious subgroup of suicidal events and the meta analysis where the data was combined across studies. I think that—if I were doing or if I had a chance to do the presentation, that is what I would have included.

Mr. WALDEN. So the way you would have presented it would have painted a much more serious situation to that Advisory Committee than the way it was painted, when it comes to the risk of suicidality in adolescents and children? Is that accurate?

Mr. MOSHOLDER. I guess we will never know what the Advisory Committee might have made of——

Mr. WALDEN. No, no, no. The difference in the two presentations.

Mr. MOSHOLDER. I think, if I had been doing it, it would have perhaps been more obvious.

Mr. WALDEN. The chairman at the outset of this hearing thanked you on behalf of the committee for your work, and I think our country feels the same way. I know you have been honored many ways.

Somebody told me you had been selected, too, to be the ABC Person of the Week. Is there any truth to that?

Mr. MOSHOLDER. I was told that I was nominated, but I did not run.

Mr. WALDEN. Well, there is always next week, I guess.

All right. We are going to add, without objection, this newspaper article from the British Medical Journal, August 7, 2004, to the record. Without objection, so ordered.

[The newspaper article follows:]

Secret US report surfaces on antidepressants in children

Jeanne Lenzer New York

Internal memos and a secret government report about the negative effects of antidepressants in children—suppressed by the US Food and Drug Administration—have surfaced publicly.

The Alliance for Human Research Protection, a national network dedicated to ensuring ethical standards in medical research, published the documents on 26 July.

The published documents confirm earlier news accounts that a government expert with the FDA's Office of Drug Safety, Dr Andrew Mosholder, found that children taking antidepressants were twice as likely to become suicidal as children taking placebo. He reportedly urged the agency to follow the lead of British health authorities by warning doctors that the risks of the newer antidepressants, except fluoxetine, might outweigh the benefits when used in children.

The leaked documents show his data and conclusions. The FDA has subsequently acknowledged to the *BMJ* that Dr Mosholder was prevented from presenting his report at an advisory committee meeting on 2 February and was told that if he was asked any questions during the meeting he could respond to queries only by using a prepared script approved by his supervisors.

Dr Mosholder had evaluated data from 22 studies using nine drugs in 4250 children and found that 74 of the 2298 children taking antidepressants had a "suicide related event" compared with 34 of the 1952 children taking placebos.

When questioned about the decision to suppress Dr Mosholder's report, Dr Robert Temple, associate director for medical policy in the FDA's drug evaluation centre, defended the agency's actions. "We thought the analysis was premature," he told the *BMJ*.

Both the raw data and Dr Mosholder's interpretation were "imperfect" said Dr Temple, adding that some of the behaviours labelled "suicidal" were highly suspect and could have been accidents, such as a child "who hit her head with her hand." FDA officials acknowledged, however, that some cases classified as "accidental injury" could be suicide related. Because of this, the FDA has contracted with Columbia University to further study and classify events that might be considered to be suicide related.

Some of these events, he added, such as superficial cutting, "might be due to anxiety" and not represent true suicidal intent.

Dr Thomas Laughren, the FDA's team leader for psychiatric drug products, told the *BMJ* that he had reported the relative risk ratios of all the drugs evaluated at the advisory meeting and that it was Dr Mosholder's conclusions, and not the data, that were withheld.

Responding to critics who say studies of antidepressants other than fluoxetine show little or no efficacy in children, Dr Temple said absence of proof should not be interpreted to mean the drugs are ineffective.

Dr Jerome Hoffman, an epidemiologist and professor of medicine at the University of California at Los Angeles, told the *BMJ* that the flip side of Dr Temple's claim that antidepressants in children could be lifesaving is that they could be life threatening—as suggested by Dr Mosholder's report.

"Most Americans undoubtedly believe that the FDA demands reasonable evidence that a drug is safe before it is allowed to be used," said Professor Hoffman. "But this episode suggests that they reject this 'precautionary principle' in favour of the idea that no drug is dangerous unless it is 'proven' to be so."

"The FDA... attempted to silence Dr Mosholder [but] repeatedly claimed to 'support his concern' for the safety of children," added Professor Hoffman, "but this apparently didn't extend to supporting his desire to express that concern publicly. That may be the most dangerous aspect of this entire affair."

The FDA has launched a criminal investigation to find out which employees leaked Dr Mosholder's report. Meanwhile the suppression of the report has triggered Congressional investigations by Senator Charles Grassley, who has interviewed employees in the agency's Office of Drug Safety, where Dr Mosholder worked. □

Mr. WALDEN. Do you have further questions? We have been called to votes on the House floor, and it would—Mr. Stupak, do you have anymore questions for this witness at this time?

Mr. STUPAK. No. I just thank Dr. Mosholder for being here.

Mr. WALDEN. Thank you. And, Dr. Mosholder, we would like you to stay with us, even though we probably won't have you on the next panel. We would like to have you available, should there be some questions that we need to seek your expert advice on. So if you could stay with us.

We are going to recess the committee until after these votes. There are four of them, which probably tells me it will be 45 minutes before we are back here. So it is a good time for everyone to go grab a quick bite, and we will reconvene the committee immediately after those votes have concluded.

The committee is in recess.

[Brief recess.]

Mr. WALDEN. I am going to call this hearing back to order and ask our next panel of witnesses to come up: Dr. Robert Temple, Food and Drug Administration; Dr. Paul Seligman, Food and Drug Administration; Dr. Thomas Laughren, Food and Drug Administration; Dr. Tarek Hammad, Food and Drug Administration; and Dr. James Knudsen, Food and Drug Administration. Please come up to the witness table, if you would.

You are aware the committee is holding an investigative hearing and, when doing so, has the practice of taking testimony under oath. Do you have any objection to testifying under oath? Do any of you have an objection?

Let the record show they all indicated they have no objection.

The Chair then advises you that, under the rules of the House and the rules of the committee, you are entitled to be advised by counsel. Do you desire to be advised by counsel during your testimony today? Mr. Knudsen? Could you turn on your mike, sir, and then we will need you to identify your counsel. Dr. Knudsen.

Mr. KNUDSEN. My name is Dr. James Knudsen.

Mr. WALDEN. Okay. Yes, you actually have to get kind of close to that. Sorry. If you could identify for the record, Dr. Knudsen, your counsel, please.

Mr. KNUDSEN. My counsel?

Mr. WALDEN. Oh, I thought you said you wanted to be represented by counsel.

Mr. KNUDSEN. No, I did not.

Mr. WALDEN. Okay, fine. No? Okay. Dr. Temple? Dr. Laughren?

Mr. LAUGHREN. No, sir.

Mr. WALDEN. Dr. Seligman?

Mr. SELIGMAN. No.

Mr. WALDEN. Okay. So let the record show, none of them is being represented by counsel.

In that case then, would you please rise and raise your right hand, and we will take your testimony under oath. Let the record show, they all indicated yes.

[Witnesses sworn.]

Mr. WALDEN. Thank you. You may be seated.

You are now under oath, and you may now give a 5-minute summary of your written statement, and we will start with Dr. Knudsen.

Mr. WALDEN. Dr. Hammad? No opening statement. Dr. Temple? Actually, I am not sure your mike is on yet.

Mr. TEMPLE. Now?

Mr. WALDEN. There it is, sir, yes. Thank you, and welcome.

TESTIMONY OF JAMES KNUDSEN, FOOD AND DRUG ADMINISTRATION; ACCOMPANIED BY ROBERT TEMPLE, FOOD AND DRUG ADMINISTRATION; PAUL SELIGMAN, FOOD AND DRUG ADMINISTRATION; THOMAS LAUGHREN, FOOD AND DRUG ADMINISTRATION; AND TAREK HAMMAD, FOOD AND DRUG ADMINISTRATION

Mr. TEMPLE. Mr. Co-Chairman, I guess, and members of the committee, I am Robert Temple, CDER's Associate Director for Medical Policy. I welcome the opportunity to participate in this hearing on FDA's regulation of pediatric uses of anti-depressants.

My colleagues and I recognize that the entire discussion of the past year has been very painful and difficult for people—both for people whose loved ones have committed suicide while on an anti-depressant and for people whose family members are seriously depressed and are uncertain as to what they can do for them.

Today I will briefly review the importance of detecting and treating depression in children, the available treatments and recent efforts to encourage studies of drugs in children, the history of the concern, the subject of this hearing, about the possibility that anti-depressants might provoke suicidal thinking or behavior, and FDA's evaluation and data—of the data from the pediatric depression studies.

Throughout my testimony and later, I will want to emphasize an important concern that we had from the beginning of this. We were concerned that overemphasis or premature conclusion about an increased risk of suicidality related to anti-depressant use could discourage treatment of serious pediatric depression, which is a potentially life threatening condition.

At the same time, failure to take adequate note of the risk could lead to inattention to the possibility for emerging suicidality or to too casual use of the anti-depressants.

We dealt with this concern by making the public fully aware of the issue and of the data that led to our concern, but we thought it was responsible to withhold an agency conclusion about what the data showed until it had been fully evaluated.

Depression in children is a serious mental illness that affects up to 2.5 percent of children and 8 percent of teenagers. In the U.S. there are about 1600 suicides in teenagers per year, many of them in people who are diagnosed as having depression.

The difficulty of obtaining good data on the effectiveness and safety in drugs in children is well recognized. A provision of the Food and Drug Administration Modernization Act which was renewed in the Best Pharmaceuticals for Children Act in 2002 provides 6 months of patent extension to sponsors who carry out pediatric studies that have been requested by the FDA.

This provision has enormously stimulated the conduct of these studies, and it was FDA's analysis of the depression studies submitted under these laws that led to the question of whether the drugs could cause suicidality in children.

Specifically, review by Dr. Mosholder of adverse effects collected under the term emotional lability in five Paxil studies that were submitted under the Act detected an excess of such cases, some of which appeared to represent suicidal thinking or behavior in patients.

I can't emphasize too strongly that, although as you will hear there were some disagreements on our part with some of Dr. Mosholder's conclusions or whether they were right, this discovery, this observation was of immense value and has kicked this whole thing off. So let there be no question about whether that was an important observation.

A request for a more focused analysis of the Paxil suicidality data led to a further suggestion of an increased rate of suicidality in the Paxil treated patients, and this was more credible because the analysis was better than their initial one.

FDA issued a Public Health Advisory on June 19, 2003, describing the results of the Paxil evaluation and stating that, although FDA had not completed its evaluation, we recommended that Paxil not be used in children and adolescents to treat major depressive disorder.

Subsequently, the Review Division asked all manufacturers of newer anti-depressants for an analysis that was similar to what GlaxoSmithKline had done for Paxil, and this was provided by late September 2003. These reports were sent to Dr. Mosholder and were also considered by the Review Division.

On October 27, 2003, FDA issued an updated Public Health Advisory, again noting the suggestion of excess suicidality in anti-depressant treated patients and the need for further data and analysis.

The Review Division had been examining the data submitted by the sponsors, too, as had Dr. Mosholder, and had significant concerns about it. It, therefore, began in September-October 2003 to make arrangements to have the reported suicidality events reviewed and reclassified by the Columbia Department of Psychiatry.

Our concern was that the companies had cast a wide net in seeking cases of suicidality, of suicidal thinking or instances of self-harm, but not all such cases—for example, a superficial cutting—represent attempted suicide.

I also want to say that I am somewhat embarrassed about my BMJ quote from before, because at least by the time that came out, I was well aware that Dr. Mosholder had excluded cases like that. I think that reflected an earlier conversation. So there is no question that he did exclude many such things, and the banging of the head. So I feel bad about that. However, remained concerned that the cases themselves needed close evaluation, and I can talk later about how those data were collected and why we thought they needed that.

Given our conclusion that they needed to be looked at closely, we concluded that a blind expert classification of the cases was needed.

In addition, we sent the Columbia reviewers narrative descriptions of additional adverse reaction cases that had not been included by the companies, because we thought there might be excess—might be cases of suicidal behavior or thinking in there, and that proved to be correct.

It is worth emphasizing that we had no idea what the results of the reclassification would be. We didn't know whether it would strengthen the findings or weaken the findings. We had no way of knowing and no expectation, and not to state the obvious, no preference. We just wanted to get at what the right answer was.

At a February 2, 2004, Advisory Committee meeting we presented the results of the company submissions, as you have heard before, study by study, in part to make the point that the results were very variable from one study to another, and from one drug to another. But many of the drugs clearly showed an increased risk of suicidality. That's the sum of suicidal behavior and suicidal thinking.

We noted to the committee our concerns with the data submissions and explained why we considered additional review by Columbia necessary.

We also acknowledged that some in the agency thought the results were, in fact, definitive and could be a basis for change in labeling to discourage use of the drug, except for Prozac, in children.

Although no specific question was put about this to the committee, discussion indicated that they clearly understood the agency's reservations, and they in fact expressed doubt that anything arising from this kind of data collection would be useful, a conclusion that they modified at the most recent Advisory Committee.

The Advisory Committee recognized that, whatever the relationship of anti-depressants to suicidality, it was perfectly clear even then that the period after initiation of treatment for depression was of great concern and that physicians needed to be warned about this, the need to be careful and make close observations.

On March 22, we asked manufacturers of anti-depressants to add warning language to their labeling and issued a third Public Health Advisory describing our request. The new warning emphasized the critical importance of observing newly treated patients for emerging suicidality or other problems.

All manufacturers added this warning to their labeling by late summer. We have no received the reclassified cases from Columbia and analyzed the data.

The analysis by Dr. Hammad was presented to the Advisory Committee on September 13, 2004. The analysis included the study you have heard about, the TAD study, a new study of Prozac carried out by the National Institutes of Mental Health.

The analysis showed that, as a group, the anti-depressants studied, both SSRIs and the so called atypicals, increased the risk of suicidality. There was variation from drug to drug and variation from study to study, but the roughly twofold increased risk was reasonably consistent across drugs. As has been pointed out, there were no actual suicides in these trials.

At the September 13-14 Advisory Committee meeting, the combined Pediatric and Psychopharm Drugs Advisory Committees agreed with FDA's conclusions that the data in aggregate indicated an increased risk of suicidality in pediatric patients, and made several critical recommendations.

First, they believed the conclusion should apply to all of the studied drugs, even though it was more prominent in some than others. They also strongly urged that we apply it to any new anti-depressant and to the older anti-depressants, including the tricyclics. They thought that partly because the logic seemed to be that this is a property of anti-depressants, and they were quite concerned that people would be driven to the tricyclics, which are rather more dangerous.

They did not believe the anti-depressants, other than fluoxetine,should be contraindicated in children, and repeatedly expressed concern that these drugs may be valuable even if that has not been shown, and they were quite aware that it had not yet been shown.

They strongly supported a patient and family directed Med Guide which we had suggested to them, and two-thirds of them thought the new warning information should be boxed.

On September 17 we announced publicly that we generally support the recommendations and had begun working on new labeling to reflect that. The term generally applies only to the thought that we are going to read closely what they said collectively about the boxed warning, and think about it.

Obviously, two-thirds of them thought that was reasonable, but the discussion indicated concern that over-discouraging use was potentially very dangerous, too, and they wanted a balance. So we are going to be thinking about that.

I appreciate the opportunity to present these remarks, and I look forward to your questions.

I am aware that you have also invited Dr. Russell Katz to appear here this morning. Unfortunately, he is not able to attend because a member of his family is having surgery today. He will be happy to answer any questions you have for him in writing or speak with your staff at a later date. Thank you.

Mr. WALDEN. We appreciate that, Dr. Temple. We were aware of that, obviously, too, and did not want to interfere in his very difficult time.

[The prepared statement of Robert Temple follows:]

PREPARED STATEMENT OF ROBERT TEMPLE, DIRECTOR, OFFICE OF MEDICAL POLICY, CENTER FOR DRUG EVALUATION AND RESEARCH, U.S. FOOD AND DRUG ADMINISTRATION

INTRODUCTION

Mr. Chairman and Members of the Subcommittee, I am Dr. Robert Temple, Director, Office of Medical Policy for the Center for Drug Evaluation and Research (CDER) at the U.S. Food and Drug Administration (FDA or the Agency). We appreciate the opportunity to discuss FDA's review of the safety and efficacy concerns in anti-depressant drugs for use in pediatric populations.

BACKGROUND ON DEPRESSION

Depression is a serious mental illness that affects the way nearly 19 million adult Americans feel, think, and interact. While everyone experiences occasional sadness, particularly in response to loss or adversity, a person with depression has persistent symptoms that can significantly interfere with their ability to function. People with depression cannot merely "pull themselves together" and get better. Depression cannot be willed or wished away.

The two most severe types of clinical depression are major depressive disorder (MDD) and bipolar depression, which is the depressed phase of bipolar disorder. Within these types, patients experience variations in the severity and persistence of mental symptoms associated with these disorders. A person experiencing MDD suffers from, among other symptoms, a depressed mood or loss of interest in normal activities that lasts most of the day and nearly every day, for at least two weeks. Such episodes may occur only once, but more commonly occur several times in a lifetime. People with bipolar disorder cycle between episodes of major depression, similar to those seen in MDD, and highs known as mania. In a manic phase, a person might act on delusional grand schemes that could range from unwise business decisions to romantic sprees. Both MDD and bipolar disorder can lead to suicide. The treatment of the two conditions is quite different. In general, anti-depressants alone are not an appropriate treatment for bipolar disorder.

DEPRESSION IN THE PEDIATRIC/ADOLESCENT POPULATION

According to a 2000 National Institute of Mental Health (NIMH) Fact Sheet on Depression in Children and Adolescents, depression affects up to 2.5 percent of children and about eight percent of adolescents in the United States. These disorders often go unrecognized by families and physicians because behaviors associated with depressive disorders may be seen as normal mood swings typical of a particular developmental stage. In addition, health care providers may be reluctant to prematurely "label" a young person with a mental illness diagnosis.

At the February 2, 2004, meeting of FDA's Psychopharmacologic Drugs Advisory Committee (PDAC), Dr. Cynthia Pfeffer of Cornell University addressed the issue of pediatric depression and its treatment. She noted that pediatric depression is very common and often recurrent, is often accompanied by very poor psychosocial outcomes for children and adolescents, and is associated with high risk for suicide and substance abuse. She reported that in 2001, about 1,600 15 to 19-year-olds committed suicide in the U.S. Suicide is the third leading cause of death in the U.S. in this age group and accounts for more deaths in this age group than all other major physical conditions combined.

At that meeting, Dr. David Shaffer of Colombia University reported on rates of suicidal ideation (thinking about suicide) and suicide attempts. He obtained his information from large community studies, particularly the Youth Risk Behavior Study (YRBS), a study carried out by the National Center for Health Statistics. In this study, officials from the National Center interviewed a broad population of between 15,000 and 20,000 high school students every two years using self-reporting measures. Based on this data, it was determined that suicidal ideation in high school students is extraordinarily common. Almost 20 percent of American high school students think about suicide. Suicide attempts are also very common. Experts report that the overall rate is about nine percent. Only about a quarter of these attempts are brought to medical attention. It is widely recognized that adolescents are frequently reluctant to disclose suicidal thoughts or even suicide attempts to parents or others. There are about 4,000 female suicide attempts for every female suicide death, and about 400 male attempts for every male death.

Dr. Shaffer also showed rates of pediatric suicide over several decades. The rate has fallen by about 25 percent over the last decade, the period in which the use of anti-depressants has grown steadily. This association does not prove that the increasing use of anti-depressants is the cause of the decline in suicide, but it is at least suggestive.

DRUGS FOR TREATING DEPRESSION

Existing anti-depressant drugs influence the levels of one or both of two neurotransmitters in the brain: serotonin and norepinephrine. Older medications—tricyclic anti-depressants (TCAs) and monoamine oxidase inhibitors (MAOs)—affect the activity of both of these neurotransmitters. The disadvantage of the older medications is that they can be difficult to tolerate due to significant side effects. MAO use may also be subject to dietary and medication restrictions. TCAs and MAOs are of limited value in the pediatric population because of serious, potentially life-threatening adverse events. These include tachycardia, convulsions, and shock-like coma. Moreover, TCAs are a potential tool for adolescents attempting to commit suicide because overdose can cause serious and protracted cardiac arrhythmias.

Newer medications, such as the selective serotonin reuptake inhibitors (SSRIs), have fewer side effects than the older drugs, making it easier for people to continue treatment. They have become very widely used to treat depression, especially in the pediatric population. FDA approved Prozac, the first SSRI, for adults, in December 1987, and for children in January 2003. Experts believe that SSRI drug products work by increasing the level of the hormone serotonin in the brain. There were no approved drugs for the treatment of depression in children before the January 2003 Prozac approval.

ANTI-DEPRESSANT TREATMENT AND SUICIDALITY

Suicidality in the context of treating patients with depression and other psychiatric illnesses has been a genuine concern and a longstanding topic of debate. In fact, for many decades, anti-depressant labeling carried the following standard language under the "Precautions" section of the label alerting clinicians to the need to closely monitor patients during initial drug therapy due to concern for the possible emergence of suicidality:

> Suicide: The possibility of a suicide attempt is inherent in major depressive disorder and may persist until significant remission occurs. Close supervision of high-risk patients should accompany initial drug therapy. Prescriptions for [name of drug] should be written for the smallest quantity of tablets consistent with good patient management, in order to reduce the risk of overdose.

This standard precaution statement did not explicitly warn of the possibility that anti-depressant drug products have a causal role in the emergence of suicidality early in treatment. Several mechanisms have been proposed to explain the clinical observation that some depressed patients being treated with anti-depressants, particularly early in treatment, have an increase in suicidality. In September 1991, FDA convened a meeting of the PDAC to discuss this issue. At that meeting, Dr. Martin Teicher, a psychiatrist from Harvard Medical School, proposed various mechanisms to explain the emergence of suicidality early in treatment of depression:

- Roll back phenomenon: anti-depressants with prominent energizing effects might actually increase suicidal behavior in severely depressed patients who are suicidal but also have psychomotor retardation and are thus inhibited from acting on their suicidal thoughts.
- Paradoxical worsening of depression: in rare cases, the patient's depressed mood might actually worsen as a result of anti-depressant treatment.
- Akathisia (inability to sit still): some anti-depressants are associated with akathisia, which might lead to suicidal behavior in certain depressed patients.
- Induction of anxiety and panic attacks: some anti-depressants may induce anxiety and panic attacks, and these might lead to suicidal behavior in certain depressed patients.
- Stage shifts: anti-depressants may lead to switching the patient from depression into mixed states in bipolar depressed patients, possibly leading to suicidality.
- Insomnia: insomnia associated with certain anti-depressants might lead to suicidal behavior in certain depressed patients.

While all of these theories have some plausibility, it is difficult to know whether these mechanisms are real. In addition, proposing a mechanism is quite different from actually demonstrating that there is a causal association between anti-depressant use and suicidality. It might be possible to demonstrate that anti-depressants cause an increase in suicidality through randomized clinical trials, but these trials would need to be quite large because suicidality is not common. It might be possible to pool results of many trials, but if this involves results from studies of different drugs, the question remains whether some drugs could behave differently from others. Furthermore, assessing this risk in uncontrolled data is particularly difficult because depression itself causes suicidality. In any given case, one cannot usually distinguish whether the suicidality occurred because of the drug or despite it.

ANTI-DEPRESSANT-INDUCED SUICIDALITY IN ADULTS

Thus, the question of whether anti-depressants can provoke suicidality has been the subject of considerable discussion. With regard to the adult population, the debate intensified in 1990 when Dr. Teicher and several colleagues published a paper describing six adult patients with depression who, in their view, became suicidal because of treatment with Prozac. This paper and subsequent discussions led Eli Lilly, the manufacturer of Prozac, to conduct new analyses of data from their controlled trials for Prozac to look for suicidality. These events also led FDA to fully re-evaluate its spontaneous reports database to determine whether we could observe a signal of increased risk.

During a September 1991 PDAC meeting, family members raised concerns about suicide by loved ones whose deaths they attributed to Prozac. Representatives from FDA, NIMH and Lilly also gave presentations. FDA gave an update on the very substantial number of spontaneous reports of suicidality in association with Prozac use, but also noted the marked increase in reporting following the publication of the Teicher paper and the publicity about the paper. A representative from NIMH gave their perspective on the issue, essentially making the case that depression is a serious disorder that itself is associated with suicidality, and arguing that the data available to date did not support the view that anti-depressants further increase the risks of suicidality in this population. Finally, Lilly presented the results of its analysis of data pooled over its extensive clinical trials, revealing no signal of increased suicidality in association with the use of Prozac. Following these presentations, a majority of the Advisory Committee members concluded that there was no clear evidence of an increased risk of suicidality in association with Prozac, and did not recommend any changes to Prozac labeling.

Over the next several years, researchers accumulated additional data as new anti-depressant drugs came to market. All of these additional data related to the treatment of adults. In recent years, several groups have conducted pooled analyses of data on completed or attempted suicides from these studies in an effort to identify a possible signal of risk from active treatment. They have also searched for risk signals from patients assigned to a placebo group, since some have challenged the use of placebo controls in a disease with potentially serious outcomes. Arif Khan, a psychiatrist from the Northwest Clinical Research Center, and other researchers published a paper in 2000 based on adult data obtained from FDA reviews. Dr. Khan concluded that the risk of completed suicide was the same, regardless of treatment assignment. A similar study reached the same conclusion. FDA researchers also analyzed completed suicides in 234 randomized controlled depression trials of 20 anti-depressant drug products. Based on all our analyses to date of these data, we reached a similar conclusion: there does not appear to be an increased risk of completed suicide associated with assignment to either active drug or placebo in adults with MDD.

ANTI-DEPRESSANTS AND SUICIDALITY IN PEDIATRIC PATIENTS

Whether anti-depressant drug use causes suicidal thinking or behavior in pediatric patients (or adults) is a critically important question that we must answer in a careful, thoughtful manner. A premature conclusion or emphasis in either direction could have adverse consequences for those who are suffering from depression. Missing or understating a signal of increased risk of suicidality could result in greater reassurance than is warranted about the safety of these drugs, insufficient attention to the patients being treated, and perhaps too casual use of the drugs. On the other hand, overstating the risk could result in overly conservative use of these drugs or excluding their use for the pediatric population, and inadequate treatment of a potentially fatal condition. Below we discuss the origins of the concern that anti-depressants could provoke suicidal ideation in children.

USE OF ANTI-DEPRESSANTS IN THE PEDIATRIC POPULATION

Many people have expressed concern about pediatric use of products approved for MDD in adults where clinical trials in children were negative. Prozac is the only product for which efficacy has been established sufficiently to meet FDA's standards for approval in the pediatric population. To date, clinical trials evaluating six other current generation anti-depressants approved for adults have not met FDA's standards for establishing efficacy in the child/adolescent population. Nevertheless, there is widespread belief among treating physicians that these products do in fact work and that the "negative" results are in fact inconclusive. Negative trials are not necessarily informative in MDD trials because they may be an indication of inadequate trials rather than evidence of benefit.

Because Prozac is the only product for which efficacy has been establish for treatment of pediatric/adolescent MDD, it is often the first product prescribed by a physician. However, in 30-40 percent of cases, Prozac does not work for the patient. In such cases, it is standard care for physicians to prescribe one of the other current generation anti-depressants approved for adults. The older medications, tricyclic anti-depressants (TCAs) and monoamine oxidase inhibitors (MAOIs), have not been approved for use in pediatric/adolescent population. Moreover, as noted previously, they are of limited value in the pediatric population because of serious, potentially life-threatening adverse events. They may cause life-threatening arrhythmias in overdose or even at normal doses in individuals who are unable to efficiently metabolize these drugs.

FDAMA AND BPCA STIMULATE NEW PEDIATRIC SUICIDALITY DATA

The question of suicidality arose in the course of FDA's review of clinical trials of anti-depressants in children. When Congress enacted the FDA Modernization Act (FDAMA) in 1997, it provided incentives to manufacturers to conduct pediatric clinical trials. Section 111 of FDAMA authorized FDA to grant additional marketing exclusivity (known as pediatric exclusivity) to pharmaceutical manufacturers that conduct studies of their drugs in pediatric populations. To qualify for pediatric exclusivity, sponsors must conduct pediatric studies according to the terms of a Written Request from FDA and submit the results of those studies in a new drug application or supplement. Congress renewed this authority in 2002, in the Best Pharmaceuticals for Children Act (BPCA).

BPCA contains important, new disclosure requirements. For studies other than those submitted under the BPCA, the Agency generally may not publicly disclose information contained in investigational new drug applications, unapproved new drug applications, or unapproved supplemental new drug applications. Only after a new drug application or supplemental new drug application is approved can the Agency make public certain summary information regarding the safety and effectiveness of the product for the approved indication. However, section 9 of BPCA regarding the dissemination of pediatric information gives the Agency additional disclosure authority and differs from FDA regulations that generally preclude the Agency from disclosing to the public information in an unapproved application. BPCA requires that, no later than 180 days after the submission of studies conducted in response to a Written Request, the Agency must publish a summary of FDA's medical and clinical pharmacology reviews of those studies. Moreover, we must publish this information regardless of whether the action taken on the pediatric application is an approval, approvable, or not-approvable action. Thus, although under FDAMA information on pediatric studies conducted in response to Written Requests is not available until after the supplemental application is approved, under BPCA, a summary of FDA's medical and clinical pharmacology reviews of pediatric studies, conducted in response to a Written Request issued under BPCA, is publicly available irrespective of the action taken on the application.

BPCA WRITTEN REQUESTS FOR ANTI-DEPRESSANTS

Prior to the enactment of BPCA, under the pediatric exclusivity authority of FDAMA, FDA issued seven Written Requests to manufacturers of drugs approved for the treatment of depression (Prozac, Zoloft, Remeron, Paxil, Celexa, Serzone, and Effexor). The sponsors of three of these drugs (Prozac, Zoloft, and Remeron) performed the studies and submitted the reports of their studies before FDAMA expired on January 1, 2002 (and thus, before BPCA took effect). The manufacturers of two of these drugs, Prozac (which has been approved for the treatment of pediatric depression) and Zoloft (which was studied but not approved for the treatment of pediatric depression) received pediatric exclusivity for having conducted studies. The third sponsor, the manufacturer of Remeron, did not receive pediatric exclusivity. Under FDA's general disclosure provisions regarding the availability of data and information in approved applications, information on the approved pediatric use of Prozac is publicly available at: http://www.fda.gov/cder/foi/nda/2003/18936s064_Prozac.htm. Just as it has for other product approvals, FDA posted this information because we granted approval for Prozac for use in treating pediatric depression. The pediatric data for Zoloft and Remeron would not normally be available for public disclosure because their pediatric supplements have not yet been approved. However, FDA nonetheless asked the sponsors to allow us to make summaries of these studies public. The sponsors agreed to our request and summaries are now available on FDA's website at: http://www.fda.gov/cder/pediatric/Summaryreview.htm.

Following enactment of BPCA in January 2002, FDA determined that the provisions of this new law should apply as broadly as possible to outstanding Written Requests for which studies had not yet been submitted. In a July 2002 letter, the Agency notified drug sponsors with outstanding Written Requests issued under FDAMA that FDA considered those Written Requests to be reissued under BPCA. In its July 2002 letter, FDA further advised manufacturers that any studies submitted in response to the reissued Written Requests would be subject to the terms of the BPCA, including, among other things, the provisions governing public availability of study summaries. However, the Written Requests for three anti-depressants (Paxil, Celexa, and Serzone) were not considered as reissued under BPCA in July 2002 because the manufacturers had already submitted their pediatric studies to the Agency before FDA issued its July 2002 letter (albeit after BPCA was enacted). Therefore, FDA considered the studies for Paxil, Celexa, and Serzone, to have been submitted under FDAMA; did not consider their Written Requests to be reissued, and did not apply the public disclosure provisions of BPCA to these studies. Nonetheless, the Agency has received permission from the sponsors of these drugs to post summaries of the safety and effectiveness reviews of their pediatric studies on FDA's website, and this information appears at: http://www.fda.gov/cder/pediatric/Summaryreview.htm.

Only one of the outstanding and reissued Written Requests under BPCA was for studies relating to the treatment of pediatric depression. This Written Request was for Effexor. FDA granted pediatric exclusivity for this product and posted the study summaries on the FDA Pediatric Summary Review website, according to the requirements of BPCA. No new Written Requests for anti-depressants have been issued since the passage of the BPCA.

We want to emphasize that although these anti-depressants have all been shown to be effective in adults, in its Written Requests FDA asked manufacturers to conduct two pediatric studies because we knew from experience that it is very difficult to show the effectiveness of anti-depressants in children. In all studies submitted in response to Written Requests, no completed suicides occurred in the trials. Nonetheless, FDA reviewers of these Written Requests identified a suicidality concern during the course of their review.

RESULTS OF THE PAXIL WRITTEN REQUEST

FDA has been reviewing the results of anti-depressant studies in children since June 2003 after an initial report on studies with paroxetine (tradename, Paxil) appeared to suggest an increased risk of suicidal thoughts and actions in the children given Paxil, compared to those given placebo. During the review of the supplemental new drug application submitted by GlaxoSmithKline (GSK) for the use of Paxil in children, FDA reviewers noted a greater number of adverse events coded under the term "emotional lability" in patients treated with Paxil compared to the placebo group. FDA reviewers in the Division of Neuropharmacological Drug Products (DNDP) of FDA's CDER noted this in some, but not all, of the Paxil studies. The reviewers also noted that the actual events coded under this term included suicidal thoughts and attempts as well as a wide range of other events.

In an effort to better understand these events and to focus on suicidal thoughts or behavior, DNDP asked the sponsor to reanalyze its data and better characterize the adverse events identified under the term "emotional lability." This FDA request resulted in additional work by GSK and a report on suicidality, submitted first to the UK (UK), and, shortly thereafter, to FDA.

GSK APPROACH TO ACCUMULATING PAXIL SUMMARY DATA

GSK's re-analysis of the Paxil data focused exclusively on placebo-controlled trials (of which there were six). This has been FDA's focus as well. As noted earlier, in their original pediatric supplement, GSK classified adverse events suggestive of suicidality (as well as various other behavioral events) under the general term "emotional lability." In response to our request for a separate approach to better identify events that suggested suicidality, GSK conducted searches to find events of potential interest. GSK's adverse event data was in an electronic file that allowed them to search for text strings that suggested suicidality, e.g. "overdose," "suic," "hung," "cut," etc. The company conducted a blind evaluation of all events detected by this text search to select those considered possibly suicide-related. A subset of these events that could represent self-harm was then classified by GSK as suicide attempts. GSK's examination of events was limited to those occurring within 30 days of the patient's last dose.

GSK submitted its report to FDA on May 22, 2003. This report suggested an increased risk (Paxil vs. placebo) of various thoughts and behaviors coded as events considered "possibly suicide related." In addition, there was a suggestion of increased risk for the subgroup of events that met the sponsor's criteria for "suicide attempts." The signal for increased risk was clearest in 1 of the 3 trials involving pediatric patients with MDD.

It is important to note that these analyses were difficult because investigators used a large variety of terms to describe what might have been suicidal behavior and provided variable amounts of detail when identifying these events. The standard assessments of depression used to evaluate effectiveness all had an item indicating suicidal thoughts, and an evaluation of these scales showed no increased suicidality compared to placebo. However, the trials were not designed to focus on the question of suicide risk with drug treatment. To address this concern, we plan to develop guidance for subsequent trials that will lead to a standard nomenclature and assessment by investigators.

INITIAL RESPONSE TO SIGNAL OF INCREASED RISK OF SUICIDALITY FOR PAXIL

The reaction to the GSK report by the Medicines and Healthcare Regulatory Agency (MHRA) in the UK was to issue a public statement explicitly stating that

Paxil "should not be used in children and adolescents under the age of 18 years to treat depressive illness," and to institute a labeling change contraindicating Paxil in pediatric MDD.

On June 6, 2003, Dr. Russell Katz, the director of DNDP, asked the Office of Drug Safety (ODS) to perform a consult review of the newly submitted GSK safety data. Dr. Katz requested that ODS assign Dr. Andrew Mosholder as the primary reviewer for the consult because Dr. Mosholder had previously been involved in reviewing data on the safety and efficacy of anti-depressants and had generated the original request to GSK. On June 19, 2003, FDA issued a public health advisory stating that: "Although FDA has not completed its evaluation of the new safety data, FDA is recommending that Paxil not be used in children and adolescents for the treatment of [major depressive disorder]."

FDA also requested data similar to that submitted by GSK from the manufacturers of eight other anti-depressant drugs that were studied in children. On July 22, 2003, the Agency sent requests for data to the manufacturers of the following drugs: Prozac, Zoloft, Luvox, Celexa, Wellbutrin, Effexor, Serzone, and Remeron. In those letters, we asked manufacturers to identify suicide-related events for their pediatric studies in a blinded manner using two search strategies. We modeled our request to these manufacturers on the approach used by GSK, and asked manufacturers to conduct an electronic search for text strings relevant to suicidality similar to the approach employed for Paxil. We also asked manufacturers to blindly search narrative summaries for any serious adverse events to identify additional instances of "suicide-related events."

FDA RE-REVIEW OF DATA FROM PEDIATRIC SUPPLEMENTS FOR OTHER ANTI-DEPRESSANTS

While waiting for the various manufacturers of anti-depressants other than Paxil to respond, we went back to the adverse event data in the pediatric supplements for the other eight drugs to re-examine the question of suicidality. Our major question was whether there were other anti-depressants with possible signals of increased risk for suicidality, as was observed for Paxil.

There were several limitations to this re-examination. First, the methods for detecting and coding events were not standard across these studies. Second, because we wanted to have categories similar to those used for the Paxil data for purposes of comparison across drug programs, we classified events described in the adverse event listings for these drug programs into two categories: "possibly suicide-related" and "suicide attempt." One obvious flaw in this approach was that FDA's reviewer was not blinded during this reclassification process. Nevertheless, we believed this re-examination of summary data might shed some light on the possibility of signals emerging from other anti-depressant programs. We discovered that there were signals of increased risk of suicidality for patients assigned to drugs other than Paxil. We also found that the findings were not consistent across the studies, even for individual drugs.

AUGUST 2003 EFFEXOR LABELING CHANGE AND FDA'S RESPONSE

While we were beginning to receive responses to our requests for summary data from the sponsors for the other anti-depressants, Wyeth Pharmaceuticals, the manufacturer of Effexor and Effexor XR, decided to make labeling changes for its products to address reports of suicidality and hostility. Sponsors have the authority to make changes to strengthen labeling to address safety issues without prior FDA approval. This action was based on the company's re-analyses of data from the Effexor pediatric trials. The labeling change was the addition of a statement to the "Usage in Children/Pediatric Use" section in the "Precautions" section of the label to note increased reports of hostility and suicidality. This labeling change was accompanied by an August 22, 2003, "Dear Health Care Professional" letter noting the findings and noting that these products are not recommended for use in pediatric patients.

In September 2003, the UK MHRA issued a regulatory response on Effexor similar to its response to the report on Paxil suicidality data. It issued a public statement advising prescribers against the use of Effexor for the treatment of pediatric MDD. This statement was accompanied by a labeling change to contraindicate the products for that pediatric indication. FDA did not take any specific regulatory action on Effexor because we viewed the data as preliminary. Like data for other anti-depressant drug products, it required a more detailed review.

SEPTEMBER 2003 FDA INTERNAL REGULATORY BRIEFING

An important milestone in our consideration of the pediatric suicidality data was the September 16, 2003, internal briefing for upper level CDER management. This briefing occurred at a time when we only had a preliminary review of the summary data for Paxil and a crude internal re-analysis of suicidality data from the other pediatric supplements. We had not yet received and reviewed the requested new analyses from all the sponsors of pediatric drugs.

There were several agreements reached at this meeting, including two that were of particular importance for our further plans to address this issue. We recognized that we had cast a very broad net to attempt to capture events of potential interest for possible suicidality. This was appropriate, but it meant that individual cases needed closer examination to determine what they actually represented. Our first conclusion was that it would be useful to try to have all events of potential interest blindly reclassified by outside experts in suicidality in order to have greater confidence in what the signals represented. This conclusion eventually led to the Columbia Classification Project, described in greater detail below. Second, because it was apparent that there was inconsistency in the signals of suicidality among the individual studies of the various drugs, we also concluded that it would be useful to attempt to obtain patient-level data sets for all of these trials. This would permit analyses that are more refined and allow adjustments for potentially important covariates. These agreements strongly influenced the subsequent course of our efforts to better understand these data.

RESPONSES TO FDA'S REQUEST FOR SUMMARY DATA FOR OTHER ANTI-DEPRESSANTS

The responses to FDA's request for summary data for all of the anti-depressants arrived by late September 2003. These responses were received within DNDP and forwarded to Dr. Mosholder in ODS as they arrived, over roughly a six-week period. Unfortunately, as we began reviewing these responses, it became clear that different sponsors had interpreted the July 22, 2003, request differently. This caused us to doubt whether all eight manufacturers used similar approaches in selecting, classifying, and presenting cases of suicidality for review. There was also a concern, due to the methods used by the manufacturers to search their database, about the possibility that manufacturers had not captured all adverse events of potential interest.

This impression was confirmed when we spoke to individual manufacturers about their approach to our request. In retrospect, the algorithm we had provided to search for potential events and select patients experiencing those events was not sufficiently detailed to result in a common understanding. This discovery presented a major hurdle in our evaluation of these data, because we needed to have confidence in the thoroughness and uniformity of the methods used to gather and classify these cases. We realized that we would need to be more certain that manufacturers captured all relevant cases, and that the relevant cases were appropriately classified.

Greater certainty on this point was necessary to accurately assess the ability of these drugs to provoke suicidality. For example, we did not receive complete descriptions of how manufacturers conducted searches or why manufacturers included or excluded individual cases. In at least one case, the search for and classification of cases was not conducted in a blind manner to avoid bias. In another case, what appeared to be a strong signal in our preliminary analysis of the previously submitted data became a weak signal on re-analysis by the manufacturer. In all, we concluded that we needed to better understand the classification and analysis process.

FDA DECISION ON INDEPENDENT RECLASSIFICATION OF CASES

FDA also was concerned about case definition and selection by manufacturers in response to our July 22, 2003, letters. We noted substantial differences across different drug products in the selection of cases included as suicide attempts. Some sponsors decided to include essentially all captured events as suicide attempts, even though there was clearly not enough information in some of the cases to justify such a classification.

For example, there was concern about a number of the adverse events classified under the category "possibly suicide related." In one case, a young girl slapped herself on the face and researchers coded this as a suicide attempt. A number of other events coded as "suicide attempts" involved children who had engaged in superficial cutting behavior and children who had ingested small numbers of pills in sight of parents. Such events, while of concern in their own right, would not necessarily be an indication of suicidal behavior.

This confirmed the view reached tentatively at our September 2003 internal regulatory briefing of the need to have potential events blindly reclassified by an independent group. Although we briefly considered doing this internally, we rejected this idea because FDA did not have the expertise in suicidality to conduct such a large reclassification effort. Furthermore, most employees who might logically participate in such an effort had already seen many of the cases. These reviewers could also be biased because they were aware of the treatment assignment (drug or placebo).

FURTHER REQUESTS FOR DATA/INITIATE THE "COLUMBIA" STUDY

Thus, we began to look outside the Agency and initiated a series of discussions with outside experts. Although we found several experts interested in such an effort, there remained the problem of who could coordinate this work and establish methods and criteria for reclassification.

Columbia University not only had well-recognized expertise in adolescent suicidality, but also had developed an approach to classifying events that possibly were representative of suicidality, and this approach precisely fit our needs. We conducted extensive discussions with this group in order to establish a contract to accomplish this reclassification of cases and to work out the details of a standard approach to finding all relevant cases and setting up categories for the reclassification effort that would meet our needs.

Additionally, as we reviewed the summary data provided by the various sponsors in response to our July 22, 2003, letters, we again noted an inconsistency in results across trials, even within individual programs, that we had observed in our re-review of the pediatric supplements. To further address this issue, on October 3, 2003, DNDP requested patient-level data sets from all manufacturers of the nine anti-depressant drugs. The availability of these more detailed data has permitted FDA to perform a more refined analysis, taking into consideration possible imbalances across study groups in these trials. In order to ensure that we had a complete capture of all relevant events that might possibly be related to suicidality for these trials, we issued follow-up requests to our

JULY 2003 LETTERS; THESE REQUESTS WERE MADE ON NOVEMBER 24 AND DECEMBER 9, 2003.

This complete set of narratives was sent to Columbia University for review by a panel of international pediatric suicidality experts. This group was assembled to undertake a blinded review of the reported behaviors using a rigorous classification system.

FDA'S OCTOBER 2003 UPDATED PUBLIC HEALTH ADVISORY AND TALK PAPER

FDA issued an updated Public Health Advisory and Talk Paper on October 27, 2003, based on our assessment of the pediatric suicidality data at that time. Although we indicated that preliminary data suggested an excess of reports of suicidality for several anti-depressant drugs, we noted the need for additional data and analysis. We also noted that we intended to bring this issue to an advisory committee meeting. We advised caution in the use of any of these drugs in treating pediatric MDD, and reminded prescribers of the standard language already in anti-depressant labeling alerting clinicians to the need for close supervision of high-risk patients, particularly during initial onset of drug therapy.

DECEMBER 2003 UK MHRA ACTION ON ANTI-DEPRESSANT TREATMENT OF PEDIATRIC MDD

The UK MHRA made a public announcement on December 10, 2003, indicating that, in addition to its earlier statements regarding the contraindications of Paxil and Effexor in pediatric MDD, it was now also contraindicating all SSRI anti-depressants except Prozac for this condition. This announcement noted that the risk to benefit profile could not be assessed for Luvox, and that, the risk to benefit profile is favorable in pediatric MDD for Prozac only. Serzone and Wellbutrin are not approved drug products in the UK. Remeron is an approved product in the UK, but MHRA has offered no specific comment on the pediatric data for this drug.

FDA'S FEBRUARY 2, 2004 ADVISORY COMMITTEE MEETING

FDA uses advisory committees to gain expert advice about scientific and public health issues and/or regulatory decisions. In preparing for an advisory committee meeting, scientific team leaders, supervisors and managers—seasoned regulatory scientists with drug development and public health expertise—exercise scientific judgment in synthesizing issues to be brought before advisory committees. This process is designed to ensure that an advisory committee considering an issue is provided with sufficient data and information to fully discuss the issues.

While CDER was conducting its more in-depth review of the data from the pediatric clinical trials, planning was also under way to hold a meeting of the PDAC on

February 2, 2004. Because the BPCA mandates a review of the post-marketing safety data for products that have been granted pediatric exclusivity, this meeting was convened to review the post-marketing safety reporting for a number of products (not limited to anti-depressants). One of the drugs scheduled for discussion at the February 2, 2004, Advisory Committee meeting was Paxil.

In planning for the discussion of the safety of the use of Paxil in children, the Agency initially intended to broaden the PDAC meeting to include a discussion of the Agency's review of the safety concerns arising from the data on the use of anti-depressants in children, as these concerns were clearly of public interest. However, as the reviews and meeting planning progressed, it became clear that the additional analyses of the data from the clinical trials of anti-depressants in children, particularly the Columbia analysis, would not be completed in time to present the Agency's final assessment of these data at the Advisory Committee meeting.

The Agency decided to proceed with the plans to discuss the post-marketing safety data for Paxil at the meeting, to brief the Advisory Committee on the Agency's progress in evaluating data from the clinical trials of anti-depressants in children, and to solicit advice and comment regarding the Agency's plans for further analyses. The plan included returning to the Advisory Committee for another meeting once the Agency's more definitive analyses of the clinical trial data were complete. This would allow us to solicit Advisory Committee input before taking further regulatory action.

While CDER was moving ahead with plans for the February 2, 2004, Advisory Committee meeting, Dr. Mosholder was nearing completion of his review of the data from the clinical trials provided in response to our July 22, 2003, request. Based on his review, he believed that the available data were sufficient to reach a conclusion about an association between the use of anti-depressants and suicidality in children and to recommend additional regulatory action, without the need for the more in-depth case classification or analyses that had already been initiated by DNDP. Dr. Mosholder shared his conclusions with his supervisors and with the DNDP/ODE I review team involved in reviewing this issue. The review team and Dr. Mosholder's direct supervisors did not agree that the available data were sufficient to reach a conclusion and believed that definitive action should await the re-analysis by Center staff using the Columbia data. There was a discussion within the DNDP/ODE I review team, as well as higher CDER management including Drs. Katz, Laughren, and Temple, as to whether

Dr. Mosholder's scientific and regulatory conclusions on the data should be presented in some form at the February meeting, given that they did not represent the Agency's (but rather an individual staff member-s) determination; it was concluded that they should not be.

However, at the February 3, 2004, meeting, Dr. Laughren did present the data that led Dr. Mosholder to his conclusions, although not in detail. These data plainly showed an excess of suicidality in individual studies and across the studies as a group.

Dr. Laughren also explained the Agency's reservations about the classification.

Dr. Katz also acknowledged in his presentation to the Advisory Committee that some reviewers had reached a conclusion that the data were sufficient to conclude that there was a link between anti-depressant use and suicidality in children. The Agency did not present Dr. Mosholder's conclusion in detail because of concerns that this would have given his determination the appearance of an Agency position before the Agency had made such a determination. This could have been harmful to the public health because it might have led patients who were actually benefiting from the use of these drugs to inappropriately discontinue therapy with potentially dire consequences, or to avoid treatment when it might be the best option.

Senior CDER staff believed that the best way to serve the public health on this very complex and important issue was to: 1) disclose the available publicly releasable safety data during the Advisory Committee meeting; 2) describe the limitations of those data in supporting a definitive conclusion; and, 3) describe the Agency's plans to further evaluate the data. The Agency realized its responsibility to the public to find the right answer to this question. A premature conclusion that these drugs are harmful (when used in the pediatric population) that does not hold up during a more careful review would be a disservice to the public health given the serious and potentially life-threatening nature of severe depression. This is of particular concern since there are no acceptable therapeutic alternatives for health care providers and their pediatric patients with depression.

CDER'S DECISION-MAKING PROCESS ON SAFETY ISSUES

CDER's decision-making process is designed to ensure that regulatory actions or policy formulation take into consideration an array of perspectives and concerns designed to advance public health. The process requires that primary reviewers, team leaders, supervisors, and managers work together effectively.

In the free and open discussion of CDER issues within a scientific and regulatory environment, we expect differing professional judgments/opinions. Individual employees are strongly encouraged to discuss their views with co-workers. A number of opportunities are available to discuss and resolve scientific differences and enhance decision-making. These include meetings among review teams, meetings with the supervisory and management chains within the Center and Agency, meetings with sponsors, CDER regulatory briefings and Advisory Committee meetings.

It is never the goal of these discussions to pressure or convince reviewers to reach any particular conclusion, or to reach a different conclusion that they have already reached, but only to provide a forum for a free exchange of views by all. After considering all of the relevant data and arguments, individual reviewers are expected to write reviews that reflect their best judgment. If their supervisor disagrees with their conclusions and/or recommendations, the supervisor documents the disagreement, and the resolution of the disagreement, in the official administrative file on a matter.

FDA'S MARCH 2004 ADVISORY: NEW WARNING STATEMENT IN LABELING

At the February 2, 2004, Advisory Committee meeting, experts raised concerns about the possible relationship between anti-depressant drug products and suicidal behavior and suicidal ideation and supported a labeling change to warn of possible suicidality. On March 22, 2004, FDA responded to these concerns by issuing a Public Health Advisory and asked manufacturers of Prozac, Zoloft, Paxil, Luvox, Celexa, Lexapro, Wellbutrin, Effexor, Serzone and Remeron to include a warning statement in their labeling recommending close observation of adult and pediatric patients treated with these drugs for worsening depression or the emergence of suicidality.

In this statement, the Agency informed the public that symptoms such as anxiety, agitation, panic attacks, insomnia, irritability, hostility, impulsivity, akathisia, hypomania, and mania have been reported in adult and pediatric patients who are being treated with anti-depressants for MDD. We warned that patients who experience one or more of these symptoms might be at an increased risk for worsening depression or suicidality. The Agency pointed out that we did not know whether the drugs increased suicidality but warned that medications may need to be evaluated and perhaps discontinued when symptoms are severe, abrupt in onset, or not part of the patient's presenting symptoms. FDA urged health care providers to instruct patients, their families, and their caregivers to be alert for the emergence of agitation, irritability, and the other symptoms described above, as well as the emergence of suicidality and worsening depression, and to report such symptoms immediately to their health care provider.

"COLUMBIA" STUDY RESULTS

The Columbia group submitted its completed review to FDA in July 2004. FDA then developed its analysis of the pediatric suicidality data based on the case classifications provided by Columbia University. While there were findings among these data suggestive of an increased risk of suicidality for some of these drugs, inconsistencies remained in the results, both across trials for individual drugs and across drugs. Thus, an overall interpretation of these findings represented a substantial challenge to the Agency. The Agency brought these findings to the Psychopharmacologic Drugs and Pediatric Advisory Committees in September 2004 for further consideration.

FDA'S AUGUST 2004 ADVISORY: AGENCY PLAN TO PRESENT DATA TO ADVISORY COMMITTEES

As part of its commitment to keep the American public fully informed about the status of its review of data concerning the use of anti-depressants in pediatric patients, on

August 20, 2004, FDA informed the public of its detailed plan to present new data to the Psychopharmacologic Drugs and the Pediatric Advisory Committees. This new data, which FDA posted on its website, included the Agency's interpretation and analyses of pediatric suicidality data based on information obtained from the Columbia Study. In addition, the Agency sought advice on appropriate regulatory actions, such as labeling changes to ensure that the labels of anti-depressants used in pediatric patients reflect the most recent information obtained from current studies and analyses.

As we noted previously, FDA also announced that it posted additional summaries on its web site of pediatric efficacy studies for drugs that have been studied for depression in pediatric patients. These summaries are for Paxil, Celexa, Serzone, Zoloft and Remeron. Although specific new labeling language has yet to be developed, FDA will work to assure that the labels of the anti-depressants used in pediatric patients reflect the most recent information obtained from these studies and analyses.

FDA'S SEPTEMBER 13-14, 2004 ADVISORY COMMITTEE MEETING

On September 13 and 14, 2004, a joint meeting was held between the Psychopharmacologic Drugs and Pediatric Advisory Committees to consider the occurrence of suicidality in the course of treatment of pediatric patients with various anti-depressants. The primary focus of FDA's presentations at the September 2004 meeting was to provide committee members with (1) a detailed description of FDA's approach to evaluating and analyzing the pediatric suicidality data, and (2) the results of this work. The Agency also included presentations on related studies, in particular, several pertinent epidemiological studies and TADS (Treatment of Adolescents with Depression Study). Committee members heard presentations by both FDA staff and experts in pediatric suicidality from the academic community outside of FDA.

The overall consensus of the committee was an endorsement of FDA's approach to classifying and analyzing the suicidal events and behaviors observed in the controlled clinical trials. Committee members expressed their view that the new analyses increased their confidence in the results. Further, the committee members concluded that the finding of an increased risk of suicidality in pediatric patients applied to all the drugs studied (Prozac, Zoloft, Remeron, Paxil, Effexor, Celexa Wellbutrin, Luvox and Serzone) in controlled clinical trials. In addition, the members:

- recommended that the products not be contraindicated in this country because the Committees thought access to these therapies was important for those who could benefit;
- recommended that the results of controlled pediatric trials of depression be included in the labeling for anti-depressant drugs;
- recommended that any warning related to an increased risk of suicidality in pediatric patients should be applied to all anti-depressant drugs, including those that have not been studied in controlled clinical trials in pediatric patients, since the available data are not adequate to exclude any single medication from an increased risk;
- reached a split decision (15-yes, 8-no) regarding recommending a "black-box" warning related to an increased risk for suicidality in pediatric patients for all anti-depressant drugs; and
- endorsed a patient information sheet ("Medication Guide") for this class of drugs to be provided to the patient or their caregiver with every prescription.

FDA'S SEPTEMBER 17 ANNOUNCEMENT REGARDING SSRIS

On September 17, FDA announced that the Agency generally supports the recommendations made to the Agency by the Psychopharmacologic Drugs and Pediatric Advisory Committees regarding reports of an increased risk of suicidality (suicidal thoughts and actions) associated with the use of certain anti-depressants in pediatric patients. FDA has begun working expeditiously to adopt new labeling to enhance the warnings associated with the use of anti-depressants and to bolster the information provided to patients when these drugs are dispensed.

EFFECTIVENESS DATA FOR ANTI-DEPRESSANTS IN PEDIATRIC MDD

To date, much of the focus has been on pediatric suicidality and the safety of anti-depressant drug products. However, it is also important to consider the efficacy data for these drugs because a risk-benefit assessment is important to clearly understand the benefit side of this equation. Of the seven products studied in pediatric MDD (Prozac, Zoloft, Paxil, Celexa, Effexor, Serzone and Remeron), FDA's reviews of the effectiveness data resulted in only one approval (Prozac) for pediatric MDD. (In January 2003, FDA approved Prozac for the treatment of children and adolescents ages 7 to 17 for depression and obsessive-compulsive disorder.)

Overall, the efficacy results from 15 studies in pediatric MDD do not support the effectiveness of these drugs in pediatric populations. It is understandable that people might conclude that these data show that the drugs, except for Prozac, have no benefit in pediatric MDD. We think that conclusion is premature, however.

There are many reasons, other than lack of effectiveness, for studies to fail to show benefit. This phenomenon is a particular problem in depression, and even more so in pediatric depression.

To begin with, in adult MDD programs for drugs approved for this indication, the overall failure rate for studies that appear in every respect to be adequate trials is about 50 percent. This indicates that showing effectiveness in depression is not easy. In fact, because we expected this difficulty, our Written Requests to sponsors asked for two studies, not the one that would have been more typical.

Additionally, the history of pediatric MDD studies with the tricyclic anti-depressants (TCAs) is uniformly negative. This finding may have several possible explanations, including flaws in study design or conduct, or the possibility that TCAs simply do not work in pediatric MDD. It is also possible, however, that there is even greater heterogeneity among pediatric patients who meet criteria for MDD than is true for adults. If true, this would also work against study success in pediatric MDD.

Finally, the context in which sponsors conducted these studies may not have been ideal. Sponsors do not need positive results when conducting a study in response to a Written Request in order to gain exclusivity. The studies simply must be conducted according to the terms of the Written Requests, and the results submitted to meet deadlines specified in those requests. We are not suggesting that sponsors of these studies did not design and conduct them with good intent and according to high standards. We merely point out that the failure of a drug registration trial to show a drug effect represents a more significant loss for the sponsor (i.e., the non-approval of the drug) than the failure of a study in response to a Written Request. We do not know whether this could have influenced the conduct of the study in subtle ways that might have worked against getting a positive result, e.g., in recruitment of patients. As an example of how our thought process has changed since the time we issued the Written Requests, if we were to make a Written Request today for an anti-depressant, we would ask that the trial include a Prozac arm as well as placebo to confirm the ability of the study to demonstrate effectiveness. .

Nevertheless, the failure of most of these programs to show a benefit in MDD heightens the concern about the drugs ability to induce suicidality. The burden is clearly upon those who believe these drugs do have benefits in pediatric MDD to design and conduct studies that are capable of demonstrating such benefits. The problem for practitioners is what to do in the face of the uncertainty. Practitioners must consider the generally negative findings in the context of several other facts.

In all but one of the failed drugs, there were only two studies in pediatric MDD. For the remaining failed drug, there were three pediatric MDD studies. Among the failed drugs, there was one drug where one of the two studies was positive (Celexa), and two others (Zoloft and Serzone) where the results, while negative by our usual standards, were at least trending toward positive in one of the two studies.

It has been observed that the published literature gives a somewhat different perspective, suggesting more positivity in two of these programs. A published paper describes one of the Paxil studies as positive on most of the secondary endpoints, while acknowledging that it failed on the primary endpoint. Another paper describes the Zoloft program as positive, based on a pooling of two similarly designed studies that, when looked at individually, failed. As noted, except for Prozac, we do not believe effectiveness has been shown for any agent in pediatric MDD.

CONCLUSION

FDA was the first to identify a concern about suicidality in several of the submitted pediatric studies. We evaluated the data closely and raised serious questions about its adequacy. We then took the initiative to acquire further relevant data from sponsors and used expertise outside the Agency to access the reports of suicidality thoroughly. FDA's assessment on this issue is designed to achieve the most scientifically rigorous review possible. The Columbia University classification project has provided the Agency with a credible basis for analyzing the risks of these drug products.

The results of pediatric depression studies to date raise very important problems. First, the poor effectiveness results, except for Prozac, make it very difficult for practitioners to know what to do to treat a very serious, life-threatening illness. While we believe that these drugs may be effective in children, studies have not shown this to be true. Second, and of equal importance, the analyses we initiated in 2002 appear to show that the drugs in the pediatric controlled depression trials can lead to suicidal behaviors or thinking. While no suicides occurred in the trials, suicides certainly have been reported in treated patients, and the devastating results of these suicides were a critical part of the February 2, 2004, Advisory Committee meeting.

FDA generally supports the recommendations that were recently made to the Agency by the Psychopharmacologic Drugs Pediatric Advisory Committees regarding reports of an increased risk of suicidality associated with the use of certain anti-depressants in pediatric patients. FDA has begun working expeditiously to adopt new labeling to enhance the warnings associated with the use of anti-depressants and to bolster the information provided to patients when these drugs are dispensed.

Thank you for inviting us today to discuss this important subject. We would be glad to answer your questions.

Mr. WALDEN. Dr. Laughren, do you have an opening statement, sir?

Mr. LAUGHREN. No, I don't.

Mr. WALDEN. Okay. Dr. Seligman?

Mr. SELIGMAN. No, I don't.

Mr. WALDEN. Thank you. Well, we appreciate all of you here today to share with us this information as we continue to look at what happened in this area and maybe what needed to happen, and where we are today and where we will be when the FDA makes it decision relative to the Advisory Committee's recommendations.

Dr. Knudsen, could you turn in our big binder there to Tab 71 and 72? While you are looking at that, these are the two versions of a letter under your signature sent to Pfizer Pharmaceuticals on March 19, 1996, Tab 71 and 72.

Tab 71 has a FAX cover page filled out in someone's handwriting to Martha Brumfield of Pfizer from James Knudsen. The top of that page indicates it was sent at 10:18 and shows FDA Neuropharm on it as well.

Does this appear to be your handwriting on the FAX cover sheet, sir?

Mr. KNUDSEN. It does appear to be.

Mr. WALDEN. It does. Okay. The letter attached to this FAX has lots of typographical errors in it as well as different fonts being used for various words. If you would turn to Tab 72, it appears to be the same letter in substance as Tab 71. However, the typos are removed, and the font is consistent. The letters alone have a different FAX time Sent stamp on them, and show them coming from a different section of FDA. Yet does the signature on both these letters appear to be yours?

Mr. KNUDSEN. Tough question, isn't it? They appear to be, but then again—yes, they appear to be. Back in 1996 when I was—my penmanship may have been a bit better than now. It varies somewhat. But I will answer the question as it appears to be. I have to equivocate a week bit, just because of the duration of time and the instability of my penmanship.

Mr. WALDEN. All of our penmanship tends to suffer with age, sir.

Mr. KNUDSEN. Thank you so much.

Mr. WALDEN. Was it your practice to send a draft letter to a pharmaceutical company requesting information, then resend a cleaned-up version later on, though? Would you have sent it as a draft and then send a different version later?

Mr. KNUDSEN. No, I don't—I mean, once again I have to preface a statement by, regrettably, this was done in 1996. So it is somewhat precarious for me to forage around in the limited gray matter that is available to answer that concretely.

Mr. WALDEN. Is it a practice you recall doing throughout your career? Do you usually send a draft and then another?

Mr. KNUDSEN. I do not—no, I do not usually send a draft and another. That's correct.

Mr. WALDEN. I mean, this wouldn't be a normal practice, I wouldn't think.

Mr. KNUDSEN. No. That's correct.

Mr. WALDEN. Okay. I don't know. I mean, I'm not the best speller in the world, but——

Mr. KNUDSEN. Well, quite frankly, I chatted with this—I mean, last week I talked with the subcommittee staffers, and I was rather appalled at what—with the typographical mistakes. I am rather fastidious most of the time. There are periods whereby I could deviate from that, but I mean, this is—this being Tab 71 is a mess. Draft or otherwise, I wouldn't be sending it to Martha, best I can recall anyway.

Mr. WALDEN. I understand that. Do you have any explanation for the fact that two versions of this letter exist?

Mr. KNUDSEN. No, but I suspect others do. I am unable to come up with an explanation.

Mr. WALDEN. Were you able to find this letter in the files at FDA?

Mr. KNUDSEN. I checked—no, to answer your question. I did check the document room. My own files are in—not trying to generate excuses, but they are in boxes which I invite you to my office and it is extremely difficult to even find a box. But they are all there. We are getting ready to relocate. So maybe with another 40 days and 40 nights I could find it.

Mr. WALDEN. Well, should there have been a copy of this letter in the NDA files?

Mr. KNUDSEN. I would—yes, and I would have kept a copy myself in my Certraline file. I keep everything.

Mr. WALDEN. Your files are in boxes?

Mr. KNUDSEN. I as unable to locate it in the document room——

Mr. WALDEN. Right.

Mr. KNUDSEN. [continuing] when I was there. I checked in a cursory way in my office, just trying to find the Certraline file that I have. In fact, I did find the Certraline file, parts of it, but I could not locate this particular document.

Mr. WALDEN. Where did you obtain a copy of your March 19, 1996, letter, and which version did you see?

Mr. KNUDSEN. I obtained two copies, one from the Division.

Mr. WALDEN. The Division?

Mr. KNUDSEN. HFD, the Division I am in, the day before I left to go to Maine. I took it with me, in addition to other things, other documents, and then the subcommittee members sent via Federal Express another document. I mean the same one.

Mr. WALDEN. Another copy of that same document?

Mr. KNUDSEN. Yes, sir. Yes, sir.

Mr. WALDEN. And where did the agency get the version they sent to you?

Mr. KNUDSEN. I did not inquire.

Mr. WALDEN. Dr. Temple, do you know?

Mr. TEMPLE. I could be wrong about this. My understanding is that Dr. Knudsen got a copy of the letter from the committee. Maybe I'm wrong about that.

Mr. KNUDSEN. Yes, I just said that.

Mr. TEMPLE. And that we never were able to find it in our files and got it from Pfizer.

Mr. WALDEN. There you go. So you had to go to Pfizer to get it?

Mr. TEMPLE. Yes.

Mr. WALDEN. That's what you provided to the committee. Right?

Mr. TEMPLE. I'm not sure, but we could not—what I am sure of is that we were unable to find a record of this letter anywhere in our files. That, I am sure of. I am not sure about the rest.

I should say that it is unusual. Letters don't ordinarily go out under a medical officer's signature. They would ordinarily go out under Dr. Katz's signature or Dr. Lieber's or whoever was in charge at the time, and a copy would be in the New Drug Application, in the file. So this was unusual.

Mr. WALDEN. All right. Dr. Knudsen, was it your practice as a medical review officer in 1996 to directly correspond with a pharmaceutical company on a matter you were reviewing, and then request information or did you need to apprise any of the supervisors of your request for additional information from the pharmaceutical company?

Mr. KNUDSEN. It was not my practice to do so.

Mr. WALDEN. So you would have—was it your practice to tell your colleagues or supervisors that you were seeking such information from a pharmaceutical company?

Mr. KNUDSEN. Correct, 86 to 95 percent of the time. There is always a slight opportunity for me to—I mean, once again, I mean, I answered the question as best I could that it is not my practice to do so. In fact, I received my copy from the Division via—of course, I guess the Division received it from Pfizer. I wasn't aware of that. I had no need to question that anyway. I just wanted to take some materials with me to Maine.

Mr. WALDEN. Isn't it a requirement of FDA regulations these types of correspondent documents be kept on file by the agency?

Mr. KNUDSEN. Yes.

Mr. WALDEN. All right. And yet in this case, that doesn't appear to be what happened. Right?

Mr. KNUDSEN. That is correct.

Mr. WALDEN. All right. In these letters, you state "We note that there appears to be an increased frequency of reports of suicidality in pediatric adolescent patients exposed to Certraline compared to either placebo or Certraline treated adult OCD patients. If this is, in fact, the case, what would be a plausible explanation?" That is what is in the letter that you signed or you think you signed and sent to Pfizer.

You asked for summary tables from Pfizer to compare data from adult and pediatric patients in their data base. Is it fair to say that you wrote this letter to Pfizer because you noticed an increase in suicide related behavior in the pediatric OCD trials relative to the rates in the adult trials, and that that was of concern to you? Is that why you wrote this letter to Pfizer?

Mr. KNUDSEN. Yes.

Mr. WALDEN. All right. And was it of enough concern that you wanted answers from the company?

Mr. KNUDSEN. Correct.

Mr. WALDEN. And approximately 10 days after you sent this letter to Pfizer, you complete a safety update to Zoloft. We have put selected pages of your safety review at Tab 81, 81, if you want to refer to that, sir.

In your safety update you note on page 15 that, "In the small pediatric adolescent pool population of OCD patients, the incidence of suicidality in the Certraline treated patients was fivefold greater than the adult OCD Certraline treated patients."

You go on to note that 4 of 6 Certraline pediatric patients had comorbid depression and, "Depression is an important risk factor for suicide." You then cite an article published in the Journal of American Academy of Child and Adolescent Psychiatry that indicated—that also noted the same phenomenon with kids being treated with Prozac.

What did you do other than note these concerns in the safety update? Where did you take it from here?

Mr. KNUDSEN. I was trying to see whether or not that was instrumental in my sending the letter to Pfizer, just to garner some additional information. This was March 28, 1996. The letter to Pfizer was October, was it?

Mr. WALDEN. I think the letter to Pfizer, you will see, is dated March 19.

Mr. KNUDSEN. March 19, before.

Mr. WALDEN. So like 9 days later——

Mr. KNUDSEN. Well, in fact, in reviewing the NDA, this was a final document that was signed off, the one that—the document in Tab 81. So prior to finalizing this document, Tab 81, I found this information to be—at the time anyway, certainly of concern to me to make some further inquiries to Pfizer, and realizing, of course, when I finalize this document, I believed that Pfizer had not responded yet to this.

Mr. WALDEN. That would be correct, based on the timeline I have seen. But 9 days before you wrote to Pfizer asking for this additional information, why didn't you include in this update the fact that you were awaiting additional information from the company to explain the fivefold increase? Would that have been a prudent thing to do?

Mr. KNUDSEN. Yes, it would have been.

Mr. WALDEN. Well, my time has expired. I will now recognize the ranking member of the subcommittee at this time, the gentlelady from Colorado.

Ms. DEGETTE. Thank you very much. Dr. Temple and Dr. Laughren, I am wondering if you can tell me, knowing what you know today, do you believe that Dr. Mosholder's initial conclusions about the increased risk of suicidality exists in pediatric populations taking anti-depressant medication to treat MDD? Dr. Temple?

Mr. TEMPLE. The reanalysis that Columbia did, did not change the overall direction of the results. So——

Ms. DEGETTE. So your answer would be yes?

Mr. TEMPLE. Would be yes. Dr. Hammad's analysis and Dr. Mosholder's are slightly different analyses, but in fact the relative proportions of suicidality are similar to what Dr. Mosholder found.

Ms. DEGETTE. What about you, Dr. Laughren?

Mr. LAUGHREN. Yes, I agree. The relative risk for both analyses is roughly twofold. So it is essentially the same. There are some differences across drugs. The signal gets a little stronger for some drugs, a little weaker for others, but overall I agree that it is roughly the same result.

Ms. DEGETTE. There was about 8 months between his findings and when, I think, the FDA took action. I guess my question to both of you: Do you wish that the agency would have taken him more seriously and allowed him to present the findings so that we could have warned parents and physicians about the increased suicidality rates instead of waiting these 8 months?

Mr. TEMPLE. Let me say a few things. Our concern, as I said before, was that the action we take be based on the best possible data. Let me describe the kind of data we had here.

The usual way we expected to evaluate increased suicidal risk is by looking at the scales that patients in trials are given that ask them how suicidal they are. Dr. Laughren in his comments on Dr. Knudsen's review points out that we are going to have more data on this question.

Those analyses revealed nothing in any of these trials. There was no increased suicidality by that measure. What we got was something unexpected, namely the adverse reaction reports, when interpreted, when translated, revealed an excess of these suicidal behaviors. What we had very little experience with was what those things mean.

We thought, as we looked at them, that somebody—that people expert in interpreting these behaviors needed to look at them. Dr. Mosholder specifically in his review says he did not try to reevaluate each of these cases, because he was no longer blinded. That conclusion——

Ms. DEGETTE. But Dr. Mosholder also said that he only looked at the most—I'm not a researcher, but he only looked at the most serious cases and, in fact, Dr. Temple, you yourself in your opening statement said that the comment you had made about the face slapping you now regretted that, because he didn't take those things into account.

Mr. TEMPLE. Let me explain. He had—in response to the concern that these cases might not be a true bill, might not be what they seemed to be, he offered several approaches. One was to only look at the serious cases. That is clear, and you can see in his review, if you look at the cases that were included and not included, that many of the trivial cases were excluded by the decision to look only at the serious cases. That is perfectly true.

There were, however, additional cases where you didn't know what they meant, and he was in no position to reevaluate them. Let me just——

Ms. DEGETTE. I apologize, but they only give me 10 minutes. So if you can make your answer concise, I would appreciate that.

Mr. TEMPLE. Okay. I wanted to explain one other point about it.

Ms. DEGETTE. Very briefly.

Mr. TEMPLE. He also said that, if there is noise in the system, if it is inaccurate, that would tend to hide a finding rather than to create one, and that is true.

What is also true, however, is if there was a bias toward interpreting certain things that the drugs do, like agitating people or making them hostile, as suicidality, that could give you the wrong picture. It could cause you to think there were suicidal events when, in fact, they were not.

That is why we thought we needed an independent look at these cases in——

Ms. DEGETTE. Okay. But at the time that Dr. Mosholder came up with his findings, there was already the British study that had come out earlier that year.

Mr. TEMPLE. No, the British were using the same data we were.

Ms. DEGETTE. Right, but they had concluded this increased risk of suicidality.

Mr. TEMPLE. But we don't know that they——

Ms. DEGETTE. But I mean there were two.

Mr. TEMPLE. Let me make it clear. There was nothing wrong with Dr. Mosholder's analysis, the ratios he designed, any of those things. That is not——

Ms. DEGETTE. Well, right. In fact, it has now turned out he was completely right.

Mr. TEMPLE. No, that is not at issue. What was at issue was what the cases were, whether they really showed suicidality, and to answer that question you either have to look at them closely or decide that they could not have been biased.

Ms. DEGETTE. Well, let me ask you this. In the spring or summer of 2003, Wyeth came to the FDA, and they wanted on their own—we heard this in the last hearing—to strengthen warnings on Efexir, and the FDA asked them not to do that. Is that right?

Mr. TEMPLE. Not quite. They were allowed to do that, and they did it until we created a new stronger warning or—you can call it strong or not—a different warning in march of 2004. That warning was in the warning section. It prominently said you really need to watch patients, and we thought that was a more trenchant warning. That was in response to the Advisory Committee.

Ms. DEGETTE. Okay. Now do you think that the FDA is going to adopt this most recent recommendation about the black box warnings?

Mr. TEMPLE. Our public statement said that we were going to do all the things they said. We want to think about the conversation they had about the black box. It is true it was 15 to 8, but there were a lot of people that said a lot of things.

You know, I don't want to——

Ms. DEGETTE. Does that mean no?

Mr. TEMPLE. No, it absolutely doesn't mean no. It means we haven't finished our decision yet. We want——

Ms. DEGETTE. Well, what is the FDA's goal with respect to labeling of these anti-depressants for off-label use for pediatrics? What is the goal at this point, knowing the information you know about increased risk of suicidality?

Mr. TEMPLE. Well, we are unquestionably going to explain that the drugs themselves appear to be—are associated with or cause an increased risk of suicidality. That is a given. The only question is what form it will take.

The discussion the Advisory Committee had was——

Ms. DEGETTE. What kinds of forms do you have that you can take with it?

Mr. TEMPLE. Oh, you could put a warning—I mean, the alternative, you could put a warning in dark print, something like that, or you can put it in a box. Those are probably the two choices.

Ms. DEGETTE. So the choice would be to put it on the bottle. No?

Mr. TEMPLE. No, no.

Ms. DEGETTE. To put it on the box?

Mr. TEMPLE. Well, a box warning is the very first thing you read in the label.

Ms. DEGETTE. Right. Open it up.

Mr. TEMPLE. A warning comes a little bit later. Those are prominent, too, and we sometimes do one and sometimes do the other. The particular——

Ms. DEGETTE. If there is a black box, that has to be in the advertising, too. Right? So if Zoloft has an ad, it has to have a warning, may cause suicidality in pediatric use, or something like that.

Mr. TEMPLE. Yes. The contents of the black box would have to appear, but——

Ms. DEGETTE. It seems to me you would want to do that.

Mr. TEMPLE. Wait, wait, wait. The content of the warning would have to be there, too.

Ms. DEGETTE. Well, sure. I understand, but that's the effect of a black box versus some of these other warnings. Right?

Mr. TEMPLE. No. The requirement for advertising is you have to balance the information. If there was a prominent dark print box, that would have to be there, too. I'm not trying to discourage a black box. I am just trying to reflect the fact that people who spoke to us were concerned that people who were at risk of killing themselves would not be treated if we scared people too much.

I'm not saying I agree with that. We put the idea of the black box before the committee. You know, we are not shrinking from it, but they said multiple things.

Ms. DEGETTE. Well, I would imagine you would share my concern. My concern is that off-label prescription of these nonapproved drugs for pediatrics with, at best, no effect on these depressed kids and, at worst, increased risk of suicidality will continue unabated. I would assume that is the FDA's role to decide that. Right?

Mr. TEMPLE. One of the problems with off-label use and not having enough data is that you don't know what the answer is. The Advisory Committee—many, many people said we know how the studies came out; they are not impressive; they weren't able to show effectiveness. But they clearly were concerned that maybe as a second line drug these drugs probably should be available and probably worked in people.

That is not the same as knowing, because we know the studies largely failed.

Ms. DEGETTE. I think we can probably all agree that it would help to have more clinical trials in this area, would it not?

Mr. TEMPLE. Yes, but they—Again, I am talking for them. I am not telling you what we decided to do. They were very concerned that we would scare people so much that people who didn't respond to, say, Prozac wouldn't use it or would be afraid to use it, and they were afraid of the consequences. They were worried about them.

You know, these are expert people who treat these conditions. They know a lot more about it than I do.

Ms. DEGETTE. Can I just ask you a question. Do you think it would be a good idea if we had more clinical trials so we could get more data on what the effects of these anti-depressants are, or should we just rely on faith?

Mr. TEMPLE. Oh, no, we live by getting more data. We can't always manage to get it.

Ms. DEGETTE. Can you require more clinical trials as part of your ongoing effort?

Mr. TEMPLE. That is going to be an interesting question. We have a number of thoughts about how to do further studies, which I would use up your 10 minutes if I told you, but I would be glad to.

Ms. DEGETTE. It's okay. It's already over.

Mr. TEMPLE. No, we think there needs to be more data. For example, we were very impressed with the TAD study. It was a very informative study done by NIMH. We are going to be talking with them, see if we can convince them to do some more stuff.

Ms. DEGETTE. Great. Now what about the companies? Are you going to require—what we learned in the last hearing: Pharmaceutical companies are making millions and millions of dollars from this off-label prescription of these anti-depressants.

Would it be reasonable for the FDA to require further studies by the companies?

Mr. TEMPLE. It is reasonable, and whether we can—well, there is a question of our authority. Whether we will be able to require further studies when they will perfectly happily say we think it is a settled question, we don't want the drug used in children—we are perfectly happy to say safety and effectiveness in children hasn't been demonstrated, and they are perfectly happy to say that, as you pointed out.

Ms. DEGETTE. Because they can still sell these drugs.

Mr. TEMPLE. Whether we will be able to persuade them to do more studies is not known to me. We definitely——

Ms. DEGETTE. Well, can't you hold the pediatric exclusivity stick over their head?

Mr. TEMPLE. Unfortunately, no. They have done what they were supposed to do under the law. They have done the trials we asked for, and pediatric exclusivity has been now granted.

Ms. DEGETTE. So if you have these recalcitrant drug companies who are refusing to do more studies because they can just blithely say, well, we don't like this off-label use anyway, we don't——

Mr. TEMPLE. To be fair, they haven't refused yet.

Ms. DEGETTE. Okay.

Mr. TEMPLE. I'm not optimistic. That's all.

Ms. DEGETTE. They might agree to do it, but if not, it would seem to me it would be in the FDA's interest then, and this is within the FDA's authority, to require the strongest possible warnings so that doctors and parents understand the risk to pediatric patients.

Mr. TEMPLE. There is no question there is going to be a strong warning. The other thing is we suggested to the committee that there ought to be patient labeling, a so called Med Guide, and they totally agreed with that.

We also told them that we didn't think a Med Guide works unless you create what is called unit of use packaging, so that it is always handed out, and I am on lengthy record as saying we are going to require that, which we will. But we did all of those things. It needs to be a strong warning.

Ms. DEGETTE. And staff points out to me, the FDA could counterindicate this drug and stop it form being prescribed, period.

Mr. TEMPLE. Well, we couldn't. They could still prescribe it. We don't control what people do. The Advisory Committee was unequivocal, voted overwhelmingly and uniformly that they did not think a contraindication was appropriate, for the reasons that I have just given. They think, without data, without evidence that these drugs actually work, they think they need to be available.

Ms. DEGETTE. Excuse me, sir. Let me just say, it seems like circular reasoning. We don't have the data to say what we should do, but we can't make them get the data. So we are just going to go along. I would suggest we work together. Do you need statutory changes, whatever you need? We need to get a grasp on this, and I think part of it is getting more data.

My time has long expired. Thanks for your comments.

Mr. TEMPLE. Can I throw one more thing out? The data were not uniformly negative. There was one positive trial with a drug called Cetalopram, and there were a couple of trials that were close, not entirely negative.

So it is not out of the question that these drugs can be shown to work.

Mr. WALDEN. Are you talking about efficacy or suicidality?

Mr. TEMPLE. Efficacy.

Mr. WALDEN. Well, I am going to go to Mr. Ferguson in a second. But you could also require that the trials that show no efficacy be published. Right? Be printed? Doctors could be notified? Couldn't you require that?

Mr. TEMPLE. That is a difficult question. Published? Absolutely not. We have no control over publication.

Mr. WALDEN. I'm sorry. I used the wrong term. Couldn't you require that on a label it says no efficacy?

Mr. TEMPLE. I believe we can, yes.

Chairman BARTON. Would the gentleman yield before you go to Mr. Ferguson? I just want to follow up on that question very briefly.

Mr. WALDEN. Certainly, Mr. Chairman.

Chairman BARTON. Dr. Temple, is the FDA now changing its criteria for approval to say, if it can be shown that it is not out of the realm of question that it might be shown to work, that you are going to approve it? I've never heard such a——

Mr. TEMPLE. We are not approving it. I am trying to reflect the views of the experts we had on our Advisory Committee.

Chairman BARTON. I understand that.

Mr. TEMPLE. They know perfectly well that these drugs have not been shown, according to our standards, to work. There is no question about it. I totally agree with that conclusion. That is not the same as knowing they don't work, and they were frightened at the prospect that people would not be able to use the drugs in——

Chairman BARTON. I understand that.

Mr. TEMPLE. That's all.

Chairman BARTON. One reason your agency has such high esteem in the public is because, almost without exception, all the time drugs or medical devices don't get approved until it has been shown without a shadow of a doubt that they do work unless it is some cancer therapy or orphan drug where you develop some sort of an informed consent that the situation is so dire that the patient is going to die unless almost a Biblical miracle occurs.

That statement you just said, to just cavalierly say, well, we can't really say that in some cases it might work, just boggles my mind.

Mr. TEMPLE. I'm obviously not communicating. There is no question that these drugs have not met the standard for approval. I don't want to approve them. I cherish the standard. I think the 1962 Act was one of the greatest pieces of legislation in all the world's history.

That is not the same as saying that anyone who uses a drug off-label is doing the wrong thing. The requirement for approval has to meet—there is a threshold set for approval, and I think that is entirely appropriate. I value it enormously, and I don't even believe it doesn't apply in orphan drug cases, in cancer drugs either.

But the fact is that data comes in a smear, in a range, and what may not be anywhere close to what we would need for approval may inform some people or convince them that they ought to give something a try. I'm just saying that is a fact. I am not saying it is a good thing or a bad thing.

What I am saying is that our Advisory Committee was uniformly concerned that people who hadn't responded appropriately to Prozac would have nothing available when they were deeply depressed, suicidal, and the like. That seems a legitimate concern, too.

That is not talking about making the drug——

Chairman BARTON. I will do this on my own time.

Mr. WALDEN. But don't virtually every single clinical trial show there is no efficacy for these drugs in kids and adolescents? Isn't Prozac like the only one that shows that for kids and adolescents, that there is any efficacy?

Mr. TEMPLE. The results are certainly discouraging. Prozac was three for three.

Mr. WALDEN. No, no. How many studies that have been done in children and adolescents for this range of drugs showed they had efficacy for kids?

Mr. TEMPLE. Not counting Prozac, I assume.

Mr. WALDEN. Count Prozac. I don't care. How many studies have been done——

Mr. TEMPLE. Three Prozacs, one Cetalopram. There is a study of Paxil in which all of the endpoints except their primary endpoint were successful. Some people would think that shows something. We wouldn't. We wouldn't buy it.

Mr. WALDEN. So you don't buy it.

Mr. TEMPLE. I don't buy it.

Mr. WALDEN. All right.

Mr. TEMPLE. Certraline published a report that said we work when you throw our two studies together. We don't buy that, but it is a trend in the right direction. It is not zero, and——

Mr. WALDEN. When it is combined, but not a stand-alone, and I thought your own agency rejected that.

Mr. TEMPLE. That is what I said. We do not believe that they have shown effectiveness. Absolutely not. That is the wrong analysis. I am just saying that is not proof that it doesn't work. I am obviously not making myself clear. I don't want to approve these drugs.

What the Advisory Committee expressed concern about was that in a world of uncertainty, they thought that you need to be able to think about using them in someone who hadn't responded to anything else and who had no other choices. I am not here to say that is a stupid thing to do. Those are knowledgeable advisors.

Mr. WALDEN. Yield to the gentleman from New Jersey.

Mr. FERGUSON. Thank you, Mr. Chairman. Dr. Temple, thank you and your colleagues for being here today. We appreciate you answering many, many questions that are very important questions.

I may have missed it if someone else asked this question. But can you tell me why Dr. Mosholder did not present at the February 2 meeting?

Mr. TEMPLE. Yes. We thought that the—let me just try to think what you've heard and what you haven't heard. Our concern was that there was uncertainty about what the cases that went into his analysis meant. They were collected from adverse reaction reports that were not particularly designed to look at suicidality, and determining whether a given clinical picture represents suicidality is not entirely simple.

The people at Columbia specialize in trying to sort those things out, and we were aware of that. Our concern was not with the analysis that Dr. Mosholder did, which was perfectly right, but with the very cases that went into the analysis and whether they were credible instances of suicidality.

So we arranged well before that meeting, the Advisory Committee meeting, and well before his final report, we arranged for Columbia to blindly review each of the cases and reclassify them. We didn't want to present what appeared to be an FDA conclusion at the February 2004 Advisory Committee.

Mr. FERGUSON. Certainly, he would be capable of explaining that himself, though, wouldn't he?

Mr. TEMPLE. Well, no. He believed the analysis was fine. You know, people can probably disagree about this. We didn't think he was wrong. We thought it wasn't ripe yet. So for us to—you know, for us to go up and say, oh, he's all wet, that wouldn't have been appropriate, and it is not that we thought it was wrong. We thought the cases needed to be looked at before conclusions should be reached.

Mr. FERGUSON. Isn't that the role of the Advisory Committee, is to gather information like this and analyze it and make a recommendation? Did you think they would be confused? Are they an easily confused group?

Mr. TEMPLE. The Advisory Committee was in no position to review each of the cases. We had no capacity to ask them to do that. That would have, you know, taken them months. When we discussed this matter with them, they clearly sympathized with the need to find out what these cases meant. We didn't get a vote. So I can't prove what they thought, but they understood the problem perfectly well, and expressed no dissatisfaction with it.

In fact, at the most recent Advisory Committee meeting, they said the review by Columbia was very impressive, that the data looked better than they could have imagined, and expressed sort of gratitude that they had something they could readily work with.

Mr. FERGUSON. Wouldn't the committee be equipped to analyze the arguments? Isn't that what they are supposed to do?

Mr. TEMPLE. Well, that's sort of what I am saying. It wasn't a matter of making arguments. We didn't have a counter-argument. We didn't think that Dr. Mosholder's review was wrong. What we thought was that the basis for doing the review, for creating the numbers, was imperfect, because the cases hadn't been analyzed——

Mr. FERGUSON. And the Advisory Committee couldn't possibly understand that?

Mr. TEMPLE. Well, I think they did understand it, and they nodded in agreement. But they didn't vote on it. We didn't ask them to vote.

Mr. FERGUSON. They didn't hear his side. He never got to present on February 2.

Mr. TEMPLE. Well, let me make it clear. What——

Mr. FERGUSON. They had information withheld from them.

Mr. TEMPLE. What Dr. Laughren showed was the results of each of the trials, many of which showed more suicidality in the treated group than the other group. Now he didn't show exactly Dr. Mosholder's data or the cumulative data, but it was easy to see, and we emphasized this in the professional advisory that we sent out, that there was more suicidality in the treated group in many of the studies.

So they knew what the issue was perfectly well, and they also heard from Dr. Laughren what our reservations about the data were.

Mr. FERGUSON. I am not at all satisfied with the reason why Dr. Mosholder was somehow blocked from presenting on February 2, for the record. Let me move on.

I'd like to go to Tab 40 in the committee's binder. This is the minutes from the February 2 meeting. Tab 40 is the minutes. I want to go to the top of the last page of Tab 40.

Mr. TEMPLE. Hang on.

Mr. FERGUSON. Sure.

Mr. TEMPLE. Top of the last page?

Mr. FERGUSON. The last page of Tab 40, and I am quoting. The text states: "The committee advised the FDA to inform the public and health care workers, including pediatricians and family practitioners"—it goes on—"of the level of concern regarding possible harm to a minority of children on anti-depressants and the signs associated with the side effect."

It is clear that the Advisory Committee wanted you to inform the public about the risk to children, not the risk to the general population but specifically the risk to children, as reflected in these minutes. Is that correct? Do you agree with that? That is what the minutes say.

Mr. TEMPLE. Yes, but I guess we interpreted that as——

Mr. FERGUSON. I am real short on time.

Mr. TEMPLE. Okay. We put a warning that applied to both adults and children.

Mr. FERGUSON. Right. The Advisory Committee seemed to indicate—they were specific to children, not the general public. That is what it says. That is what the minutes say. Right? Why didn't you issue an advisory specific to the side effects in the pediatric population?

Mr TEMPLE. Because the same side effects occur in adults. Remember, this—we did not write a conclusion that the drugs increased the risk of this, because we thought that was premature, and the committee didn't tell us otherwise. But the possibility that people being given these drugs get worse when they are given them is a phenomenon that has been observed in both adults and children. We thought the warning should apply to anybody being started on these drugs.

Mr. FERGUSON. But if the committee says in their quotation, in the quote from the minutes, from your minutes, the possible harm to a minority of children on anti-depressants and the signs associated with the side effect, why not issue a warning specific to children?

Mr. TEMPLE. Even though we thought the same warning should apply to adults?

Mr. FERGUSON. Why not? What's the harm? Why not?

Mr. TEMPLE. Well, in the labeling what would we say about adults?

Mr. FERGUSON. We consider children and adults different in all sorts of ways. You do, too. The side effects in children are different from the side effects in adults. Right?

Mr. TEMPLE. Yes. This was a statement——

Mr. FERGUSON. There is a reason we test on pediatric. There is a reason we do tests on kids and different tests on adults. We don't extrapolate one to the other necessarily.

Mr. TEMPLE. Right, but——

Mr. FERGUSON. We do tests on both.

Mr. TEMPLE. But the potential for getting worse when you are starting therapy is a phenomenon of both adults and children.

Mr. FERGUSON. Okay. Are the side effects different in children and kids—between children and adults?

Mr. TEMPLE. Well, we now think that they are, because we have seen no increase in suicides in adults with a very large data base, but we now believe there is an increase in suicidal thinking and behavior in children. But that is what we know now, and the new labeling will surely say that.

Mr. FERGUSON. Okay. I am going to keep going, because we are kind of getting fuzzed over here. To me, it is mystifying that, given this information, that you would not have issued—particularly, because this is what the Advisory Committee seemed to be saying, that you wouldn't have issued a warning specific to kids. Let me move on.

The minutes go on to note that the committee is concerned that the public does not know that a strong majority of randomized controlled trials of SSRIs do not demonstrate superiority over placebo in the treatment of major depression in children and adolescents.

Did you address this concern publicly and through a labeling change?

Mr. TEMPLE. We did not introduce a labeling change. All the labeling——

Mr. FERGUSON. Why not?

Mr. TEMPLE. Well, what the labeling all says is that safety and effectiveness in children has not been demonstrated, and the new warning moves that statement forward to the warning language.

Mr. FERGUSON. What warning?

Mr. TEMPLE. The warning that all of the drugs got in March—sorry, after the Advisory Committee meeting.

Mr. FERGUSON. You're talking about the March 22?

Mr. TEMPLE. We asked for it in March. It was all implemented by about August, I think.

Mr. FERGUSON. Okay. Which is Tab 44. So it just seems to me that the agency first tries to determine what information that the Advisory Committee can handle, for instance pulling Dr. Mosholder, not allowing him to present his data and information to the committee, and then when they make a recommendation, when the Advisory Committee makes a recommendation, you disregard the recommendations that they make.

Mr. TEMPLE. I don't agree that we disregarded it. The third paragraph of the thing you just showed me says that anxiety, agitation, panic attacks, etcetera, have been reported in adult and pediatric patients being treated with anti-depressants. I mean, adults are people, too. We thought this is a risk that applies to all people who are started on an anti-depressant.

Mr. WALDEN. Would the gentleman yield?

Mr. FERGUSON. I will yield. I am mystified that, given what is going on with this issue, that you seem to be incapable or refuse to decipher the difference between effects on kids and effects on adults. I will yield to the gentleman.

Mr. WALDEN. Really, I think, what you are asking is: If you knew it affected children and adults, but you also knew it affected kids more than adults.

Mr. TEMPLE. We didn't think we knew that at the time.

Mr. FERGUSON. And worse, more and worse.

Mr. WALDEN. Dr. Mosholder indicated that in his study. This came out—when did this come out, 2004? This came out in February 2004. Right? You own agency began flagging this in 1996 and 1997.

Mr. TEMPLE. We did not think it had been established—again, you have heard the debate about that. Obviously, Dr. Mosholder thought it was well established. We did not think it was established that there was a special risk in children, but we knew that both adults and children started on therapy, early in therapy, can have all these things, including increased suicidality. That is what we wanted to warn about.

We did not say at this time that there was an increased risk in children.

Mr. WALDEN. Are you acknowledging that there is an increased risk in adults?

Mr. TEMPLE. Increased risk compared to no treatment?

Mr. WALDEN. Right.

Mr. TEMPLE. No. We don't know that.

Mr. WALDEN. So there is no increased risk of suicidality in adults who are on anti-depressants in the trials?

Mr. TEMPLE. We have done analyses of suicides now, and we don't see anything like that. Dr. Mosholder presented at the last Advisory Committee an analysis of the Paxil adult data using exactly the same approach that was used in the children. That showed no increase in suicidality in the adults. So at this time, that appears to be different, but it remains true that, whether there is an increase or not, increased suicidal behavior and thinking does occur early in therapy.

Mr. FERGUSON. Mr. Chairman, could I reclaim the time that I don't have left for one more question?

Mr. WALDEN. Yes, sure.

Mr. FERGUSON. I want to just go to one more, Tab 49, which is your statement, the FDA's statement from September 16 on the recommendations of the Psychopharmacologic Drugs and Pediatric Advisory Committees. These are the recommendations from September.

Mr. TEMPLE. I'm sorry. Which am I looking at now?

Mr. FERGUSON. Tab 49.

Mr. TEMPLE. Forty-nine? Sorry. Okay.

Mr. FERGUSON. My question is: Given the fact that, in my estimation, you seem to have, No. 1, tried to control the information that the Advisory Committee was getting; No. 2, seemed to disregard the Advisory Committee's recommendations that they made back in February.

What assurance do we have that these recommendations from September will be followed or adopted?

Mr. TEMPLE. Well, you have the statement about what we are going to do, and in a couple of weeks you will see the labeling change.

Mr. FERGUSON. No, no, no, no. The statement says the FDA general supports the recommendations that were recently made. That is—I mean, my gosh, this is Washington. That could mean anything.

Mr. TEMPLE. Well, let me make it clear. We had some discussion of this before we came in. The only thing we want to think further about is the box, for reasons that I explained before and would be glad to explain again. All the rest of the recommendations are——

Mr. FERGUSON. I heard the conversation about the box.

Mr. TEMPLE. All the rest of them are clearly going to be implemented. We, frankly, suggested half of them.

Mr. FERGUSON. Okay. You said in the New York Times on September 14, "I think we now—I think that we now all believe that there is an increase in suicidal thinking and action that is consistent across all the drugs." And you have the Advisory Committee saying 15 to 8 that they think the black box is a good idea.

I mean, that is almost the override of a veto. I mean, 15 to 8 is substantial. What is left? What is the problem?

Mr. TEMPLE. Well, you have to have been to a lot of Advisory Committees to notice this, but as much as anything else, you want to hear the words people use to explain why they think what they think and what the reservations are. All I am saying is we are going to look at what those are.

I am not predicting that we won't buy the black box. My guess is we probably will, but we owe the people who spoke and tried to advise us a look at what they said.

Mr. FERGUSON. If there is a vote on another issue that is 15 to 8, is it generally adopted or is it something that is not adopted or do you kind of think about it for a little while longer?

Mr. TEMPLE. Yes, that is a very hard thing to answer, but divided committees recommending approval or not approval—when it is reasonably close, we don't necessarily go by the majority, you know. You sort of have to read what people say and——

Mr. FERGUSON. Is 15 to 8 reasonably close?

Mr. TEMPLE. Well——

Mr. FERGUSON. That is a whitewash.

Mr. TEMPLE. There is no question the majority of the people thought that it ought to get a box, and they overcame in recommending that their concern that use of the drugs would be over-discouraged.

Mr. FERGUSON. Recommending a black box is a pretty big deal. That is not taken lightly. Right?

Mr. TEMPLE. We understand it. One of the questions we asked them is should we put a black box on it. We put it on their table so that we could hear their opinion, and we wanted their opinion and their discussion on the pros and cons, and how they came to pro, in spite of certain reservations and concerns is extremely informative.

Mr. FERGUSON. You have almost a two to one vote on a—you don't see a black box on too many drugs.

Mr. TEMPLE. You see them on a fair number. We are not saying that we don't want to do it or don't plan to do it. We just owe that one some thought. That's all.

Mr. FERGUSON. I'm done. Thank you. I yield back.

Mr. WALDEN. Thank you. I now turn to the gentleman from Michigan, Mr. Stupak, for questions.

Mr. STUPAK. Thank you, Mr. Chairman. This black box—where is it going to go?

Mr. TEMPLE. Black boxes are always the first thing in labeling.

Mr. STUPAK. Where is the label? Is that for health care professionals or do people get a chance to see that?

Mr. TEMPLE. Sorry. The label refers to the package insert that is written for physicians.

Mr. WALDEN. Mr. Stupak, I erred. I was committed to the chairman to go to him, because he has to go to mark-up.

Mr. STUPAK. That's all right.

Mr. WALDEN. Could you——

Mr. STUPAK. Go ahead, Joe.

Mr. WALDEN. Mr. Chairman.

Mr. STUPAK. But let me just clarify that. That black box only goes to physicians. It doesn't go to the general public?

Mr. TEMPLE. Right. There will be an equivalent emphasis in the patient labeling, what is called a Med Guide, that we were also very strongly advised to create. So that will be very prominent in that form, too.

Chairman BARTON. I apologize for going out of order, but we've got a mark-up on the waste bill upstairs. I thank the courtesy of Mr. Stupak.

Dr. Temple, have you ever run for any political office?

Mr. TEMPLE. No.

Chairman BARTON. Do you follow Presidential politics?

Mr. TEMPLE. Oh, yes.

Chairman BARTON. Okay. You are aware there is going to be a debate next week between President Bush and Senator Kerry.

Mr. TEMPLE. So I've heard.

Chairman BARTON. How would you feel if you were really looking forward to that and at the last moment the news reported that it had been decided that Senator Kerry couldn't represent himself in the debate, that Congressman Joe Barton had been appointed to represent Senator Kerry's views in the debate with President Bush about who is qualified to be the next President of the United States?

Would you think that was a fair thing to do or an unfair thing to do?

Mr. TEMPLE. Unfair thing to do.

Chairman BARTON. Unfair thing to do. So when the decision was made that Dr. Mosholder could not present his findings last February, nobody was allowed to even hear what his findings were, but that when it was finally decided that his findings could be presented last week or the week before last, somebody else did it, and somebody else did it who probably disagreed with his findings. Was that fair or unfair?

Mr. TEMPLE. He presented his findings. He compared his findings with the new findings.

Chairman BARTON. Oh, Dr. Mosholder did present his—I was told he did not.

Mr. TEMPLE. Well, the primary analysis was done by Dr. Hammad on the new data, but what Dr. Mosholder did was show how the analyses were similar and different.

Chairman BARTON. Well, now I want to be fair. When I'm wrong, I'm wrong. I was told that Dr. Mosholder did not get to present his own findings. That is apparently not true?

Mr. TEMPLE. When do you mean now?

Chairman BARTON. Well, there have been two Advisory meetings, one last February that I——

Mr. TEMPLE. Oh, I think I misunderstood you. In the most recent Advisory Committee——

Chairman BARTON. There have been Advisory——

Mr. TEMPLE. A couple of weeks ago.

Chairman BARTON. There was an Advisory at the beginning of this year in February. Then there was another Advisory just a couple of weeks ago. Isn't that correct?

Mr. TEMPLE. Yes. At the February meeting, he did not present his analysis. If that is what you mean, that is true. That is what we talked about.

Chairman BARTON. Well, at that meeting did anybody present any of his findings?

Mr. TEMPLE. I see. I understand. That sort of depends on what you mean. The results of the numbers, the number of adverse—of suicidality events were shown, study by study, not Dr. Mosholder's analysis, by Dr. Laughren. I mean, these are the data that we had that were submitted to us. Those were presented. They showed an excess in some studies, not an excess in other studies, and they did not——

Chairman BARTON. Which meeting are you talking about?

Mr. TEMPLE. The February 2004 meeting.

Chairman BARTON. But he was not there?

Mr. TEMPLE. He was there, but he didn't present the results.

Chairman BARTON. He was there, but he wasn't allowed to speak.

Mr. TEMPLE. Yes.

Chairman BARTON. Publicly allowed to speak.

Mr. TEMPLE. He presented other data, but he didn't present the—he didn't present the analysis of the controlled trials in depression.

Chairman BARTON. Well, I would argue that that was unfair. Now let's fast forward to a couple of weeks ago. There was another Advisory meeting. Was he allowed to present there?

Mr. TEMPLE. Yes.

Chairman BARTON. Unencumbered?

Mr. TEMPLE. Unencumbered.

Chairman BARTON. Okay. So then I was misinformed on that. I was told that he was not allowed at the second meeting to present, that his data was presented, I believe, by Dr. Laughren. That was at the first one? Okay. Well, then I was misinformed.

Mr. TEMPLE. At the first one Dr. Laughren presented somewhat different data that were basically derived from the same data bases. We didn't try to present Dr. Mosholder's views. We just tried to show why we were worried about these things in the first place.

Chairman BARTON. Well, my main point, and I think it is still valid: If somebody is viewed as credible, which Dr. Mosholder was initially when he was appointed, when he was still in the Pharmacological Neuropharm Directorate. He was picked to do the review, apparently because they felt he was the best qualified. Now I understand that he later got transferred to a different division or different directorate.

Mr. TEMPLE. He moved voluntarily. We didn't want him to go.

Chairman BARTON. Okay. He moved voluntarily. Anyway, he was no longer in that group.

Mr. TEMPLE. We consider that a loss for us.

Chairman BARTON. Okay. Well, we agree on that. We agree on that. You know, if he was the one who was picked to do the initial review, he should be the one that is picked to do the presentation of the data. We, I think, all agree up here that the impression is that he wasn't allowed to present, because higher-ups disagreed with him and wanted to muzzle him.

Mr. TEMPLE. Well, what higher-ups thought was that the data weren't ripe for presentation, because they needed the analysis of the cases by the Columbia group, and you know, it is always a difficulty when there is disagreement about something like that. But the people at the next level have responsibility for making that decision.

We thought it was potentially dangerous for the community to present prematurely what appeared to be an FDA conclusion. You know, I am positive people can argue that judgment, but that is what the judgment was.

Chairman BARTON. Well, we all agree that the best advocate for a position is normally the person who is actually most responsible for developing the position. You agreed with me that Senator Kerry would be a little hacked off if Joe Barton got to present his position, because if I was doing the presenting and I say, now this is what Senator Kerry said but this is really what I think ought to be, you know, and every time President Bush said something, I'd say, well, I have to oppose that, but you know, really I do agree with you, it wouldn't be a very good debate.

Mr. TEMPLE. This may be more nuance than is safe, but it wasn't that we disagreed with him. What we thought was that the data weren't ready. So what I didn't want to do——

Chairman BARTON. Why wouldn't you let the Advisory Committee—it's not like you are making a presentation to the unwashed like Members of Congress. You are making the presentation to a technical advisory committee of experts that you yourself—not you personally perhaps, but the FDA has picked.

They certainly ought to be able to determine the nuances of the data and, if they are really on their toes, they are going to ask him a lot of very pointed questions trying to pick out any flaws in his presentation.

Mr. TEMPLE. We could probably have done that and offered our own critique and then let them choose. What we were worried about, you know, for better or for worse, is that it would appear to be an FDA conclusion and that we thought it was premature, and we thought that was not the right thing to do and was potentially a bad thing for the community.

I think Dr. Laughren has been trying to—can I let him?

Mr. LAUGHREN. Can I just try and clarify?

Chairman BARTON. Yes, sir. This is an open hearing. We are not going to muzzle anybody.

Mr. LAUGHREN. Okay. You know, let me just say, first of all, that we fully appreciate Dr. Mosholder's role in this. As Dr. Temple pointed out, he was the one who discovered the signal initially, the potential signal in the Paxil pediatric supplement back in 2002, and alerted us to this problem with the way the data were coded that led to the report from Glaxo in May 2003. And everyone agrees that he was the right person to begin looking at those data.

What he did, he looked at the Paxil summary report, which was the first one. In the meantime, he began looking back at the pediatric supplements for the other drugs while we were waiting for data from the other drugs and made a very important contribution at the internal regulatory briefing in September.

The focus—our focus changed dramatically over the course of the fall, as we started looking at the cases and recognized that there might be a problem in understanding—in whether or not they all represented suicidalities. That was one major theme we were pursuing.

We were also concerned about case finding. We recognized, as again we started looking at these documents, that we may not have gotten all the cases, and that is why late in the year we issued additional requests for more cases from the companies.

A third theme that we were pursuing was getting what is called patient level data so that we could try and understand the striking differences between trials.

So this was our focus, and gradually it became clear that we were going to have to do our own analysis of the data, based on this more complex dataset. That is why Dr. Mosholder's role changed during that period of time. So——

Chairman BARTON. Are you saying he wasn't competent to do that?

Mr. LAUGHREN. No, I'm not—well, I'm not saying that. We had the expertise to deal with——

Chairman BARTON. Who is we?

Mr. LAUGHREN. Well, the Neuropharm Division, in particular the safety team, Dr. Hammad.

Chairman BARTON. And Dr. Hammad is not in the direct line. He is kind of a staff auxiliary advisory to the main chain of command in the Center. Is that not correct? I mean, his job is to kind of double check everybody else?

Mr. LAUGHREN. No, no, no. He did the primary analysis, the definitive analysis that we presented to the Advisory Committee last week.

Mr. TEMPLE. There is a group called the Safety Group in Neuropharm that specializes in doing safety analyses, and he is a member of that group. He, too, is actually moving to the Office of Drug Safety.

Chairman BARTON. But Dr. Hammad's—I looked at a flow chart to try to figure out who everybody is, and my understanding is, of the group that is here, Dr. Temple is the biggest dog and is an Associate Director, and Dr. Laughren reports directly to you, and Dr.——

Mr. TEMPLE. Well, Dr. Katz who couldn't be here is the Division Director, one of three in the office that I run.

Chairman BARTON. You report to him. Right?

Mr. TEMPLE. He reports to me, and Dr. Laughren reports to Dr. Katz.

Chairman BARTON. And Dr. Hammad is in a staff group that is not in the direct chain. Is that correct?

Mr. TEMPLE. No. Well, there's two Psychopharm groups, one of which is headed by Dr. Laughren, and there is a safety group that reports the same way as Dr. Laughren does, to Dr. Katz, and Dr. Hammad is in that group.

Chairman BARTON. Okay. Well, I have kind of gotten off on a rabbit trail here. My time has expired. Let me refocus this again to the members of this subcommittee who have really no ax to grind except that we want the very best for the American people, and in this particular case we don't want children taking anti-depressant drugs if there appears to be quite a bit of evidence that, not only does it not help them, in some cases it actually hurts them, increases the risk of suicidality.

Time after time in reviewing the documents and reviewing the transcripts and the testimony, you know, it really does appear to me that the FDA has gone out of its way to short circuit the findings of Dr. Mosholder and create this counter-argument that you epitomized earlier when you said, well, if there is some evidence that it might help some people some of the time, why should we stop it, which seems to me exactly contrary to what the normal FDA standard is, that if you can't show that it helps a lot of people all the time, we shouldn't allow it.

Mr. TEMPLE. I was trying to describe what our Advisory Committee of people in the field who actually do this were worried about.

Chairman BARTON. I am just really puzzled about that.

My last thing, again back on Dr. Mosholder: Is it true that, when ABC contacted him to say that they were considering him for man of the week, that higher-ups at FDA tried to stop that? Is there any truth to that?

Mr. TEMPLE. I have no idea. I can't imagine that we would try to stop it, but I do imagine that it might have to get cleared, something like that. But I have no knowledge of this.

Chairman BARTON. Would Mr. Mosholder—you are still under oath. Do you know for a fact if anybody at FDA, when you were asked to be man of the week for ABC, either did not clear that or tried to prevent that?

Mr. MOSHOLDER. Actually, I had a conversation about that with Dr. Seligman, whose chair I just took, and Dr. Seligman had some reservations about it. In my mind, too, was at that time I had been asked to be a witness at this hearing, and I had some concerns about whether it would be unseemly, because being person of the week involves an on-air interview, whether that would be unseemly coming just a few days before this hearing.

Chairman BARTON. So who withdrew? Did you withdraw?

Mr. MOSHOLDER. I withdrew. Yes.

Chairman BARTON. You withdrew. You didn't—I am going to ask Dr. Seligman as soon as he retakes his seat what is concerns were.

Dr. Seligman, we just heard from Dr. Mosholder that, after talking to you, he withdrew from consideration for ABC man of the week, which I would think would be something the FDA would want, that they would want their employees being men and women of the week to show that they are doing good deeds for the American people.

What were the concerns that you expressed to him about that?

Mr. SELIGMAN. I congratulated him for his selection.

Chairman BARTON. That is not expressing a concern.

Mr. SELIGMAN. No, I know. I am just telling you what the nature of our conversation was. I just expressed the same concern that I express over any interaction with the media, which is to make sure that was careful and thoughtful in his presentation and that things he said were, you know, succinct so that it potentially could not be taken out of context.

Chairman BARTON. So did you encourage him to go forward or did you encourage him to withdraw?

Mr. SELIGMAN. I did neither. I did neither encourage him nor discourage him.

Chairman BARTON. Okay. Well, if ABC is listening, I would encourage ABC to nominate Dr. Mosholder for man of the week, because I think he is doing the kind of things that we want our researchers and evaluators to do. So for what it is worth, the chairman of Energy and Commerce Committee that has jurisdiction over the FDA thinks that would have been an excellent selection.

Mr. WALDEN. And Telecommunications.

Chairman BARTON. My time has way expired. So with that, I yield back.

Mr. WALDEN. Thank you, Mr. Chairman. Now I again appreciate the courtesy extended by the gentleman from Michigan, and we look forward to your questions. Mr. Stupak.

Mr. STUPAK. Thank you. Dr. Temple, you said the black box warnings goes to health care professionals hearing this and not to the public. Are you going to do an informed consent on this drug?

Mr. TEMPLE. The Advisory Committee didn't vote on that question, but talked about it and did not think that was appropriate. The problem here is that——

Mr. STUPAK. So are you going to do an informed consent or not?

Mr. TEMPLE. Well——

Mr. STUPAK. Yes or no?

Mr. TEMPLE. I don't think that is fully settled, but I would say probably not.

Mr. STUPAK. So wc don't get the black box warning. There is no informed consent. How are people out here going to know what is going on with these drugs?

Mr. TEMPLE. Sorry, I missed the first part of your sentence.

Mr. STUPAK. There is no black box warning that people will receive. There is no informed consent. How are they going to know that these drugs are not effective and increases possibility of suicide behavior?

Mr. TEMPLE. Well, patients will—with unit of use packaging, every patient who gets the drug gets the patient labeling, so called Med Guide. That will have a very prominent statement—whether we box it or not, I think that hasn't been determined yet; we don't necessarily——

Mr. STUPAK. You are going to put the Med Guide, which is supposed to be in very plain, simple English—you are going to put that into every packet?

Mr. TEMPLE. Yes.

Mr. STUPAK. Every one?

Mr. TEMPLE. Every one.

Mr. STUPAK. Is the pharmacist going to have to dispense it or is it going to be in every one?

Mr. TEMPLE. No. We despair of success when the pharmacist has to dispense it.

Mr. STUPAK. Beg pardon?

Mr. TEMPLE. We don't think it is successful if the pharmacist has to do it. That is why we create—that is why we insist, in some cases anyway, on unit of use packaging. Unit of use packaging means——

Mr. STUPAK. Right. Familiar with it. You indicated that—we have heard testimony the last couple of times that everyone was quick to say there were no suicides in clinical trials. Is that correct? Yes or no? You can't shake your head.

Mr. TEMPLE. I'm sorry. Yes.

Mr. STUPAK. Okay. So where did you get the information on the suicides then?

Mr. WALDEN. Just for our audience, we are being called for one vote. We will wait, though, a few minutes, and then we will recess while we make that one vote. Then we will come back. Oh, is it two votes? Okay. Well, we will do the same drill.

Mr. TEMPLE. There were no suicides in the 4,000 or so patients who were in the controlled trials—in the pediatric trials.

Mr. STUPAK. Correct.

Mr. TEMPLE. In the much larger data bases that have been carried out in adults, there were suicides, and we have compared the frequency of suicides on-treatment and off-treatment in those. There, it comes out even. That is our suicide data.

Mr. STUPAK. So your suicide data would be coming from reports from the drug manufacturers then, right, or unless it is voluntarily——

Mr. TEMPLE. No. These are results of trials. There have been a lot of trials altogether. So we have 30-40,000 people. Dr. Hammad can tell us how many.

Mr. STUPAK. So the suicides were found in the adult population. You extrapolated that to make some kind of conclusions as to children?

Mr. TEMPLE. No. We have reached the conclusion about adults. We don't know that adults and children are the same. As I said, when Paxil data in adults were examined in exactly the same way as they were examined in children, and the children's analysis showed a clear excess of suicidal behavior and thinking, no similar excess was seen in adults.

I don't have a good explanation for that. I don't know why that should be true, but that is what the result is so far.

Mr. STUPAK. If you have no suicides in the clinical trials, do you have suicides in your adverse events file?

Mr. TEMPLE. Yes.

Mr. STUPAK. With children?

Mr. TEMPLE. Oh, yes.

Mr. STUPAK. And what percentage are reported?

Mr. TEMPLE. Well, we have no idea.

Mr. STUPAK. Wasn't it true that with your adverse events report, only about at most 10 percent are ever reported?

Mr. TEMPLE. That is a figure commonly given, but we don't know what the right answer is.

Mr. STUPAK. In fact, FDA has used that figure many times, somewhere between 1 percent and 10 percent.

Mr. TEMPLE. We have used that figure to try to make rough estimates, but that is not the same.

Mr. STUPAK. What you have is only 10 percent of what may actually be out there. We can't say with certainty, but based upon, again, extrapolation of the data, it is basically 10 percent of the known number.

So when you do your black box warning, are you going to use the word rarely, that suicide behavior, suicide thoughts, suicide ideation, suicides may rarely occur with the use of these anti-depressants in young people?

Mr. TEMPLE. No. The results of the trials would not support the term rare. Dr. Hammad estimated—well, it is roughly, just roughly, 2 percent in people who get placebo and about 3.5 or 4 percent in people who get the drug. That doesn't meet anybody's test for rare.

The excess risk is in the neighborhood of 2 to 3 percent. I think that is the figure Dr. Hammad gets. So that would not be called rare.

Mr. STUPAK. When will you end your conversations about the black box?

Mr. TEMPLE. Really, within a few days, we will reach a decision.

Mr. STUPAK. Right. You have stated in your testimony, the little bit I have been in—we have a mark-up going on upstairs; so I am running back and forth between the two. You have stated in your testimony that thus far these anti-depressants in children, "doesn't work; do not meet the standards for approval; results are discouraging." Then why does the FDA allow these anti-depressants be given to children under the age of 18?

Mr. TEMPLE. Well, we don't allow it. The labeling all says, except for Prozac, that safety and effectiveness——

Mr. STUPAK. Are you telling this committee, if the FDA put on the thing that says not to be distributed to children under 18, you don't have that authority? You can't do that?

Mr. TEMPLE. Not to be distributed?

Mr. STUPAK. Not to be filled by pharmacists.

Mr. TEMPLE. We could, for example, contraindicate the use in people under 18.

Mr. STUPAK. Yes, you could.

Mr. TEMPLE. We could. We were advised by our committee in the strongest way—this was not 15 to 8——

Mr. STUPAK. This was the Advisory Committee. Right?

Mr. TEMPLE. Right.

Mr. STUPAK. You don't listen to advisory committees if you don't want to anyway. Take Accutane. We have been waiting for 4 years for certification and registry. Four years, we still don't have it. After two advisory committees tell you do it, we are still waiting 4 years later.

The FDA does what it wants. Now the bottom line here——

Mr. TEMPLE. I have to protest. We take—I can't speak to the case you are referring to here. We take——

Mr. STUPAK. The bottom line is you have the authority.

Mr. TEMPLE. We could seek to contraindicate their use.

Mr. STUPAK. Then if it doesn't work and increases the possibility of suicidal behavior in people under the age of 18, why don't you do it? Aren't you supposed to protect the safety and welfare of the American people?

Mr. TEMPLE. Yes, and we are not sure that your proposal or your suggestion would protect the American public. It might harm them.

Mr. STUPAK. Well, let me just read you here. This was an article handed out earlier today. This is the San Francisco Chronicle, I think it was, the article. It says on paragraph, column four, first paragraph: "But this episode suggests that they"—being the FDA—"reject the precautionary principle in favor of the idea that no drug is dangerous unless it is proven to be so."

Mr. WALDEN. I believe that is the British Journal.

Mr. STUPAK. The British Journal? Okay. So in other words, shouldn't you err on the side of caution when you are talking about increased possibility of suicidal behavior in young people, especially when the drugs thus far has not shown to be effective in the treatment of depression?

Mr. TEMPLE. Well, like the Advisory Committee, I believe we have to think about a whole bunch of things. There are—I don't want to make more of this than they deserve, but it is very clear that the suicide rate in adolescents has been declining for the last 10 years, the period in which these drugs were started.

Mr. STUPAK. But you can't give the anti-depressants credit for that, because you have said that they are not effective in that.

Mr. TEMPLE. No. I have not said that they are not effective, and it is very important to recognize the distinction.

Mr. STUPAK. Wait a minute. You're saying now they are effective in treating depression in young people?

Mr. TEMPLE. No. What I said is that they have not been shown to our satisfaction to be effective. That is, they haven't been shown in well controlled studies to do the things that you are supposed to do to be considered effective. But we know from depression trials in adults that lots of drugs that work can't show that they are effective every time.

In fact, more than 50 percent of all trials in adults fail. Why they seem to fail so much in children, we don't know. It could be they really don't work.

Mr. STUPAK. You don't know.

Mr. TEMPLE. We don't know.

Mr. STUPAK. For all indications right now, we know they don't work. We know they increase suicide behavior. Then why don't you not allow the drugs be prescribed to children under 18 until you do know—until you do know? Isn't it more harm to these people who may be of fragile mind, suffering from depression, to give them something like Paxil, which is supposed to make them feel better, and it really doesn't? Isn't the mind then saying, geez, I had a little hope here; you gave me this prescription, and I would be better. It doesn't work. In fact, it is not being effective. Aren't you really putting that person at risk, at a greater risk with a false hope that you are giving them?

Mr. TEMPLE. Having untreated depression is risky, too, and we don't know——

Mr. STUPAK. Absolutely.

Mr. TEMPLE. We can't know. You can't do mortality studies here. No one will let you do them. We don't know whether you would be worse off or better off. The Advisory Committee was quite convinced, but I am not going to tell you they had data to work from. They didn't. They were quite convinced that there are many people who are suicidal because of their disease who would be made worse off.

I am not telling you that they know that to be true. I am not telling you that is evidence. I am not telling you that should lead to a claim in labeling. But I don't dismiss it out of hand either.

Mr. WALDEN. If I could interrupt just a second, Mr. Stupak. Are you able to come back after the votes?

Mr. STUPAK. Sure.

Mr. WALDEN. In which case I would extend you another 5 minutes after the votes. We are probably down to about 7 minutes or so to go over to vote. What I would like to do is recess the committee, return, and then I will return to you for further questions, if that is appropriate.

The committee will stand in recess, and we would request our witnesses to stay here as well. Thanks.

[Brief recess.]

Mr. WALDEN. If I could have our witnesses return to the table, we will get started here in just a moment. I am going to call the Committee on Oversight and Investigations back to order.

When we left for the vote, Congressman Stupak had the floor, and we are extending you another 5 minutes for your continuing line of questions. So the Chair would recognize the gentleman from Michigan.

Mr. STUPAK. Thank you, Mr. Chairman.

Dr. Temple, in response to one of the questions by someone up here, they were asking about the studies, and you said there were some studies you could not publish concerning the anti-depressants.

Mr. TEMPLE. I said we can't force people to publish things.

Mr. STUPAK. But can you publish them?

Mr. TEMPLE. Well, let me describe what we can and can't do. When we approve a new drug or a supplement to a new drug, our reviews and things like that are all made public. They are put on our website. If we do not approve——

Mr. STUPAK. Your reviews, but not the studies?

Mr. TEMPLE. Our reviews, not the studies. But our reviews are quite detailed. I would modestly say there are at least as informative as a publication in a journal, as a rule.

Mr. STUPAK. Okay. So these are all approved. All these anti-depressants are approved drugs. If another study comes out, do you get that study? Do you receive that study?

Mr. TEMPLE. Like if they do another study, they must be reported in annual reports, but unless they show something bad, they don't have to be—not much has to be done with them. If they show something dangerous, then they have to be reported to us promptly.

Mr. STUPAK. So they are found in what is called the Annual Progress Report or another one they call it is the Investigative Drug Brochure. Correct?

Mr. TEMPLE. Well, that is for a drug that——

Mr. STUPAK. That is for an IND. Right?

Mr. TEMPLE. Yes.

Mr. STUPAK. Okay. In the Annual Progress Report—that is just a summary of what they did. Right? A summary of these studies, the drug companies send it to you: Here's what we have done in the past year; here is where reference to our pill has showed up in a medical journal, or something like that.

Mr. TEMPLE. They may actually put the reprints, but I wouldn't want to boast too much about how useful those documents are to us.

Mr. STUPAK. What if the company fails to leave out part of the critical point that you are looking for, that something would be dangerous, such as causing suicide or affecting the central nervous system. They don't put it in their annual report.

Mr. TEMPLE. Well, if we somehow become aware of it, we can bring various legal actions against them. You have to tell us about things like that. There are examples where delays in reporting to us have resulted in criminal penalties of various kinds.

Mr. STUPAK. Okay.

Mr. TEMPLE. Of course, we do have to find out about it.

Mr. STUPAK. Sure. Let me ask you this question. Is it true that the FDA published its Public Health Advisory with a recommended label change about worsening depression and suicidality in patients treated with anti-depressants on March 22, 2004?

Mr. TEMPLE. Yes.

Mr. STUPAK. Okay. And who wrote the text of that label change?

Mr. TEMPLE. Wow. Let me ask Dr. Laughren, because he and his people would have had a major role in that.

Mr. LAUGHREN. The initial draft of the label change came out of the Division, but there were a number of other groups within the agency who had input into that, including people in Office of Drug Safety, Office of Pediatrics and Counterterrorism.

Mr. STUPAK. Well, let me ask you this then. Who would have been the person to sign off? Who gives it final signature? I know you have these initial drafts.

Mr. TEMPLE. I mean, something like that goes through parts of the Commissioner's office for final sign-off.

Mr. STUPAK. Okay. So Dr. Crawford would be the guy who would sign off on it eventually then?

Mr. TEMPLE. I can't say that, but someone in the Commissioner's office would.

Mr. STUPAK. If you compare the text that the FDA approved for the labels of anti-depressants on March 22, 2004, and what is on the labels of the anti-depressants today, would they be the same?

Mr. TEMPLE. It depends on how the Public Health Advisory is written. Sometimes they are written before——

Mr. STUPAK. I am talking about the March 22, 2004 Public Health Advisory. Look at Tab 44. That might help a little bit here.

Mr. TEMPLE. They wouldn't necessarily be the same. You are writing in a different way. You are trying to communicate a little more in the Public Health Advisory.

Mr. STUPAK. Well, explain this to me. Look at Tab 44.

Mr. TEMPLE. They shouldn't be in major——

Mr. STUPAK. March 22, 2004, says, and I am quoting: "Health care providers should carefully monitor patients receiving anti-depressants for possible worsening of depression and suicidality, especially at the beginning of therapy or when the dose either increases or decreases. Although FDA has not yet concluded that these drugs cause worsening depression or suicidality, health care providers should be aware that worsening of symptoms could be due to the underlying disease or might be a result of drug therapy."

But now the actual labels say this—that is approved by the FDA. It says, "Patients with major depressive disorder, both adult and pediatric, may experience worsening of the depression and/or the emergence of suicidal ideation and behavior (suicidality), whether or not they are taking anti-depressants medications, and this risk may persist until significant remission occurs. Although there has been a longstanding concern that anti-depressants may have a role in inducing worsening of depression and the emergence of suicidality in certain patients, a causal role for anti-depressants inducing such behaviors has not been established. Nevertheless, patients being treated with the anti-depressants should be observed closely for clinical worsening and suicidality, especially at the beginning of the course of drug therapy or at a time the dose changes."

This is just one example of how March 22, 2004, labeling warning label text is different from the labels we see on the drugs today, and there is actually another one. My question is, why is the March 22 language published on your website not good enough to make it to the labels for the doctors? If you have already weakened your March 22 recommendation—I believe you have—how can we trust that you won't have strong, clearly worded labels on the package that demonstrate the lack of efficacy and the increase of risk with these drugs?

See what I am saying. March 22 you had pretty strong warning. That is on your website. Now what we see on the package is completely different.

Mr. TEMPLE. I guess I think the labeling language is of similar strength, although the words are somewhat different. They both emphasize monitoring. They both emphasize that you can get much——

Mr. STUPAK. See, here's our problem. Most of us up here aren't doctors. We looked at it. We read it, and we can't—we think it is less. We think it is weaker, and then you tell us you are going to do this black box warning, which the patients and families aren't going to get, and the first notice they are going to get about they are not being effective and may actually increase suicidal behavior is when they open up their package, because in there is going to be a Med Guide.

Isn't that a little bit too late? They have already had their prescription. They already had it filled. They are already there. They got it. They've spent the money. Now after all this, now you are going to tell them, hey, wait a minute, before you do this you ought to know this.

That is our concern up here. Sounds like we got the horse before the cart, the cart before the horse, whatever you want to call it. Ain't right.

Mr. TEMPLE. That's a different question. That is why we made sure that the Committee discussed the question of whether there ought to be some attempt to give something out beforehand. The difficulty with those, and we do do it sometimes, mostly in relation to fetal abnormalities where the urgency seems maximal, is that how you structure that, how you get these into the office, how you get them discussed adequately, given the current situation on how long people spend, is not so clear.

Mr. STUPAK. Right. When you discuss these, it is between the FDA and the drug company. Is anyone there representing the people, the patients, a public citizen or anyone like that at these discussions that you are having on black box and all that?

Mr. TEMPLE. Well, these discussions aren't being held with the drug companies either. We are going to propose labeling. Then maybe after that——

Mr. STUPAK. And then you go back and forth?

Mr. TEMPLE. Maybe, but——

Mr. STUPAK. No, no, you do, every one of them. I have never seen a drug company yet accept a first recommendation you made on labeling.

Mr. TEMPLE. Well, we didn't—I mean, Tom would know best, but I don't know how much difficulty we had with the one in March.

Mr. STUPAK. Let's go back to my original question. See, the confusion with your March 22, what you have on the website, people get it after they purchase drug. Why don't we just go to an informed consent? I would strongly urge you go to informed consent before you ever even get this, when you start treating with these doctors, that clearly spells out like a Med Guide would that here is what we find. And if it changes, we can change that informed consent.

I don't want a voluntary one, because half the doctors don't give it. We want a mandatory informed consent, especially when dealing with young kids.

Mr. TEMPLE. To do that, you also have to have a completely separate distribution system. It has to be shipped directly to the doctor or something like that. It is——

Mr. STUPAK. I know doctors are busy, but if you tell them it is a mandatory informed consent and then they are practicing improperly, they would do it.

Mr. TEMPLE. May be. I think what the people on the committee thought was that the burdensomeness of it would interfere more than they wanted with the appropriate use of the drugs. That doesn't mean we can't consider this further, but that is what they thought. They did talk about this a fair amount.

Mr. STUPAK. I would encourage you to do the informed consent, and thank you for the extra time.

Mr. WALDEN. You are welcome. Thank you for your participation.

Dr. Knudsen, if you would turn to Tab 73, please, sir. Do you recall ever getting this response from Pfizer? I note it says a desk copy to you on the bottom of the second page, I believe.

Mr. KNUDSEN. I did not—I don't recall getting the response from Pfizer that addressed that request that I had of them to provide additional information. Once again, just because I don't recall doesn't—let's see.

Mr. WALDEN. Had you gotten an official company response to the question about suicidality, what would have been your protocol in reviewing that response?

Mr. KNUDSEN. Yes. I would have read it and ascertained whether or not they answered the questions posed to them, whether or not they answered the questions adequately, and often indicated what we—well, NAI, no action indicated, signed my name.

I am not saying I did it for this one, because I do not recall anything from them.

Mr. WALDEN. Right. I understand.

Mr. KNUDSEN. But that is how I have done it in the past.

Mr. WALDEN. Were you able to find any memo in the Zoloft files you looked at, at the agency or in your own files, evidencing that you or anyone else within the agency actually reviewed Pfizer's response?

Mr. KNUDSEN. No.

Mr. WALDEN. Had you been satisfied with Pfizer's response, would you have most likely written a memo to that effect, had you been satisfied with their response?

Mr. KNUDSEN. It is conceivable.

Mr. WALDEN. I think your mike got turned off there, sir.

Mr. KNUDSEN. I may have put a No Action Intended—indicated, excuse me. But, yes, I——

Mr. WALDEN. I mean, you would have written some response.

Mr. KNUDSEN. Yes. Yes.

Mr. WALDEN. So would you have let your supervisor know that you had reviewed and received the company's response to a safety question you posed? Is that standard operating procedure?

Mr. KNUDSEN. I would have put my response in the box, yes.

Mr. WALDEN. The box?

Mr. KNUDSEN. Well, the mailbox for my supervisor.

Mr. WALDEN. Okay. Thank you. Who was your supervisor at the time?

Mr. KNUDSEN. Dr. Laughren.

Mr. WALDEN. Okay. Dr. Laughren, do you recall ever reviewing Pfizer's response on this issue of suicidality in kids?

Mr. LAUGHREN. Not at that time. I have looked at it subsequently.

Mr. WALDEN. And that was because of the hearing coming up here?

Mr. LAUGHREN. I just learned about it as a result of document exchanges and what-not. We did not have the letter that Dr. Knudsen sent to Pfizer in our files. I believe we had to get that from Pfizer.

Mr. WALDEN. That is our understanding. But we are talking about Pfizer's response to that letter.

Mr. LAUGHREN. Right, right.

Mr. WALDEN. But you didn't have either one, is what you are saying. Is that in part because you don't have a record retention policy? Dr. Temple, what is your policy for saving documents like this?

Mr. TEMPLE. Materials that are—go ahead.

Mr. LAUGHREN. We did have the May—was it May 28, the date of the receipt?

Mr. WALDEN. Yes, May 28, 1996.

Mr. LAUGHREN. We did have that in our files. What we did not have is the letter that Dr. Knudsen sent back in March. We didn't have a copy of that letter in our files.

Mr. WALDEN. Oh, I see. But you did have Pfizer's response?

Mr. LAUGHREN. It was in our files. But there was no indication that it had been reviewed.

Mr. WALDEN. I see. And you hadn't reviewed it prior to the committee bringing this to your attention?

Mr. LAUGHREN. There wouldn't have been any reason for it to have come to me, ordinarily.

Mr. WALDEN. Unless he had referenced it to you.

Mr. LAUGHREN. Unless he had given it to me. Right.

Mr. WALDEN. All right, and there is no record of that. Okay. But I guess the question is: Now you have reviewed it, do you think it raises serious safety concerns?

Mr. LAUGHREN. No. It basically provides additional information that supports the view that I expressed in my October—I think it was October 25, 1996, memo where I commented on the issue that Dr. Knudsen raised in his March review. It basically supports that view.

Mr. WALDEN. And what he raised at that time was a serious safety concern, wasn't it?

Mr. LAUGHREN. Well, he raised a concern that there might be a signal of increased risk of suicidality in pediatric patients relative to adults, but if you have seen my October 25 memo, I believe I fully addressed that. I mean, there were a couple of issues there.

No. 1, he was comparing risk of suicidality in adult patients who had been scrupulously screened out for not having depression with a group of children, many of whom had primary depression. So it was not, in my view, a reasonable comparison.

Mr. WALDEN. all right. If you would turn to Tab 75, we will send the book of tabs back your way. This is a memo that you authored on October 25, 1996. Subject line is: You note that "a concern about the possibility of a signal of emergent suicidality, suicide attempts, gestures or ideation association with Certraline used in pediatric patients was raised by Dr. Knudsen in his 3/28/96 safety review." In your memo you did not mention the fact that Dr. Knudsen requested and received additional information from the company. Why is that? You had no idea?

Mr. LAUGHREN. Because, obviously, I didn't know about it.

Mr. WALDEN. Okay. As you know, the company's response was May 1996, and so over 4 months before you write this memo. So this memo gets written. This is in the file somewhere in theory, because it is there today, and nobody reviewed it?

Mr. LAUGHREN. Well, again I said, now that I became aware of it very recently, I have reviewed it; and as I say, it supports—sorry?

Mr. WALDEN. It doesn't raise serious——

Mr. LAUGHREN. Well, it answers the questions that Dr. Knudsen raised in his letter to the company. It provides additional data and, having looked at those data, it supports the conclusion that I am reaching in my memo, that there is no signal.

I mean, really, the only data in that final safety update that Dr. Knudsen reviewed back in 1996 that is relevant are the controlled trials data for that one study in pediatric OCD. That was roughly—that was the study that we have subsequently reviewed, roughly 100 patients in drug, 100 patients in placebo. There is one suicidality event. That occurs in a placebo patient.

That is really the only data there that are directly pertinent to the question.

Mr. WALDEN. Let me just read the final paragraph of this memo. It is Tab 75. This is the one that you wrote to file. It says: "In summary, I don't consider these data to represent a signal of risk for suicidality for either adults or children. Supplements are planned for both depression and OCD in pediatric patients, and when we have more complete data, including Ham-D data, we can look more critically at this issue using the now standard approach of comparing the proportions of drug and placebo exposed patients who show worsening on Item 3, suicidality item of the Ham-D during treatment. At the present time, current labeling simply notes Zoloft has not been adequately evaluated for safety and effectiveness in pediatric patients."

So you are saying that you are going to look at additional studies. Right?

Mr. LAUGHREN. Well, basically, what I am saying here is that we would likely look at the Ham-D item. Every one of these depression rating scales that is used in evaluating—they are often used in OCD trials as well. They have a standard suicide item. In the case of the Ham-D it is the Item 3.

Dr. Hammad as part of his review of these pediatric suicidality data did look at the item scores. He looked at two measures of the item scores, both——

Mr. WALDEN. But that was when?

Mr. LAUGHREN. Well, that was recently.

Mr. WALDEN. Right. What happened between 1996 and recently? Did the agency look more critically at this issue? Did you put this in the pediatric trials for anti-depressants for kids, the written request?

Mr. TEMPLE. No. They all do that, though. They all do a Ham-D.

Mr. WALDEN. Well, that is not my question. My question——

Mr. TEMPLE. No, no. It did——

Mr. WALDEN. Now wait a minute. Dr. Temple, did the FDA specifically in your written request ask for exploration of this question, suicidality?

Mr. TEMPLE. The answer is we did not. But again——

Mr. WALDEN. Why?

Mr. TEMPLE. At the time we issued—prepared and issued the written request, obviously, it was not an issue that was prominent in our thinking. Again, keep in mind, up until this point we had never seen a signal for suicidality in the adult data.

Mr. WALDEN. But doesn't this memo indicate that this is something you needed to look at?

Mr. LAUGHREN. I did consider, and again, as I am saying, looking at the data that were available in this safety update, there was no signal for suicidality in children. The signal that emerged for Zoloft in pediatric patients came later. It came in the depression trials.

There was one study here, only one study,an OCD trial. There was no signal in that trial.

Mr. WALDEN. All right. But your memo says, when we have more complete data, including Ham-D data, we can look more critically at this issue. How did you look more critically at the issue? How did you go about getting more data?

Mr. LAUGHREN. We have looked more critically very recently, looking——

Mr. WALDEN. Very recently?

Mr. LAUGHREN. Very recently.

Mr. WALDEN. See, I am looking at this gap between 1996-97 when some of these issues began to be raised by various people in FDA.

Mr. LAUGHREN. Well, raised but also addressed. There is no signal in these data.

Mr. TEMPLE. The first real signal came when Dr. Mosholder evaluated the Paxil data.

Mr. WALDEN. And when was that?

Mr. LAUGHREN. That supplement came in, in probably the spring of 2002, and he finished his review in the fall of 2002, and that is when we——

Mr. WALDEN. Didn't we already go through this with Mr. Mosholder on a 1997 memo where this was also raised as an issue?

Mr. LAUGHREN. Not suicidality. That was agitation and, by the way, that information got into labeling. That is included in the labeling for Luvox. There was no issue of suicidality raised in Dr. Mosholder's review.

Mr. WALDEN. So from 1997 to 2002, how did the agency look more critically at the data?

Mr. LAUGHREN. We had no—again, up until the time that Dr. Mosholder reviewed the Paxil pediatric supplement in 2002, we had no reason to do anything more. There was no signal.

Mr. TEMPLE. Can I also repeat a distinction I made earlier? We thought at the time—and you can see that in Dr. Laughren's memo—that looking at the suicide item on a Ham-D or the equivalent in a pediatric score would be the way to find suicidality. That is plainly not true, because you don't see, as Dr. Hammad's review showed—you don't see any increase in that item even in the trials that show the increased suicidality.

What turned out to be the place to look, which we didn't know, was in the adverse reaction reports, and I would say we don't know why that is. Why, if you are not feeling more suicidal, do you have more suicidal events? I don't think we know the answer to that. But it is very clear now that the way to look for suicidal ideation is to, in a more structured and better way that we have probably done up to now, look at those events that may represent suicidal behavior or thinking, and that the——

Mr. WALDEN. There is a March 1991 article, a case study called Emergence of Self-Destructive Phenomena in Children and Adolescents During Fluoxetine Treatment.

Mr. LAUGHREN. Is that the King article?

Mr. WALDEN. I am sorry?

Mr. LAUGHREN. I am sorry. Is that the King article?

Mr. WALDEN. I believe it is, yes, sir.

Mr. LAUGHREN. Right, and that is reporting on individual cases. Those are not controlled trials data.

Mr. WALDEN. Is this a peer reviewed study? Is this in Journal of American Academy of Child and Adolescent Psychiatry?

Mr. LAUGHREN. It very likely is. It came out around the same time as the Teicher article reporting on a series of, I believe, six adults being treated with fluoxetine. Again, it is a suggestion that there might be something, but it is far from, in any sense, definitive.

Again, we had been systematically looking at the adult data for almost that entire decade, you know, looking at both suicide item scores, looking at event data, and more recently had begun to accumulate the completed suicides in adults, had not seen a signal. So there was no particular reason why that issue should have been on our radar screen.

Mr. WALDEN. Okay. So, basically, you had no reason in these trials to even look for it, is what you are telling us? When you put out the written request——

Mr. LAUGHREN. They were looked at in the routine ways. Adverse events were reported, and the item data were collected. Again, a signal did emerge in the Zoloft data later on with the two pediatric trials in depression, but even that wasn't recognized until—actually, Dr. Mosholder was the medical officer who reviewed that supplement initially. He did not observe a signal for suicidality. it is only when he went back during the summer of 2003 and looked at—relooked at the same data that a weak signal emerged.

Mr. WALDEN. Dr. Temple, did you have the authority to ask the companies to look at this, to keep better data so you could, in your written request to them?

Mr. TEMPLE. Let me be clear. You always measure the standard suicide scores, and we have the capacity to look at those. That is what you do in all these studies. It is how you measure improvement.

So every time you do these studies, you get a suicidality score, and we look at it. There isn't anything the company has to do except give us the data. What we could have thought—what we conceivably could have asked but didn't know to ask was a better, more structured, more careful look at events that might or might not represented suicidality, but we didn't know to do that.

Mr. WALDEN. But didn't Dr. Laughren say that in the depression trials you should look more critically?

Mr. TEMPLE. We were looking at the items in the Ham-D score, and nobody saw anything. It shouldn't surprise us that we didn't see it, because in the very data that have created the signal we are worried about now, you don't see any increase in the pediatric version of a Ham-D. That is not where it shows up, for some reason.

Mr. WALDEN. I guess, as I have listened to this, and I have sat through these hearings a long time, the picture that begins to emerge in my mind isn't a pretty one, because it is one that says you are worried less about suicidality than in continuing to allow physicians to prescribe a drug that most studies show at best has no effect in treating depression in kids and adults.

Mr. TEMPLE. I don't agree that that is our conclusion. We spent tremendous resources and devoted tremendous effort to evaluate the suicidality question.

Mr. WALDEN. Well, when Dr. Mosholder does the review and says I am spotting something here that is very troubling, when you are dealing with drugs in kids that virtually every trial shows have no effect and Dr. Mosholder is finding some link to suicide, you—well, it seems to me, my opinion is you ended up on the side of let them prescribe it, because they might be okay; we don't necessarily agree Mosholder has got this right; we are going to go run it out somewhere else and see, and take that risk.

Mr. TEMPLE. We didn't think we were letting them prescribe it or not letting them prescribe it. The question we were trying to face was do we have enough information to say there is increased suicidality in children given these drugs. That is what we were grappling with.

Mr. WALDEN. You have said earlier today that you didn't want to discourage the prescribing of these off-label, because they may work in some people.

Mr. TEMPLE. That is a different question. We thought that it was very important to get the right answer on this question. That is correct.

Mr. WALDEN. Well, I will tell you, I guess that is where we are just going to agree to disagree maybe, but if I had to err and I saw a sign from one of my top scientists that I handpicked to take a look at this and who I have a great respect for, and he came back and said I have looked at the data and I am seeing a link to suicide in kids, I'd say we better err on the side of caution here. And maybe you got to go peer review it, but meanwhile since most of these drugs don't show any efficacy in kids, let's err on the side of against suicide.

Mr. TEMPLE. But we put out several public announcements saying that you should be careful and that we are worried about this. We didn't change the label, though. That is correct.

Mr. WALDEN. I have way overrun my time. Thanks for your patience. I yield to the ranking member, Mr. Deutsch.

Mr. DEUTSCH. Dr. Temple, in an earlier point there was a discussion regarding this issue of different sort of contraindications for children versus adults, and you are saying that it applies to both—you know, no separation of warning. At what point is a recommendation that there be a separate warning? Are there separate warnings—I mean, how atypical is this? Is this the process? Is this the procedure? Are there cases where you do have separate warnings?

Mr. TEMPLE. Well, the warning language that will describe the now documented increased—now we believe it is documented. Maybe someone else thought it was documented before. What we now believe is the documented increase in suicidality in children. That will be a separate statement, because we don't think such a——

Mr. DEUTSCH. What tips it to make that difference, the separation?

Mr. TEMPLE. Well, it isn't so much the separation, but we now——

Mr. DEUTSCH. Well, the dual warning.

Mr. TEMPLE. Well, we now believe—we have not seen such a thing in adults. As I mentioned before, Dr. Mosholder presented an analysis on Paxil that quite clearly does not show that finding in an adult population, using the same methods that showed it in pediatrics.

So you need a special warning on that subject for children, because they are the ones who get that reaction. The warning in March was about pay attention to people when you are starting therapy. That is still a good warning for everybody. That still applies to everybody.

Mr. DEUTSCH. I guess the question I am trying to get at is at what point do you tip the balance and then say a separation for children?

Mr. TEMPLE. I don't think it is a balance. I think, as soon as you have information that says children are different, you do it.

Mr. DEUTSCH. And are you looking for that information or is it just——

Mr. TEMPLE. Well, one of the points of doing studies in children is that very point, to see if they respond differently.

Mr. DEUTSCH. Right, but is that only done in terms of, you know, the incentives that we have put on in terms of increased exclusivity based upon that issue?

Mr. TEMPLE. The usual request for data, written request for data, includes a request for studies of effectiveness, pharmacokinetic studies because that can be something, and a safety study . That is what they usually consist of.

Mr. DEUTSCH. Right, but generally those safety studies don't break out children. So that——

Mr. TEMPLE. Sorry. This is for a written request on gaining pediatric exclusivity.

Mr. DEUTSCH. Right.

Mr. TEMPLE. So that is only children.

Mr. DEUTSCH. Right. Right, but if it is a pediatric exclusivity, then you would have that. But outside of that, a pediatric exclusivity, then you would have no information.

Mr. TEMPLE. Outside of that, it is extremely hard to get any studies in children. That is why we have the Best Pharmaceuticals for Children Act, because children—well, it is extremely unusual, and most people would say it is not appropriate, to start studies of children before you have the drug properly worked up in adults. There's a lot of nervousness about, you know, children can't give consent and so on.

So it has always been true, whether we have the Best Pharmaceuticals for Children Act or before, that we expected the pediatric studies to be done afterward.

Mr. DEUTSCH. If I can switch to Dr. Seligman, I have a series of questions, but I want at least to open it up and give you an opportunity, because my understanding, this has not been brought up at this point, which is the investigation regarding—I guess in response to the San Francisco Chronicle article detailing the FDA's decision to remove Dr. Mosholder's presentation.

If you can at least give us your perspective of why that investigation began and the appropriateness of that investigation.

Mr. SELIGMAN. Certainly. Both prior to and subsequent to the publication of two articles in the San Francisco Chronicle, a number of staff in the Office of Drug Safety approached me raising a concern of the possibility that there may have been an inappropriate disclosure of confidential information to the reporter at the San Francisco Chronicle.

Upon receipt of that information, as you have in your book, I forwarded those concerns on to the Office of Internal Affairs at the FDA.

Mr. DEUTSCH. Did you result in finding who had leaked the information?

Mr. SELIGMAN. I'm sorry?

Mr. DEUTSCH. Did you find out who leaked the information?

Mr. SELIGMAN. No, I did not.

Mr. DEUTSCH. If you can turn to Tab 65, an e-mail dated February 20, 2004, from yourself to Horace Coleman and Thomas Doyle at the Office of Internal Affairs in which you outline your reasons for initiating this investigation. You attached an article, the San Francisco Chronicle article.

I assume you are familiar with the article. Is that correct?

Mr. SELIGMAN. Yes, I am.

Mr. DEUTSCH. Your e-mail states that a member or members of the staff of the Office of Drug Safety may have inappropriately disclosed information of a sensitive matter.

Were staff members of the Office of Drug Safety the only people with access to the information contained within the newspaper article?

Mr. SELIGMAN. No, they were not.

Mr. DEUTSCH. But you were only concerned with the activities of your staff?

Mr. SELIGMAN. No, I was not.

Mr. DEUTSCH. Then why is the memo only talking about the staff of the Office of Drug Safety?

Mr. SELIGMAN. Only members of the Office of Drug Safety raised the concern to me that such information had been improperly disclosed.

Mr. DEUTSCH. Why would that be?

Mr. SELIGMAN. Because I am their direct supervisor.

Mr. DEUTSCH. Right, but if you are asking Internal Affairs to be looking for a leak in your office—I mean, the leak would only be within that particular group of people?

Mr. SELIGMAN. I don't believe I stated that I thought the—that is correct. I did say that I am concerned that a member or members of the staff of the Office of Drug Safety may have inappropriately disclosed information. I did state that, although in my interview with the Office of Internal Affairs, I did point out that there were clearly others who had access to such information as well.

Mr. DEUTSCH. If you turn back to Tab 66, the report of the investigation, on page of that report it notes that you named five employees of the ODS who had been called at home by Waters. How did you know that these five individuals had been called at home?

Mr. SELIGMAN. They either came to me or they reported such to my deputy, Dr. Anne Trontell, who informed me of that information.

Mr. DEUTSCH. And apparently another ODS employee, David Bram, merely because he had been very vocal in the past regarding the scientists' findings being suppressed—did you call—again, is that—we are trying to understand why—I mean, were you suspicious of people within your own group for any particular reason because of actions like that?

Mr. SELIGMAN. As I indicated in the interview, the investigator asked me whether there were people of whom I had particular concern in the office, and I indicated as such, that there were such individuals.

Mr. DEUTSCH. If you turn to the conclusions on page 6, you will note the initial conclusion was that no evidence was found that classified or proprietary information from the FDA was released. In fact, the release of the classified or proprietary information is the only basis to initiate an investigation into a leak. Is that correct?

Mr. SELIGMAN. That is correct.

Mr. DEUTSCH. So let me just again follow up on Tab 69. The fourth page of that exhibit is headed by the date 5/7/04. This is a document which Horace Coleman of the Office of Investigation noticed that he is closing the case, and further noticed that he had to ask you to contact Dr. Mosholder to assure him that he was not a specific target of this investigation, that OIA found no evidence to indicate that classified or proprietary information had been released and that OIA was closing the investigation.

Why did Mr. Coleman need to have you assure Dr. Mosholder that he had not been the target of this investigation?

Mr. SELIGMAN. I don't know the answer to that question, but I did reassure Dr. Mosholder of that fact.

Mr. DEUTSCH. On that same page, Dr. Coleman notes that he had advised you that he would also contact the CDR Director Galson to advise him of the above information. Since Galson had left the office to attend an awards ceremony, he would be requesting his director, Terry Vermelion, to reach out and debrief Director Galson.

This raises several questions. What was the urgency to get this information to Galson?

Mr. SELIGMAN. I have no—I don't know the answer to that question.

Mr. DEUTSCH. And what about the propriety to initiating an investigation? Whom did you talk to in CDER and what were their opinions about your proposed actions?

Mr. SELIGMAN. I took these actions independently. I informed Dr. Galson, who is indeed my supervisor, that I was considering such action, but received no direction from him, one way or the other, as to whether I should take it. He was the only person with whom I discussed these matters.

Mr. DEUTSCH. Who did you keep informed regarding the progress of the investigation?

Mr. SELIGMAN. The only time I received any information about the progress of the investigation was at the conclusion of the investigation on May 10 when I met with Agent Coleman and Kurisky who provided me the report and debriefed me on the investigation.

Mr. DEUTSCH. One final question. This summary report, also Dr. Hammad's reanalysis and its comparison to Dr. Mosholder's original work was widely reported in the press before FDA released any of the information publicly.

My understanding is you did not initiate an investigation into these leaks and, if not, why not?

Mr. SELIGMAN. I did not report those allegations to the—I did not—that is correct. I didn't mention that to the Office of Internal Affairs.

Mr. DEUTSCH. Why was that different than the earlier release?

Mr. SELIGMAN. Probably no different than the earlier release.

Mr. DEUTSCH. I mean, there is no basis for the difference? The original investigation is technically considered a criminal investigation. I mean, is it just by whim that we start criminal investigations? I mean, is there some basis of differentiating?

Mr. SELIGMAN. This is not treated as a whim. I take, and I imagine everyone at the agency takes the protection of proprietary information and trade secret information very seriously. When allegations of such are brought to my attention, I——

Mr. DEUTSCH. Let's be very specific, though. The Mosholder thing didn't involve proprietary information.

Mr. SELIGMAN. As it turned out, that is correct.

Mr. DEUTSCH. Right, but even the allegation, even the report wasn't proprietary.

Mr. SELIGMAN. The allegation had to do with inappropriate disclosure of——

Mr. DEUTSCH. Yes, but not proprietary.

Mr. SELIGMAN. That is correct. Inappropriate disclosure of confidential information. That is correct.

Mr. DEUTSCH. I mean, I am just going to ask one more time and give you a chance to maybe try to be clearer or think again. But why were these two leaks treated differently?

Mr. SELIGMAN. I can't explain why they were treated differently.

Mr. DEUTSCH. And it was your decision to treat them differently.

Mr. SELIGMAN. It was probably my oversight in the latter circumstance to treat it differently, yes.

Mr. DEUTSCH. Thank you.

Mr. WALDEN. Dr. Seligman, can we go to this affidavit again.

Mr. SELIGMAN. Certainly. What tab was that?

Mr. WALDEN. This is troubling just in—this is the one that I think is Tab 57, I believe, sir. Now walk me through again. What was the reason for, and who would have suggested that Mr. Mosholder modify this?

Mr. SELIGMAN. I wasn't involved in that at all.

Mr. WALDEN. Who was?

Mr. SELIGMAN. I would have to turn to Dr. Mosholder for that. I wasn't involved in the discussion or consideration of this affidavit.

Mr. WALDEN. Okay, but this is an affidavit that was provided to you. Right? The original affidavit?

Mr. SELIGMAN. The affidavit did appear in the May 10 report. That is the first time that I saw it.

Mr. WALDEN. All right. So it was an official affidavit. It comes to your—it is part of your investigation. Right?

Mr. SELIGMAN. It was part of the Office of Internal Affairs investigation Mr. WALDEN. I'm sorry. All right, part of the Office of Internal Affairs.

Mr. SELIGMAN. I did not conduct any such investigation.

Mr. WALDEN. All right. So I guess what I am trying to figure out with this affidavit is what was the need to—who can answer why this affidavit would need to be altered to be presented to somebody else?

Mr. TEMPLE. I don't think anyone at the table can. It was my understanding that a letter or something like that has been sent to the committee explaining all that. Am I mistaken?

Mr. WALDEN. All right. If there is nobody here that can address that, I believe we do have a letter. I just remain concerned about it is all. I was hoping to dive in a little deeper on it, because it is sort of——

Mr. TEMPLE. I am sure, if after looking at our response the committee has more questions, we will be glad to answer them.

Mr. WALDEN. I appreciate that, Dr. Temple. Dr. Hammad, would you agree that, with only 400 or so person years of exposure that FDA cannot rule out that there is a risk of suicidal behavior of one out of 100? I'll make you a deal. You turn your mike on, and I will repeat the question. There we go.

Would you agree that, with only 400 or so—we are talking about the pediatric clinical trials. Would you agree with only 400 or so person years of exposure that FDA cannot rule out the possibility there is a risk of suicidal behavior of one out of 100?

Mr. HAMMAD. Actually, I did not deal with the person years. I used the individuals as the unit of analysis. So I can't answer the question, because I did not analyze it.

Mr. WALDEN. Dr. Mosholder, would you mind returning, and perhaps you could help us on this question. I appreciate your long day here, sir.

Here's the deal. You have 10 million prescriptions for anti-depressants written on an annual basis for children in the United States, and so how many person years of exposure would you estimate this prescription volume represents?

Mr. MOSHOLDER. Well, 10 million prescriptions, just a very rough rule of thumb, one would figure a month per prescription is usual practice. So that would be 10 million months divided by 12. So I guess that is something like 800,000 person years, if my arithmetic is correct.

I think you may be referring to a calculation that was in my March consult report, if I may. If that is in this binder, perhaps I can refer to it.

Mr. WALDEN. Yes, sure. I think it was in your presentation, too, the PowerPoint presentation that is dated September 13, 2004. It is one of the slides there. Reference is 406.9 patient years.

Mr. MOSHOLDER. Oh, yes, that is correct. Having observed no actual suicides in that amount of person time, there is a way to calculate sort of the upper limit of what a true number of suicides might be expected, which I did in my March consult. If it is in the binder, I can probably find that.

Mr. WALDEN. We are going to see if we can't find it in the binder. It looks like there are 74 sponsored defined suicide related events, 54 serious, it says on your slide. But again we are trying to find the right tab in our binder of documents. Tab 53, I am told.

Mr. MOSHOLDER. Oh, yes. These are my slides from last week. The calculation I was referring to, I think I can find in the March consult document, which I think may address your question.

Mr. WALDEN. Well, I'll tell you. Why don't we go to this question, the one that is more recent, dealing with the 400. I guess the question is: Would you agree that with only 400 or so person years of exposure that FDA cannot rule out there is a risk of suicidal behavior of 1 out of 100?

Mr. MOSHOLDER. I am not sure I——

Mr. TEMPLE. You don't mean suicidal behavior. You mean suicide.

Mr. MOSHOLDER. Do you mean—yes, that was my question.

Mr. TEMPLE. Suicidal behavior, we know, occurs at 2 percent in the control group and about 4 percent in the treated group. So as Dr. Hammad showed, there is a 2 to 3 percent frequency of that. I think you must be referring to how sure can you be that there are no suicides, and the answer is, with that exposure, you don't have much information on that.

Mr. MOSHOLDER. Yes. If I can refer to my March consult, which is Tab 29, page 20 at the top paragraph, this is a calculation I did based on some statistical assumptions. The upper one-sided 95 percent confidence limit for the actual rate given in observation——

Mr. WALDEN. Dr. Mosholder, can I interrupt you a second, sir. What page in that document are you referring to?

Mr. MOSHOLDER. Page 20.

Mr. WALDEN. Page 20. Thank you. Okay, and where are you on that page?

Mr. MOSHOLDER. The top paragraph on that page, I think, is maybe pertinent to your question.

Mr. WALDEN. Okay. Go ahead and read that for us, would you.

Mr. MOSHOLDER. Yes. What it says is that the upper 95 percent confidence limit, as we say, for an actual rate in the population given an observation of zero suicides out of 407 patient years of exposure is 1 in approximately 136 patient years, the point being not the numbers so much, but just to illustrate that 407 patient years, as we reckon these things, doesn't—it only goes so far in reassuring about whether or not there is a risk of actual suicide as opposed to suicidal behavior, which we have already established is increased.

Mr. WALDEN. So, basically, 400 patient years is not a very long time for the kind of research you need or the data you need?

Mr. MOSHOLDER. Well, the real question here, one of the limitations of all this is that the real issue is whether there is an impact on suicide, not just suicidal behaviors, and we don't have enough information to really address that as adequately as one would like.

Mr. WALDEN. But there could be a risk of death?

Mr. MOSHOLDER. There could be——

Mr. WALDEN. You can't rule that out either.

Mr. MOSHOLDER. There could be. The clinical trials aren't long enough in exposure to give us a precise risk estimate.

Mr. WALDEN. But you do know from the data we have that there is a higher risk of suicidality. Correct?

Mr. MOSHOLDER. That is true.

Mr. WALDEN. Okay. All right. Dr. Temple, on page 4 of your testimony you state, the pediatric suicide rate, "has fallen about 25 percent over the last decade, the period in which the use of anti-depressants has grown steadily. This association does not prove that the increasing use of anti-depressants is the cause of the decline in suicide, but it at least is suggestive." However, according to the slide presentation by Dr. Diane Wiskausky of FDA's Office of Drug Safety before the September 2004 Advisory Committee meeting, the increasing use of anti-depressants and decreasing suicide may simply co-exist and may not relate at all to each other. Her slide states that correlation does necessarily imply causality, and that numerous factors may be coincidental, not causal.

Dr. Temple, did you ever have a discussion on ecological association with Dr. Wiskausky?

Mr. TEMPLE. Well, we talked a little at meetings about this. I don't think I had a particular discussion, and I don't disagree with the assertion that these kind of data are hard to interpret. There could be other factors. But these were presented to us at an Advisory Committee by people who thought that there weren't any obvious other explanations, and it is something to be considered.

I would never allege that that is proof. It is not a controlled trial. You can't do controlled trials of that, but it is what you got. And it also doesn't seem to be going up, which is not a trivial matter either, because the drug use has been going through the roof, as people have pointed out.

Mr. WALDEN. If that is all the case then, why would the Europeans suddenly find there are problems?

Mr. TEMPLE. Well, I don't think the Europeans found anything that we didn't find also. In fact, they used our data. The question is what to do about it. What they decided to do about it was tell everybody to start with Prozac and, if that doesn't work, only experts should use the other drugs.

You know, it depends on the arrangements you have, whether experts are available, and a lot of other things. That determines what you do.

One of the major concerns of our advisors was that people who aren't really knowledgeable about these drugs are using them, and that is one of the reasons, you know, all these warnings go in there. One of the hopes—there is sort of pro and con here. One of the hopes is that it will scare people who aren't very qualified into sending people to doctors who are.

Nonetheless, the same figures, I understand, are seen in Europe, too, that the rate is declining.

Mr. WALDEN. But they prescribe a far lower percentage, do they not, among this class?

Mr. TEMPLE. Yes, they do. That is correct.

Mr. WALDEN. Do you know the difference?

Mr. TEMPLE. No, I wouldn't have those figures.

Mr. WALDEN. I thought I had heard it was like 1/6 of what we do in young people.

Mr. TEMPLE. That could certainly be.

Mr. WALDEN. That would tend to lend some credence to Dr. Wiskausky, her comment that it may not be causal.

Mr. TEMPLE. Well, or it could mean they are better at picking the people who really can benefit.

Mr. WALDEN. I see.

Mr. TEMPLE. One of the concerns that was expressed. There isn't any doubt that people—almost everybody thinks the drugs are used casually for people who really probably don't need it, and if there is a risk of making people worse, there may be no compensating benefit in those people. So that is a legitimate worry.

Mr. WALDEN. Just seems like, when these concerns have been raised, again it seems like effort by the FDA hasn't been to put that word out. You've really erred on the side of caution in terms of putting any word out there that there may increased rates of suicidality, and yet when the studies are there that show these may be no more effective than sugar pills, that doesn't seem to be something that gets put out there much. I just—I don't get it.

The Chair recognizes the gentleman from Michigan, Mr. Stupak.

Mr. STUPAK. Thank you, Mr. Chairman. On the last document you just showed from Diane Wiskausky—this was shown at last week's Advisory Committee hearing—underneath there it mentions a patient level controlled observation study, the Jick, et al., study. Is that Dr. Jick from Saskatchewan, Canada? Do you know?

Mr. TEMPLE. No. I think he operates out of Seattle.

Mr. STUPAK. Okay. I was interested in your conversation when you were going back and forth with the Chair on, you call it, suicidality scores or signals, and you were saying, not that Dr. Mosholder was wrong, but you were looking at different signals, and there's different signals to look at, and you mentioned the Hamilton-D scale, Hamilton depression scale, Ham-D you called it. Okay? Remember that?

Mr. TEMPLE. Yes.

Mr. STUPAK. Earlier today when Dr. Mosholder was testifying, I had a couple of exhibits there. One was pharmacology/toxicology consultation from September 2001, and that was on Accutane, but they related to an SSRI. Remember that discussion?

Mr. TEMPLE. Yes.

Mr. STUPAK. Then I had the PET scan which, again with Accutane at 4 months, showed a decrease in the brain in the frontal orbital lobe. You remember that?

Mr. TEMPLE. I remember that. Not that I know how to read those.

Mr. STUPAK. I'm not asking you to read it. But that study showed that the 17-year-old was noted by her family and clinician to have behavioral disturbances and dropped out of school. She did not, however, have a clinically significant increase in depression as measured by the Hamilton depression scale. Even though we can see a physical change in the brain, the Hamilton-D scale did not pick it up, but the PET scan picked up.

Are we maybe looking at the signals?

Mr. TEMPLE. Maybe Tom knows the answer to this. I don't know how well any particular brain lesion or finding has been correlated with depression. The world is full of people who are trying to do that, to try to pick out who is going to be a responder and things like that. But I don't know that literature. So I don't know whether there is a credible PET scan that indicates depression or anything like that.

Mr. LAUGHREN. I am not an expert in that area, but from what I know, most experts agree that we don't understand—we really don't understand the pathophysiology of depression or any other psychiatric illness. But what I wanted to come back to is this issue of whether or not the Ham-D, as it is currently used, or any other depression rating scale, is an adequate instrument for assessing suicidality.

I think that is one of the things that we have learned here, and one future direction in which we are moving and trying to greatly improve our ability to do ascertain it for suicidality. This is one of the things that we hope to come out of this collaboration with Columbia University.

The one thing that they have done is help us in classifying more appropriately and rationally events, but the other thing that was apparent in these trials is that it appeared patients were not asked all the right questions.

Mr. STUPAK. Well, isn't the questions on the Hamilton-D scale the same?

Mr. LAUGHREN. No, no. Again, there is no clear instruction on these instruments as to what sort of follow-up questions should be asked if a patient responds positively. That is something that Columbia is working on, developing an instrument that gives clinicians very clear instructions about how to follow up if there——

Mr. STUPAK. Sure, but the point here is the patient, whether you want to believe the PET scan or not, had social behavior, like dropping out of school and behavioral disturbances, but one of the scales you used, the Hamilton-D scale, to judge depression didn't pick it up, which would indicate—which would indicate either the person didn't tell the truth when they did the testing on the Hamilton-D scale and is good enough to fool the clinician and everything, or does it really beg to another question that maybe there really is something going on here in the brain with these SSRIs that we are not picking up and we never thought of before.

That's the only question. I am putting forth another possibility here, because the jury is still out, as you keep saying, and if the jury is still out, I think you ought to start looking at other factors, because obviously you guys are missing something.

I think Dr. Mosholder, more or less, said that. You didn't want to believe his stuff. So you went to a different set of signals, and those set of signals, at least according to the little bit I have seen from this one study, can be fooled.

Have you ever thought about bringing in outside experts other than just the FDA, like a workshop to bring in other experts and see what is happening with the orbital frontal cortex, which is an area we know mediates depression, or the hippocampus with retinoids and all these other things, and the SSRIs. Have you thought about bringing in outside experts, outside the FDA, to take a look at this data and ask them their suggestions on how do we get to this problem, which we don't seem to have a good answer for?

Mr. LAUGHREN. It is undoubtedly true that our understanding of depression and other psychiatric illnesses is in its infancy. We really do not understand them at a biological level. There is a lot of work going on. You know, it is something that we would hope in the future to have a better understanding of.

There is a lot of work going on, trying to identify various genetic markers and other things that might help us make distinctions among people who clinically all look the same.

I mean, that is one of the problems, is that you have a number of people who all have the same—roughly the same clinical state, but they may have different underlying pathophysiologies, and that may explain why some respond to drugs differently than others, both in a positive sense and in a negative sense. We just don't understand this.

Mr. STUPAK. Absolutely. So that is why I am asking, have you brought in different people for a workshop or a study to look at this anti-depressant, this SSRI, to see what are we missing here? Do we have different ideas on how best to explore it, to measure it, test it, to do some studies?

Mr. TEMPLE. Tom is going to know this better. There are just constant workshops on these very questions, some of them devoted to——

Mr. STUPAK. Okay. But I am asking about SSRIs. Have you done that, like you have done for Accutane and some of these others? Have you done that? That's what I am asking.

Mr. TEMPLE. You mean to see if there is something about the effects on the brain of SSRIs that would tell you something? Is that the specific question?

Mr. STUPAK. No. The question was: On SSRIs have you brought in to do a workshop to try to figure out maybe what else—are we just missing something, just kick it around with the experts, whether it is the talk about SSRIs, the effect on hippocampus where we know there is depression, the frontal orbital cortex where we know it mediates depression, different ideas other than—you know, we all, even Members of Congress, believe it or not, get rigid in our thinking, and sometimes we don't think outside the area and bring i n other experts to help us out.

Have you done that in this problem which has confronted you on these anti-depressants? That's all the question is. No trick, just a simple question.

Mr. TEMPLE. I'm sure Tom would know better. There are constant workshops on every neurologic disease and every psychiatric disease you can name on these very subjects. They must, by definition, deal with the question of whether the drugs work differently and things like that.

I mean, I don't go to those workshops, but the people in the Division regularly would. The interest in those things is partly because people, as Tom said, hope to find out who is a responder and who is not, who gets toxic and who doesn't, and it is partly because people hope to be able to choose drugs to develop better on the basis of the effects on some of these markers.

So there is a tremendous amount of interest in it. But I can't speak to SSRIs particularly.

Mr. STUPAK. Okay. Let me ask you this, Dr. Temple, just a couple of quick questions here. My time is almost up. I want to ask a couple of series of questions on the pediatric exclusivity.

As I understand it, there's 293 written requests that have been written by the FDA for products to be studied in children. Of these 393, studies have been submitted on over 110 products. How many of these studies were efficacy studies?

Mr. TEMPLE. I am just not going to know the answer to that. In neurology——

Mr. STUPAK. Do you require efficacy studies on all drugs? Do you require efficacy study? No?

Mr. TEMPLE. Not necessarily.

Mr. STUPAK. Why not?

Mr. TEMPLE. There are some kinds of drugs where the pediatric request is based on what you call a pharmacologic effect. For example, if you wanted to see whether a beta blocker works in children, you might look at heart rate, if that was thought to be relevant, for example, for protection against arrhythmias. That is a judgment call.

In psychiatric disease, there is no marker like that. So I am quite positive that everyone of them called for efficacy studies.

It is worth noting that the written requests in depression always called for at least two studies, because we know it is so hard to do. The written request in other things, like obsessive compulsive disease, sometimes have only called for a single study.

Mr. STUPAK. So you don't know how many efficacy studies were done of these 293 studies. Right?

Mr. TEMPLE. I don't. I may have some notes on it. I will keep looking.

Mr. STUPAK. We will put it in writing to you, because we would really like to know that.

Mr. TEMPLE. Okay, that's fine.

Mr. STUPAK. Of those for which efficacy studies were done, how many showed they were not effective, that there was no efficacy?

Mr. TEMPLE. Yes. I'm not going to know that either, but we can get you the answer.

Mr. STUPAK. It would be interesting, because we are working on some legislation on pediatric exclusivity.

If efficacy is shown, is this then added to the label of the drug in pediatrics?

Mr. TEMPLE. At least usually, and we can get you numbers on how many have had——

Mr. STUPAK. And if efficacy is not shown in a pediatric study, is that added to the label?

Mr. TEMPLE. Well, we are in the process of changing our view on that. Historically——

Mr. STUPAK. Up until today, before you change you mind, was efficacy—if efficacy was not established, was that put on the label?

Mr. TEMPLE. Usually not.

Mr. STUPAK. So we give them the good news but not the bad news.

Mr. TEMPLE. Well, the reason, which you have heard me say before, is that failing to show something in a trial doesn't mean that it doesn't work. This is not related to the pediatric setting particularly.

Mr. STUPAK. Sure.

Mr. TEMPLE. However, in reconsidering this, what we have come to think is that, really, the whole point of the Best Pharmaceuticals for Children Act is to find out if what you know—mostly—mostly—is to find out if what you think you know about—what you know about adults is applicable to children, and it is more relevant than usual to say, hmm, I didn't see anything in children. We are intending to put——

Mr. STUPAK. When you are talking about adults and children, dosage has a lot to do with that, too, does it not?

Have you done any dosage studies on the SSRIs ?

Mr. TEMPLE. No. The substitute for dosage studies—and it is not an adequate substitute—is to look at the pharmacokinetics and at least try to get close on the blood levels. Dose response information in a disease that is hard to study at all is murderously difficult to get.

Mr. LAUGHREN. Actually, I have one comment on the question of SSRIs and dose and exposure. Actually, the written request for the Luvox application was specifically focused on looking at pharmacokinetics, because what we found—the company had already done the efficacy trial even in advance of the written request. They had done the one study that we actually talked about earlier.

What they had shown is that the drug appeared to work in children, but there were also adolescents in that trial. It did not work. So we asked them as part of the written request to go back and look at exposure, and that helped us to understand possibly why that trial had failed to show efficacy in adolescents.

Mr. STUPAK. Well, our concern is, being the policymakers and writing the Best Pharmaceuticals—I didn't write it, thank God. But in 1997 when we did it, and again in 2001, the Best Pharmaceutical Act, we were told efficacy would be labeled. Now you are telling us, up until today, it has not been labeled.

That was one of the big contentions on this committee. If you are going to give people the good news, you also have to give them the bad news.

Mr. TEMPLE. Just let me be sure I understand. You were told that, if the studies were negative, that would go in?

Mr. STUPAK. That would go in?

Mr. TEMPLE. That would go into the labeling.

Mr. STUPAK. Of course, you shouldn't label before you give the patent extension, so people know what the heck is going on. But we don't do that either.

Mr. TEMPLE. We have pretty much decided to do that. So it is a little late, but we are going to do that.

Mr. STUPAK. We are not a little late. FDA is a little late, since 1997.

Mr. TEMPLE. That is what I said. We are a little late.

Mr. STUPAK. Okay. I thought you said it is a little late now. All right. Probably got time to vote.

Chairman BARTON. Is the gentleman through? Okay. The Chair would recognize himself for what he hopes to be the last 10 minutes. I'm sure you all are glad to hear that.

We want to thank you all for being here this afternoon. It has been a long day, and I appreciate your patience. I have just 2 or 3 questions, and then a wrap-up.

I am going to direct some of these questions to Dr. Knudsen—Is it Knudsen or K-nudsen? Knudsen? Sure. Okay. You've got to push that little button there.

Now I know that some of this ground has been plowed before, but I wasn't here when it was plowed. So I apologize if we have gone over this.

You are aware that your letter of March 19, 1996, was not in the FDA file. I think you are also aware now that there are two versions of the letter that wasn't in the file, one apparently a typographically incorrect that was sent at 10:18 on March 19, 1996. The other was sent at 12:10.

I believe you told the staff that you have no recollection of these letters. Is that correct or incorrect?

Mr. KNUDSEN. That is correct.

Chairman BARTON. So once you saw the letters, did that revive any memories of them?

Mr. KNUDSEN. No.

Chairman BARTON. What were you involved in, in March 1996, that would have caused you send these letters to the Pfizer Corporation?

Mr. KNUDSEN. I was involved in the review of the OCD NDA Supplement for Certraline.

Chairman BARTON. Which is an anti-depressant?

Mr. KNUDSEN. That is correct.

Chairman BARTON. And they were attempting to have it approved for use in adults or in adolescents?

Mr. KNUDSEN. Treatment of OCD in adults, I believe.

Chairman BARTON. And you—were you the reviewer of that application or were just asked to comment on it by somebody that was reviewing the application?

Mr. KNUDSEN. I was the reviewer of the supplement or the OCD supplement submitted by Pfizer—for Certraline by Pfizer.

Chairman BARTON. Taking aside the point that the letter wasn't in the file, and apparently you didn't have a copy in your personal files, the substance of the letter is that it appears—and I will read the last paragraph: "We note"—These are your words: "We note that there appears to be an increased frequency of reports of suicidality in the pediatric/adolescent patients exposed to Certraline compared to either placebo or Certraline treated with adult OCD patients. If this in fact the case, what would be a plausible explanation?"

So even though you have no recollection, you apparently were looking at some data that caused you to think that, if this particular drug was used, it would increase suicidality in the pediatric population, which is a serious concern. Would you agree with that?

Mr. KNUDSEN. Yes.

Chairman BARTON. Now once you sent the letter, apparently you and everybody at FDA forgot about it. Is that true or not true?

Mr. KNUDSEN. I want to back up a second. I commented upon the fact that I did not recall at the time—since it was 1996 this letter was generated, I personally do not recall information back that length of time. Even with looking at the letter, you asked if I generated the letter or if I recall generating the letter. In fact, as I said, I do not recall writing the letter.

It does not mean that I did not. I simply do not recall. I understand. But 1996, for me—even yesterday is a little difficult to remember sometimes. But 1996, quite frankly, as I told the subcommittee folks who called me in Maine, much to my chagrin, I simply do not recall writing that letter. I may have.

Chairman BARTON. You do recall that you were involved in the review of an application for the drug.

Mr. KNUDSEN. That is correct, although that is a bit different than generating and writing a letter and not—I just——

Chairman BARTON. Well, but this isn't a run of the mill application. Your last paragraph is pretty important. "There appears to be an increased frequency of reports of suicidality in the pediatric/adolescent patient exposed to Certraline compared to either the placebo or the Certraline treated with adult OCD patients."

That is a pretty important finding or pretty important question. Yet once you sent the letter off, which nobody at the FDA kept any copies of, everybody forgets about it until 8 years later or 6 years later.

Mr. KNUDSEN. Well, in fact——

Chairman BARTON. You can't even remember writing the letter.

Mr. KNUDSEN. Well, I mean, how many people in this room, I would like to ask, can remember writing letters in 1986? This is purely speculative, and I am not going to speculate. I cannot recall writing the letter.

The point of fact is it is a very important issue. I may have written it. For simplicity, I will say I did write it, and because I was very much concerned about this issue when I reviewed the OCD——

Chairman BARTON. You are missing my point. Nobody is challenging whether you wrote the letter or not. Now if you want to—you know, you said it looked like your signature, so you probably did or you did. You will stipulate. I could care less.

What I am concerned about, that we have a drug that is being used in adolescents to treat depression and, according to whoever wrote this letter, there appears to be an increase in suicidality. Now that is an important thing, and nobody at the FDA did anything on it for 6 years. That is pretty important.

Mr. TEMPLE. That is not entirely correct. Dr. Laughren reviewed——

Chairman BARTON. It is more correct than incorrect.

Mr. TEMPLE. Dr. Laughren reviewed the data that was the basis for that letter, wrote a memo.

Chairman BARTON. Well, you all didn't even find a copy, and now we got two different copies from the drug manufacturer, and we get—when we asked about document retention policy—you don't have access to this, because it didn't come in until today.

It is an e-mail that was sent today to the young lady to my right, and it says, "FDA does not have a specific regulation that governs the record retention of NDA files and drug master files."

It is pure serendipity that the manufacturer kept a copy.

Mr. TEMPLE. I think the problem was that the letter never went into appropriate channels. That is why it was never seen.

Chairman BARTON. Well, it is not stamped. There is no stamp that it was.

Mr. TEMPLE. It didn't go to Dr. Laughren. It didn't get into the file. That is why nobody knows it was there.

Chairman BARTON. Do you think you should have a document retention policy? Do you think that something like this should have gone through channels, that somebody at your level or some level should have checked into it and done something before 6 years later?

Mr. TEMPLE. Of course.

Chairman BARTON. Yes or no?

Mr. TEMPLE. Of course, it should have gone through channels.

Chairman BARTON. And you think something should have been followed up on this?

Mr. TEMPLE. Had anybody known about it and seen the result, yes, of course. But I do want to point out that the basis for that letter was reviewed by Dr. Laughren a couple of months later, and his conclusion was that there was no signal there.

Chairman BARTON. Beg your pardon?

Mr. TEMPLE. His conclusion was that there was no signal there, that the analysis was invalid. I believe the letter never should have been sent. It doesn't make any sense.

Chairman BARTON. In spite of all the studies that have been done since then—and correct me if I am wrong. We have looked at 15 studies. Twelve of the 15 have shown no effect, no efficacy. Some of those have shown an increase in suicidality, and in spite of that, you say this letter shouldn't have been sent?

Mr. TEMPLE. This letter reported that there was an increased risk of suicidality in children compared to adults.

Chairman BARTON. Let's be fair. It says there appears to be.

Mr. TEMPLE. Okay.

Chairman BARTON. He is just questioning. Even though he has developed amnesia, at the time he was doing his job, and he was saying that somebody needs to check—well, he didn't say that. He just says what are your comments on it. Now once he wrote it, he forgot he wrote it. He didn't keep a record of it, and it was forgotten about.

Mr. TEMPLE. Right. The——

Chairman BARTON. Now this gentleman to your right, Dr. Laughren, says that he reviewed this letter?

Mr. TEMPLE. No, not the letter, the review that led to the letter.

Mr. LAUGHREN. I would like to clarify.

Chairman BARTON. All right. So you reviewed the same data.

Mr. LAUGHREN. No, no. Let me explain. Dr. Knudsen wrote a review of March 1996 around the same time that he sent the letter. He raised the concern in his review, and I responded to that concern in a memo that I wrote to the file later that year.

It is true—I mean, there is no question. This is a failure in our document flow. However, the response that Pfizer sent in response to his letter in May of that same year——

Chairman BARTON. The response is in the file. Isn't that correct?

Mr. LAUGHREN. That response apparently is in our file. I have since—I agree that it is years later, but I have recently looked at it. It is completely consistent with the conclusion that I reached in the memo that I wrote in October of the same year, in October 1996.

So it is true, you know, this is a document failure. No question about it.

Chairman BARTON. Well, it is more than document failure.

Mr. LAUGHREN. No, no. There is no signal there. There is just no signal there. There is no signal in those data.

Mr. TEMPLE. The analysis included three uncontrolled trials and one controlled trial in excessive compulsive disease. In the OCD trial there was one suicidality case in the placebo group and none in the treated group.

The comparisons are entirely invalid. The letter should not have been sent.

Mr. LAUGHREN. Yesterday I spoke to someone completely independent, an epidemiologist in our Division, the head of the safety team, about these data just to get another view on this, and she completely agreed with me, that looking at those data that Dr. Knudsen looked at back in 1996, there is no signal for pediatric suicidality. None.

Chairman BARTON. But nobody did that. You all didn't even look at the data.

Mr. TEMPLE. No, he did.

Mr. LAUGHREN. I did.

Mr. TEMPLE. He looked at the data that Dr. Knudsen had placed in his review, not the letter. We didn't know about the letter.

Chairman BARTON. Well, let me ask another, because I don't follow the—I am not a medically trained person.

This particular drug—in 1996 was it being prescribed off-label for adolescents?

Mr. LAUGHREN. I can't answer that. It probably was.

Chairman BARTON. It probably was?

Mr. LAUGHREN. The point of this——

Mr. TEMPLE. But it is not for depression.

Mr. LAUGHREN. Right. This study was for—sorry.

Mr. TEMPLE. This was for a different condition.

Mr. LAUGHREN. This study was for obsessive compulsive disorder in kids.

Chairman BARTON. But it leads to an increase in—it could—it appears that there could be, "that there appears to be an increased frequency of reports of suicidality."

Mr. TEMPLE. Yes, that is what it says, but——

Chairman BARTON. That was in 1996. This is 2004. It is 8 years ago. If it was prescribed to 10,000 children and 100 of them committed suicide because they took it, I think something should have been done.

Mr. TEMPLE. That would be a bad thing. This provides no signal that that is a risk. There is no signal in those data. In the controlled trial there were more suicidality——

Chairman BARTON. What did—apparently, what the FDA—I've got some other questions, but apparently what the FDA did about this, this gentleman or others looked at this data and said we don't see a problem there. And so you did nothing. You did absolutely nothing.

Mr. TEMPLE. I don't understand. There was no signal.

Chairman BARTON. Well, you know what I would have done?

Mr. TEMPLE. What would you have done?

Chairman BARTON. I would have gone in and done some more trials. I might have even told the drug manufacturers not to let it be—strongly encourage them not to prescribe it off-label. I might have erred on the side of safety and prudence and said let's don't take a chance. That's what I would have done.

Mr. TEMPLE. So in response to a study that showed more suicidality in the placebo group than in the treatment group, you would have done more studies? I don't think I understand.

I understand why the words—this looks like it might be a signal—would be distressing, but that was a wrong interpretation of the data.

Chairman BARTON. Well, even Dr. Laughren said—and again this is a memorandum. It is Tab 75 dated October 25. This is apparently after he had reviewed the data. He says, "I don't consider these data to represent a signal of risk for suicidality for either adults or children. Supplements are planned for both depression and OCD in pediatric patients, and when we have more complete data, including Ham-D data, we can look more critically at this issue using the now standard approach of comparing the proportions of drug in placebo exposed patients to show worsening on Item 3, which is the suicidality item, to the Ham-D during the treatment." So even he said that there should be something done.

Mr. TEMPLE. Well, those things were done, but we now have exquisite evidence that looking at the Ham-D doesn't work.

Chairman BARTON. Well, I am going to, unfortunately, have to run and vote.

Should FDA develop a document retention policy for NDAs and drug master files? Yes or no? You have none now.

Mr. TEMPLE. Well, I believe we have one, but we will——

Chairman BARTON. Well, your e-mail says you don't.

Mr. TEMPLE. We don't have a rule.

Chairman BARTON. If you don't, should you?

Mr. TEMPLE. Yes.

Chairman BARTON. What did the British see when they pulled these things off the market that you didn't see, that FDA didn't see?

Mr. TEMPLE. You mean when they wrote their thing contraindicating it?

Chairman BARTON. Yes, sir.

Mr. TEMPLE. It is a different interpretation of the same data. I don't know why they reached that conclusion. One reason might be that they are less inclined to use these drugs in the first place. Why that is, I can't say.

Chairman BARTON. All right. I am going to thank you gentlemen. There will be further questions for the record, and we are going to adjourn this hearing.

[Whereupon, at 5:46 p.m., the subcommittee was adjourned.]

[Additional material submitted for the record follows:]

Tab	Document Description	Date
	Mosholder SSRI Studies	
1	Email: From Katz to Mosholder re: please do consult on paxil/ssri's	June 3, 2003
2	Email: From Laughren re: how Neuropharm first aware of Paxil/suicidality issue	June 3, 2003
3	Formal Request for Consultation by Neuropharm to ODS re: Mosholder	June 5, 2003
4	Email: From Mosholder to Katz/Laughren et al re: questioning Paxil suicidality data	June 19, 2003
5	Email: coding dictionary for Paxil peds MDD supplemental NDA	June 23, 2003
6	Email: FW: Pamer to Mosholder re: Suicide-related terms in WHO-ART/Paxil	June 24, 2003
7	Email: From FDA Ombudsman RE: SSRI complaints and a heads-up	August 18, 2003
8	Memo: Consult by Mosholder: Suicidality in pediatric clinical trials with paroxetine and other antidepressant drugs	September 4, 2003
9	Email: From Mosholder to Paul David re: Zoloft's JAMA study and "spin"	September 16, 2003
10	Email: From Katz to Mosholder re: "superb" presentation at regulatory meeting	September 17, 2003
11	Email: From Katz to Willey re: no Paxil consult presented at Oct. Ped. Adv.C.Mtg	October 2, 2003
12	Email: Meeting on Pediatric Suicide Patient Narratives/Columbia group identified	October 28, 2003
13	Email: Dianne Murphy/John Jenkins re: Discussion about not presenting Paxil data in Oct	December 10, 2003
14	Email: Mosholder Consult: Suicidal events in pediatric clinical trials of antidepressants sent to M. Avigan for review	December 17, 2003
15	A. Mosholder Draft Consult on all SSRI's with Mark Avigan handwritten "great job"	Nov/Dec 2003
16	Email: From Laughren to Katz and Temple Re: Mosholder not presenting	December 21, 2003
17	Email: FW: Pediatric MDD Suicide Planning Mtg	December 18, 2003
18	Email: From Katz to Mosholder re: presentation	January 6, 2004
19	Email: Mosholder's Draft Slide Presentation RCT data for Feb. 2 AC mtg	January 7, 2004
20	Email: From Mosholder to Dubitsky re: Katz et al asking him to "bow out"	January 9, 2004
21	Email: From Trontell to Mosholder re: suggested alternative language to consult	January 20, 2004
22	Email: From Willy to Mosholder re: Mosholder informing her of Waters call	January 23, 2004
23	Email: From Mosholder to Trontell and Willy re: Feb 2 preparing answers to q's	January 28, 2004
24	Email: Mosholder to Willy re: finalizing consult and attaching consult	January 29, 2004
25	Several versions of Proposed Agenda for February 2 mtg	February 2, 2004
26	Agenda For February 2, 2004 (1) by T. Laughren	February 2, 2004
27	Agenda For February 2, 2004 (2)	February 2, 2004
28	Email: From Mosholder to Willy re: Labeling issues and DFS consult	February 10, 2004
29	Memo: Mosholder consult Final: Trontell & Avigan cover memos attached	March 15, 2004
30	Meeting Reminder - Subject: Adult MDD Suicide Data Discussion	May 28, 2004
31	Interim Results of the Analysis of Pediatric trials by Tarek Hammad	July 19, 2004
32	Memo: Mosholder Follow up Consult/ Trontell cover memo	August 16, 2004
	FDA Documents	
33	CDER 2002 Report to the Nation - Mission of CDER	2002
34	Letter from HHS to Glaxo re: Pediatric Exclusivity Request (sample)	April 28, 1999
35	Letter from GSK to FDA (Katz) re: submission of pediatric suicide analysis	May 22, 2003
36	GSK's analysis of pediatric suicidality data - Submitted to the FDA w/letter	May 22, 2002
37	FDA Talk Paper June 2003 regarding the anti-depressants Paxil for pediatric population	June 19, 2003
38	FDA Draft Meeting Minutes re: Sept. 16 Paxil briefing by A. Mosholder	September 16, 2003
39	FDA Talk Paper October 2003: FDA issues Public Health Advisory Entitled: Reports of Suicidality in Ped. Patients Being Treated with Antidepressant Meds	October 27, 2003
40	Summary Minutes of the Psychopharmacologic Drugs Advisory Committee Mtg.on Feb. 2, 2004	February 2, 2004

Tab	Document Description	Date
41	HHS letter to Wyeth re: remove hostility labeling and add new class labeling	March 19, 2004
42	HHS letter to Glaxo re: new Written Request pursuant to BPCA	July 2, 2002
43	HHS letter to Glaxo re: additional "emotional liability" info	October 10, 2002
44	FDA Public Health Advisory March 2004 Subject: Worsening depression and suicidality in patients being treated with antidepressant medications	March 22, 2004
45	Wyeth Response to HHS March 19, 2004 letter; keeping hostility w/added sentence	April 2, 2004
46	HHS Letter to the Committee re: suppression of Dr. Mosholder's consult	April 14, 2004
47	HHS Memorandum by Laughren re: Overview of September 13 & 14, 2004 Advisory Committee meeting and Neuropharm's actions to date	August 16,2004
48	FDA - CDER Joint Meeting - Questions and Issues	September 13-14, 2004
49	FDA Statements on Recommendations of the Psychopharmacologic Drugs and Pediatric Advisory Committees	September 16, 2004
50	HHS Letter to Kenneth R. Bonk - Wyeth Pharmaceuticals Re: Labeling Changes	May 1, 2004
51	FDA Letter to Wyeth re: No inclusion of negative efficacy pediatric clinical trials	no date
52	Hammad Presentation at September Pediatric Advisory Committee	September 13, 2004
53	Mosholder Presentation at September Pediatric Advisory Committee	September 13,2004
	OIA Investigation	
54	Email: From Mosholder to Trontell and Willey re: why he continued to look at data after regulatory briefing with attached emails	January 28, 2004
55	Email: As we discussed--OIA written statement	May 3, 2004
56	Email: Abridged Written Statement for tomorrow's meeting with Senate Finance Committee - 8:53 AM	May 4, 2004
57	Email: From Katz to Mosholder re: Katz's edits to statement 2:37pm	May 4, 2004
58	Email: From Mosholder to Katz et al re: "uncomfortable" with changes 3:17pm	May 4, 2004
59	Email: From Meister to Mosholder re: notification OIA investigation is closed	May 11, 2004
60	A. Mosholder Written Statement for OIA	May 2004
61	Whistleblower Fact Sheet Given to A. Mosholder	March 3, 2004
62	Written Administrative Statement Signed by A. Mosholder	March 3, 2004
63	Email: From Mosholder to ODS ees re: OIA investigation into leak	March 3, 2004
64	Email: From Meister to Mosholder re: meeting on Mon. at 1 p.m	April 29, 2004
65	Email: From Seligman to Coleman and Doyle re: Inappropriate Disclosure	February 10, 2004
66	FDA Memo: Report of Investigation on the CDER, Office of Drug Safety E-mail	March 10, 2004
67	Mosholder Statement to OIA	March 15, 2004
68	Katz Statement to OIA	May 6, 2004
69	FDA Memo: OIA Investigative Report in Response to Request of Senate Chairman Grassley	June 1, 2004
70	Email: From Mosholder to Trontell, Avigan and Willy re: Feb 2 AC meeting/letter from Rob Waters, freelance reporter	January 27, 2004
	Documents Raising Suicidality Concerns in Children	
71	Letter from Dr. James Knudsen to Pfizer re: explain increase in suicidality in OCD pediatric trials vs. adults	March 19, 1996
72	HHS letter to Brumfield	March 19, 1996
73	Pfizer's Response to Knudsen 3/19/96 letter - re: Suicidality in OCD pediatric trials (Selected pages)	May 28, 1996
74	HHS Memorandum by Laughren re: Recommendation for Approval Action for Zoloft (sertraline) for Obsessive Compulsive Disorder	September 30, 1996
75	HHS Memorandum by Laughren re: Comment on data in the pediatric OCD database re: suicidality raised in Knudsen's 3/28/96 safety review	October 25, 1996

Tab	Document Description	Date
76	HHS Memorandum by Paul Leber re: : Zoloft OCD Approval Action Memorandum	October 25, 1996
77	Review and Evaluation of Clinical Data - Sponsor Solvay Pharm. Drug: Fluvoxamine maleate (Luvox) by Mosholder (Selected Pages)	August 27, 1996
78	Review and Evaluation of Clinical Data - Sponsor Solvay Pharm. Drug: Fluvoxamine maleate (Luvox) by Mosholder re: mania reports in kids	February 12, 1997
79	Luvox Label (Selected Pages)	September 28, 2004
80	Laughren Memo: Recommendation of Approvable Action for Luvox (fluvoxamine) for Pediatric OCD	November 14, 1996
81	Review and Eval. Of Clinical Data - Zoloft - Reviewer Knudsen (Selected Pages)	March 28, 1996
	MHRA	
82	Public Health Link - To: Directors of Public Health of PCTs re: warnings of SSRI's in Kids	December 10, 2003
	Docs from 9/9/04 O&I Hearing	
83	Article: "Efficacy of Paroxetine in the Treatment of Adolescent Major Depression: A Randomized, Controlled Trial," Keller, et al. J.AM. ACAD. Child Adolesc. Psychiatry	July-01
84	Dear Healthcare Letter - Re: Pediatric Use of Effexor	August 22, 2003
85	Article: "Efficacy of Sertraline in the Treatment of Children and Adolescents with Major Depressive Disorder," Wagner et al. (JAMA)	August 27, 2003
86	Sample Written Request for Pediatric Study on Antidepressants	no date
87	FDA PowerPoint - Re: Drug Utilization for Antidepressants Among Children & Adolescents	February 2, 2004
	Miscellaneous	
88	Dingell Letter to FDA	September 14, 2004
89	Grassley Letter to FDA	June 16, 2004
90	Hammad Analysis (Selected Pages)	August 16, 2004
91	New York Times Article: F.D.A. Links Drugs to Being Suicidal - Harris	September 14, 2004
92	Wall Street Journal Article: FDA: Antidepressants Appear to Raise Juvenile Suicide Risk - Dooren	September 13, 2004

Mosholder, Andrew D

From: Katz, Russell G
Sent: Tuesday, June 03, 2003 9:24 AM
To: Mosholder, Andrew D
Subject: RE: Paxil and pediatric suicidality

Tab 1

Andy-

Thanks a lot. We'll send over a formal consult ASAP.

Rusty

-----Original Message-----
From: Mosholder, Andrew D
Sent: Tuesday, June 03, 2003 8:56 AM
To: Katz, Russell G
Cc: Willy, Mary E
Subject: RE: Paxil and pediatric suicidality

Hello, Rusty,
Yes, I would be interested in working on this consult. I've confirmed my availability to do so with my team leader, Mary Willy (I'm cc-ing her on this reply).
As I recall, a number of the other SSRI pediatric supplements showed signals for behavioral adverse events. But these were mainly events such as agitation and hypomania, not self-injury (unless, as you suggest, they were similarly obscured by inappropriate terminology).
Regards
Andy

> -----Original Message-----
> **From:** Katz, Russell G
> **Sent:** Monday, June 02, 2003 4:12 PM
> **To:** Mosholder, Andrew D
> **Subject:** Paxil and pediatric suicidality
>
> Andy-
>
> Hi, hope you are well.
>
> We have recently become aware of a presumed association
> between Paxil and suicidality in pediatric patients. We
> received a call from the EMEA a little over a week ago. A
> Dr. Raines told us that the company (GSK) had submitted data
> that demonstrated that use of Paxil in kids was associated
> with increased suicidality compared to placebo, and that the
> company proposed labeling changes; I believe she also said
> that it was in the news, and it was a big issue. Tom and I
> told her that the company had not informed us of any of this,
> and we agreed to look into it.
>
> It turns out that the sponsor was in the process of
> submitting to us a partial response to a question we asked in
> the Approval letter for the pediatric use (you, you may
> recall, were the reviewer). Specifically, we had asked them
> to further elaborate the events subsumed under the preferred
> term "Emotional Lability". We have received this partial
> response, and almost all of these events related to
> suicidality. The bottom line is that when data from the
> controlled trials in depression, OCD, and Social Anxiety are

> pooled, for "possible suicide related" events occurring
> during treatment or within 4 days after discontinuation, the
> rate is 0.14/patient-year on drug, and 0.05/patient-year on
> placebo, p=0.02. We have some problems with the methodology
> they used to capture cases, but this is the major finding,
> and it has us worried. The sponsor has not proposed labeling
> changes, and makes a feeble attempt to dismiss the finding.
> We are also awaiting the submission of what the sponsor
> submitted to the UK.
>
> We want to move quickly to evaluate this signal. We are
> planning to look at the NDAs for the other SSRIs to see
> whether or not similar events are being hidden by various
> inappropriate coding maneuvers, but we'd also like to compare
> the drugs in other meaningful ways if we can. We also want
> to call the sponsor very soon and ask some questions about
> their methodology.
>
> We want to send a consult over to you folks, and ask that you
> be assigned the project. Given your history with this
> application and this general issue, we think you would be the
> right person to help us think about the best way to approach
> the data in the other NDAs (and their sponsors), as well as
> to provide ideas for further sources of potentially relevant
> data and possible approaches to better evaluate this signal
> study (e.g., insurance claims databases, etc.). Anyway, I
> wanted to run this by you to see if you have any strong
> objections to being fingered as the guy to do this; if you're
> OK with it, we'll send a formal consult request. Also, we'd
> like you to be in on the phone call, if possible. Of course,
> we recognize that we'd need to get you the submission pronto.
>
> Hope you can do this; if you could let me know soon, either
> way, that'd be great.
>
> Thanks,
> Rusty

Mosholder, Andrew D

Tab 2

From: Laughren, Thomas P
Sent: Tuesday, June 03, 2003 12:53 PM
To: Nighswander, Robbin M
Cc: Katz, Russell G; Racoosin, Judith A; Dubitsky, Gregory M; Mosholder, Andrew D; David, Paul A
Subject: RE: reminder-weekly report

Robbin,

On 6-23-03, Rusty and I first became aware of concerns in the UK about an increased risk of suicidal ideation in pediatric patients taking paroxetine, based on results of new analyses of safety data from a pool of 6 pediatric studies (3 in MDD, 2 in OCD, and 1 in social anxiety disorder). These analyses were actually done in response to requests (included in our 10-10-02 approvable letter the Paxil pediatric supplement) for a more detailed breakdown of events subsumed under the broad heading, "emotional lability;" in particular, we were interested in analyses focusing on events considered to represent suicidality. These results had been sent to the MHRA (UK) before being sent to FDA, due to a difference in the timing of submissions. We have now received these data (in a submission dated 5-22-03, but not received until 5-28-03), as a partial response from GSK to our approvable letter for the Paxil pediatric supplement. These analyses suggest an excess risk of suicidality in patients taking Paxil compared to those taking placebo. The submission to the UK had also included draft labeling to describe this risk, however, I have been informed by David Wheadon, M.D., of GSK, that the MHRA has stated its intent to contraindicate paroxetine in pediatric major depressive disorder, on the basis of these data along with the negative results in the pediatric major depressive disorder studies. GSK does not agree, and they are currently negotiating with the UK and other European regulatory agencies. GSK intends to fully respond to the 10-10-02 approvable letter for the Paxil pediatric supplement by the third week of June, and this will include proposed labeling to address this risk, but also new language regarding the OCD claim in peds. Since the original review of the Paxil supplement, as well as the reviews of most other pediatric supplements for SSRIs, was done by Andrew Mosholder, M.D., and these requests were a direct result of Dr. Mosholder's review, we have submitted a consult to ODS and have asked that this consult be assigned to him in his new position in ODS. We seek his advice on further analysis and interpretation of the Paxil results, as well as more general advice on what might be done to reconsider the pediatric databases for other SSRIs. In addition, we would be interested in his thoughts on further studies that might be done to better understand this signal, e.g., a cohort study using claims based data, perhaps looking at hospitalization for suicidality as an endpoint.

Tom

-----Original Message-----
From: Nighswander, Robbin M
Sent: Tuesday, June 03, 2003 11:52 AM
To: Katz, Russell G; Laughren, Thomas P
Subject: FW: reminder-weekly report

Rusty and Tom:

Although I included a brief description in last weeks report, as you can see, John would like a longer summary. Last weeks report is attached.

Thanks

Robbin

<< File: OND1 Weekly Report May 28 2003.doc >>

Tab 3

DEPARTMENT OF HEALTH AND HUMAN SERVICES PUBLIC HEALTH SERVICE FOOD AND DRUG ADMINISTRATION	REQUEST FOR CONSULTATION
TO (Division/Office): **Mail: ODS (Room 15B-08, PKLN Bldg.)**	FROM: **HFD-120/Division of Neuropharmacological Drug Products**

DATE	IND NO.	NDA NO.	TYPE OF DOCUMENT	DATE OF DOCUMENT
6-5-03		**20-031/SE5-037**	**Minor Amendment**	**5-22-03**

NAME OF DRUG	PRIORITY CONSIDERATION	CLASSIFICATION OF DRUG	DESIRED COMPLETION DATE
Paxil (paroxetine HCl) Tablets		**Selective Serotonin Reuptake Inhibitor (SSRI)**	

NAME OF FIRM: GSK

REASON FOR REQUEST

I. GENERAL

- NEW PROTOCOL
- PROGRESS REPORT
- NEW CORRESPONDENCE
- DRUG ADVERTISING
- ADVERSE REACTION REPORT
- MANUFACTURING CHANGE/ADDITION
- MEETING PLANNED BY
- PRE--NDA MEETING
- END OF PHASE II MEETING
- RESUBMISSION
- SAFETY/EFFICACY
- PAPER NDA
- CONTROL SUPPLEMENT
- RESPONSE TO DEFICIENCY LETTER
- FINAL PRINTED LABELING
- LABELING REVISION
- ORIGINAL NEW CORRESPONDENCE
- FORMULATIVE REVIEW
- OTHER *(SPECIFY BELOW)*:

IV. DRUG EXPERIENCE

- PHASE IV SURVEILLANCE/EPIDEMIOLOGY PROTOCOL
- DRUG USE e.g. POPULATION EXPOSURE, ASSOCIATED DIAGNOSES
- CASE REPORTS OF SPECIFIC REACTIONS (List below)
- COMPARATIVE RISK ASSESSMENT ON GENERIC DRUG GROUP
- REVIEW OF MARKETING EXPERIENCE, DRUG USE AND SAFETY
- SUMMARY OF ADVERSE EXPERIENCE
- POISON RISK ANALYSIS

COMMENTS/SPECIAL INSTRUCTIONS:

We have received a partial response (5-22-03) from GSK to our approvable letter for the Paxil pediatric supplement, including results of new analyses of safety data from a pool of 6 pediatric studies (3 in MDD, 2 in OCD, and 1 in social anxiety disorder). These analyses were in response to requests in our 10-10-02 approvable letter for a more detailed breakdown of events subsumed under the broad heading, "emotional lability;" in particular, we were interested in analyses focusing on events considered to represent suicidality. These analyses have been done, and they suggest an excess risk of suicidality in patients taking Paxil compared to those taking placebo. Since the original review of the Paxil supplement, as well as the reviews of most other pediatric supplements for SSRIs, was done by Andrew Mosholder, M.D., and these requests were a direct result of Dr. Mosholder's review, we ask that this consult be assigned to him. We seek his advice on further analysis and interpretation of the Paxil results, as well as more general advice on what might be done to re-evaluate the risk of suicidality in the pediatric databases for other SSRIs. In addition, we would be interested in his thoughts on epidemiological studies that might be done to better understand this signal, e.g., a cohort study using insurance claims based data, perhaps looking at hospitalization for suicidality as an endpoint.

If you have any questions, please feel free to contact the Safety Group Team Leader, Dr. Judith Racoosin (x4-5505), or the Project Manager, Mr. Paul David (x4-5530).

SIGNATURE OF REQUESTER	METHOD OF DELIVERY (Check one) MAIL HAND
SIGNATURE OF RECEIVER	SIGNATURE OF DELIVERER

This is a representation of an electronic record that was signed electronically and this page is the manifestation of the electronic signature.

/s/

Russell Katz
6/6/03 12:39:48 PM

Mosholder, Andrew D

From: Mosholder, Andrew D
Sent: Thursday, June 19, 2003 4:30 PM
To: Katz, Russell G; Laughren, Thomas P; Andreason, Paul J; Stasko, Robert; Racoosin, Judith A; David, Paul A
Subject: Paroxetine suicidality data in 4-11-02 submission

Tab 4

Hello all,

During today's meeting there were some questions about exactly what data the sponsor provided on this topic, and why we asked for what we requested in the approvable letter. This prompted me to look back at the approvable letter, the original ISS for the supplement (which is still available via the EDR) and my clinical review from last October.

The sponsor did provide a line listing of all patients with serious adverse events (ISS Table 7.8) for both drug and placebo. This table showed suicide attempts such as overdoses coded as "emotional lability," which is how we knew that was being done. Using Table 7.8, I noted in my review that there was a higher rate of suicidality-related serious adverse events for paroxetine than for placebo in the acute trials, but that this was not statistically significant.

Additionally, the sponsor provided a line listing for all adverse events coded as "emotional lability," "hostility," or "agitation" (ISS Table 6.14). Although it included nonserious events as well as serious, it did not include placebo patients, only paroxetine patients. This table also showed suicide attempts coded as emotional lability.

As a result of this situation, we asked for the following in the approvable letter:

> Table 6.14 in the ISS listed paroxetine treated patients who experienced adverse events coded under the terms hostility, emotional lability or agitation. However, the table did not include placebo patients, nor did it include psychiatric adverse events that were coded under other terms. Please prepare an expanded version of this table, including all psychiatric and behavioral adverse events, and also those that occurred among placebo patients...

We also asked GSK to provide a rationale for their coding of suicide attempts as emotional lability.

Also, the data from the Social Anxiety Disorder trial was still blinded when the supplement was submitted.

I hope this historical information is helpful.

-Andy

Mosholder, Andrew D

Tab 5

From: Mosholder, Andrew D
Sent: Monday, June 23, 2003 10:24 AM
To: Racoosin, Judith A
Subject: RE: coding dictionary for paxil peds MDD supplemental NDA

Hi Judy,

Here's what is says in the Paxil pediatric supplement ISS, section 6.3.1.

> AEs were coded from the verbatim terms provided by the investigators by using the World Health Organization Adverse Reaction Terminology (WHO ART) codelist. These terms were then mapped to Adverse Drug Experiences Coding System (ADECS) classification to provide body system and preferred term. The ADECS is a COSTART based dictionary. Gender specific events were tabulated separately from gender non-specific events to allow percentages to be corrected for gender. As stated previously, the coding process differed between the acute clinical studies and acute clinical pharmacology Study 715 (i.e., for Study 715, terms were not mapped to ADECS). Therefore, body system and preferred terms will differ between these studies.

Of course, study 715 is not relevant here.

-Andy

\> -----Original Message-----
\> **From:** Racoosin, Judith A
\> **Sent:** Monday, June 23, 2003 10:14 AM
\> **To:** Mosholder, Andrew D
\> **Subject:** coding dictionary for paxil peds MDD supplemental NDA
\>
\> Hi Andy,
\> Do you know which coding dictionary was used for the paxil
\> peds MDD supplemental NDA? You have probably already told me,
\> but I just can't recall.
\>
\> thanks
\> Judy

Mosholder, Andrew D

From: Pamer, Carol
Sent: Tuesday, June 24, 2003 9:13 AM
To: Racoosin, Judith A
Cc: Mosholder, Andrew D; Singer, Sarah J
Subject: FW: Suicide-related terms in WHO-ART?

Tab 6

Clear Day Bkgrd.JPG

From our coding guru, Sally Singer.

Carol

-----Original Message-----
From: Singer, Sarah J
Sent: Tuesday, June 24,2003 9:10 AM
To: Pamer, Carol; Goetsch, Roger A; Piazza Hepp, Toni D
Cc: Lu, Susan
Subject: RE: Suicide-related terms in WHO-ART?

Hi Carol,
I have an old COSTART manual; SUICIDE ATTEMPT did exist. The manual has a COSTART to WHOART translation table which states that SUICIDE ATTEMPT also existed in WHOART.
-Sally

-----Original Message-----
From: Pamer, Carol
Sent: Tuesday, June 24, 2003 9:07 AM
To: Goetsch, Roger A; Piazza Hepp, Toni D; Singer, Sarah J
Cc: Lu, Susan
Subject: Suicide-related terms in WHO-ART?

Good morning--

A question has come up about the way that suicides/suicide attempts were coded in a recent NDA supplement. Apparently the company chose a term like "emotional lability" when in actuality most were suicide attempts. They used WHOART and COSTART as their dictionaries (see below), and a dictionary I am not familiar with, ADECS. We are talking about GSK and Paxil pediatric supplement. FYI. How can we verify that WHOART has a specific term for suicide/attempts? I don't have a copy of a WHOART reference, if there is one around here. It would also be helpful to have someone verify for me that COSTART has Suicide Attempt and perhaps others for the same. Too many brain cells have come and gone for me since the era of COSTART!!

Thanks!

Carol

AEs were coded from the verbatim terms provided by the investigators by using the World Health Organization Adverse Reaction Terminology (WHO ART) codelist. These terms were then mapped to Adverse Drug Experiences Coding System (ADECS) classification to provide body system and preferred term. The ADECS is a COSTART based dictionary. Gender specific events were tabulated separately from gender non-specific events to allow percentages to be corrected for gender. As stated previously, the coding process differed between the acute clinical studies and acute clinical pharmacology Study 715 (i.e., for Study 715, terms were not mapped to ADECS). Therefore, body system and preferred terms will differ between these studies.

Tab 7

From: Rumble, Warren F
Sent: Monday, August 18, 2003 1:56 PM
To: Woodcock, Janet; Galson, Steven; Henderson, Deborah J; Roberts, Khyati N; Katz, Russell G; Temple, Robert; Behrman, Rachel E; Raczkowski, Victor F; Marks, Norman S
Subject: SSRI complaints and a heads-up

Hello Everyone,

I want to briefly alert you all about the numerous concerns I receive on the adverse events associated with the SSRIs. My most frequent drug complaints are on these drugs and the letters I get are very detailed and quite scary. I pasted at the end of this note my most recent consumer letter.
The most frequent problems I hear about are suicide or attempted suicide, akathisia, and the struggle to get off the drugs.
My most significant contact was by a person whose teenage son committed suicide and now her goal is to petition various parties (manufacturers, FDA, Congress, Grand Juries) to investigate:

> Eli Lilly's suppression of the truth that these drugs cause suicide and suicidal ideation,
>
> GSK's and Wyeth-Ayerst's false advertising that only drug abusers are at risk of physical and psychological dependence, and withdrawal problems when tapering back or discontinuing Paxil and Effexor.

What is quite noteworthy here is that the person, [redacted], claims to have 11K signatures on the petitions. In my correspondence with her, I suggested that she encourage signers to report their adverse events to our MedWatch system so we could analyze the reports for possible labeling changes. I have attached her most recent e-mail to me that includes the web text letter (quite sophisticated) to the President and to Sen. Hatch. The letter includes links to the petitions. We may get a Congressional on it some day.
Thanks
Warren

Letter Received
rom Senator O..

Good day. am not one who ordinarily writes to anyone about such things, but this I feel is important. I reads a newspaper article yesterday about the potential dangers of Paxil in children and teens. It was quite disturbing and yet I believe incomplete. I was on Paxil several years ago for depression. I was about 44 at the time. I had not ever considered suicide until I was on this drug for several weeks. The day my husband and son found me in the closet taking 2 and 3 pills with a sip of wine and repeating the process over and over until they found me, I realized something was terribly wrong. I remember thinking this would end it all and that would be that. Fortunately, I stopped taking Paxil and life was good again. I was even able to work through my depression without the "help" of drugs. Not too many months ago, I again found myself in a state of depression. Again I was prescribed Paxil. Not giving any thought to the past occurrence, I began taking it. For a while it seemed to be helping. Then low and behold I found myself thinking such things as, if I pull in front of that truck, if I take all of these pills, etc., etc. I remembered the last time I was on this drug. I stopped taking it. And again, thoughts of suicide have disappeared. What really prompted me to write this, however, was a conversation I had with a new friend yesterday. We were discussing the article when she confided in me that her husband committed suicide 6 years ago after he began taking Paxil. Is it coincidence? I am beginning to fear not. What may be good for some may be fatal for others. How do we determine the difference? Thank you for your time. Please feel free to contact me at my e-mail address if you have any questions, or if I can be of any further assistance concerning this potential hazard.

MEMORANDUM

Tab 8

DEPARTMENT OF HEALTH AND HUMAN SERVICES
PUBLIC HEALTH SERVICE
FOOD AND DRUG ADMINISTRATION
CENTER FOR DRUG EVALUATION AND RESEARCH

PID#	D030341
DATE:	September 4, 2003
FROM:	Andrew D. Mosholder, M.D., M.P.H., Epidemiologist
THROUGH:	Mark Avigan, M.D., Acting Director Division of Drug Risk Evaluation, HFD-430
TO:	Russell Katz, M.D., Director Division of Neuropharmacological Drug Products, HFD-120
SUBJECT:	Consult: Suicidality in pediatric clinical trials with paroxetine and other antidepressant drugs Drugs: paroxetine, sertraline, venlafaxine, fluoxetine, fluvoxamine, citalopram, nefazodone, mirtazapine

*****NOT TO BE USED OUTSIDE OF FDA WITHOUT PRIOR CLEARANCE BY IMS HEALTH AND ADVANCEPCS*****

EXECUTIVE SUMMARY

At the request of the Division of Neuropharmacological Drug Products (DNDP), recently submitted data on adverse events involving suicidal ideation and self injury from the paroxetine pediatric development program were reviewed. These data indicate an association of paroxetine treatment with suicidal ideation and behaviors in acute treatment settings, although the degree of association varied according to trial (study 329 having the largest relative risk) and indication (most, but not all, of the suicidal adverse events occurred in depression trials). Almost all of the events occurred in adolescents. Events were categorized by the sponsor as either "possibly-suicide related," which included both suicidal ideation and self-injurious behaviors, or as "suicide attempts," which were frank self-injurious acts and were thus a subset of the broader category of possibly suicide-related events. Stratified analysis by study yielded a relative risk of 2.6 for possibly suicide-related events (95% confidence interval 1.2-5.9). Consistent with this, the relative risk for the more narrowly defined category of suicide attempts was approximately 2, but was not statistically significant.

This finding prompted an examination of the data on suicidality and suicide attempts from other pediatric psychopharmacology clinical trials. Data on adverse events from pediatric clinical trials with seven other drugs were reviewed and combined for analysis with the paroxetine data. These drugs were the selective serotonin reuptake inhibitors (SSRIs) sertraline, fluoxetine, fluvoxamine, and citalopram; and the atypical antidepressants nefazodone, venlafaxine, and mirtazapine. There were a total of 20 acute treatment placebo-controlled trials with these 8 drugs. In these trials, there were 40 suicide attempts (defined as any self-injurious behavior) among 2213 drug-treated subjects, and 13 suicide attempts among 1901 placebo-treated subjects. A stratified analysis yielded a relative risk for suicide attempts of 2.5 (95% confidence interval 1.4-4.6) with active drug treatment in these short-term trials, relative to placebo. As with paroxetine, depression trials had more such events than trials in other psychiatric indications. For each individual drug, the aggregated data from trials in depression showed that possibly suicide-related adverse events were more numerous on active treatment than on placebo, and for no drug did the data suggest a protective effect. This finding suggests that the association with suicidality observed for paroxetine may be a class effect, rather than a unique effect of paroxetine.

DNDP has asked the sponsors of 8 other psychiatric drugs to search their pediatric trial databases and furnish data on suicidality that will be comparable to the data submitted for paroxetine. These new data will also include person-time of exposure so that rates of events may be calculated. When this data is received it will be possible to perform a more definitive meta-analysis. However, if the results from this preliminary analysis are substantiated, there will be broad implications for the pharmacological management of pediatric depressive disorders.

This consult covers the following topics. A background section discusses the regulatory history of the paroxetine pediatric development program, the history of the controversy over whether certain antidepressant drugs promote suicidal behavior in adults, and adolescent suicide. Next, the paroxetine pediatric clinical trial data on suicidal adverse events provided by the sponsor is summarized, along with some additional exploratory analyses. Following this is a discussion of whether epidemiological methods might be applied to study this issue further. The final section of the consult is a survey and meta-analysis of suicidal adverse events from other pediatric development programs for antidepressant drugs.

BACKGROUND

Regulatory history

GlaxoSmithKline (GSK) submitted a pediatric supplement for paroxetine HCl (Paxil) on 4-11-02 (NDA 20-031, supplement 37), and in exchange received pediatric exclusivity for the compound. DNDP issued an approvable letter for this supplement 10-10-02, and the letter included a request for additional information about behavioral adverse events in the pediatric clinical trials. In response, GSK analyzed the incidence of suicide attempts and suicidality in the trials, and submitted this information to FDA on 5-22-03. The analyses showed a statistically significant association of suicidality with paroxetine treatment relative to placebo. These data were also submitted to the UK Medicines and Healthcare Products Regulatory Agency (MHRA), and on 6-10-03 the MHRA issued a statement contraindicating paroxetine in the treatment of pediatric depression. On 7-14-03 the Marketed Health Products Directorate of Health Canada posted a similar warning.

DNDP consulted ODS to obtain assistance with (1) analyzing and interpreting the paroxetine data, (2) examining other pediatric antidepressant clinical supplements for the presence of comparable signals, and (3) exploring whether any epidemiological data sources might be available to confirm or refute the signal.

Regulatory status of antidepressant drugs for pediatric use

Currently, fluvoxamine, sertraline, fluoxetine (all SSRIs) and clomipramine (a tricyclic antidepressant compound) are indicated for pediatric obsessive compulsive disorder (OCD).

Fluoxetine was recently granted an indication for pediatric major depressive disorder, but no other drugs are presently indicated for pediatric depression; pediatric exclusivity supplements submitted for mirtazapine, venlafaxine, sertraline, citalopram, paroxetine and nefazodone failed to demonstrate efficacy in pediatric major depressive disorder. Parenthetically, it should be noted that off-label use of selective serotonin reuptake inhibitors (SSRIs) to treat pediatric depression has been endorsed in practice guidelines for child psychiatrists[1] and in the recent report by the U.S. Surgeon General on mental health[2], along with use of non-pharmacological treatments such as cognitive-behavioral therapy.

Suicidality and antidepressant drugs

For over a decade there has been controversy over whether some antidepressant drugs, particularly fluoxetine and the other SSRIs, can induce suicidality. A full review of this issue is beyond the scope of this consult, but a few points will be summarized herein.

In 1990, Tiecher et al. published a case series describing six patients who developed intense suicidal ideation during treatment with the selective serotonin reuptake inhibitor (SSRI) fluoxetine.[3] Similar events were subsequently reported in pediatric patients.[4] To address concerns about fluoxetine treatment precipitating suicidality, Lilly, the manufacturer of fluoxetine, performed a meta-analysis of their fluoxetine clinical trial database, which showed that there was no increase in suicidal acts among fluoxetine-treated patients compared to placebo-treated patients.[5] The issue of fluoxetine-associated suicidal behavior was considered at a meeting of FDA's Psychopharmacological Drugs Advisory Committee on 9-21-91; the committee concluded that the evidence for such an association was not credible. More recently, one author has linked suicidality to use of the SSRI sertraline.[6] A study in the U.K. using the General Practice Research Database during the period 1988-93 did find a somewhat higher rate of suicide among fluoxetine users compared to users of other antidepressants.[7] However, these data were from a clinical setting and were not randomized, and the authors attributed the imbalance in suicide rates to selection bias. In 2000, the U.K. Committee on the Safety of Medicines (CSM) re-considered the issue of SSRI-induced suicidality.[8] They noted that anecdotal reports continued to suggest such a link to fluoxetine, although data from epidemiological studies and clinical trials have failed to confirm this; the CSM also noted that "the risk of suicide may increase in the early stages of treatment with any antidepressant."

Some authors have conducted meta-analyses of suicidality in antidepressant clinical trials to address a somewhat different concern; i.e., whether randomization to placebo confers a greater risk of self-harm. Khan and associates analyzed clinical trial data from the development programs for 5 recently marketed antidepressant compounds (the SSRIs sertraline and paroxetine, and the atypical antidepressants nefazodone, mirtazapine, and bupropion), comprising a total of 19,639 subjects worldwide.[9] The authors determined rates for completed suicides and suicide attempts on active drug treatment and placebo, using both open label and randomized, double-blind data from studies in depression and other indications. Their results showed incidence rates for completed suicide per 1000 person years of exposure in clinical trials of 8.4, 6.9, and 3.6, for investigational drugs, active controls and placebo, respectively. The authors also determined incidence rates for suicide attempts; per 1000 person years, these were 28.1, 34.3, and 27.0 for investigational drugs, active controls, and placebo, respectively. In a similar study, Storosum et al. examined registration dossiers for 9 antidepressants submitted to the regulatory agency for the Netherlands.[10] Analysis of 77 short-term studies involving a total of 12,246 patients showed similar incidences of suicide attempts (approximately 0.4%) and completed suicides (approximately 0.1%) for patients receiving placebo or active drugs. DNDP has also performed a meta-analysis of suicides in randomized controlled trials of antidepressant drugs.

This analysis showed no differences in suicide rates for active drugs versus placebo, after the rates were adjusted for relevant covariates (age, gender, inpatient versus outpatient setting, and foreign versus North American location of the trial).[11]

Adolescent suicide

In 2000, intentional self-harm was the third leading cause of death for individuals aged 15-24 years in the U.S. (following accidental deaths and homicides), and accounted for more deaths than any natural cause.[12] The overall suicide rate for individuals aged 15-19 years was 8.2 per 100,000 in the year 2000, with the rate for males almost five times higher than that for females.[13] The rate for younger persons was much lower, at 0.8 per 100,000 for individuals aged 5-14 years.

Estimates of the number of suicide attempts and the proportion of attempts that are successful vary, however. A work group of the American Academy of Child and Adolescent Psychiatry estimated that roughly 2 million adolescents attempt suicide annually nationwide. Of these 2 million, an estimated 700,000 receive medical care because of the attempt, and approximately 2000 succeed in their attempt (i.e., roughly 1 in 1000 attempts are successful). The publication did not describe how the work group arrived at these figures.[14] In a recent review of the topic, Maris gave a somewhat lower estimate of 100-200 adolescent suicide attempts for every completed adolescent suicide, although the author sited no specific source of this information.[15] The Centers for Disease Control (CDC) has estimated the rates of self-inflicted injuries treated in emergency rooms from the National Electronic Injury Surveillance System (NEISS).[16] The majority of these injuries were suspected to be suicidal in nature, although documentation of this was lacking in many cases. The estimated number of emergency department visits for self-inflicted injuries among individuals in the U.S. aged 15-19 years was 51,526 in the year 2000, representing a rate of 259 per 100,000. In contrast to completed suicide, for which the rate is higher in males, the larger proportion of non-fatal self-inflicted injuries occurred among females; in fact, the self-inflicted injury visit rate for females aged 15-19 years was the highest for any age and gender subgroup. Of note, the rate for ages 10-14 years, at 70 per 100,000, was much lower than the rate for the older adolescents. Comparing the rate for 15-19 year olds to the previously noted rate of completed suicides for the same age group (259 per 100,000 versus 8.2 per 100,000) yields a ratio of approximately 30 emergency department visits for self-inflicted injuries for each completed suicide in the 15-19 year age group. An additional estimate of the ratio of attempts to completed suicides is available from the Oregon Adolescent Suicide Attempt Data System (ASADS). In Oregon, hospitals are required to report adolescent suicide attempts to this database, and during the period 1988-1993 there were 31 reported adolescent suicide attempts for every completed suicide in the same age group.[17]

It has been proposed that recent declines in adolescent suicide rates are related to more widespread use of antidepressant medications. Gould et al. observed that the male adolescent suicide rate peaked at a rate of approximately 20 per 100,000 per year in 1988, but then began to decline in the early nineties. They proposed that one of the most likely explanations for this decline is the increased use of antidepressant medication among adolescents during this time period.[18] The use of antidepressant medications by adolescents has indeed increased significantly; Olfson and colleagues reported data from the National Medical Expenditure Survey and the Medical Expenditure Panel Survey showing that between 1987 and 1996, the prevalence of antidepressant medication use among adolescents aged 15-18 increased fourfold, reaching 2% by 1996.[19] Hall and associates studied the correlation between suicide rates in individuals over age 15 years and prescribing of antidepressant medications in Australia, stratified by age and gender subgroups.[20] Increased usage of antidepressant medication was correlated with declines in suicide rates; however, it appeared that this correlation was most evident among older age groups. In a similar analysis, Isacsson examined trends in Sweden for suicide rates and antidepressant prescribing.[21] During recent years there was a negative correlation between suicide rates and antidepressant sales; however, this correlation was not observed in young females (aged 15-29), or females older than 75 years.

SUMMARY OF THE PAROXETINE PEDIATRIC TRIAL DATA ON SUICIDALITY

(Sources of information: NDA 20-031, supplement 37 submitted 4-11-02; additional data submitted to NDA 20-031 on 5-22-03, 6-13-03, 6-16-03, 6-20-03, 6-23-03, 6-30-03, 7-14-03, 7-17-03; spreadsheet summarizing cases prepared by Dr. Judy Racoosin of DNDP)

Pediatric development program for paroxetine

The pediatric development program for paroxetine comprised 6 randomized, double blind, placebo controlled studies. These studies are summarized in the following table. (Data from two uncontrolled trials, an open label pediatric trial and a pediatric pharmacokinetic study, are not included in the analyses to be described.) The sample sizes shown are from the study reports where available (there is no study report for study 676). In some cases it will be seen that these sample sizes differ slightly from those in the sponsor's safety analyses submitted in May and June of this year, perhaps because of differences in defining the samples for safety versus efficacy analyses.

Table 1. Randomized, double blind studies in the paroxetine pediatric development program

Indication	Study	Age range (yrs)	N	Description
SAD	676	8-18	Paroxetine 165, placebo 157	Randomized, double blind, placebo controlled, parallel group, 16-week trial; paroxetine 10-50 mg/day versus placebo
MDD	329	12-18	Paroxetine 93, placebo 87, imipramine 95	Randomized, double blind, placebo controlled, parallel group, 8 week trial; paroxetine 20-40 mg/day versus placebo; continuation phase allowed for up to 6 months of additional double blind medication; 13 U.S. sites.
MDD	377	12-19	Paroxetine 181, placebo 93	Randomized, double blind, placebo controlled, parallel group, 12 week trial; paroxetine 20-40 mg/day versus placebo; 33 non-U.S. sites
MDD	701	7-17	Paroxetine 104, placebo 102	Randomized, double blind, placebo controlled, parallel group, 8 week trial; paroxetine 10-50 mg/day versus placebo; n=203 children and adolescents; 40 sites in U.S. and 1 in Canada
OCD	453	6-18	Double blind phase: paroxetine 95, placebo 98	Randomized, double blind, placebo controlled, 16 week relapse prevention trial; 16 week open label treatment with paroxetine followed by randomization of responders to placebo or paroxetine 10-60 mg/day; 26 sites in U.S.
OCD	704	6-17	Paroxetine 98, placebo 105	Randomized, double blind, placebo controlled, parallel group, 10 week trial; paroxetine 10-50 mg/day versus placebo; 37 sites in U.S. and 2 in Canada

Abbreviations: MDD Major Depressive Disorder; SAD Social Anxiety Disorder; OCD Obsessive Compulsive Disorder

Case definition

In the original pediatric exclusivity supplement, GSK used the WHO adverse event term "emotional lability" to code suicidal ideation and suicide attempts, but there were other types of behavioral events that were also coded to that term, making the data difficult to interpret. Accordingly, GSK adopted a special search strategy for the more recent analyses of suicidality. The methodological details for these searches can be found on pages 2-3 and 14-15 of GSK's 5-22-03 submission. An electronic search identified adverse events from placebo controlled pediatric trials for which the verbatim adverse event terms suggested a self-injury or suicide attempt. Specifically, verbatim adverse event terms with the following text strings were selected: attempt, cut, gas, hang, hung, jump, mutilat, overdos, self damag, self harm, self inflict, self injur, shoot, slash, suic. Also selected were any events with preferred terms of overdose or intentional overdose (i.e., accidental overdose was not selected). To distinguish suicide attempts from suicidal ideation, event descriptions that also included verbatim terms such as "thought," "threat," or "tendency" were considered "possibly suicide-related," while events that did not include such descriptors were considered suicide attempts.

The sponsor also submitted narrative descriptions of these cases. Review of the narratives revealed several cases that could arguably have been classified differently. However, the number of such cases was small, and because the sponsor's selection of cases was done in a manner that was automated and blind to treatment assignment, I have chosen not to reclassify any of the designated cases in a post-hoc fashion.

Calculation of incidence[1]

GSK included all of the 6 randomized placebo-controlled trials in their analysis. The sponsor also determined person time for each treatment group, and stratified the data by study and by age group (children < 12 years old and adolescents ≥12 years old). They calculated the incidence of all "possibly suicide-related" events as well as the incidence of suicide attempts, which are a subset of the former category. Events occurring up to 30 days after the end of treatment were included. At the request of DNDP, to insure consistency, events and person-time from the continuation phase of study 329 were excluded in the final analysis. (Since this phase was a blinded continuation of treatment for patients who had improved during the acute treatment phase, the data might not be comparable to that from the acute phase of the trial.)

The following table summarizes the results of these analyses, submitted by GSK on 6-30-03, in Attachment 3 of that submission. There were a total of 32 "possibly suicidal related events" and 21 suicide attempts in these clinical trials (there were no completed suicides). The sponsor performed statistical testing of the comparisons between paroxetine and placebo using Fisher's exact test, and the comparisons with p-values ≤ 0.05 are indicated.

---

[1] Grateful acknowledgment is made to Dr. Yi Tsong of the Office of Biostatistics for providing consultation on this section.

Table 2. Summary of "possibly suicidal related events" and suicide attempts in paroxetine pediatric placebo-controlled trials, including events within 30 days follow-up after treatment									
Indication	Study	Paroxetine		Placebo		Possibly suicidal related events		Suicide attempts	
		N	Pt-yrs	N	Pt-yrs	Paroxetine N (%)	Placebo N (%)	Paroxetine N (%)	Placebo N (%)
MDD	329	93	13	88	13	8 (8.6)*	1 (1.1)	5 (5.4)	0
MDD	377	181	41	95	21	9 (5.0)	4 (4.2)	8 (4.4)	4 (4.2)
MDD	701	104	16	102	17	3 (2.9)	2 (2.0)	2 (1.9)	1 (1.0)
MDD Total		378	70	285	51	20 (5.3)	7 (2.5)	15 (4.0)	5 (1.8)
OCD	453	96	22	98	19	0	0	0	0
OCD	704	99	19	107	22	1 (1.0)	0	0	0
OCD Total		195	41	205	41	1 (0.5)	0	0	0
SAD	676	165	51	157	47	4 (2.4)	0	1 (0.6)	0
Grand Total		738	162	647	139	25 (3.4)**	7 (1.1)	16 (2.2)†	5 (0.8)

Abbreviations: MDD Major Depressive Disorder, OCD Obsessive Compulsive Disorder, SAD Social Anxiety Disorder, Pt-yrs patient-years of exposure
*p-value = 0.04 versus placebo
**p-value < 0.01 versus placebo
†p-value = 0.05 versus placebo

Totaling data from all trials, the relative risk for possibly suicide-related events is 3.1 (95% confidence intervals 1.4-7.2, EpiInfo2000 software).

From the data in Table 2 the incidence rates for possibly suicide-related events and suicide attempts may be calculated, and these data are shown below. Instead of rates per patient year as shown in the sponsor's analysis dated 6-30-03, here the incidence rates are shown per 100 patient years. There are some slight differences from the sponsor's calculations, most likely due to rounding.

Table 3. Incidence rates of suicide-related adverse events in paroxetine pediatric clinical trials					
Indication	Study	Incidence/100 pt yrs of possibly suicide-related events		Incidence/100 pt yrs of suicide attempts	
		Paroxetine	Pbo	Paroxetine	Pbo
MDD	329	61.5	7.7	38.5	0.0
MDD	377	22.0	19.0	19.5	19.0
MDD	701	18.8	11.8	12.5	5.9
MDD total		28.6	13.7	21.4	9.8
OCD	453	0.0	0.0	0.0	0.0
OCD	704	5.3	0.0	0.0	0.0
OCD total		2.4	0.0	0.0	0.0
SAD	676	7.8	0.0	2.0	0.0
Grand total		15.4	5.0	9.9	3.6

Instead of calculating a simple total of the numbers of events and numbers of patients across all studies, an alternative method is to use a Mantel-Haenszel stratified analysis to combine studies as separate strata, yielding an overall relative risk estimate. This approach is considered appropriate when the data from individual strata are heterogeneous, as is the case here. The Mantel-Haenszel weighted relative risk calculations were performed with the EpiInfo2000 software and are shown below.

Event	Mantel-Haenszel relative risk (95% confidence interval)
Possibly suicide-related events	2.64 (1.19-5.85)
Suicide attempts	2.13 (0.83-5.47)

Another analytic method makes use of person time in the denominator. Guess and colleagues devised a computer "shareware" program to estimate relative risk from a group of studies where the denominators are in units of person-time.[22] Using this software program, a combined relative risk (i.e., incidence rate ratio) was calculated with Fisher binomial confidence limits, considering each study as a separate stratum. The results are shown below.

Event	Mantel-Haenszel incidence rate ratio (95% confidence interval)
Possibly suicide-related events	2.69 (1.17-7.78)
Suicide attempts	2.15 (0.78-7.98)

Thus, the relative risks are somewhat lower with stratified calculations, which are less sensitive to outliers (such as study 329) than a simple totaling of data from all studies. However, the risk ratio is still statistically significant for the category of all possibly suicide-related events. For suicide attempts, the relative risks are not statistically significant, but the point estimates are consistent with the relative risk for the broader category. Note that the relative risks do not differ much according to whether the numbers of patients or patient exposure years are used in the denominators. Because the average duration of treatment was approximately equal for drug and placebo patients, accounting for duration of treatment has little effect on the values of the relative risks.

Rating scale assessments of suicidality during MDD trials

The depression symptom rating scales employed in the MDD trials all included items on which the investigator rated the subject's degree of suicidality. GSK analyzed these data from the suicidality items of the rating scales employed in the trials (i.e., Hamilton Depression Scale (HAMD) item 3, Montgomery Asberg Depression Rating Scale (MADRS) Item 10, and Children's Depression Rating Scale (CDRS) item 13). The proportion of patients developing suicidal ideation during treatment as documented on the rating scale items was approximately the same for the paroxetine and placebo treatment groups. However, examination of the data for the subjects identified as having suicide-related adverse events showed that there was poor correlation between the occurrence of a suicidal adverse event and an increase in the suicidal rating scale item for that same subject. Among the explanations for this were the presence of suicidality at baseline in many cases (which excluded the patients from the analysis), and the absence of a rating at the time of the suicidal adverse event.

Subgroup and other exploratory analyses

Below I will summarize some of the descriptive and subgroup analyses that have been done in an effort to better understand this finding.

Dose

All trials used a flexible dose design. The dose ranges allowed are shown below, along with the duration of double blind treatment.

Study	Dose range (mg/day)	Duration (weeks)
676	10-50	16
329	20-40	8
377	20-40	12
701	10-50	8
453	10-60	16 open/16 double blind
704	10-50	10

Plasma drug concentration sampling was performed in clinical trials 676, 701 and 704. These data had not been analyzed at the time the sponsor submitted the pediatric supplement, however.

To examine the potential influence of dose on these events, it may be useful to consider the two trials with the largest numbers of events on paroxetine treatment, studies 329 and 377. In Study 329, there were 6 paroxetine patients who developed suicidal events while on active treatment; the mean dose for these 6 patients was 22 mg and the mean duration of treatment was 25.5 days. According to the study report, of the three possible paroxetine doses (20, 30 and 40 mg/day), the most frequently administered dose was 20 mg (the mean dose was not provided).

In Study 377, there were 7 paroxetine patients who developed suicidal events while on active treatment, and the mean daily dose and duration of exposure for these patients were 29 mg and 59 days, respectively. The mean dose on active treatment for this trial was 24 mg.

Duration of treatment

GSK reported in their 5-22-03 submission that the mean time to event for subjects developing suicidality was 54 days for paroxetine and 61 days for placebo; thus, there was no apparent relationship with duration of treatment. There was possibly a relationship to discontinuation of treatment, however (please see below).

There were 16 paroxetine patients and 7 placebo patients who had events during active treatment. The time to onset for these events is shown in the figure below. No discernable pattern is evident with respect to the timing of these events, although the numbers of cases are small.

Figure 1. Week of onset of possibly suicide related events during active treatment

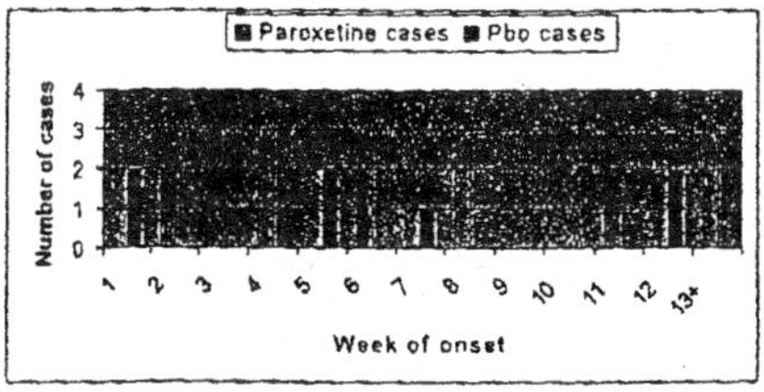

Study

It can be seen from Tables 2 and 3 that study 329 stands out as having the largest differential in suicidal adverse events between drug and placebo, one that is in fact statistically significant. There was also an imipramine arm in that trial, and the incidence of suicidality among patients receiving imipramine was intermediate between the incidence for placebo and that for paroxetine (3 of the 95 imipramine patients experienced possibly suicide-related events, and 1 imipramine patient attempted suicide). No particular investigator or site in study 329 was over-represented among the reports of suicidal events in that trial, according to the site-specific data submitted 7-15-03. Although the incidence of events in the paroxetine arm is the highest seen in this set of trials, the incidence for the placebo arm is lower than in the other MDD trials. The majority of events among paroxetine patients (6 of 8) in study 329 occurred on treatment, and two occurred after treatment discontinuation. As noted previously, the mean dose for the 6 patients on paroxetine was 22 mg, not very different from the modal dose of 20 mg in the trial. One might ask whether the level of severity of depression was more severe among the subjects of study 329 compared to the other trials; however, each MDD trial employed a different depression rating scale, making comparisons across trials difficult. On balance, no obvious factor accounts for the fact that the highest relative risk was observed in study 329.

It may be instructive to examine the relative risks observed for the three depression trials separately. The following shows the relative risk for possibly suicide-related adverse events by study, calculated using the EpiInfo2000 software Fisher's Exact test.

Table 4. Relative risk by study for possibly suicide-related events in MDD trials

Study	Relative risk, possibly suicide-related events	95% CI
329	7.6	0.97 – 59
377	1.2	0.4 - 3.7
701	1.5	0.3 - 8.6

While the relative risk estimates are discrepant, the confidence intervals for the relative risk estimates are wide and overlapping, owing to the small number of events in each study.

It may also be useful to calculate the relative risk excluding study 329 as an outlier. The following table displays the relative risks obtained with and without data from study 329.

Table 5. Relative risks obtained with or without data from Study 329

Event	Including Study 329	Excluding Study 329
Mantel-Haenszel relative risk (95% confidence interval)		
Possibly suicide-related events	2.64 (1.19-5.85)	1.94 (0.80-4.72)
Suicide attempts	2.13 (0.83-5.47)	1.35 (0.49-3.75)
Mantel-Haenszel incidence rate ratio (95% confidence interval)		
Possibly suicide-related events	2.69 (1.17-7.78)	1.95 (0.74-6.29)
Suicide attempts	2.15 (0.78-7.98)	1.35 (0.43-5.06)

This shows that the relative risk estimates omitting data from study 329 are still consistent with drug effect, but are lower and are no longer statistically significant.

With respect to study 453, data from that trial could reasonably have been omitted from these analyses on the basis that it was a relapse prevention study and not an acute treatment study. However, since there were approximately the same number of patients and patient exposure years for both paroxetine and placebo, but no events in either group, the data from the double blind phase of this study has virtually no effect on the overall relative risk estimates. It should be noted, however, that there were 7 patients with serious adverse events involving suicidality during the open label paroxetine run-in phase of this trial that was not included in the above analysis, and 5 of these patients were withdrawn from the trial. Speculatively, this may have resulted in a selection bias, to the extent that patients who successfully completed the open label phase and progressed to randomization may have been those less prone to become suicidal.[23]

Severity of depressive symptoms

Studies 329 and 377 had the largest number of events on paroxetine and may provide insight into the influence of the level of depressive symptoms. In study 329, baseline HAMD total scores were available from narrative summaries for 6 of the 8 paroxetine patients with events, and the mean score among these patients was 20. This is comparable to the mean baseline HAMD score of 19 for both the paroxetine and placebo treatment arms. The sponsor provided the HAMD scores obtained near the time of the event for five of these patients; the change from baseline was worse for two patients, improved for two patients, and unchanged for one patient. In study 377 the MADRS was used to assess depression; the mean baseline MADRS score for the 9 paroxetine patients with events was 27, which is comparable to the mean baseline score of 26 for all paroxetine patients. Among these 9 patients, the MADRS rating near the time of their event was improved from baseline for 4, worse for 4, and unchanged for 1.

Age

Of the 32 suicidal adverse events from the final analysis, only one occurred in a patient under 12 years of age (an 11-year old female patient receiving paroxetine in MDD study 701 experienced suicidal ideation). Thus, the absolute incidence of these events is higher in the adolescent-only subgroup of patients than in the total sample. However, because the vast majority of events occurred in adolescents, the paroxetine:placebo risk ratios for the adolescent patient subgroup differ only marginally from those for the entire sample of subjects. It should be noted, however, that in the open label paroxetine treatment phase of study 453, 4 of the 7 patients with serious adverse events involving suicidal ideation were under 12 years of age; however, these events were not part of the analysis described above, since they occurred during uncontrolled treatment.

To illustrate, the following table displays the adolescent-only subgroup analysis for all MDD trials. The incidence rate ratio is approximately 2 for both types of events, which is consistent with the data from all ages combined, but the adolescent incidences for both paroxetine and placebo are higher than those for the entire sample shown in Table 3.

Table 6. Incidence of events in MDD trials, adolescent patients only

Event	Incidence per 100 person years in adolescent subjects	
	Paroxetine	Placebo
Possibly suicide-related events	31	16
Suicide attempts	24	12

Finally, the largest discrepancy between paroxetine and placebo was observed in study 329, and without this trial the risk is not statistically significant. However, in no trial was a protective effect observed.

Usage data for paroxetine in the pediatric population[2]

An estimate of the number of dispensed paroxetine prescriptions was obtained from IMS Health's National Prescription Audit *Plus*™ (NPA *Plus*™). This estimate includes information from chain, independent, and food stores, long term care facilities, and mail order houses. According to NPA *Plus*™, in 2002 paroxetine was the most frequently prescribed antidepressant drug in the U.S., with an estimated 26.9 million prescriptions for paroxetine dispensed nationwide. Demographic information on paroxetine users was obtained from the National Disease and Therapeutic Index ™ (NDTI™), IMS Health's survey of approximately 2,000-3,000 office-based physicians in the continental United States. This survey provides statistical information about diagnoses, patients, and treatment patterns. According to the National Disease and Therapeutic Index™ (NDTI™) of IMS Health, an estimated 9.3% of all paroxetine use in 2002 was recommended to patients under 20 years of age, in approximately equal proportions by gender. Focusing on the adolescent age group, which is more relevant to the issue of suicide attempts, 7.9% of the total for all ages was for patients aged 12-19 years. Applied to the NPA Plus™ data for total prescriptions dispensed, this 7.9% represents approximately 2.1 million prescriptions for paroxetine in the 12-19 year old age group in 2002. According to the NDTI™ data, the estimated use of paroxetine to treat patients between 12 and 19 years of age increased by 78% between 1997 to 2002.

Data on pediatric use of paroxetine was also obtained from the AdvancePCS database. AdvancePCS is a pharmacy benefit management (PBM) company, currently covering 50 million individuals and processing 300 million prescription claims annually. All dispensed prescriptions paid for by the PBM are captured for each patient, across all prescribers and pharmacies. The demographics of the population covered in the AdvancePCS database appear to be similar to the U.S. population overall. In the AdvancePCS system, paroxetine is the second most commonly dispensed antidepressant for pediatric use, after sertraline. From the AdvancePCS database it is possible to distinguish between patients initiating paroxetine treatment and those refilling prescriptions for continued treatment. If one defines new treatment with paroxetine as a prescription dispensed to a patient who did not have a paroxetine prescription in the preceding 3 months, then in 2002 the majority of paroxetine prescriptions fell into this category (502,160 prescriptions out of a total of 688,552 prescriptions for all ages). Of these 688,552 total paroxetine prescriptions, 30,891 (4.5%) were new prescriptions for patients aged 12-19 years.

Extent of public health impact

To estimate the potential public health impact of this putative effect, it is necessary to make projections based on the clinical trial data. As an estimate of person-years of exposure, using the average length of prescription of one month (Advanced PCS), the number of dispensed paroxetine prescriptions would be equivalent to 177,000 person-years of exposure to paroxetine among adolescent patients nationwide last year. Based on NDTI™ data for the past 2 years, it appears that approximately 40% of adolescent use of paroxetine is for depressive disorders, although the diagnostic information in the NDTI™ data is not always precise. Applied to the

[2] Provided by Gianna Rigoni, Pharm.D., M.S., Division of Surveillance, Research and Communication Support. See Memorandum dated 6-26-03, PID# D030341.

estimate of 177,000 person-years, this would mean approximately 71,000 person-years of paroxetine use for adolescent depression. From table 6, the incidence rate difference for suicide attempts between paroxetine and placebo (i.e., the attributable risk) observed in the MDD trials is 12 per 100 person-years of exposure to paroxetine. If one projects this estimate of the attributable risk to the estimated national use of paroxetine for adolescent depression, there would be an excess of approximately 8,500 suicide attempts annually among adolescents attributable to paroxetine exposure. The severity of self-injury would likely vary considerably, although as previously discussed, a small but difficult to estimate proportion of these attempts would be expected to be successful. Of course, this estimate is very crude, and requires making the untestable assumption that the attributable risk observed in short term clinical trials is applicable to chronic use of the drug in the population. Also, this estimate is not adjusted for gender differences. However, it does illustrate that there are a large number of patients at risk, if this is a real drug effect.

Alternatively, one could assume that the risk only applies to the initial stage of treatment with paroxetine, and thus estimating the impact in the general population would require knowing how many new adolescent patients are started on paroxetine for the treatment of depression. In the MDD clinical trials, the incidence of suicide attempt was 4.0% for paroxetine and 1.8% for placebo, from Table 2 above. This yields an attributable (i.e., placebo-subtracted) risk of 2.2%. As noted above, 4.5% of paroxetine prescriptions in AdvancePCS were new prescriptions for patients aged 12-19 years. Applying this percentage to the 26.9 million estimated national number of prescriptions from NPA *Plus*™ yields an estimate of 1.2 million adolescents initiating treatment with paroxetine in 2002. (For comparison, the total U.S. population aged 10-19 years is approximately 41 million.[24]) Assuming that 40% of the use is for depression (as stated above), this would represent approximately 480,000 new paroxetine prescriptions for the treatment of depression in adolescents. Applying the attributable risk of 2.2% (i.e., the excess risk of suicide attempts with paroxetine compared to placebo that was observed in short-term clinical trials) to the 480,000 new courses of treatment yields an estimate of 10,600 episodes of self-injury associated with paroxetine use. This may be an overestimate since the 2.2% attributable risk was cumulative for trials that were somewhat longer than one month. Also, all of the aforementioned caveats apply equally to this estimate as well.

FEASIBILITY OF PHARMACOEPIDEMIOLOGICAL STUDIES[3]

In the agency's Adverse Event Reporting System (AERS) database, there were a total of 100 reports involving paroxetine use by patients under age 17 that were possibly related to suicide, and of these, 16 were fatal. (These counts are for the entire duration of paroxetine's marketing, but are uncorrected for duplicate reports.)[4] It was decided not pursue further analysis of spontaneous reporting data; in situations where the event of interest is associated with the disease under treatment even in the absence of drug exposure, spontaneous reports are not likely to be informative.

We consulted with Dr. Wayne Ray, a CERTS Principal Investigator at Vanderbilt University Medical Center in Nashville TN, regarding the feasibility of studying this issue with the Tennessee Medicaid claims database. He did not believe such a study would be feasible because of the difficulty in ascertaining suicide attempts in such a database; there is apparently little uniformity in the diagnostic codes that may indicate a suicide attempt. While ascertainment of

---

[3] Grateful acknowledgment is made to Drs. David Graham, Cynthia Kornegay and Parivash Nourjah of ODS for their help with this section.

[4] AERS data provided by Carol Pamer, R.Ph., ODS

completed suicides is much more reliable, adolescent suicides are sufficiently rare that it would be very difficult to accrue a meaningful number of cases. We also investigated the feasibility of approaching this issue using two databases maintained by the Centers for Disease Control (CDC).[25] The National Hospital Ambulatory Medical Care Survey (NHAMCS) collects data on ambulatory patients and emergency room patients from a sample of general hospitals. The National Electronic Injury Surveillance System (NEISS), jointly operated by the CDC and the Consumer Product Safety Commission, obtains data from a sample of 100 hospital emergency departments. Although both NHAMCS and NEISS capture suicide attempts, neither one reliably records the medications used by the patient at the time of the emergency department visit; thus, neither would be suitable for studying an association of paroxetine treatment with adolescent suicide attempts. It is possible that the U.K. General Practice Research Database (GPRD) might be employed to study this question, but FDA at the moment has no formal mechanisms for collaborating with the GPRD. On balance, there is no source of epidemiological data that would be readily available to FDA to study the association of paroxetine treatment with adolescent suicide attempts.

OVERVIEW AND META-ANALYSIS OF DATA ON SUICIDALITY FROM OTHER PEDIATRIC DEVELOPMENT PROGRAMS

In order to examine whether this apparent increase in suicidal behaviors with pediatric use of paroxetine is unique to paroxetine or may occur with other drugs as well, the pediatric development programs for seven other antidepressant and anti-OCD drugs were reviewed. Acute treatment trials ranging from 8-16 weeks in duration were selected for analysis. A brief summary of the clinical trial programs for these drugs, and the available data on self-injurious behaviors follows. The sources for these data were the designated NDA submissions and their corresponding clinical reviews.

Sertraline (NDA 19-839)

The supplement for pediatric OCD indication (S-017) was submitted 12-19-96 and included a single randomized, double blind trial, study 498. In this trial, one placebo patient experienced suicidal ideation. The pediatric exclusivity supplement (S-044, submitted 12-14-01) included two identical randomized, placebo controlled depression studies, protocols 1001 and 1017. The two studies were considered as a single trial for safety analyses. From the table of adverse events (Table 6.2.1 of the combined study report) there were 5 suicidal events with sertraline and 2 with placebo; these events were all considered serious adverse events, and were described in the section of the study report dealing with serious adverse events.

Fluvoxamine (NDA 20-243, supplement 06, submitted 12-21-95)

There was a single randomized, controlled trial supporting the pediatric OCD indication, study 114; one fluvoxamine treated patient in the trial experienced suicidal ideation.

Fluoxetine (NDA 18-936, supplement 63, submitted 9-14-00)

This supplement included two randomized, placebo controlled pediatric depression trials (studies HCJE and X065), and one randomized, placebo controlled OCD trial, study HCJW. The sponsor's Integrated Summary of Safety included a special analysis of suicide attempts. For this, the sponsor conducted a search of the clinical trial database both by examination of serious adverse events and adverse dropouts, and by electronic search for key words in the adverse event verbatim descriptions that suggested suicidal behavior. Final determination of whether the event was a suicide attempt was made by a child psychiatrist blind to treatment assignment. This search showed a total of 3 suicide attempts among fluoxetine patients and 1 in a placebo patient. In the analysis that follows, I used the sponsor's counts of 3 suicide attempts with fluoxetine and 1 with placebo. I note that there were 3 additional adverse events (one with fluoxetine and two with placebo) coded as "intentional injury" but these were apparently not judged to be suicidal. The sponsor did not perform a corresponding search for instances of suicidal ideation without self-injury, but I found no adverse events coded under the term suicidal ideation. (An additional clinical trial in adolescents with depression, study HCCJ, was prematurely stopped and therefor was not included in the sponsor's Integrated Summary of Safety database. Although this trial was stopped after only 40 patients were enrolled, there were 2 suicidal events each for drug and placebo, a comparatively high frequency. I have omitted this trial from the meta-analysis.)

Venlafaxine (NDA 20-151, supplement 024, submitted 9-25-02)
This pediatric exclusivity supplement included two placebo-controlled depression trials, studies 382 and 394, as well as two placebo controlled generalized anxiety disorder (GAD) trials, studies 396 and 397. The sponsor included in the Integrated Summary of Safety a description of events that were considered suicide attempts or suicidal ideation, and I relied upon these descriptions as the source of information regarding the adverse events of interest. The sponsor did not describe how these events were identified from the safety database, however. There were a total of 11 events for venlafaxine and 3 for placebo.

Nefazodone (NDA 20-152 supplement 032, submitted 4-16-02)
This pediatric exclusivity supplement included two randomized, placebo controlled depression trials, studies 141 and 187. In study 187 there was one adverse event of suicide attempt and one adverse event of overdose; from the line listing of adverse events these events were reported simultaneously in the same nefazodone-treated patient, and so were taken to represent a single event (suicide attempt).

Mirtazapine (NDA 20-415 supplement 011, submitted 05-01-01)
The pediatric exclusivity supplement for mirtazapine included two identical placebo-controlled studies, and for the safety analysis the data from these trials was combined. No adverse events in these trials were coded as suicide attempts or suicidal ideation, but from the narrative description of serious adverse events, there was one suicide attempt and one event of suicidal ideation among patients treated with mirtazapine.

Paroxetine: For consistency, I have omitted the data from study 453, the relapse prevention trial in OCD. As noted above, this study contributed no events.

Citalopram (NDA 20-822 supplement 016, submitted 4-18-02)
There were two pediatric randomized, double blind, placebo controlled trials in patients with MDD, studies CIT MD 18 and 94404. In study CIT MD 18 there were two adverse events coded as suicidal tendency; one citalopram treated patient (193/22) cut himself, and one placebo patient (519/13) dropped out for suicidal ideation. In the non-U.S. study 94404 there were 19 adverse events coded as suicide attempts; however, the study report noted that some of these were actually suicidal ideation rather than self-injury. I reviewed the line listing for adverse events (Appendix II.6) and from the verbatim descriptions classified 13 of the 19 events as actual self-injury (11 occurred with citalopram treatment and 2 with placebo treatment). Two of the citalopram treated patients had events after the end of double blind treatment (but within 30 days of discontinuing). In the study report for study 94404 the sponsor noted that there was no difference between citalopram and placebo with respect to the items assessing suicidality on the depression rating scales (Kiddie-SADS-P and MADRS). The sponsor also noted that approximately 30% of the subjects in the study had a history of a suicide attempt, and 14% of the subjects were inpatients at the time of enrollment. However, it was not stated what proportion of

the subjects who had self-injurious behaviors during the study were among those with a history of suicide attempt, or were inpatients.

Methods for meta-analysis

From the available information as suicidal adverse events in these trials, events were categorized as either suicidal ideation or self-injurious behavior. For purposes of consistency with GSK's analysis for paroxetine, instances of suicidal ideation and overt self-injury were combined in the category "possibly suicide-related events," and instances of actual self-injury were designated as "suicide attempts." Thus, the category of "suicide attempts" is a subset of the broader category "possibly suicide-related events." Relative risks were calculated using crude totals and also using a Mantel-Haenszel calculation stratified by study. Comparisons between drugs were made by subgrouping MDD study data for individual drugs.

Results

There were a total of 20 acute treatment placebo-controlled trials with these 8 drugs. In these trials, there were 40 suicide attempts (defined as any self-injurious behavior) among 2213 drug-treated subjects, and 13 suicide attempts among 1901 placebo-treated subjects. The table below displays the counts of events by individual drug and trial, for 8 different pediatric development programs.

Table 7. Suicidal adverse events in short-term, randomized, double blind, placebo controlled trials from eight pediatric antidepressant development programs

Drug	Indication	Study	N		Possibly suicide-related events		Suicide attempts	
			Drug	Placebo	Drug N (%)	Placebo N (%)	Drug N (%)	Placebo N (%)
Paroxetine	MDD	329	93	88	8 (8.6)	1 (1.1)	5 (5.4)	0
	MDD	377	181	95	9 (5.0)	4 (4.2)	8 (4.4)	4 (4.2)
	MDD	701	104	102	3 (2.9)	2 (2.0)	2 (1.9)	1 (1.0)
	OCD	704	99	107	1 (1.0)	0	0	0
	SAD	676	165	157	4 (2.4)	0	1 (0.6)	0
Sertraline	MDD	1001/1017	189	184	5 (2.6)	2 (1.1)	2 (1.1)	2 (1.1)
	OCD	498	92	95	0	1 (1.1)	0	0
Venlafaxine	MDD	382	80	85	5 (6.3)	2 (2.4)	2 (2.5)	2 (2.4)
	MDD	394	102	94	5 (4.9)	0	3 (2.9)	0
	GAD	396	80	84	0	0	0	0
	GAD	397	77	79	1 (1.3)	1 (1.3)	0	1 (1.3)
Fluvoxamine	OCD	114	57	63	1 (1.8)	0	0	0
Mirtazapine	MDD	003-045	170	88	2 (1.2)	0	1 (0.6)	0
Fluoxetine	MDD	HCJE	109	110	0	1 (0.9)	0	1 (0.9)
	MDD	X065	48	48	2 (4.2)	0	2 (4.2)	0
	OCD	HCJW	71	32	1 (1.4)	0	1 (1.4)	0
Nefazodone	MDD	141	102	99	0	0	0	0
	MDD	187	184	94	1 (0.5)	0	1 (0.5)	0
Citalopram	MDD	CIT-MD-18	89	85	1 (1.1)	1 (1.2)	1 (1.1)	0
	MDD	94404	121	112	14 (11.6)	5 (4.5)	11 (9.1)	2 (1.8)

The overall relative risks for all suicidal events and self injury were calculated in two ways, from a simple total (crude relative risk) and from a stratified analysis with each study as a stratum. The results are shown below.

Table 8. Overall relative risk for suicidal events, pediatric antidepressant trials

Event	Crude relative risk (95% confidence interval)	Mantel-Haenszel weighted relative risk (95% confidence interval)
Possibly suicide-related events	2.71 (1.64-4.46)	2.70 (1.65-4.43)
Suicide attempts	2.64 (1.42-4.93)	2.50 (1.35-4.64)

These results indicate an association of both types of events with active drug treatment relative to treatment with placebo. Note that the stratified calculation does not differ greatly from the crude relative risk calculation.

Next, the data were subgrouped according to indication. Table 9 summarizes the data by indication, pooling across drugs.

Table 9. Suicidal adverse events by Indication

Indication	GAD	MDD	OCD	SAD	Total
Total of Drug N	157	1572	319	165	2213
Total of drug possibly suicide-related events	1	55	3	4	63
Total of Drug suicide attempts	0	38	1	1	40
Total of Pbo N	163	1284	297	157	1901
Total of Pbo possibly suicide-related events	1	18	1	0	20
Total of Pbo suicide attempts	1	12	0	0	13

The weighted relative risks for these events in MDD trials and trials in other indications are shown below in Table 10.

Table 10. Relative risks for suicidal events in pediatric trials, by indication

MDD trials	
Event	Mantel-Haenszel weighted relative risk (95% confidence interval)
Possibly suicide-related events	2.58 (1.54-4.35)
Suicide attempts	2.57 (1.36-4.85)
Non-MDD trials	
Possibly suicide-related events	3.87 (0.79-18.87)
Suicide attempts	1.62 (0.12-22.63)

The relative risks for possibly suicide-related events and suicide attempts in trials for indications other than MDD are also greater than one, but have wide confidence intervals compared to the values for MDD trials because these events were less frequent in non-MDD studies.

To assess the impact of the location of the trial (i.e., North America versus outside North America), the MDD studies were classified according to whether they were conducted entirely in the U.S. and Canada or they included overseas sites. Two MDD trials were conducted entirely outside the U.S. (paroxetine study 377 and citalopram study 94404), and the sertraline MDD protocol 1001/1017 included a mixture of U.S. and non-U.S. sites. Excluding these three protocols from the analysis yielded the following results (Table 11). As shown, the association is stronger in the North American trials, but is still somewhat evident in the smaller group of trials with non-North American sites.

Table 11. Relative risks in MDD trials by location

U.S./Canadian MDD trials	
Event	Mantel-Haenszel weighted relative risk (95% confidence interval)
Possibly suicide-related events	3.67 (1.58-8.51)
Suicide attempts	4.09 (1.34-12.48)
MDD trials including non-North American sites	
Possibly suicide-related events	1.97 (1.01-3.86)
Suicide attempts	1.93 (0.88-4.22)

From Table 9 it can be seen that both the majority of patients and the majority of events are from studies of MDD. Also, every development program except that for fluvoxamine included at least two trials in MDD. Accordingly, in order to explore the question of whether these drugs differ in respect to the association with suicidality, comparisons between drugs were made within MDD trial data. For these comparisons, data was totaled across all MDD trials for each drug; i.e., a weighting procedure by study was not employed. The difference in the percentage of patients experiencing events between drug and placebo was calculated, along with 95% confidence intervals for the drug-placebo difference. This allowed calculations for drugs with zero events in the placebo group, which would have prevented expressing the data as a relative risk. The calculations were performed with Stata 7.0 software.

Figure 2 displays the results for possibly suicide-related events. A value of zero in this analysis represents equivalent risk, less than zero a protective effect of the drug, and greater than zero a risk associated with drug treatment. Although the degree of separation between drug and placebo varies, the numerical values for all drugs exceed zero, and for no drug are the data consistent with a protective effect. The drug-placebo difference for the pooled data (not weighted by study) is statistically robust (p-value = 0.0005).

Figure 2. Placebo-subtracted percentage of patients with possibly suicide-related events in pediatric MDD trials, with 95% CIs

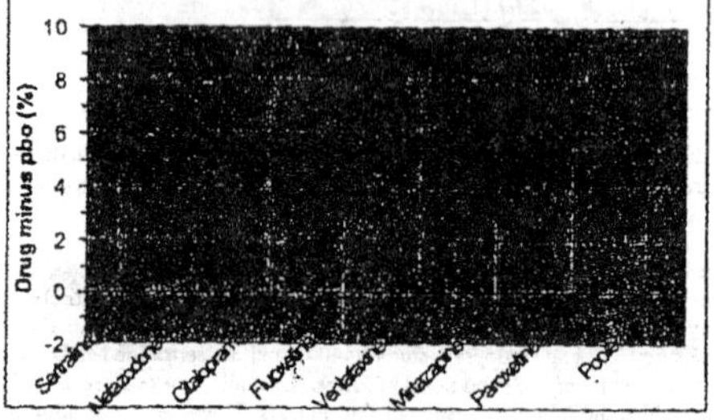

Figure 3 displays a similar analysis for suicide attempts.

Figure 3. Placebo-subtracted percentage of patients with suicide attempts, pediatric MDD trials, with 95% CIs

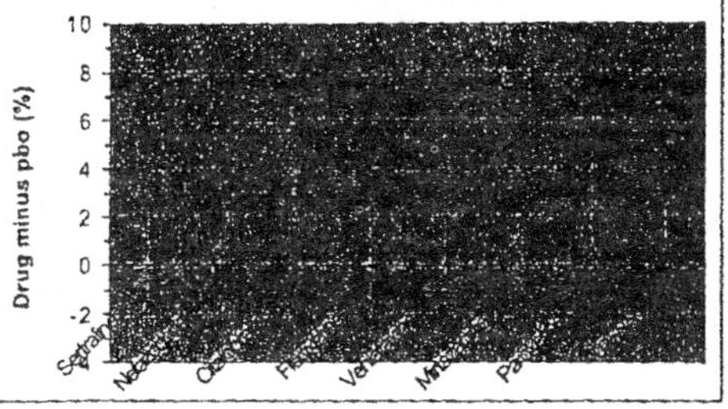

The events were less frequent than for the broader category of suicidality shown above, and hence the confidence intervals are wider. There is also more variability across drugs in the magnitude of the differences between drug and placebo. In this case, citalopram stands out with the largest difference between drug and placebo. This reflects the relatively large number of events in study 94404, which, like study 329 for paroxetine, stands out as showing a large attributable risk (see table 7). As with study 329, there is no immediately obvious explanation for this, although it is true that study 94404 was unusual by virtue of including inpatients. Overall, the pooled data (unweighted by study) are consistent with an association between active drug treatment and suicide attempts, and the difference is statistically robust (p-value = 0.0024).

DISCUSSION AND CONCLUSIONS

The pediatric clinical trial data for paroxetine indicate an association between paroxetine treatment and suicidality (i.e., suicidal ideation and suicide attempts) during acute treatment. A preliminary meta-analysis of data from pediatric development programs for other antidepressant drugs suggests that this association may be a class effect and not confined to paroxetine. Furthermore, the magnitude of the association is non-trivial (i.e., relative risk greater than 2). What is not known is whether there is a constant hazard; i.e., whether the elevated risk persists as long as pediatric patients are taking the drug, or whether it is limited to the early stages of treatment. Conceivably there might even be a protective effect of the drug with long-term use, as some authors have suggested (see above). Accordingly, it might be worthwhile to examine data on suicidal adverse events from long term pediatric studies with these drugs, if such data are available. Typically, however, longer-term studies have been open label (with the exception of a few relapse-prevention studies), and so there would be the problem of finding an appropriate comparison group. In these pediatric supplements, there were only 2 long term controlled trials, study 453 with paroxetine, and study HCJE's relapse prevention segment with fluoxetine.

This meta-analysis should be regarded as preliminary because of several limitations. Although the intent was to be consistent with the methods employed by GSK in their analysis of the paroxetine data, nonetheless, different sponsors employed different methods of ascertainment and classification of suicidal adverse events in the various clinical trials. Also, the influence of dosage was not considered in this analysis; however, the flexible-dose design of the majority of these pediatric clinical trials (i.e., subjects were not randomized to their dosages) would tend to make data on dose at the time of the event relatively uninformative. Additionally, although the data used were limited to short-term trials, duration of treatment at the time of event was not analyzed. Also, this analysis did not attempt to address the influence of drug withdrawal for the other compounds.

On 7-22-03 DNDP sent requests for data on suicidality in pediatric trials to the sponsors of the relevant antidepressant drugs; their responses should provide data on these adverse events that is generated with consistent definitions and search strategies, and will include exposure data in units of person-time. These data will make a more definitive meta-analysis possible. It should also be more feasible to assess the influence of factors such as duration of treatment, dosage, and medication withdrawal from the data that will be supplied in these responses. However, if the preliminary findings are substantiated, this will have broad implications for the pharmacological management of pediatric depressive disorders.

Andrew D. Mosholder, M.D. M.P.H.
Epidemiologist

Mary Willy, Ph.D.
Team Leader

References

[1] American Academy of Child and Adolescent Psychiatry. Practice parameters for the assessment and treatment of children and adolescents with depressive disorders. J Am Acad Child Adolesc Psychiatry 1998; 37(10 supplement)63S-83S.
[2] U.S. Department of Health and Human Services. Mental health: a report of the Surgeon General. Rockville, MD: 1999. Accessed at http://www.surgeongeneral.gov/library/mentalhealth/home.html
[3] Tiecher MH, Glod C, and Cole JO. Emergence of intense suicidal preoccupation during fluoxetine treatment. Am J Psychiatry 1990;147:207-210.
[4] King RA, Riddle MA, Chappell PB et al. Emergence of self-destructive phenomena in children and adolescents during fluoxetine treatment. J Am Acad Child Adolesc Psychiatry 1990;30:179-186
[5] Beasley CM, Dornseif BE, Bosomworth JC, Sayler ME, Rampey AH, Heiligenstein JH, Thompson VL, Murphy DJ, Masica DN. Fluoxetine and suicide: a meta-analysis of controlled trials of treatment for depression. BMJ 1991;303:685-92.
[6] Healy D. Emergence of antidepressant induced suicidality. Primary Care Psychiatry 2000: 6:23-28.
[7] Jick SS, Dean AD, Jick H. Antidepressants and suicide. BMJ 1995;310:215-8.
[8] Committee on Safety of Medicines. Current problems in pharmacovigilance 2000;26:11-12.
[9] Khan A, Warner HA, Brown WA. Symptom reduction and suicide risk in patients treated with placebo in antidepressant clinical trials: an analysis of the Food and Drug Administration database. Arch Gen Psychiatry 2000; 57:311-317.
[10] Storosum JG, van Zwieten BJ, van den Brink W, et al. Suicide risk in placebo-controlled studies of major depression. Am J Psychiatry 2001; 158:1271-1275.
[11] Hammad TA, Mosholder A, Boehm G, Racoosin JA, Laughren T. Incidence of suicide in randomized controlled trials of patients with major depressive disorder (abstract). International Society of Pharmacoepidemiology annual meeting, Philadelphia PA, August 2003.
[12] Minino AM and Smith BL. Deaths: preliminary data for 2000. National Vital Statistics Reports, Volume 49, No. 12, October 9, 2001; accessed at http://www.cdc.gov/nchs/data/nvsr/nvsr49/nvsr49_12.pdf
[13] National Center for Health Statistics. Health, United States, 2002 With Chartbook on Trends in the Health of Americans. Hyattsville, Maryland: 2002. Accessed at http://www.cdc.gov/nchs/data/hus/tables/2002/02hus047.pdf
[14] American Academy of Child and Adolescent Psychiatry. Practice parameter for the assessment and treatment of children and adolescents with suicidal behavior. J Am Acad Child Adolesc Psychiatry 2001; 40 (7 supplement):24S-51S.
[15] Maris RW. Suicide. Lancet 2002;360:319-26.
[16] CDC. Nonfatal self-inflicted injuries treated in hospital emergency departments—United States, 2000. Morb Mortal Wkly Rep 2002;51:436-8.
[17] CDC. Fatal and nonfata suicide attempts among adolescents: Oregon, 1988-1993. Morb Mortal Wkly Rep 1995;44:312-314.
[18] Gould MS, Greenberg T, Velting DM, Shaffer D. Youth suicide risk and preventive interventions: a review of the past 10 years. J Am Acad Child Adolesc Psychiatry 2003; 42:386-405.
[19] Olfson M, Marcus SC, Wiessman MM, and Jensen PS. National trends in the use of psychotropic medications by children. J Am Acad Child Adolesc Psychiatry 2002;41:514-521.
[20] Hall WD, Mant A, Mitchell PB, et al. Association between antidepressant prescribing and suicide in Australia, 1991-2000: trend analysis. BMJ 2003;326:1008-1013.
[21] Isacsson G. Suicide prevention—a medical breakthrough? Acta Psychiatr Scand 2000;102:113-117.
[22] Guess HA, Lydick EG, Small RD, Miller LP. Epidemiologic programs for computers and calculators. Exact binomial confidence intervals for the relative risk in follow-up studies with sparsely stratified incidence density data. Am J Epidemiol 1987;125:340-7.
[23] Personal communication from Dr. Cathy Petersen of Health Canada to Dr. Thomas Laughren of DNDP.
[24] U.S. Census Bureau July 1, 2002 Population Estimates, accessed at www.census.gov
[25] For a description of these databases see www.cdc.gov

This is a representation of an electronic record that was signed electronically and this page is the manifestation of the electronic signature.

/s/

Andy Mosholder
9/5/03 08:44:02 AM
DRUG SAFETY OFFICE REVIEWER

Mark Avigan
9/5/03 08:54:10 AM
DRUG SAFETY OFFICE REVIEWER

Rappaport, Bob A; Shames, Daniel A; Simon, Lee; Smith, Nancy D (CDER); Soreth, Janice M; Talarico, Lilia; Throckmorton, Douglas C; Trontell, Anne E; West, Robert L
Subject: Regulatory Briefing - Paxil SPECIAL
When: Tuesday, September 16, 2003 2:00 PM-4:00 PM (GMT-05:00) Eastern Time (US & Canada).
Where: CDER OCD LAPTOP; CDER EOS PROXIMA; CDER WOC2 6FL-G Conf Room

NDA 20-031/S-073
Paxil (paroxetineHCl) Tablets
This supplement provides for controlled clinical studies in children and adolescents with major depressive disorder (MDD) and obsessive compulsive disorder (OCD). The controlled studies in the pediatric population with MDD demonstrated that pediatric patients who received Paxil had a higher incidence of suicidal ideation/attempts. This supplement received an approvable action on October 10, 2002. GlaxoSmithKline has not submitted a complete response to this action letter.

Andy

Tab 9

> -----Original Message-----
> **From:** David, Paul A
> **Sent:** Wednesday, August 27, 2003 10:00 AM
> **To:** Mosholder, Andrew D
> **Subject:** RE: JAMA article on Zoloft in pediatric depression
>
> Thanks for the reprints Andy. It made for some interesting
> reading. I forwarded them to the peds suicide team as well
> as the psych reviewers.
>
> I've been working with Jennifer Mercier on the Regulatory
> Briefing, and she is going to get back to me in a few days
> with the date. I believe that you are Tarek will be presenting.
>
> We're also starting to get responses from our pediatric
> suicide data request letters, and I believe that Judy is
> going to talk to you about looking at the data. I'm
> receiving lots of desk copies so it should not be a problem
> to forward the submissions to you.
>
> -Paul
>
> -----Original Message-----
> **From:** Mosholder, Andrew D
> **Sent:** Wednesday, August 27, 2003 9:30 AM
> **To:** David, Paul A
> **Subject:** JAMA article on Zoloft in pediatric depression
>
> Hi Paul,
> I downloaded the JAMA articles referred to in today's Daily
> Clips. Please share with anyone else over their who's interested.
> As you recall, we turned down this supplement because each
> trial by itself failed. This article combines the two trials
> to show a statistically significant effect. I don't see
> where they've said that the individual trials failed and they
> had to pool them to have a result. Instead, the authors tout
> the combined analysis for having a large sample size...talk
> about spin!
> Andy
>
> << File: Varley editorial JAMA.pdf >> << File: Wagner et al
> JAMA.pdf >>

Mosholder, Andrew D

From: Katz, Russell G
Sent: Wednesday, September 17, 2003 8:31 AM
To: Mosholder, Andrew D
Subject: yesterday's reg briefing

Tab 10

Andy-

I had to run out of the meeting yesterday to go to my next meeting, but I just wanted to thank you for a superb presentation (not to mention all the work that went into it). I believe everyone was duly impressed, as they should have been. What the next step is, I don't know yet, but we'll probably get together soon to figure it out. I believe the charge from the group was to "get to the bottom of this", so I guess that's what we'll do.

Anyway, we'll be in touch, but thanks again for all the work and the presentation-it was great.

Rusty

Mosholder, Andrew D

Tab 11

From:	Willy, Mary E
Sent:	Friday, October 03, 2003 7:42 AM
To:	Avigan, Mark I; Mosholder, Andrew D
Subject:	FW: October Pediatric Advisory Subcommittee discussion

FYI

Mary Willy, PhD
Office of Drug Safety
(301) 827-3175

-----Original Message-----

From:	Katz, Russell G
Sent:	Thursday, October 02, 2003 4:18 PM
To:	Willy, Mary E
Cc:	Laughren, Thomas P; Racoosin, Judith A
Subject:	RE: October Pediatric Advisory Subcommittee discussion

Mary-

I thought we had already decided that presenting the data in October is inadvisable. We recognize that some folks outside the division have concluded that there is enough of a signal already established to make some sort of a meaningful statement about the data, but we haven't, and we think that publically presenting part of the data in its current state has the great potential to be misleading and uninformative. I recognize that people want to inform the Committee, but we think it's not a good idea at this time. A simple statement that we're working on it (I recognize that many find this unsatisfying), or some slightly expanded version of this, would be best, from our point of view.

Let me know what you think.

Thanks,
Rusty

-----Original Message-----

From:	Willy, Mary E
Sent:	Thursday, October 02, 2003 2:48 PM
To:	Katz, Russell G; Racoosin, Judith A; Laughren, Thomas P; Andreason, Paul J; Murphy, Dianne; Murphy, Shirley; Cummins, Susan; Iyasu, Solomon; Trontell, Anne E; Avigan, Mark I; Seligman, Paul
Cc:	Mosholder, Andrew D; Willy, Mary E; Pamer, Carol
Subject:	October Pediatric Advisory Subcommittee discussion

Andy and I had a follow-up discussion this morning about the October Pediatric Advisory Subcommittee. Since we are obligated to discuss paroxetine, we wonder if it there might be some benefit to providing the committee members with an update of the paroxetine/ suicidiality issue (first half of Andy's analysis in his Sept 5, 03 consult that addresses paroxetine). Andy (or someone else) could give a brief review of the analysis (with appropriate caveats) and a description of the plan for further analysis. This would provide the committee members an update and also let them know in some detail what remains to be done. Let us know if you think this is desirable and if you would like us to prepare a short summary slide presentation.

Mary Willy, PhD
Office of Drug Safety
(301) 827-3175

Mosholder, Andrew D

Tab 12

From: Mosholder, Andrew D
Sent: Tuesday, October 28, 2003 12:06 PM
To: Willy, Mary E
Subject: Meeting on Pediatric Suicide Patient Narratives

Hi Mary. Here's the report on this meeting.

Tom has identified a group at Columbia University, led by Kelly Posner and Larry Greenhill, that has done studies of suicidal behavior, and has an algorithm for classifying cases according to the following categories.

1. Actual attempt
2. Interrupted attempt (e.g., the patient was discovered tying a noose)
3. Hospitalization for suicidal ideation
4. Emergency department visit for suicidal ideation

This group is apparently willing to review all 130+ cases for the agency at no charge. This is probably by far the most expedient way to get the cases reviewed by the Feb meeting, and so Neuropharm is going to pursue this.

The Columbia group excludes non-suicidal self injury, even if deliberate, but that could be another category. We would probably collapse categories 3 and 4.

I believe I argued successfully for not discounting cases of non-suicidal deliberate self-injury altogether, so that those cases can be preserved for a separate analysis. I also did my best to point out that the new analysis has to be viewed in the context of our previous analyses, and that these are all simply different ways of looking at the same dataset. I also pointed out that the more categories we have, the fewer events in each category, and thus the less statistical power.

For the purpose of this exercise, we are going to ask all the sponsors to send narratives for the cases they excluded (some have done this already, which is why the number of narratives is higher than the number of suicide-related events).

Neuropharm is optimistic that the covariate analysis can be completed by Feb 2.

-Andy

> -----Original Appointment-----
> **From:** David, Paul A
> **Sent:** Friday, October 24, 2003 7:05 AM
> **To:** David, Paul A; Laughren, Thomas P; Racoosin, Judith A;
> Mosholder, Andrew D; Chiao, Evelyn
> **Cc:** Stasko, Robert; Dubitsky, Gregory M
> **Subject:** Pediatric Suicide Patient Narratives
> **When:** Tuesday, October 28, 2003 10:30 AM-11:30 AM (GMT-05:00)
> Eastern Time (US & Canada).
> **Where:** CDER WOC2 4FL-E Conf Room
>
> Follow-up meeting to our 10-21-03 meeting
> ***********
> Internal meeting to discuss the following:
> 1) logistics of extracting the narratives from the
> submissions responding to our first pediatric suicide data
> request letter
> 2) redacting the narratives
> 3) setting up a definition(s) of pediatric suicidality
> 4) selection of participants to review blinded narratives

Tab 13

From: Murphy, Dianne
Sent: Wednesday, December 10, 2003 7:17 PM
To: Jenkins, John K; Galson, Steven; Woodcock, Janet; Henderson, Deborah J; Kweder, Sandra L; Oliva, Armando; Hess, Maureen; Lemley, Lee; Martin, Terry; Crescenzi, Terrie L; Goldkind, Sara; Iyasu, Solomon
Cc: Temple, Robert; Katz, Russell G; Axelrad, Jane A; Murphy, Shirley; Roberts, Rosemary
Subject: RE: FYI: Drugs for depressed children banned in the U.K.

John,
Did not mean to imply that. Was simply providing as background for the very discussion you are suggesting, as the companies did know about the October meeting. We are very cognizant of needing to inform companies when we are reporting on their AE's to the AC. I will have to check, but GSK may have been notified of our intent to discuss Paxil's AE's at the October meeting and then we removed it from the FR and discussion. Cannot recall for certain the sequence of events and think we should find out what we have done already. I agree that does not negate the need to inform re the February meeting. Am trying to put the picture in context of previous activities for those who were not previously involved.
Dianne

-----Original Message-----
From: Jenkins, John K
Sent: Wednesday, December 10, 2003 6:28 PM
To: Murphy, Dianne; Galson, Steven; Woodcock, Janet; Henderson, Deborah J; Kweder, Sandra L; Oliva, Armando; Hess, Maureen; Lemley, Lee; Martin, Terry; Crescenzi, Terrie L; Goldkind, Sara; Iyasu, Solomon
Cc: Temple, Robert; Katz, Russell G; Axelrad, Jane A; Murphy, Shirley; Roberts, Rosemary
Subject: RE: FYI: Drugs for depressed children banned in the U.K.

Dianne

Not sure I understand your point. The issues I am raising relate to ensuring that we follow proper procedures with regard to presentation of data from unapproved supplements in a public meeting so that we do not violate our disclosure rules and also to ensure that sponsors are provided a reasonable opportunity to present their views on the data at the meeting. I am not suggesting we not have the meeting.

John

-----Original Message-----
From: Murphy, Dianne
Sent: Wednesday, December 10, 2003 2:56 PM
To: Jenkins, John K; Galson, Steven; Woodcock, Janet; Henderson, Deborah J; Kweder, Sandra L; Oliva, Armando; Hess, Maureen; Lemley, Lee; Martin, Terry; Crescenzi, Terrie L; Goldkind, Sara; Iyasu, Solomon
Cc: Temple, Robert; Katz, Russell G; Axelrad, Jane A; Murphy, Shirley; Roberts, Rosemary
Subject: RE: FYI: Drugs for depressed children banned in the U.K.

I see we are having a meeting tomorrow about this issue.

Pasted below is the information from the transcripts of the last Pediatric Advisory Subcommittee in October, where we were suppose to report on Paxil and did not. It states that we are not reviewing a certain product, even though it was mandated we were to do so, because of issues that need further assessment. I then quote the October 2003 Talk Paper stating FDA is issuing a Public Health Advisory concerning reports of suicidality in pediatric patients being treated with antidepressant medications for major depressive disorder. The Talk Paper specifically mentions Paxil and also includes it in the list of 8 drugs that are named in the Talk Paper and the Health Advisory. The committee is told that FDA is deferring review of any of the products in this class until the February 2nd AC.

RE FYI Drugs for depressed children banned in the U.K. .txt

This is being provided as some of the background activity that has already occurred relevant to this issue.

Transcript copy:
Before we move into the presentation by Dr. Iyasu and the division on the product safety update on the products that have been granted exclusivity, I needed to tell the committee that there is a product that was to be -- its due date was for this meeting. Let's put it that way. And to bring your attention to an FDA talk paper that was released this week in case you did not see that. The talk paper is that FDA issues public health advisory reports of suicidality in pediatric patients being treated with antidepressant medications for major depressive disorder. I wanted you to know that FDA -- I'm going to read from this just so you'll know why we're moving some of these products to the next meeting that will occur in February.

FDA has completed a preliminary review of reports for eight antidepressant drugs -- I'm not going to list them all -- all studied under the pediatric exclusivity provisions of FDAMA. We note to date that the data do not clearly establish an association between the use of these drugs and increased suicidal thoughts or actions by pediatric patients. Nevertheless, it is not possible at this point to rule out an increased risk of these adverse events for any of these drugs, including Paxil, which was the subject of an FDA talk paper on June 19th, 2003.

Because of this issue, we are deferring review of any of the products in this class until February, of which I hope many of you have already been notified about the date of February 2nd, those of you on the Pediatric Advisory Subcommittee. In order to promote a public discussion of the data and pertinent regulatory actions, FDA has scheduled a meeting on February 2nd, 2004 before the Psychopharmacologic Drugs Advisory committee and the Pediatric Subcommittee of the Anti-Infective Drug Advisory Committee. So that is information to you why we may not be presenting products in this area that may have -- indicate that we should be discussing them because we will be delaying that until February.

That is all the housekeeping that I needed to do. Thank you very much.

-----Original Message-----
From: Jenkins, John K
Sent: Wednesday, December 10, 2003 8:03 AM
To: Galson, Steven; Woodcock, Janet; Henderson, Deborah J; Kweder, Sandra L; Oliva, Armando; Hess, Maureen; Lemley, Lee; Martin, Terry
Cc: Temple, Robert; Katz, Russell G; Axelrad, Jane A; Murphy, Dianne; Murphy, Shirley; Roberts, Rosemary; Jenkins, John K
Subject: FW: FYI: Drugs for depressed children banned in the U.K.
Importance: High

Steven and others

See the attached. The UK is apparently banning the use of all SSRIs other than Prozac in patients under the age of 18. This is a significant extension of their prior ban on Paxil and Efexor. I'm sure this will get press attention here in the US. We should alert the press office and do any necessary alerts. I think that Russ Katz should be our spokesperson on this issue. As you know, we are planning an AC meeting on this issue in early February. Some issues came up yesterday about the planning for the meeting with regard to our plans to present the clinical trial data for the unapproved supplements. I spoke with Jane and Russ about these issues and I will arrange for a meeting/telecon for tomorrow to sort these out. Basically, the issues revolve around our plans to present unblinded Paxil clinical trial data and to what degree GSK has been offered the opportunity to submit a briefing package and to make a presentation at the meeting (also the issue of whether we need their approval to present their data in public on this safety issue). The other issue relates to our plan to present the data from the other drugs in a blinded fashion and what our obligations are under the law with regard to protecting confidential information from disclosure and what role the sponsors of these drugs should be offered in the meeting.

Tab 14

-----Original Message-----
From: Mosholder, Andrew D
Sent: Wednesday, December 17, 2003 3:50 PM
To: Avigan, Mark I
Cc: Willy, Mary E; Trontell, Anne E
Subject: Consult: Suicidal events in pediatric clinical trials of antidepressants (follow-up to September consult)

consult
12-17-03.doc

Hello Mark,
This is ready for your sign-off. It's a follow-up to the previous consult on this topic.
Mary, I added one sentence about how Lilly did not follow-up patients after the fluoxetine clinical trials, as per our discussion; otherwise it's the same document that you OK'd.
Anne, fyi, this is the consult Mary and I were referring to today.

Thanks all,
Andy

MEMORANDUM

DEPARTMENT OF HEALTH AND HUMAN SERVICES
PUBLIC HEALTH SERVICE
FOOD AND DRUG ADMINISTRATION
CENTER FOR DRUG EVALUATION AND RESEARCH

PID# D030341

DATE:

FROM: Andrew D. Mosholder, M.D., M.P.H., Epidemiologist

THROUGH: Mark Avigan, M.D., Director
Division of Drug Risk Evaluation, HFD-430

TO: Russell Katz, M.D., Director
Division of Neuropharmacological Drug Products, HFD-120

SUBJECT: Suicidality in pediatric clinical trials with paroxetine and other antidepressant drugs: Follow-up to 9-4-03 consult

Drugs: paroxetine, sertraline, venlafaxine, fluoxetine, fluvoxamine, citalopram, nefazodone, mirtazapine, and bupropion

EXECUTIVE SUMMARY

This consult is a follow-up to the previous consult on this topic, dated 9-5-03. As described in that consult, GlaxoSmithKline (GSK) performed an analysis of suicidal behaviors in their paroxetine pediatric clinical trial database, and found that there was a statistically significant increase in suicide-related adverse events for paroxetine-treated subjects compared to placebo. The method GSK used for their analysis involved an electronic search of the adverse event data for certain events that might have represented suicidal behaviors, followed by a blinded review of these events to select those that appeared to be probably related to suicide. In July 2003, the Division of Neuropharmacological Drug Products (DNDP) requested the sponsors of the other antidepressant drugs to replicate GSK's analysis in their own pediatric clinical trial databases. This consult summarizes the results of these analyses for 22 short-term placebo-controlled trials involving 9 different antidepressant drugs.

These trials included a total of 4250 pediatric subjects, 2298 treated with active drug and 1952 treated with placebo. There were 108 patients with suicide-related events (74 on active drug and 34 on placebo); 78 of these adverse events were serious (54 on active drug and 24 on placebo).

Considering individual development programs separately, the data for venlafaxine and paroxetine showed a statistically significant increase in suicide-related events relative to placebo. Additionally, on one measure (the incidence rate difference for serious suicide-related events) the data for citalopram approached statistical significance (p-value = 0.063). The relative risks for suicide related events with two compounds, fluoxetine and mirtazapine, were below one, consistent with a protective effect. However, the mirtazapine relative risk estimate of 0.5 was based on a very small number of events and had very broad confidence intervals. The relative risk of suicide-related events for fluoxetine was 0.9 (95% confidence limits 0.3-2.3). (For all the other drugs, the relative risk estimates were greater than one.)

Overall, comparing active drug treatment to placebo, there was an association of suicide-related events (incidence rate difference 0.08/year, p-value = 0.002) and serious suicide-related events (incidence rate difference 0.06/year, p-value = 0.006) with active drug treatment. This association was observed principally in major depressive disorder (MDD) trials, where the relative risk was 1.80 (95% confidence limit 1.18—2.74) and the attributable risk (drug rate minus placebo rate) was 0.10 per patient-year of exposure to drug (p-value = 0.013). For serious suicide-related events in MDD trials, the relative risk was 1.94 (95% confidence interval 1.18–3.18), and the attributable risk was 0.085 events per patient-year of exposure to drug (p-value = 0.015), equivalent to approximately 1 excess serious suicide-related event per 12 years of drug treatment. For non-MDD trials, the data also showed a higher rate of events with active drug treatment, but the attributable risk for serious events was much smaller than for MDD trials (0.01/year), and the data were not statistically significant.

There are a number of limitations to this analysis, the chief among them being that the clinical trial data are limited to short-term use of these drugs. Unfortunately, there are not comparable data available regarding safety and efficacy of long-term use of these drugs in pediatric patients.

At the present time, a number of additional steps are under way to enhance the quality of the data for the assessment of this signal. These initiatives include arranging for a blinded review of the clinical trial cases by suicidology experts at Columbia University, requesting additional details on how each sponsor conducted their analysis, and obtaining electronic clinical trial datasets for each study to permit a more sophisticated statistical analysis.

However, while these efforts will yield valuable information, particularly at the level of the data for individual trials and drugs, in my view it is unlikely that the new information will alter the basic finding of an association of suicide-related events and serious suicide-related events with active treatment. This is because of the strength of the observed association and the statistical robustness of the overall finding. Also, it seems less likely that misclassification or failure to identify relevant events would produce a false positive signal; rather, those types of errors tend to weaken a signal. Only systematic bias could be reasonably expected to yield a false positive signal of this magnitude, and that seems unlikely.

Given this signal of an important risk, which is on the order of one serious suicide-related event per 11 years of active treatment for MDD, the fact that off-label use of this class of drugs in pediatric patients is extremely widespread, the probability that these additional analyses will take many months to complete, and the observation that the risk appears greatest for the off-label treatment of MDD, I recommend that the agency take active steps at the present time to warn patients and health care providers of the risk of off-label use of these compounds, and to minimize their off-label use for MDD.

BACKGROUND

This memorandum is in follow-up to our consult to DNDP dated 9-5-03. On May 22 of this year, GlaxoSmithKline submitted an analysis of adverse events related to suicidal behaviors in pediatric trials of paroxetine (Paxil, NDA 20-031). The sponsor performed this analysis by conducting an automated, electronic search of the safety database from their pediatric trials for adverse event terms that would suggest suicidal behaviors. This analysis showed a statistically significant increase in such behaviors with paroxetine treatment, compared to placebo. The consult of 9-4-03 reviewed these data, and also provided a preliminary analysis of data from seven other pediatric development programs for other antidepressant drugs. Overall, there was a statistically significant increase in suicidal adverse events for active drug treatment compared to placebo, similar to the findings from the paroxetine trials. These findings were discussed at a CDER Regulatory Briefing held on 9-16-03.

However, this preliminary review of pediatric trials with the other antidepressant drugs was limited to a manual search of the reports submitted to FDA. In order to provide a meaningful comparison to the paroxetine findings, the Division of Neuropharmacological Drug Products requested the sponsors of eight other drugs (sertraline, venlafaxine, fluoxetine, fluvoxamine, citalopram, nefazodone, mirtazapine, and bupropion) to conduct a search of their databases similar to the analysis performed by GlaxoSmithKline. All of the 8 sponsors responded to this request within the next few months. The purpose of this memorandum is to summarize the findings reported in those submissions.

With respect to pediatric indications for the antidepressant drugs, clomipramine, fluvoxamine, sertraline and fluoxetine are approved for pediatric obsessive compulsive disorder. (Clomipramine is an older tricyclic compound that was not part of this analysis.) For pediatric major depressive disorder, the only drug approved is fluoxetine. Appendix table 5 presents a summary of the efficacy results from placebo-controlled trials with the aforementioned drugs, along with the regulatory status of the drugs for pediatric use.

METHODS

The sponsors of the aforementioned 8 drugs all received identical information request letters from DNDP dated 7-22-03. The letters asked for the following analyses for all randomized, placebo-controlled trial involving pediatric subjects (the indented text below is reproduced from the letters):

> The identification of the following events should be done blinded to treatment to avoid bias. All adverse events occurring within 30 days of the last dose of drug should be included in the search.
>
> "Suicide-related events" should be identified using the following algorithm:
> • Any events coded to preferred terms that include the text strings "suic" or "overdos"
> • Exclude "accidental overdose" cases
> • Regardless of the preferred term to which the verbatim term is mapped, all verbatim terms should be searched for the following text strings: "attempt", "cut", "gas", "hang", "hung", "jump", "mutilat-", "overdos-", "self damag-", "self harm", "self inflict", "self injur-", "shoot", "slash", "suic-"
> • Any terms identified by this search because the text string was a substring of an unrelated word should be excluded (for example, the text string "cut" might identify the word "acute")
> • In addition to the algorithm above, narratives of all serious adverse events (SAEs) should be reviewed (in a blinded fashion) to identify any additional cases of suicidality or self- harm. In particular, SAEs related to mania and hostility should be examined closely for suicidality or self-harm.
> • Any death found to be due to suicide or overdose should be included (if not already identified by the previous search methods).
>
> We are also interested in an analysis of suicide attempts. "Suicide attempts" are a subset of the "suicide-related events" identified above; they should be identified using a blinded hands-on review of the records of all patients identified by the above algorithm as having a "suicide-related event". For the purposes of this analysis, any case in which the patient exhibited self-injurious behavior should be considered as a suicide attempt. Any case in which the patient's suicidal ideation did not lead to self-injurious behavior should be excluded from this subset.
>
> Separate analyses should be performed for the group of "suicide-related" events and the group of "suicide attempts". Both the risk (# of events/# of patients) and the rate (# of events/person-time exposure) should be presented by treatment group. All treatment groups should be presented, including active controls. If

a study has a blinded extension phase, events identified while the patient is in that extension phase should be excluded.

In addition to presenting the overall risks and rates across all indications and within each indication, the following stratified analyses should be performed:
• Child (<12) vs. Adolescent (>= 12).
• On-therapy vs. On-therapy + 30 days.
• Within each indication, data from each trial should be presented separately.

Also requested were detailed clinical data about the patients identified as having suicidal events, in the form of narrative summaries and tabulations.

The analyses submitted by each sponsor are summarized herein. A brief description of the relevant pediatric clinical trials is presented for each drug. Also, Appendix table 3 lists each pediatric subject having a suicide-related event.

Although I reviewed all the narrative summaries of the identified adverse events, I have not reclassified any events myself; the sponsors maintained the blind on treatment when they categorized these events, and this is obviously not possible for me. Instead, I have simply noted the few cases where in my opinion a different classification of the event might reasonably have been made. For a few patients who experienced more than one event of interest, I have chosen to count each patient only once in the analysis, at the time of their first event; their subsequent events are described under "Comments" in appendix table 3. Also described under "Comments" are any other adverse events that were prominently associated with the suicidal events. For a few of the clinical development programs, there were a sufficient number of cases to warrant a discussion of possible contributing clinical factors such as dose and duration of treatment, and I have included those details where appropriate.

Also included is a summary analysis of the clinical trial data, both overall and by drug and indication, with statistical testing. This analysis examines the question of the association of these events with active drug treatment in two ways: by calculation of the attributable risk (more precisely, the incidence rate difference between drug and placebo), as well as the relative risk (i.e., incidence rate ratios for drug:placebo). All statistical calculations were performed with Stata version 7.0 software. (Grateful acknowledgement is made to Dr. Yi Tsong of OPSS for his comments on the statistical methods.)

RESULTS

Including the previously reviewed data on paroxetine, this analysis comprised a total of 22 randomized, placebo-controlled trials with 9 different antidepressant drugs in the pediatric population. A total of 2298 pediatric subjects were exposed to active drug, for a total of 406.9 patient-years; for placebo, there were 1952 subjects exposed for a total of 347.6 patient-years. (One trial, Study 329 for paroxetine, included an imipramine arm as an active control, but I have omitted those data from this analysis. Also, patient-years of exposure were not available for the single trial with bupropion.)

The sponsors identified a total of 108 patients with suicide-related events in these trials, 74 on active drug and 34 on placebo. There were no completed suicides. All 83 patients with suicide-related events described in the previous consult were included among these 108 patients. Seventy-eight patients had events classified as serious (54 on drug and 24 on placebo), and 75 had events classified as "suicide attempts" under the method described above (with 49 suicide attempts on drug, and 26 on placebo). Appendix table 1 presents the complete data on the numbers of these events from all 22 clinical trials, and Appendix table 2 presents the derived rates of these events for each trial. Appendix figures 1-4 depict graphically the rates enumerated in Appendix table 2, for MDD and non-MDD studies. Note that the placebo rates of events vary considerably from trial to trial, even within the subgroup of MDD studies. With respect to the classification of events, discussion at the 9-16-03 CDER Regulatory Briefing and subsequently has raised questions about the appropriateness of the "suicide attempts" classification, since this category actually includes all types of deliberate self-injury. Accordingly, in the following I have chosen to emphasize the category of serious suicide-related events, rather than the category of suicide attempts, as being perhaps more clinically meaningful. The data for the category "suicide attempt" are included in Appendix tables 1 and 2 for completeness.

Overview of each sponsor's submission.

Bupropion (Wellbutrin, NDA 18-644, GlaxoSmithKline, submission dated 8-22-03)

There were no pediatric studies for the indications of major depressive disorder (MDD) or smoking cessation. There was one placebo-controlled pediatric study for the indication of attention deficit hyperactivity disorder (ADHD), as shown below. The requested electronic search of adverse event data revealed no suicide-related events in this study.

Indication	Protocol	No. of sites	Age range (yrs)	Duration (wks)	N	
					Bupropion	Placebo
ADHD	75	4	6-12	6	71	36

Thus, there are no available data on pediatric suicidality with bupropion in the relevant patient populations.

Mirtazapine (Remeron, NDA 20-415, Organon, submission dated 8-21-03 and email dated 11-24-03)

There was only one clinical protocol in the mirtazapine development program, described below; the sponsor conducted two identical studies under that protocol, which were combined for the analysis of safety information.

Indication	Protocol	No. of sites	Age range (yrs)	Duration (wks)	Dose (mg/day)	N	
						Mirtazapine	Placebo
MDD	003-045	34	7-17	8	15-45	170	88

The electronic search of the adverse events terms in study 003-045 yielded a total of 13 adverse events; these were listed in Organon's email submission dated 11-24-03. Of these 13 events, 10 were obviously not related to suicidal behaviors and were excluded, leaving 3 cases for further review; one of these cases ocurred pre-randomization and so was not part of the analysis. Additionally, a subject who was hospitalized for suicidal ideation was identified from the review of all serious adverse events (subject 0404), yielding a total of 3 cases, summarized in Appendix table 3. Note, however, that Organon excluded one of these events from the analysis: subject 0801, a 9 year old boy receiving mirtazapine treated in the emergency room for an overdose on 4 Depakote tablets. This was not considered a suicide attempt because the boy took the tablets "on a dare."

Fluoxetine (Prozac, NDA 18-936, Lilly)

N.B. The following summary is based primarily upon Lilly's submission to Health Canada dated 10-7-03, and not their submission to FDA dated 9-2-03, because Lilly discovered an additional fluoxetine-associated event while preparing their Canadian submission. For details, please refer to Lilly's correspondence dated 10-9-03.

There were four clinical trials relevant to this analysis, three in MDD and one in obsessive-compulsive disorder (OCD). Study HCCJ, a pilot study in adolescent depression, was excluded from the sponsor's Integrated Summary of Safety for the pediatric supplement, but is included in this analysis.

Indication	Study	No. of sites	Age range (yrs)	Duration (wks)	Dose (mg/day)	N	
						Fluoxetine	Pbo
OCD	HCJW	22	7-18	13	10-60	71	32
MDD	HCJE	22	8-18	19*	20	109	110
MDD	X065	1	8-18	8	20	48	48
MDD	HCCJ	1	12-17	6	20-60	21	19

*includes subacute phase (weeks 10-19), during which poorly responding patients could receive a higher dose of double-blind study medication

Lilly's search for adverse events of interest yielded a total of 220 possibly relevant events. Of these, 176 were considered obviously unrelated to the issue of suicidality and were not reviewed further (a list of these adverse events was provided by email 11-17-03, and I concur with the sponsor that none of the events involve self-harm). The remaining cases are summarized in the sponsor's table, reproduced below.

Table 1. Number of Patients per Patient Category

Patient Category	Number of Patients
1) Suicide-related events with suicide attempts (acute/subchronic phases[a])	10
2) Suicide-related events with no suicide attempts (acute/subchronic phases[a])	7
3) Accidental overdose/death	1
4) Could be suicide related, but insufficient information	3
5) Suicide-related event prior to treatment phase	14
6) Suicide-related event during extension phase	2
7) Suicide-related event that was not treatment emergent	7

[a] Defined as the acute treatment phases for Studies HCCJ, X065, and HCJW, and the acute and subchronic phases from Study Periods III through V of Study HCJE.

Lilly provided narratives on all the cases listed, in their aforementioned submission to Health Canada and also in their email submission 11-18-03. My own review of these narratives substantiated Lilly's categorization of them.

The 17 events in categories 1 and 2 above were included in the analysis; a listing of these patients appears in appendix table 3.

A few observations can be made regarding the clinical details of these cases. With respect to dose, among the 9 fluoxetine-treated subjects with suicide-related events, the daily dose at the time of event was 20 mg for 7 subjects, 30 mg for one, and 60 mg for one. Median duration of treatment for fluoxetine subjects at the time of their event was 38 days, and the corresponding median for placebo subjects was 33 days. The adolescent age category predominated; children under 12 years of age comprised 43% of the total sample of 458 clinical trial subjects, but only 3 (18%) of the 17 suicide-related events occurred in children. Of the 17 suicide-related events, 13 (76.5%) occurred in female subjects, although females comprised only 228 (49.8%) of the 458 subjects.

Regarding the relationship to drug discontinuation, only one of the events (a drug overdose by fluoxetine patient 001-6401 in study HCCJ) occurred during the 30-day follow-up period. This patient was regarded as having discontinued by virtue of being non-compliant with study medication. However, Lilly acknowledged that "events occurring after study completion were not systematically collected," and so some events in the 30-day follow-up period may have been missed.

Nefazodone (Serzone, NDA 20-152, Bristol Myers Squibb, submission dated 8-21-03)

The table below provides the details for the two randomized, placebo-controlled pediatric studies with nefazodone.

Indication	Protocol	No. of sites	Age range (yrs)	Duration (wks)	Dose (mg/day)	N	
						Nefazodone	Placebo
MDD	CN104141	15	12-18	8	100-600	95	95
MDD	CN104187	28	7-17	8	100-300 or 200-600	184 (both arms)	94

The sponsor performed the requested search and identified two suicide-related events in these trials, both occurring in nefazodone-treated patients (please refer to Appendix table 3). (In addition to these events, the sponsor reported a total of 5 suicide-related events that occurred during open label treatment with nefazodone in follow-up to study 187. However, only the two events during double-blind treatment are relevant for this analysis.)

Fluvoxamine (Luvox, NDA 21-519, Solvay, submission dated 8-22-03)

There was one randomized, placebo controlled pediatric trial with fluvoxamine, described in the table below.

Indication	Protocol	No. of sites	Age range (yrs)	Duration (wks)	Dose (mg/day)	N	
						Fluvoxamine	Placebo
OCD	114	20	8-17	10	50-200	57	63

Solvay's search of the safety dataset for this trial revealed a single suicide-related event in a fluvoxamine-treated patient.

Sertraline (Zoloft, NDA 19-839, Pfizer, submission dated 9-12-03)

There were three randomized, placebo-controlled trials in the pediatric population, summarized in the table below. In addition, Pfizer is conducting a pediatric trial in post-traumatic stress disorder, for which the treatment is still blinded. Note that there were two studies for MDD conducted under the same protocol, and these have been combined in this analysis.

Indication	Protocol	No. of sites	Age range (yrs)	Duration (wks)	Dose (mg/day)	N	
						Sertraline	Placebo
OCD	498	12	6-17	12	25-200	92	95
MDD	1001/1017	51	6-17	10	50-200	189	184

The electronic search of adverse event terms yielded 89 potential events from these trials. Pfizer's blinded review of the 89 cases identified 25 patients with possibly relevant events, and further review of these cases excluded 19 events (mostly associated with accidental injuries). This yielded a total of 9 events occurring among 8 subjects that were considered suicide-related. (My own review of the listing of these 89 events did not disclose any additional events that were obvious omissions.) In addition, Pfizer performed the requested review of all serious adverse events in these trials, yielding one additional case relevant to the analysis (subject 1001-29533-2006, who was hospitalized for suicidal ideation). Thus there were a total of 9 patients with suicide-related events. It should be noted, however, that in their submission Pfizer questioned the clinical relevance of events in two sertraline-treated patients (subject 30506-1076, with self-mutilation, and subject 6193-1022, who was hospitalized for suicidal threats), although they did not exclude these events from their analysis.

Although the number of events was probably too small for any meaningful characterizations, the median age among the 6 sertraline treated patients was 10 years, somewhat younger than seen in other development programs. These 6 subjects included 3 males and 3 females; their median dose was 100 mg/day.

There were no events reported within the 30-day period after discontinuation of study medication, and no events in the OCD trial. Of the nine events, six occurred on drug and three on placebo. Six of the nine events occurred in female subjects. With respect to age, there was a somewhat different pattern from that seen in other clinical trial programs, since four events out of the nine occurred in children rather than adolescents (one event considered a suicide attempt occurred in a 6 year old boy). The duration of treatment among the six sertraline-associated events ranged from 21 to 50 days.

Citalopram (Celexa, NDA 20-822, Forest, submission dated 8-21-03)

There were two randomized, controlled clinical trials in the citalopram pediatric development program, summarized below.

Indication	Protocol	No. of sites	Age range (yrs)	Duration (wks)	Dose (mg/day)	N	
						Citalopram	Placebo
MDD	CIT-MD-18	21 in U.S.	7-17	8	20-40	89	85
MDD*	94404	31 in Europe	13-18	12	10-40	121	112

*subjects could be inpatients or outpatients

Note that in addition to these two completed trials, the sponsor is conducting study SCT-MD-15, a randomized, double blind, placebo controlled trial of escitalopram, the s-isomer of citalopram, in children and adolescents with MDD. This trial is still blinded; the total number of subjects planned is 264, and there have been two suicide-related events thus far.

Forest made a couple of departures from the requested methods for the adverse event search. They included an analysis of 8 patients who experienced worsening of depression, but not suicidal thoughts or behaviors; all these patients were treated with placebo. These events were not included in the analysis presented here; the interested reader should refer to their submission dated 8-21-03 for details. Forest also reported that their search of all serious adverse events for events involving suicidality was not performed blind to treatment. (I reviewed the serious adverse events in these two trials myself, and although I was not blind to treatment group either, I did not find any cases that were obvious omissions. However, among the serious adverse events, there were 6 placebo-treated and 2 citalopram-treated patients in study 94404 with psychiatric hospitalizations. These events were not counted in the analysis, however, because suicidality was not specifically documented.)

In addition to the events selected for the analysis, Forest reported that the electronic search identified 11 patients with "false positives" who were excluded (please refer to the sponsor's 11-17-03 email). In addition to the electronic search, Forest conducted a manual search of all adverse events and patient narratives from the two trials, yielding 6 patients with relevant events that were not disclosed in the electronic search. This made a total of 30 patients with events. In addition, one patient who took an extra dose of medication by mistake was considered to have taken an accidental overdose (patient 485 in study 94404); this event was not included in the analysis. Two events occurred prior to randomized treatment, yielding a total of 28 patients for the analysis (please refer to Appendix table 3 for a list of these patients). Note that 27 of the 28 events were classified as suicide attempts. However, Forest indicated in an email dated 11-17-03 that six of the study 94404 patients classified with "suicide attempts" (patients 664, 693, 867, 607, 152, and 713) were so categorized simply because the recorded preferred term was suicide attempt, and not because the event description documented self-injurious behavior.

Four placebo-treated patients and four citalopram-treated patients had events during the 30-day follow-up period after the end of randomized treatment. However, two of these 4 placebo patients also had events during double blind treatment, and so are counted as having events while on-treatment. Note that patient 007 in study 94404 was actually receiving fluoxetine, not citalopram, at the time of the event during the post-study period.

The median age of the 28 patients with events was 16 years; 19 were females and 9 males. Among the 13 patients receiving citalopram at the time of their event, the median dose was 20 mg/day, and the median duration on treatment was 27 days. Forest noted that 11 of the 16 citalopram-treated patients with suicide-related events in study 94404 had a past history of suicidality.

Forest also provided an analysis of scores on the suicidality item of the depression rating scales in the two trials; i.e., the CDRS-R in study CIT-MD-18, and the K-SADS in study 94404. There was a greater improvement on the suicidality item in study CIT-MD-18 with citalopram treatment compared to placebo, and this almost reached statistical significance. However, the mean change from baseline on item IX from the K-SADS in study 94404 was approximately equal between citalopram and placebo. Details of these analyses may be found in the 8-21-03 submission.

Paroxetine (Paxil, NDA 20-031, GlaxoSmithKline)

Please refer to the consult dated 9-5-03 for details regarding the paroxetine pediatric clinical trial data. Subsequently, GSK provided the agency with a copy of their report to the Committee for Proprietary Medicinal Products of the European Agency for the Evaluation of Medicinal Products (submitted electronically to the Paxil NDA on 11-7-03). Included in this is an analysis of suicide-related events in adult trials with paroxetine that mirrors GSK's analysis of the pediatric clinical trials. The results of the adult trial analysis show essentially no difference in the rates of suicide-related events between paroxetine and placebo treatment groups, in contrast to the previously described pediatric trial data, which showed a statistically significant increase with paroxetine treatment. The sponsor's tables describing both the adult and the pediatric analyses are reproduced in Appendix figure 5.

Venlafaxine (Effexor and Effexor XR, NDAs 20-151 and 20-699, Wyeth)

There were four randomized, double blind, placebo-controlled venlafaxine trials in pediatric patients, summarized in the following table. The sponsor also reported that two additional pediatric placebo-controlled trials, one in social anxiety disorder and one in panic disorder, have been completed but are not fully analyzed yet.

Indication	Protocol	No. of sites	Age range (yrs)	Duration (wks)	Dose* (mg/day)	N	
						Venlafaxine	Placebo
MDD	382	16	7-17	8 + taper	37.5-225	80	85
MDD	394	37	7-17	8 + taper	37.5-225	102	94
GAD	396	39	6-17	8 + taper	37.5-225	80	84
GAD	397	35	6-17	8 + taper	37.5-225	77	79

*administered as Effexor XR in all trials; dosage based upon weight of subject, and tapered over ≤2 weeks following double-blind treatment

Wyeth identified 16 randomized patients with suicide-related events, along with two events that occurred prestudy and so were not counted in the analysis. Additionally, one more event was identified through review of adverse event narratives, yielding a total of 17 patients who experienced a total of 20 events of interest. Wyeth, in their analysis submitted 8-28-03, counted all 20 events, rather than simply enumerating the number of patients with events. Note that two patients were considered to have had separate events a few days apart (patients 39402-0041 and 39428-1087); after review of the narrative summaries, I have elected to count these instead as single events. A third patient also had two events, patient 38211-012, but these were separated by approximately 3 weeks and I have elected to count only the first event in the analysis that follows. Thus, the analysis shown below is based upon the number of patients with events, rather than the number of events (as in Wyeth's analysis). The listing in the appendix provides further details about the patients.

In Wyeth's analysis, the "on-therapy" period does not include the taper period, but only the period of randomized treatment during which patients received their full dose of study medication. Therefor, "on-therapy period + 30 days" does not include a full 30 days from the last dose of study medication, if the patient had a taper following the end of their study treatment. The patient-years of exposure used in the analysis include exposure during medication taper as well as time on the assigned dose of study medication. This is slightly different from GlaxoSmithKline's analysis of the paroxetine pediatric trials, in which the "on-therapy" period included the taper phase, through the last dose of study medication, and the "on-therapy + 30 days" period included a full 30 days from the last dose of study medication.

With respect to classification of events, there were some issues with the "suicide attempts" category. The reason that patient 38205-019 was not counted in the suicide attempt category for taking an overdose was unclear. Also, I was unable to verify Wyeth's count of 3 suicide attempts on venlafaxine and 2 on placebo in study 382, as shown in Table 3A of their 8-28-03 submission.

Instead, I have used the counts from Wyeth's Table 4A in that submission, "Abbreviated Table of Patient Characteristics."

The median age among the 17 patients with suicide-related events was 13 years. For the 13 venlafaxine-treated patients, at the time of the event the median dose was 112.5 mg/day, and the median duration of treatment was 24 days. Wyeth counted any events occurring within 1 day of the last full dose of study medication as having occurred on-therapy. Five of the 17 events did not occur on-therapy, 3 with venlafaxine and 2 with placebo.

Risk estimates

Analysis of attributable risk

Pooling the exposure and event data by drug and by indication provides the results shown in tables 1 and 2. Appendix figure 6 displays these same results graphically. Here, an incidence rate difference greater than zero would indicate a risk associated with active drug versus placebo, while an incidence rate difference less than zero would indicate a protective effect of the drug.

Table 1.

Attributable risks (incidence rate differences) per patient-year for suicide-related events in pediatric trials			
Drug	**Incidence rate difference, drug minus placebo**	**95% confidence interval**	**p-value**
Citalopram	**0.14**	**-0.16-0.43**	**0.374**
Fluoxetine	**-0.03**	**-0.20-0.14**	**0.737**
Fluvoxamine	**0.11**	**-0.10-0.32**	**0.485**
Mirtazapine	**-0.04**	**-0.21-0.14**	**0.691**
Nefazodone	**0.05**	**-0.02-0.12**	**0.367**
Paroxetine	**0.12**	**0.04-0.20**	**0.005**
Sertraline	**0.06**	**-0.05-0.17**	**0.327**
Venlafaxine	**0.17**	**0.02-0.33**	**0.029**
All MDD trials	**0.10**	**0.02-0.18**	**0.013**
All non-MDD trials	**0.04**	**-0.01-0.09**	**0.114**
All trials	**0.08**	**0.03-0.14**	**0.002**

Table 2

Attributable risks (incidence rate differences) per patient-year for serious suicide-related events in pediatric trials			
Drug	**Incidence rate difference, drug minus placebo**	**95% confidence interval**	**p-value**
Citalopram	**0.24**	**-0.01-0.48**	**0.063**
Fluoxetine	**-0.02**	**-0.18-0.14**	**0.775**
Fluvoxamine	**0**	**-**	**-**
Mirtazapine	**0.04**	**-0.04-0.12**	**0.654**
Nefazodone	**0.03**	**-0.02-0.08**	**0.606**
Paroxetine	**0.08**	**0.01-0.15**	**0.038**
Sertraline	**0.06**	**-0.04-0.16**	**0.276**
Venlafaxine	**0.06**	**-0.07-0.18**	**0.379**
All MDD trials	**0.09**	**0.02-0.15**	**0.015**

All non-MDD trials	**0.01**	**-0.02-0.05**	**0.498**
All trials	**0.06**	**0.02-0.11**	[redacted]

The incidence rate differences by drug for MDD trials alone are shown in Appendix tables 6 and 7. These data are displayed graphically in Appendix figure 7.

It can be seen that overall the data are consistent with an increased risk of suicidal events with active drug treatment; the comparison between active treatment and placebo for all trials pooled together is statistically significant (p-value = 0.002 for all suicide-related events, and p-value = 0.006 for serious suicide-related events). The observed incidence rate differences are larger in MDD trials (0.085/year) than in trials with other indications (0.014/year). Based on these results, the estimated excess of serious suicide-related events in MDD trials associated with active drug is 0.085/year, or approximately 1 excess serious event per 12 patient-years of active treatment compared to placebo.

With respect to individual drugs, the incidence rate differences for all suicide-related events are largest for paroxetine, venlafaxine and citalopram, reaching statistical significance for paroxetine and venlafaxine. For serious suicide-related events, citalopram showed the largest incidence rate difference, which approached statistical significance (p-value = 0.063).

Analysis of relative risk

In addition to estimating the excess risk attributable to drug, the data can also be analyzed in terms of the relative risk, or more precisely, the ratio of the incidence rates for drug and placebo. Accordingly, Mantel-Haenszel combined incidence rate ratios were calculated, stratified by study. This approach has the advantage of providing stratification by study, while the analysis of excess risk shown above simply involved summing all the relevant data without regard for differences between trials. In addition to calculating the combined incidence rate ratio, the Stata software also tests for homogeneity of the individual study ratios.

The Stata output for the "All trials" category is shown in Appendix table 3. There were two studies by themselves that showed statistically significant rate ratios for suicide-related events, paroxetine study 329 and venlafaxine study 394. No individual study showed a statistically significant protective effect.

Table 3 below displays the relative risks (more precisely, the incidence rate ratios) for suicide-related events and serious suicide-related events for each of the antidepressant drugs, and for all 21 clinical trials combined. Here placebo is the reference, and thus a value less than one indicates a protective effect of the drug, and a value greater than one a risk associated with drug treatment. For each combined incidence rate ratio calculated, statistical testing did not show a lack of homogeneity (i.e., indicating that data from the individual studies can be combined statistically).

Table 3. Combined incidence rate ratios for suicide-related events and serious suicide-related events

Drug	Number of pediatric trials	Incidence rate ratios* (95% confidence interval), by drug	
		All suicide-related events	Serious suicide-related events
Paroxetine	5	[illegible]	[illegible]
Sertraline	2	2.07 (0.52-8.30)	2.58 (0.50-13.29)
Venlafaxine	4	3.31 (1.06-10.29)	1.79 (0.52-6.18)
Fluoxetine	4	0.87 (0.33-2.28)	0.87 (0.31-2.43)
Citalopram	2	1.36 (0.64-2.91)	2.45 (0.88-6.80)
Mirtazapine	1	0.53 (0.007-41.45)	†
Nefazodone	2	†	†
Fluvoxamine	1	†	†
MDD trials	14	1.80 (1.18-2.74)	1.93 (1.18-3.18)
Non-MDD trials	7	2.34 (0.67-8.22)	1.28 (0.25-6.57)
All trials	21	1.85 (1.24-2.76)	1.87 (1.17-3.01)

†Ratio undefined due to zero events in placebo group

It will be seen that the suicide-related event incidence rate ratios for venlafaxine and paroxetine indicate an association with drug treatment, and that the corresponding confidence intervals exclude one. Overall, the incidence rate ratio of approximately 1.9 for both suicide-related events and the subcategory of serious suicide-related events indicate an association of these events with drug treatment, although rate ratios for serious suicide-related events were not statistically significant for any individual drug. Put another way, compared to placebo, treatment with active drug increased the rate of suicide-related events by an estimated 85%, and by an estimated 87% for serious suicide-related events. For the subgroup of MDD trials, the incidence rate ratios were also statistically significant, while for non-MDD trials the incidence rate ratio estimates had very wide confidence intervals.

DISCUSSION AND CONCLUSIONS

In short-term pediatric trials, antidepressant drug treatment is associated with an increase in suicidal adverse events compared to placebo. This finding is seen for both the broad category of any suicide-related event, and the more specific category of serious suicide-related events. The association is more prominent in the MDD trial data, where the relative risk of serious suicide-related events is approximately 1.9, and the attributable risk is equivalent to one additional serious suicide-related event per 11 patient-years of drug treatment. The finding appears to be statistically robust, inasmuch as the p-value for the incidence rate difference for all suicide-related events across all trials is 0.002.

With respect to individual drugs, the data for paroxetine and venlafaxine show a statistically significant increase in suicide-related events with active treatment in their pediatric development programs. Also, the incidence rate difference for serious suicide-related events with citalopram was close to statistical significance (p-value = 0.063). For fluoxetine and mirtazapine, the point estimates were consistent with a protective effect, but the confidence intervals for mirtazapine were very broad, and even for fluoxetine the confidence interval on the incidence rate ratio includes a relative risk of greater than 2. Put another way, although an increase in suicide-related events reached statistical significance for two drugs (paroxetine and venlafaxine), for no drug was a protective effect demonstrated at a statistically significant level.

This analysis has several limitations. Most importantly, it is limited to short-term trials only. Conceivably, long-term treatment in patients who have responded positively to a drug might not produce an increased risk, or might even provide a protective effect. In other words, it may not be appropriate to extrapolate a finding of a risk in short-term trials to use of the drug for long-term maintenance treatment, especially if the patients have manifested a clinical response to the drug. Unfortunately, there is very little long-term controlled pediatric trial data for antidepressant drugs, to the best of my knowledge.

Another limitation of this analysis is that although there is evidence of a class effect overall, it is difficult to know to what extent it applies to particular members of the class. Inspection of the confidence intervals for the risk estimates will show that the confidence limits for individual drugs overlap considerably. The existing clinical trial data, moreover, cannot provide a fair comparison between drugs, since the sizes of the clinical development programs and the specific indications studied vary from drug to drug.

A third limitation pertains to the difficulties in standardizing the methodology used by the nine different sponsors. Although all sponsors were given the same set of instructions in the letters issued 7-22-03, there were some discrepancies in how these instructions were applied. For example, Forest (sponsor of citalopram) performed not only the requested electronic search of all adverse event terms, but also a manual search, which yielded cases not found with the electronic search. Also, the 30-day follow-up period was interpreted differently by GSK (paroxetine) and Wyeth (venlafaxine). GSK counted followed-up time for 30 days after the last dose of study medication, and the taper phase was not part of that 30-day period. However, Wyeth began the 30-day period from the last full dose of study medication, so that the period of dosage taper was included in the 30-day follow-up time. Also, Lilly (sponsor of fluoxetine) reported that adverse event data was not consistently collected once patients discontinued their study treatment.

As Appendix figures 1-4 illustrate, there was considerable variability in the rates of these events from trial to trial, even within the same indication. This could be due to differences in the patient population (some trials included children, for example), or to differences in ascertainment of suicide-related events, or to both. This, of course, raises questions about whether it is appropriate to combine the data from different trials. The statistical testing for homogeneity of the rate ratios provided by the Stata software, however, did not reveal any statistically significant lack of homogeneity.

The increase in suicidal events was most clearly demonstrated in MDD trials. However, events with active drug treatment were more frequent than events with placebo in non-MDD trials, although the numbers are small and the risk estimates are very uncertain. Nonetheless, this leaves open the possibility of a drug-associated risk of such behaviors for non-MDD patients, although at a much lower incidence rate difference than for MDD patients.

With respect to clinical factors that might be contributory, as described in the previous consult, the paroxetine data suggested a possible role for drug withdrawal, but this pattern was not as prominent in the data for other drugs. However, this observation might point to a lack of consistency across development programs with respect to ascertainment of adverse events following the end of double-blind treatment.

The absence of completed suicides in these data is only reassuring to a limited degree. The total drug exposure time in these trials was 407 patient-years. For assessing the rate of a rare event such as completed suicide with active drug treatment, this is a relatively small data set. To illustrate, the upper confidence limit (one sided, 97.5% level) for the actual rate in the population given an observation of no suicides in 407 patient-years is 1 completed suicide in approximately 110 patient years.

In contrast to the paroxetine pediatric data, the analysis of suicide-related events in adult paroxetine trials, employing methods identical to the corresponding analysis of pediatric trial data, failed to show an increase in the rate of such events with paroxetine treatment relative to placebo. This was despite the fact that the placebo rate for these events was similar between the adult MDD trials (0.10/year) and the pediatric MDD trials (0.13/year). This suggests that adults and pediatric patients may have different responses to paroxetine with respect to suicidality.

Several steps are being taken at the moment to evaluate this signal further. First, a joint meeting of the Psychopharmacologic Drugs Advisory Committee and the Pediatric Subcommittee of the Anti-Infective Drugs Advisory Committee will be held 2-2-04 to discuss this issue. Secondly, DNDP has requested electronic data sets from the sponsors of these clinical trials that will permit a more sophisticated statistical analysis. This analysis will permit examination of a number of issues that were beyond the scope of this consult, such as adjustment for a number of relevant covariates and exploration of risk factors such as agitation and relevant family history. Thirdly, DNDP has arranged for a group of suicidology experts at Columbia University to review the clinical narrative summaries for all of the identified cases; this will permit a more sophisticated case classification, particularly with regards to whether the event was a serious suicide attempt, a gesture, or self-mutilation. Fourthly, on 11-24-03 DNDP sent a memo to all the sponsors requesting a more detailed description of the methods each sponsor used to generate the submissions reviewed in this consult, to ensure the highest possible quality of data for review by the Columbia University experts.

These initiatives should indeed provide higher-quality data for evaluation of this signal. However, in my view, the new analyses are more likely to change the findings for individual studies and drug compounds where the numbers are relatively small, than they are to alter the overall finding of an increase in suicide-related adverse events and serious suicide-related events with active drug treatment compared to placebo. There are, I believe, several reasons for this. First, the aggregate findings are statistically robust (e.g., p-value = 0.002). Secondly, the counts of serious suicide-related events are, in my view, less likely to be unstable, because of the methods routinely employed to account for serious adverse events in clinical trials, and the greater amount of clinical information that is often collected about serious adverse events compared to non-serious events. Additionally, to the extent that events have been misclassified or overlooked in the sponsor's searches, this would generally be expected to introduce "noise" that would weaken the signal and produce a false negative, not generate a false positive. Only a systematic bias that caused events in the placebo group to be missed while events in the drug group were captured would be expected to produce a false positive, and it is difficult to conceive of what could produce such a bias.

As previously noted, fluoxetine is currently the only drug approved for pediatric MDD, although several drugs are approved for pediatric OCD (see Appendix table 5). As shown in that table, all of the four pediatric OCD trials were positive and provided evidence of efficacy for approval of the drugs for pediatric OCD. This is in contrast to the experience with pediatric MDD trials, for which only 3 of the 15 trials have been judged positive, two with fluoxetine and one with citalopram.

In sum, short-term pediatric clinical trials of antidepressant drugs demonstrate an increased rate of suicidal events with active drug compared to placebo. It is important to make every effort to enhance the quality of the data contributing to this signal, and these steps are currently under way.

However, given the strength of the association shown by the present data, the clinical importance of the apparent effect (i.e., an estimated excess of one additional serious suicide-related event per 12 patient years of treatment attributable to active drug treatment), and the fact that the additional analyses are likely to take several more months while considerable numbers of pediatric patients will be exposed to these drugs, in my view an interim risk management plan to limit the exposure of the population at greatest risk is needed at this time. Specifically, this risk management strategy should be directed at minimizing the off-label pediatric use of antidepressants, particularly the use of drugs other than fluoxetine in the treatment of pediatric MDD. I recommend this approach because fluoxetine is the only drug shown to be effective in pediatric MDD in two clinical studies, with an absence of an increase in suicidal events relative to placebo.

Andrew D. Mosholder, M.D., M.P.H.
Epidemiologist

Mary Willy, Ph.D.
Epidemiology Team Leader

Appendix table 1. Summary of pediatric clinical trial data on suicidal adverse events

Drug	Indication	Study	Drug					Placebo				
			N	Patient-years	Suicide-related events	Serious suicide-related Events	Suicide attempts	N	Patient-years	Suicide-related events	Serious suicide-related events	Suicide attempts
Paroxetine*	MDD	329†	93	13	8	7	5	88	13	1	1	0
	MDD	377	181	41	9	7	8	95	21	4	4	4
	MDD	701	104	16	3	3	2	102	17	2	1	1
	OCD	704	99	19	1	1	0	107	22	0	0	0
	SAD	676	165	51	4	0	1	157	47	0	0	0
	Paroxetine Total		*642*	*146*	*25*	*18*	*16*	*549*	*120*	*7*	*6*	*5*
Sertraline	MDD	1001/1017	189	32.2	6	5	3	184	32.5	2	2	2
	OCD	498	92	18.8	0	0	0	95	19.7	1	0	0
	Sertraline Total		*281*	*51*	*6*	*5*	*3*	*279*	*52.2*	*3*	*2*	*2*
Venlafaxine	MDD	382	80	11.01	5	3	1	85	11.73	3	3	3
	MDD	394	102	15.95	7	3	3	94	15.47	0	0	0
	GAD	396	80	13.08	0	0	0	84	13.56	0	0	0
	GAD	397	77	11.63	1	1	1	79	11.44	1	1	1
	Venlafaxine Total		*339*	*51.67*	*13*	*7*	*5*	*342*	*52.2*	*4*	*4*	*4*
Fluvoxamine	OCD	114	57	9.37	1	0	0	63	9.95	0	0	0
Mirtazapine	MDD	003-045	170	24.05	1	1	0	88	12.7	1	0	1
Fluoxetine	MDD	HCJE	109	31.57	4	3	1	110	27.96	4	3	2
	MDD	HCCJ	21	2.11	1	1	1	19	2.11	1	1	1
	MDD	X065	48	6.71	2	2	2	48	5.83	2	2	0
	OCD	HCJW	71	15.12	2	2	2	32	5.98	1	1	1
	Fluoxetine Total		*249*	*55.51*	*9*	*8*	*6*	*209*	*41.88*	*8*	*7*	*4*
Nefazodone	MDD	141	95	13.6	1	0	1	95	12.5	0	0	0
	MDD	187	184	25.4	1	1	1	94	12.9	0	0	0
	Nefazodone Total		*279*	*39*	*2*	*1*	*2*	*189*	*25.4*	*0*	*0*	*0*
Citalopram	MDD	CIT-MD-18	89	12.8	1	0	1	85	12	2	0	1
	MDD	94404	121	23.5	16	14	16	112	21.3	9	5	9
	Citalopram Total		*210*	*36.3*	*17*	*14*	*17*	*197*	*33.3*	*11*	*5*	*10*
Bupropion	ADHD	75	71	**	0	0	0	36	**	0	0	0
Grand Total			**2298**	**406.9**	**74**	**54**	**49**	**1952**	**347.63**	**34**	**24**	**26**

*Paroxetine patient-years of exposure were provided only to the nearest integer **Patient-years of exposure data were not provided †Imipramine arm omitted

Appendix table 2. Rates of suicidal adverse events, per patient-year, in pediatric clinical trials

Drug	Indica-tion	Study	Drug				Placebo			
			Patient-years	Rate of Suicide-related events	Rate of Serious suicide-related Events	Rate of Suicide attempts	Patient-years	Rate of Suicide-related events	Rate of Serious suicide-related events	Rate of Suicide attempts
Paroxetine	MDD	329	13	0.62	0.54	0.38	13	0.08	0.00	0.08
	MDD	377	41	0.22	0.17	0.20	21	0.19	0.19	0.19
	MDD	701	16	0.19	0.19	0.13	17	0.12	0.06	0.06
	OCD	704	19	0.05	0.05	0.00	22	0.00	0.00	0.00
	SAD	676	51	0.08	0.00	0.02	47	0.00	0.00	0.00
Sertraline	MDD	1001/1017	32.2	0.19	0.16	0.09	32.5	0.06	0.06	0.06
	OCD	498	18.8	0.00	0.00	0.00	19.7	0.05	0.00	0.00
Venlafaxine	MDD	382	11.01	0.45	0.27	0.09	11.73	0.26	0.26	0.26
	MDD	394	15.95	0.44	0.19	0.19	15.47	0.00	0.00	0.00
	GAD	396	13.08	0.00	0.00	0.00	13.56	0.00	0.00	0.00
	GAD	397	11.63	0.09	0.09	0.09	11.44	0.09	0.09	0.09
Fluvoxamine	OCD	114	9.37	0.11	0.00	0.00	9.95	0.00	0.00	0.00
Mirtazapine	MDD	003-045	24.05	0.04	0.04	0.00	12.7	0.08	0.08	0.00
Fluoxetine	MDD	HCJE	31.57	0.13	0.10	0.03	27.96	0.14	0.07	0.11
	MDD	HCCJ	2.11	0.47	0.47	0.47	2.11	0.47	0.47	0.47
	MDD	X065	6.71	0.30	0.30	0.30	5.83	0.34	0.00	0.34
	OCD	HCJW	15.12	0.13	0.13	0.13	5.98	0.17	0.17	0.17
Nefazodone	MDD	141	13.6	0.07	0.00	0.07	12.5	0.00	0.00	0.00
	MDD	187	25.4	0.04	0.04	0.04	12.9	0.00	0.00	0.00
Citalopram	MDD	CIT-MD-18	12.8	0.08	0.00	0.08	12	0.17	0.08	0.00
	MDD	94404	23.5	0.68	0.60	0.68	21.3	0.42	0.42	0.23
Total			406.9	0.18	0.13	0.12	347.63	0.10	0.07	0.07

Appendix table 3. Listing of all patients with suicide-related events in pediatric antidepressant drug trials.

MIRTAZAPINE

Study	Indication	Patient ID	Age Sex	Treatment	Dose (mg/day) at time of event	Duration (days)	Event	Serious (y/n)	Comments
003-045	MDD	0404	15 M	Mirtazapine	15	7	Hospitalization for suicidal ideation	Y	
003-045	MDD	0801	9 M	Mirtazapine	45	52	Depakote overdose "on a dare"	Y	Excluded by sponsor
003-045	MDD	1603	12 F	Placebo	-	56	Self inflicted cuts	N	

FLUOXETINE

Study	Indication	Patient ID	Age Sex	Treatment	Dose (mg/day) at time of event	Duration (days)	Event	Serious (y/n)	Comments
HCCJ	MDD	001/6401	17 F	Fluoxetine	30	40	Overdose, details unknown; discontinued from trial	y	Patient poorly compliant with study drug
HCCJ	MDD	001-6408	13 M	Placebo	-	33	Overdose of aspirin	y	
HCJE	MDD	008-0806	15 M	Placebo	-	37	Hospitalized for suicidal ideation and self-mutilation	y	
HCJE	MDD	008/0804	15 F	Placebo	-	60	Overdose on study medication	y	
HCJE	MDD	009-0901	15 F	Fluoxetine	60	101	Self-mutilation	n	
HCJW	OCD	006-0609	15 F	Placebo	-	71	Self-injurious behavior	Y	No details provided
HCJW	OCD	013-1300	12 F	Fluoxetine	20	25	Tylenol overdose	Y	Hospitalized
HCJW	OCD	018-1811	7 F	Fluoxetine	20	60	Self-destructive cutting	y	
X065	MDD	001-2051	16 F	Fluoxetine	20	14	Multiple drug overdose	Y	Other adverse events included manic reaction
X065	MDD	001-2163	17 F	Fluoxetine	20	12	Overdose on unknown pills	Y	No psychiatric family history, no previous attempts
HCJE	MDD	004-0419	13 F	Fluoxetine	20	67	Hospitalized for suicidal ideation	Y	
HCJE	MDD	022-2216	15 F	Fluoxetine	20	38	Suicidal ideation	Y	
HCJE	MDD	003-0302	17 F	Fluoxetine	20	32	Suicidal thoughts	y	
HCJE	MDD	019-1901	11 F	Placebo	-	?	"wanting to die"	N	
HCJE	MDD	022-2203	9 M	Placebo	-	9	Suicidal ideation, intermittent	Y	Displayed self-injurious behavior during later extension phase of trial
X065	MDD	001-2052	16 M	Placebo	-	33	Suicidal ideation	Y	
X065	MDD	001-2087	14 F	Placebo	-	6	Hospitalized for suicidal ideation	y	

NEFAZODONE

Study	Indication	Patient ID	Age Sex	Treatment	Dose (mg/day) at time of event	Duration	Event	Serious (y/n)	Comments
141	MDD	3-1065	12 M	Nefazodone	600	38	Self mutilation (superficial cutting)	n	
187	MDD	18-322	13 F	Nefazodone	0	4 days post d/c	Overdose on 14 tablets of study medication	y	Hospitalized

FLUVOXAMINE

Study	Indication	Patient ID	Age Sex	Treatment	Dose (mg/day) at time of event	Duration (days)	Event	Serious (y/n)	Comments
RH1140201	OCD	65815	15 M	Fluvoxamine	200	36	Suicidal ideation	N	Self-mutilation during open label extension phase

SERTRALINE

Study	Indication	Patient ID	Age Sex	Treatment	Dose (mg/day) at time of event	Duration (days)	Event	Serious (y/n)	Comments
498	OCD	90N0242-19	12 F	Placebo	-	12	Suicidal ideation	N	
1001	MDD	29533-2006	12 M	Sertraline	100	49	Suicidal ideation	y	Hospitalized
1001	MDD	29534-1089	10 F	Sertraline	100	35	Suicidal ideation	Y	Hospitalized
1001	MDD	30506-1076	9 F	Sertraline	100	37	Self mutilation	n	Second episode of self mutilation on day 46
1001	MDD	6193-1022	10 M	Sertraline	100	21	Suicidal ideation	Y	Hospitalized. Also had mild agitation.
1017	MDD	29384-4022	16 F	Sertraline	150	50	Multidrug overdose	Y	Also noted to have restlessness
1017	MDD	30627-3095	6 M	Sertraline	100	34	Threatened to jump from vehicle, suicidal ideation	Y	Hospitalized; also experienced agitation
1017	MDD	31940-4329	17 F	Placebo	-	9	Attempted self-immolation	Y	Minor burn wounds. Subject later denied suicidality
1017	MDD	31942-4321	15 F	Placebo	-	63	Attempted suicide by hanging	Y	Second suicide attempt by overdose on day 66

CITALOPRAM

Study	Indication	Pt ID	Age Sex	Treatment	Dose (mg/day) at time of event	Duration (days)	Event	Serious (y/n)	Comments
CIT-MD-18	MDD	193	9 M	Citalopram	20	37	Cut self with knife	N	Agitation reported on previous day
CIT-MD-18	MDD	137	10 M	Placebo	-	31	Attempted to hang self	N	Personality disorder; 24 days post-tx had another suicide-related event
CIT-MD-18	MDD	519	12 F	Placebo	-	41	Severe suicidal tendency (no details)	N	
94404	*MDD*	*007*	*15 M*	*Citalopram*	-	*25 days post tx*	*Multiple drug overdose*	*Y*	*Patient had received fluoxetine X 2? days since completing trial*
94404	MDD	009	17 F	Citalopram	20	15	Hospitalized for suicidality; overdose on naproxen on day 6 of hospitalization	Y	
94404	MDD	121	18 F	Citalopram	-	12 days post tx	Overdose of chlorxazone	Y	Patient had been discontinued from study on day 8 because of abnl clinical laboratories
94404	MDD	148	17 F	Citalopram	20	47	Overdose of 4-6 citalopram tablets	Y	Made a second overdose later in trial
94404	MDD	426	14 F	Citalopram	20	70	Overdose on 11 paracetamol tablets; denied suicidal intent	Y	Event coded as medication error
94404	MDD	573	14 F	Citalopram	20	88	Intentional ingestion of cigarettes	Y	Subject was an inpatient at screening
94404	MDD	575	14 F	Citalopram	20	55	Suicidal ideation, cut arm	Y	Subject was an inpatient at screening
94404	MDD	664	15 M	Citalopram	20	10	Re-hospitalized for suicidality	Y	Subject was an inpatient at screening
94404	MDD	713	16 M	Citalopram	30	27	Re-hospitalized for suicidality	N	Subject was an inpatient at screening. No explanation for why this was not designated a serious event.
94404	MDD	715	17 F	Citalopram	20	14	Hospitalized for suicidality, cut wrists, denied suicidal intent	Y	
94404	MDD	729	16 M	Citalopram	10	63	Ingested 15 caffeine pills plus alcohol	N	Event coded as medication error
94404	MDD	761	13 M	Citalopram	-	1 day post tx	Hospitalized for suicidality, event designated as a suicide attempt	Y	Also developed agitation, mood lability
94404	MDD	776	17 F	Citalopram	-	1 day post tx	Multiple drug overdose; only dose of study medication was the previous day	Y	Subject was an inpatient at screening. Also experienced anxiety
94404	MDD	867	17 F	Citalopram	30	20	Hospitalization due to suicidal thoughts	Y	Also experienced anxiety
94404	MDD	874	17 f	Citalopram	20	13	Overdose	Y	Patient cut her wrist 4 days after overdose
94404	MDD	884	16 F	Citalopram	20	16	Hospitalized after overdose on diazepam (9 tablets)	Y	On day 22, re-hospitalized for suicidality, and on day 81, another overdose
94404	MDD	071	16 F	Placebo	-	16	Hospitalized after self-inflicted wrist laceration	Y	Re-hospitalized for suicidality on day 36
94404	MDD	152	14 F	Placebo	-	8 days post tx	Hospitalized for suicidality	Y	Treated with citalopram after hospitalization
94404	MDD	412	18 F	Placebo	-	1 day post tx	Overdose on mother's medication	Y	Also receiving oxazepam for anxiety

Study	Indication	Pt ID	Age Sex	Treatment	Dose (mg/day) at time of event	Duration (days)	Event	Serious (y/n)	Comments
94404	MDD	605	13 M	Placebo	-	35	Self mutilation (forearm)	N	
94404	MDD	607	17 M	Placebo	-	62	Suicidal ideation and tension, treated with lorazepam	N	Inpatient at screening.
94404	MDD	691	17 F	Placebo	-	29	Self mutilation (palms)	N	
94404	MDD	693	16 F	Placebo	-	2	Hospitalized for suicidal ideation	Y	Later in trial had self-inflicted scratches on arm. After completing trial, started citalopram and was re-hospitalized for suicidal ideation 8 days later
94404	MDD	787	13 F	Placebo	-	29	Self-mutilation	N	
94404	MDD	871	17 F	Placebo	-	25	Overdose on 8 tablets of tolfenamic acid	Y	

PAROXETINE (Sources: 6-16-03 submission and Excel spreadsheet courtesy of Dr. Judith Racoosin, Division of Neuropharmacological Drug Products)

Study	Indication	Pt ID	AGe	SEx	Treatment	Dose (mg/day) at time of event	Duration (days)	Event	Serious (y/n)	Comments
329	MDD	32900300313	18	M	Paroxetine	20	11	Command hallucinations, self mutilation	Y	Hospitalized
329	MDD	32900400015	16	F	Paroxetine	20	31	Mild self mutilation	N	
329	MDD	32900600038	15	F	Paroxetine	20	57	Multiple drug overdose	Y	
329	MDD	32900200245	14	F	Paroxetine	20	13	Acetaminophen overdose (27-28 capsules)	Y	Treated in emergency room and released
329	MDD	32900500250	15	F	Paroxetine	30	28	Overcompliance (by 124%) with study medication	Y	Coded as "overdose intentional." (Same patient subsequently overdosed on 20 capsules of study medication during continuation treatment.)
329	MDD	32900100065	14	M	Paroxetine	20	13	Angry outburst (with destruction of property) followed by suicidal thoughts	Y	
329	MDD	32900500333	16	F	Paroxetine	20	+4 post study	Hospitalized for severe suicidal ideation	Y	
329	MDD	32900200106	15	F	Paroxetine	40	51	Combative with mother, threatened suicide	Y	Hospitalized
377	MDD	37701100061	17	F	Paroxetine	40	75	Overdose (28 tablets of study medication)	Y	Hospitalized
377	MDD	37702400158	14	F	Paroxetine	30	86	Slapping herself in the face (automutilation)	N	
377	MDD	37702300172	16	M	Paroxetine	30	38	Overdose on 5 gm paracetamol plus 600 mg aspirin	N	Considered a non-serious event by investigator
377	MDD	37703000181	18	F	Paroxetine	40	56	Hostility, depression, writing suicide notes; possible drug abuse (cannabis)	Y	Hospitalized
377	MDD	37700900225	17	F	Paroxetine	20	78	Overdose on study medication	Y	Hospitalized
377	MDD	37704200310	15	F	Paroxetine	20	23	Self-inflicted wrist lacerations, superficial	Y	

Study	Indication	Pt ID	AGe	SEx	Treatment	Dose (mg/day) at time of event	Duration (days)	Event	Serious (y/n)	Comments
377	MDD	37705300508	14	F	Paroxetine	20	54	Cut left wrist after arguing with mother	Y	
377	MDD	37704200315	15	F	Paroxetine	20	+4 post study	Overdose on 5 acetaminophen pills and two other pills, agitation, anxiety	Y	Hospitalized
377	MDD	37704900479	17	M	Paroxetine	40	+2 post study	Suicidal ideation, irritability	Y	Hospitalized
676	SAD	67601124283	15	M	Paroxetine	30	+1 post study	Vague suicidal ideation	N	
676	SAD	67601424376	13	F	Paroxetine	40	34	Worsening panic attacks, suicidal ideation	N	
676	SAD	67610024705	16	F	Paroxetine	20	43	Self-inflicted scratch on wrist	N	
676	SAD	67610124629	14	F	Paroxetine	40	99	Threatened suicide when brother hospitalized	N	
701	MDD	70116325718	16	F	Paroxetine	50	41	Patient reported taking an overdose of 100 paroxetine tablets	Y	Overdose not confirmed by urine drug screen
701	MDD	70118025639	15	F	Paroxetine	30	+2 post study	Cut arms, overdose on acetaminophen	Y	Required ICU admission
701	MDD	70118327620	11	F	Paroxetine	20	+4 post study	Threatened to hang self	Y	Hospitalized
704	OCD	70403325513	15	M	Paroxetine	40	25	Hospitalization due to suicidal thoughts	Y	
329	MDD	32900100123	16	F	Placebo	-	45	Worsening depression, suicidal thoughts	Y	
377	MDD	37700500231	14	F	Placebo	-	31	Overdose of study medication and chlorazepate	Y	
377	MDD	37701000068	14	F	Placebo	-	83	Overdose on 21 alprazolam tablets	Y	Hospitalized
377	MDD	37702900024	17	F	Placebo	-	29	Tried to kill herself with scissors	Y	Details not provided
377	MDD	37704100294	14	F	Placebo	-	84	Overdose on 10 gm of acetaminophen	Y	Hospitalized
701	MDD	70115425768	13	M	Placebo	-	5	Wrecked parent's car and became suicidal	Y	Hospitalized
701	MDD	70118327617	12	F	Placebo	-	3	Mild self-mutilation of arms	N	

VENLAFAXINE

Study	Indication	Pt ID	AGE	Sex	Treatment	Dose (mg/day)	Duration (days)	Event	Serious (y/n)	Comments
382	MDD	38202-036	13	F	Placebo	-	+18 post tx	Angry, kicked a cabinet	Y	Resulted in ER visit
382	MDD	38204-023	11	F	venlafaxine ER	112.5	21	Suicidal ideation	N	
382	MDD	38205-008	12	M	venlafaxine ER	75	29	Suicidal ideation, auditory hallucinations	Y	Hospitalized
382	MDD	38205-019	8	F	venlafaxine ER	NA	13	Overdose on venlafaxine 300 mg	Y	Hospitalized
382	MDD	38207-008	12	M	Placebo	-	+17 post tx	Suicidal ideation, scratching on arms	Y	Hospitalized
382	MDD	38207-023	14	F	Placebo	-	3	Overdose on study medication (~8 capsules)	Y	Treated at ER and released
382	MDD	38209-020	13	F	venlafaxine ER	37.5	13	Suicidal ideation with plan to overdose	Y	Hospitalized
382	MDD	38211-012	10	F	venlafaxine ER	112.5	23	Mild self-injurious behavior	N	On day 43 of trial, hospitalized for swallowing aftershave

394	MDD	39402-0041	7	M	venlafaxine ER	75	25 and 29	Suicidal ideation, plan to stab self	Y	Hospitalized
394	MDD	39404-0126	14	M	venlafaxine ER	75	15	Suicidal and homicidal ideation	Y	Hospitalized
394	MDD	39411-0405	14	F	venlafaxine ER	150	51	Cut arm in context of family discord	N	Treated at ER and released
394	MDD	39420-0769	13	M	venlafaxine ER	225	36	Mild suicidal ideation	N	
394	MDD	39428-1087	16	M	venlafaxine ER	150	47 and 50	Rage attack, suicidal, homicidal	Y	Hospitalized; drug screen positive for PCP
394	MDD	39435-1366	17	F	venlafaxine ER	37.5	5	Mild self-mutilation	N	
394	MDD	39440-1561	12	F	venlafaxine ER	-	+6 post tx	Overdose on study medication (17 capsules)	N	Treated at ER and released. Not considered a serious event
397	GAD	39701-0012	17	F	Placebo	-	15	Overdose of 18 Excedrin PM tablets following fight with boyfriend	Y	Hospitalized
397	GAD	39710-0361	10	M	venlafaxine ER	-	+3 post tx	Suicidal (wrapped cord around neck), agitated, and physically agressive	Y	Hospitalized

BUPROPION No cases

Appendix table 4. Stata outputs for calculation of combined incidence rate ratios

Category: Suicide-related events

Study	IRR	[95% Conf.	Interval]	M-H Weight	
003-045	.5416667	.0069015	42.51311	.6486486	(exact)
1001/1017	3.09375	.5531832	31.33657	.9846154	(exact)
114	.	.0284829	.	0	(exact)
141	.	.0238036	.	0	(exact)
187	.	.01333	.	0	(exact)
329	8	1.072641	354.959	.5	(exact)
377	1.152439	.3216551	5.121634	2.645161	(exact)
382	1.818182	.3537461	11.70784	1.434783	(exact)
394	.	1.35128	.	0	(exact)
396	.	.	.	0	(exact)
397	.9166667	.0116794	71.94527	.5217391	(exact)
498	0	0	41.06291	.4871795	(exact)
676	.	.6083716	.	0	(exact)
701	1.59375	.1825649	19.08565	.969697	(exact)
704	.	.0296822	.	0	(exact)
94404	1.555556	.6472562	3.993838	4.8	(exact)
CIT-MD-18	.4615385	.0078219	8.865721	1.04	(exact)
HCCJ	1	.0127412	78.48575	.5	(exact)
HCJE	.875	.1629756	4.697789	2.133333	(exact)
HCJW	.8	.041647	47.20484	.7142857	(exact)
X065	.8571429	.0621403	11.82315	1.076923	(exact)
Crude	1.860963	1.224067	2.881543		(exact)
M-H combined	1.846414	1.235783	2.758773		

Test of homogeneity (M-H) chi2(13) = 7.76 Pr>chi2 = 0.8590

Category: Serious suicide-related events

Study	IRR	[95% Conf.	Interval]	M-H Weight	
003-045	.	.0138854	.	0	(exact)
1001/1017	2.578125	.4221158	27.07521	.9846154	(exact)
114	.	.	.	0	(exact)
141	.	.	.	0	(exact)
187	.	.01333	.	0	(exact)
329	7	.8993189	315.599	.5	(exact)
377	.8963415	.2278526	4.175488	2.645161	(exact)
382	1.090909	.1460938	8.146018	1.434783	(exact)
394	.	.3874375	.	0	(exact)
396	.	.	.	0	(exact)
397	.9166667	.0116794	71.94527	.5217391	(exact)
498	.	.	.	0	(exact)
676	.	.	.	0	(exact)
701	3.1875	.2559633	167.3341	.4848485	(exact)
704	.	.0296822	.	0	(exact)
94404	2.45	.8338509	8.690724	2.666667	(exact)
CIT-MD-18	.	.	.	0	(exact)
HCCJ	1	.0127412	78.48575	.5	(exact)
HCJE	.875	.1171794	6.533786	1.6	(exact)
HCJW	.8	.041647	47.20484	.7142857	(exact)
X065	.8571429	.0621403	11.82315	1.076923	(exact)
Crude	1.923833	1.169076	3.254079		(exact)
M-H combined	1.87431	1.165424	3.014387		

Test of homogeneity (M-H) chi2(10) = 6.38 Pr>chi2 = 0.7821

Appendix table 5. Summary of efficacy findings from eight pediatric antidepressant development programs

Drug	Indication	Approval status for pediatric use*	Study	N Drug	N Placebo	Efficacy results on primary variable
Paroxetine	MDD	NA	329	93	88	Failed (but + on secondary variables)
			377	181	95	Failed
			701	104	102	Failed
	OCD	AE	704	99	107	+
	SAD	Not submitted	676	165	157	? (not submitted)
Sertraline	MDD	NA	1001/1017	189	184	Two studies under same protocol, both failed (but + if data pooled)
	OCD	AP	498	92	95	+
Venlafaxine	MDD	NA	382	80	85	Failed
			394	102	94	Failed
	GAD	NA	396	80	84	Failed, by a small margin (p=0.09)
			397	77	79	+
Fluvoxamine	OCD	AP	114	57	63	+
Mirtazapine	MDD	NA	003-045	170	88	Two studies under this protocol, both failed
Fluoxetine	MDD	AP	HCJE	109	110	+
			X065	48	48	+
	OCD	AP	HCJW	71	32	+
Nefazodone	MDD	NA	141	102	99	Failed, by a small margin (p=0.08)
			187	184	94	Failed
Citalopram	MDD	NA	CIT-MD-18	89	85	+
			94404	121	112	Failed

* NA not approvable, AE approvable, AP approved

Appendix Table 6.

Attributable risks (incidence rate differences) per patient-year for suicide-related events in pediatric MDD trials			
Drug	Incidence rate difference, drug minus placebo	95% confidence interval	p-value
Citalopram	0.14	-0.16-0.43	0.374
Fluoxetine	-0.02	-0.21-0.17	0.829
Mirtazapine	-0.04	-0.21-0.14	0.691
Nefazodone	0.05	-0.02-0.12	0.367
Paroxetine	0.15	-0.01-0.31	0.088
Sertraline	0.12	-0.05-0.30	0.176
Venlafaxine	0.33	0.05-0.62	0.020
All MDD trials	0.10	0.02-0.18	0.013

Appendix Table 7.

Attributable risks (incidence rate differences) per patient-year for serious suicide-related events in pediatric MDD trials			
Drug	Incidence rate difference, drug minus placebo	95% confidence interval	p-value
Citalopram	0.24	-0.01-0.48	0.063
Fluoxetine	-0.02	-0.20-0.16	0.842
Mirtazapine	0.04	-0.04-0.12	0.654
Nefazodone	0.03	-0.02-0.08	0.606
Paroxetine	0.13	-0.02-0.27	0.121
Sertraline	0.09	-0.07-0.25	0.284
Venlafaxine	0.11	-0.11-0.33	0.337
All MDD trials	0.09	0.02-0.15	0.015

Appendix figure 1.

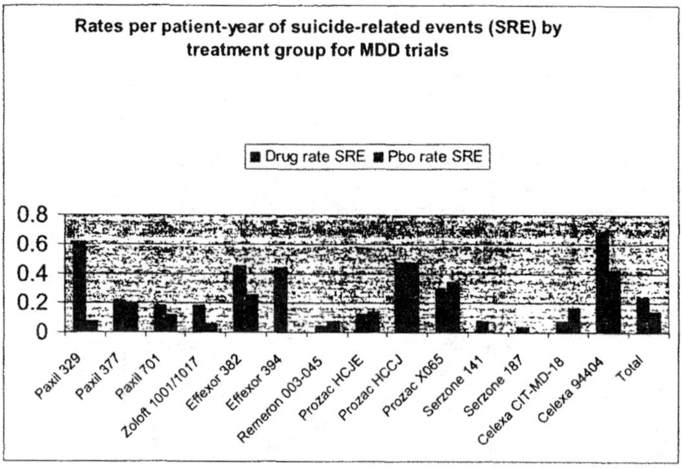

Appendix figure 2.

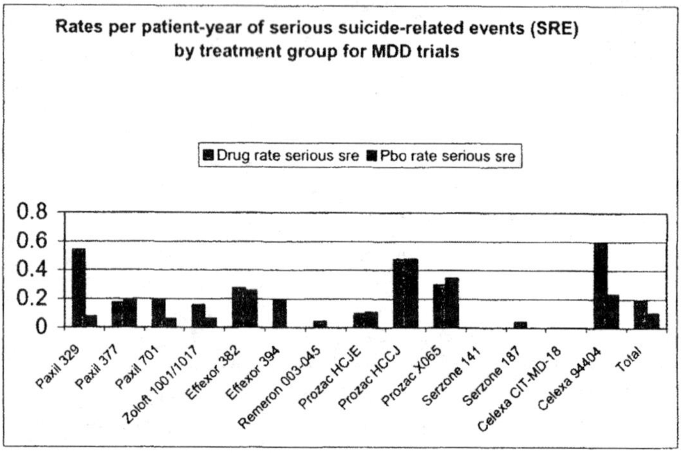

Appendix figure 3.

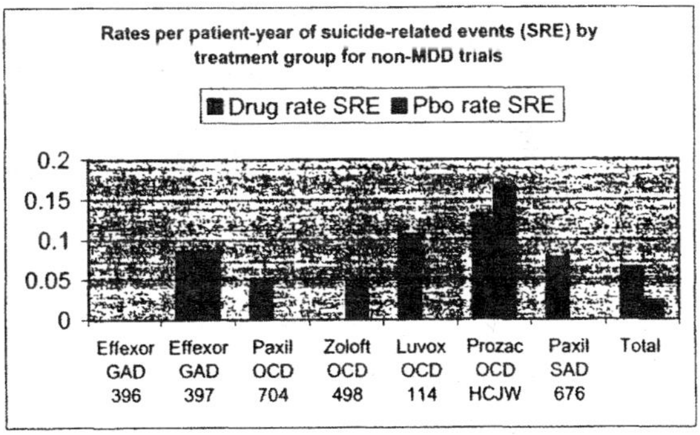

Appendix figure 4.

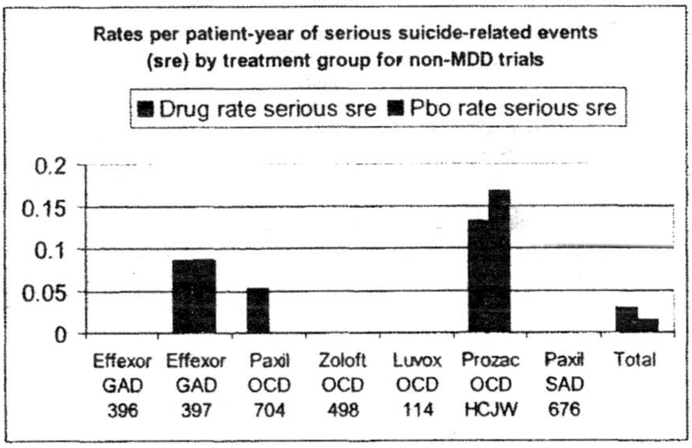

MEMORANDUM

Tab 15

DEPARTMENT OF HEALTH AND HUMAN SERVICES
PUBLIC HEALTH SERVICE
FOOD AND DRUG ADMINISTRATION
CENTER FOR DRUG EVALUATION AND RESEARCH

Andy Great Job!! See comments Mark

PID# D030341

DATE:

FROM: Andrew D. Mosholder, M.D., M.P.H., Epidemiologist

THROUGH: Mark Avigan, M.D., Director
Division of Drug Risk Evaluation, HFD-430

TO: Russell Katz, M.D., Director
Division of Neuropharmacological Drug Products, HFD-120

SUBJECT: Suicidality in pediatric clinical trials with paroxetine and other antidepressant drugs: Follow-up to 9-4-03 consult

Drugs: paroxetine, sertraline, venlafaxine, fluoxetine, fluvoxamine, citalopram, nefazodone, mirtazapine, and bupropion

EXECUTIVE SUMMARY

This consult is a follow-up to the previous consult on this topic, dated 9-5-03. As described in that consult, GlaxoSmithKline (GSK) performed an analysis of suicidal behaviors in their paroxetine pediatric clinical trial database, and found that there was a statistically significant increase in suicide-related adverse events for paroxetine-treated subjects compared to placebo. The method GSK used for their analysis involved an electronic search of the adverse event data for certain events that might have represented suicidal behaviors, followed by a blinded review of these events to select those that appeared to be probably related to suicide. In July 2003, the Division of Neuropharmacological Drug Products (DNDP) requested the sponsors of the other antidepressant drugs to replicate GSK's analysis in their own pediatric clinical trial databases. This consult summarizes the results of these analyses for 22 short-term placebo-controlled trials involving 9 different antidepressant drugs.

These trials included a total of 4250 pediatric subjects, 2298 treated with active drug and 1952 treated with placebo. There were 108 patients with suicide-related events (74 on active drug and 34 on placebo); 78 of these adverse events were serious (54 on active drug and 24 on placebo).

Considering individual development programs separately, the data for venlafaxine and paroxetine showed a statistically significant increase in suicide-related events relative to placebo. Additionally, on one measure (the incidence rate difference for serious suicide-related events) the data for citalopram approached statistical significance (p-value = 0.063). The relative risks for suicide related events with two compounds, fluoxetine and mirtazapine, were below one, ~~consistent with a~~ protective effect. However, the mirtazapine relative risk estimate of 0.5 was based on a very small number of events and had very broad confidence intervals. The relative risk

raising the possibility of a

Tab 16

From: Laughren, Thomas P
Sent: Sunday, December 21, 2003 3:35 PM
To: Katz, Russell G; Temple, Robert
Subject: Feb 2nd AC Meeting

I need to alert you to several problems that I see emerging in the planning for the Feb 2nd Peds Suicidality AC meeting.

First I want to briefly summarize the general position that I think we should be putting forward to the committees. Suicidality data from placebo-controlled pediatric studies in MDD have suggested a signal of increased risk for patients assigned to drug. However, concerns have been raised about exactly what the identified events represent and about the inconsistency of the signal across studies, even within individual programs. In order to further explore these concerns, we have embarked on two additional exploratory efforts. One is to have all the events of concern independently and blindly reclassified by a group of outside experts in adolescent suicidality. Second, we have asked for patient level data for these studies so that we can appropriately adjust for covariates of particular interest.

I believe this position accurately represents the position of DNDP, and the center. However, it clearly does not represent the position of Andy Mosholder, the medical officer from ODS who has been looking at these clinical trials data since last summer. I say this for several reasons. First, after these concerns were identified clearly in the regulatory briefing, he expressed his lack of enthusiasm for helping in this aspect of the overall effort, and instead, went off on his own to independently look at the summary data accumulating from other sponsors during September and October. I have been left on my own to follow up on the reclassification effort, including multiple contacts with drug companies to get a complete accounting of all events of interest and also all negotiations with the group from Columbia to establish a contract to have this work done. Second, now that we are at the planning stages for FDA presentations at the Feb 2nd meeting, it is clear that Andy intends to present the clinical trials data in such a manner to suggest much greater confidence in the signal than I believe is justified. I will forward to you tomorrow an outline of his planned talk that he provided for our planning meeting last Thursday (Dec 18th). I of course also had an opportunity to talk with him about his planned comments at the Dec 18 meeting. Several things are clear:

- He is planning on presenting aggregated data, both across studies within programs and across different programs.
- He has gone beyond the companies own analyses to select on his own (and completely unblinded) cases that he thinks represent true suicidality to come up with his own risk estimates.
- I believe he has relied on the On-Therapy + 30 days data, which I think are seriously flawed, since they are confounded by withdrawal events and are problematic because the approaches used in the +30 days analyses varied dramatically among the different sponsors.
- He has made clear that he intends to ask the committees if they think, based on what he plans to present, that we need go no further and can take definitive regulatory action now.

I think that all we need to do regarding these trials is present a table that I have attached

to this e-mail. This table is based on the on-therapy data for these trials, and is presented without any modifications, personal selections, etc. I think it makes several points clearly:
-These are potential signals arising from several programs.
-The signal is very inconsistent for individual studies within the various programs, with the exception of venlafaxine. For paroxetine, the RR is 1 for 2 studies, yet there is a strong signal from a 3rd study. This is also the case for sertraline and citalopram (i.e., not even a hint of an effect for 1 of the 2 studies in each of these programs, but an apparent signal for the other study). Fluoxetine is generally lacking a signal, except for suicide attempts in 1 study. There isn't much happening for either nefazodone or mirtazapine, with a weak signal for drug with nefazodone and a weak signal for placebo with mirtazapine.

I am very concerned that, if we go forward with the plan to have Andy make a presentation, I will have to spend a lot of my time undoing his presentation instead of trying to make the case for our plans for further exploration of the data. I don't think a very public fight like this will be helpful for the agency. I think I can handle all of the clinical trials issues in my presentation, including comments on efficacy that I think will put the lack of efficacy in context. I think Andy has clearly reached a conclusion about the data, and cannot be helpful in supporting our position that more work is needed.

Another concern has to do the plans by ODS to discuss the AERS data. As I've already mentioned, after extraordinary resistance, they have done the 1st 3 years analyses we insisted that they do. Paxil is clearly in the middle of the pack in these analyses, and only Prozac is an outlier. Yet, as I told you Friday, they have strongly resisted providing reporting rates. Instead, they plan to present only numerator data. They argue that the reporting rates "provide too much reassurance that there might not be a signal for Paxil (Anne Troentel's words)." They apparently are not worried that the mindless 1 year slice for Paxil might be misinterpreted.

Finally, I learned late Friday afternoon from ACS that they are rejecting Neal Ryan, a child psychiatrist from the PDAC, on the grounds that he was a co-investigator on one of the Paxil studies. He is one of our strongest members with regard to this issue, and his loss is a severe blow. I also learned late Friday that another PDAC member (and a strong advocate for a careful, rational approach to these data) may also be in jeopardy of being rejected. She is Ellen Liebenluft, a psychiatrist from NIMH with particular expertise in adolescent affective disorder. Her husband works for a law firm that does some work for drug companies. I have been informed by ACS that it is too late to approach anyone outside government at this late date, but that if I identify new government candidates by next Tuesday, there might be at least a chance of getting them cleared (a very generous offer indeed). Just as an aside, they have had all these names for clearance since April, 2003.

I need support on establishing an agenda for this meeting.

Tom

Henig, Anne M

Tab 17

‾rom: Laughren, Thomas P
ent: Friday, September 03, 2004 10:18 AM
To: Henig, Anne M; David, Paul A
Subject: FW: Pediatric MDD Suicide Planning Meeting

-----Original Message-----
From: Mosholder, Andrew D
Sent: Thursday, December 18, 2003 10:01 AM
To: David, Paul A; Laughren, Thomas P; Racoosin, Judith A; Dubitsky, Gregory M; Stasko, Robert; Andreason, Paul J; Cummins, Susan; Iyasu, Solomon; Sachs, Hari; Murphy, Shirley; Murphy, Dianne; Roberts, Rosemary; Crescenzi, Terrie L; Patel, Anuja; Addy, Rosemary; Perez, Thomas; Somers, Karen M; Goldkind, Sara; Toigo, Theresa A
Cc: Katz, Russell G; Willy, Mary E; Behrman, Rachel E; Clifford, Johanna; Trontell, Anne E; Seligman, Paul; Covington, Magdalene L; Pamer, Carol; Rigoni, Gianna; Jenkins, John K; Avigan, Mark I; Lu, Susan; Staffa, Judy A; Katz, Russell G
Subject: RE: Pediatric MDD Suicide Planning Meeting

Hello all,
As requested, I am attaching a draft outline for my presentation. I will also bring some hard copies to the meeting.
Regards,
Andy

Outline for
!-2-04.doc (24 KB)..

> -----Original Appointment-----
> **From:** David, Paul A
Sent: Monday, December 15, 2003 10:43 AM
> **To:** David, Paul A; Laughren, Thomas P; Racoosin, Judith A;
> Mosholder, Andrew D; Dubitsky, Gregory M; Stasko, Robert;
> Andreason, Paul J; Cummins, Susan; Iyasu, Solomon; Sachs,
> Hari; Murphy, Shirley; Murphy, Dianne; Roberts, Rosemary;
> Crescenzi, Terrie L; Patel, Anuja; Addy, Rosemary; Perez,
> Thomas; Somers, Karen M; Goldkind, Sara; Toigo, Theresa A
> **Cc:** Katz, Russell G; Willy, Mary E; Behrman, Rachel E;
> Clifford, Johanna; Trontell, Anne E; Seligman, Paul;
> Covington, Magdalene L; Pamer, Carol; Rigoni, Gianna;
> Jenkins, John K; Avigan, Mark I; Lu, Susan; Staffa, Judy A;
> Katz, Russell G
> **Subject:** Pediatric MDD Suicide Planning Meeting
> **When:** Thursday, December 18, 2003 1:00 PM-2:00 PM (GMT-05:00)
> Eastern Time (US & Canada).
> **Where:** CDER WOC2 3FL-C Conf Room
>
> For those of you whom wish to dial into the meeting, the
> number/passcode is below.
> DIAL-IN NUMBERS:
> USA Toll Free Number: 888-810-3946
>
> PASSCODE: 44419
>
> **
>
> Follow-up meeting to our 12/9/03 planning meeting. Revised
> agenda attached.
> << File: PDAC 2-2-04 AGENDA DRAFTED 12-11-03.doc >>

Andy Mosholder
Draft outline for 2-2-04 AC presentation
For planning meeting 12-18-03

I. Background
- A. Paroxetine pediatric supplement submitted 4-11-02
- B. Approvable letter 10-10-02 requested additional information on behavioral adverse events
- C. GSK submission of suicidal event analysis May 2003
- D. FDA talk paper regarding paroxetine 6-19-03
- E. Request for other sponsors to duplicate GSK's paroxetine analysis in their pediatric databases
- F. Wyeth DHCP letter regarding venlafaxine 8-22-03

II. Paroxetine pediatric clinical trial program-summary
- A. 6 trials
- B. efficaçy shown only in OCD

III. GSK's analysis of suicidal events
- A. Case definition
- B. Method: electronic search of adverse event data followed by blinded review of cases
- C. Results
  1. Relative risk = 2.69 (1.20-6.00)
  2. Attributable risk = 0.12 (0.04-0.20) per patient-year of treatment

IV. Exploration of possible risk factors in paroxetine data
- A. Indication (association with MDD)
- B. Gender (female > male)
- C. Association with drug discontinuation
- D. Age (adolescents > children)
- E. Absence of similar findings from adult trials

V. Pediatric clinical trials with other antidepressants
- A. Overview of clinical trials and efficacy results
- B. Method--intended to replicate GSK's paroxetine analysis -
- C. Results (blinded?) --with emphasis on serious suicide-related events
  1. By individual drug--some differences, but overlapping confidence intervals
  2. By indication--more frequent in MDD
  3. Aggregated data
     - a. Relative risk for serious events in MDD trials = 1.94 (1.18-3.18)
     - b. Attributable risk for serious events in MDD trials = 0.09 (p=0.015) (equivalent to one additional serious suicide-related event per 12 years of exposure)

VI. Limitations
- A. Limited to short-term use
- B. Difficulties classifying events
- C. Discrepancies in methods used by the various sponsors
- D. Issues in combining data from various trials and drugs

[VII. Recommendations?]

Mosholder, Andrew D

Tab 18

From:	Katz, Russell G
Sent:	Tuesday, January 06, 2004 8:07 AM
To:	Mosholder, Andrew D
Subject:	phone call

Andy-

I'd like to talk to you about your planned presentation at the Feb Advisory Committee meeting. Are you free sometime today? I have spaces in my schedule at 10 and noon (also between now and 9 this morning). I'd appreciate it if we could set something up today.

Thanks a lot,
Rusty

McCary, Barbara M

From:	Mosholder, Andrew D
Sent:	Wednesday, January 07, 2004 3:16 PM
To:	Addy, Rosemary; Murphy, Dianne; Cummins, Susan; Iyasu, Solomon; Laughren, Thomas P; Katz, Russell G; Trontell, Anne E; Seligman, Paul; Temple, Robert; Racoosin, Judith A; Willy, Mary E; Avigan, Mark I
Cc:	Mosholder, Andrew D
Subject:	Draft presentation RCT data for Feb. 2 AC mtg

Hello all,

Rusty has told me that I won't be giving the presentation of the pediatric clinical trial data at the Feb. 2 meeting as originally planned, because I've reached a somewhat different interpretation of the pediatric clinical trial data from that of DNDP, and so it would be awkward to have me present.

However, I had already drafted my slides (although they had not yet received supervisory concurrence). I am attaching them in case they are of any interest to the team. Whoever does present the clinical trial data on Feb. 2 should feel free to use any of this material that they feel is suitable.

draft
ntation RCT dat

Tab 19

Regards,
Andy

Psychopharmacologic Drugs Advisory Committee
and
Pediatric Subcommittee of the Anti-Infective Drugs Advisory Committee

February 2, 2004

Suicide-related adverse events in pediatric trials of antidepressant drugs

Andrew D. Mosholder, M.D., M.P.H.
Division of Drug Risk Evaluation

1 DRAFT

Acknowledgements

- Office of Biostatistics
  - Dr. Yi Tsong
- Division of Neuropharmacological Drug Products
  - Dr. Judy Racoosin
  - Paul David, R.Ph.
- Division of Drug Risk Evaluation
  - Mary Willy, Ph.D.

2 DRAFT

Outline

- Background
- Suicidal events in paroxetine pediatric clinical trials
- Pediatric clinical trial data on suicidal events with other antidepressant drugs
- Limitations of the data and analyses

3 DRAFT

Regulatory background

- 4-11-02: GlaxoSmithKline (GSK) submitted pediatric exclusivity supplement for paroxetine, NDA 20-031 supplement 37, for which exclusivity is granted
- 10-10-02: Approvable letter for this supplement requested additional data on behavioral adverse events in clinical trials
- 5-22-03: GSK submitted analyses of suicidal adverse events, showing a higher incidence with paroxetine than placebo

4 DRAFT

Other pediatric development programs

- In addition to paroxetine, pediatric clinical trial data is available from 7 other antidepressant development programs:

fluvoxamine	venlafaxine
sertraline	citalopram
fluoxetine	nefazodone
mirtazapine	

5 DRAFT

Summary of current regulatory status for pediatric use

- Drugs currently approved for pediatric OCD
  - clomipramine
  - fluvoxamine
  - sertraline
  - fluoxetine
- Drugs currently approved for pediatric MDD
  - fluoxetine

6 DRAFT

Paroxetine Pediatric Clinical Trial Data

Paroxetine pediatric data

- 6 randomized, placebo controlled trials (5 were included in the pediatric exclusivity supplement)
- 3 indications
- All trials used a flexible dose design
- Total N
  - 738 paroxetine
  - 647 placebo

Randomized, double blind studies in the paroxetine pediatric development program

Indication	Study	Age range (yrs)	N	Dose (mg/day)	Duration (wks)
SAD	676	8-18	Paroxetine 165, placebo 157	10-50	16
MDD	329	12-18	Paroxetine 93, placebo 87, imipramine 95	20-40	8
MDD	377	12-19	Paroxetine 181, placebo 93	20-40	12
MDD	701	7-17	Paroxetine 104, placebo 102	20-40	8
OCD relapse prevention	453	6-18	Paroxetine 95, placebo 98	10-60	16 open/16 DB
OCD	704	6-17	Paroxetine 98, placebo 105	10-50	10

Abbreviations: MDD Major Depressive Disorder, SAD Social Anxiety Disorder, OCD Obsessive Compulsive Disorder

Paroxetine: case definitions and methods

- GSK conducted an electronic search of their clinical trial database for AE descriptions included the following text:
  - attempt, cut, gas, hang, hung, jump, mutilat, overdos, self damag, self harm, self inflict, self injur, shoot, slash, suic
  - overdose other than accidental

Paroxetine: case definitions and methods

- To distinguish suicide attempts from suicidal ideation,
  - event descriptions that also included verbatim terms such as "thought," "threat," or "tendency" were designated "possibly suicide-related,"
  - while events that did not include such descriptors were designated "suicide attempts."
    - any deliberate self-injury classified as a suicide attempt

Summary of "possibly suicidal related events" and suicide attempts in paroxetine pediatric placebo-controlled trials, including events within 30 days follow-up after treatment

Indication	Study	Possibly suicidal related events		Suicide attempts	
		Paroxetine N (%)	Placebo N (%)	Paroxetine N (%)	Placebo N (%)
MDD	329	8 (8.6)*	1 (1.1)	5 (5.4)	0
MDD	377	9 (5.0)	4 (4.2)	8 (4.4)	4 (4.2)
MDD	701	3 (2.9)	2 (2.0)	2 (1.9)	1 (1.0)
MDD Total		20 (5.3)	7 (2.5)	15 (4.0)	5 (1.8)
OCD	453	0	0	0	0
OCD	704	1 (1.0)	0	0	0
OCD Total		1 (0.5)	0	0	0
SAD	676	4 (2.4)	0	1 (0.6)	0
Grand Total		25 (3.4)**	7 (1.1)	16 (2.2)†	5 (0.8)

Abbreviations: MDD Major Depressive Disorder, OCD Obsessive Compulsive Disorder, SAD Social Anxiety Disorder, Pt-yrs patient-years of exposure
*p-value = 0.04 versus placebo
**p-value < 0.01 versus placebo
†p-value = 0.05 versus placebo

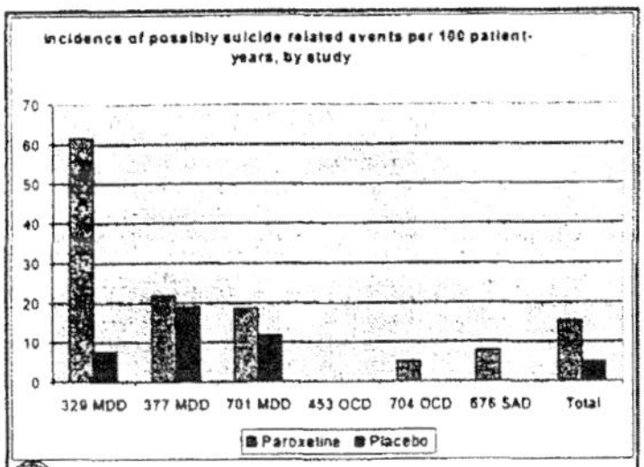

13 DRAFT

Combined results for paroxetine

Event	Mantel-Haenszel relative risk (95% confidence interval)
Possibly suicide-related events	2.6 (1.2-5.9)
Suicide attempts	2.1 (0.8-5.5)

Event	Mantel-Haenszel rate ratio (95% confidence interval)
Possibly suicide-related events	2.7 (1.2-7.8)
Suicide attempts	2.2 (0.8-8.0)

14 DRAFT

Data on suicidal ideation from rating scales used during the trials

- Suicidality rating items
  - HAM-D Item 3
  - MADRS Item 10
  - CDRS Item 13
- Paroxetine and placebo groups had similar proportions of patients with worsening on these items
- Poor correlation for individual patients between scores on these items and suicide-related adverse events
  - Possibly due to separation in time between ratings and adverse event

15 DRAFT

Comparison to adult trials

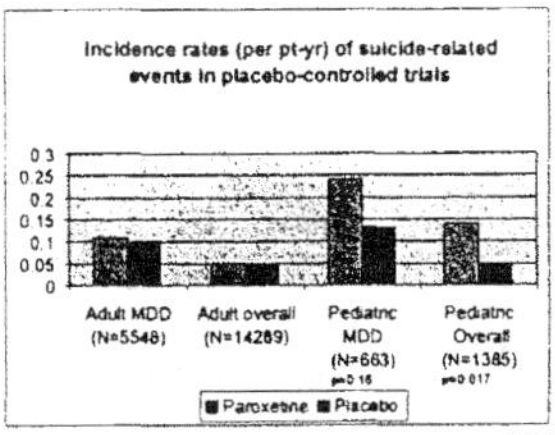

16 DRAFT

Suicide-related events: Examination of possible contributing factors

Dose	For studies 329 and 377, no apparent relationship
Duration of treatment	No apparent relationship
Age	Adolescents > children
Gender	Females > males
Drug withdrawal	Cluster of 7 events within 4 days of paroxetine d/c
Level of depression on rating scales	No apparent relationship

17 DRAFT

Pediatric Data From Other Antidepressant Development Programs

18 DRAFT

Pediatric trial data for 8 other antidepressant drugs

- On 7-22-03 the Division of Neuropharmaclogical Drug Products requested the sponsors of the following drugs to perform analyses of their pediatric trial databases comparable to the analysis GSK performed for paroxetine:
  - fluoxetine
  - citalopram
  - sertraline
  - fluvoxamine
  - venlafaxine
  - nefazodone
  - mirtazapine
  - buproprion

19 DRAFT

Suicidal events in pediatric trials with other antidepressants

- 21 clinical trials with 8 drugs
  - Bupropion: only one pilot study in ADHD, omitted
  - Acute treatment trials only (not relapse prevention trials)
  - Trials under identical protocols combined
- Total Drug N = 2227, patient-years = 406.9
  - no completed suicides
  - 74 possibly suicide related events
- Total Pbo N = 1916, patient-years = 347.6
  - no completed suicides
  - 34 possibly suicide related events

20 DRAFT

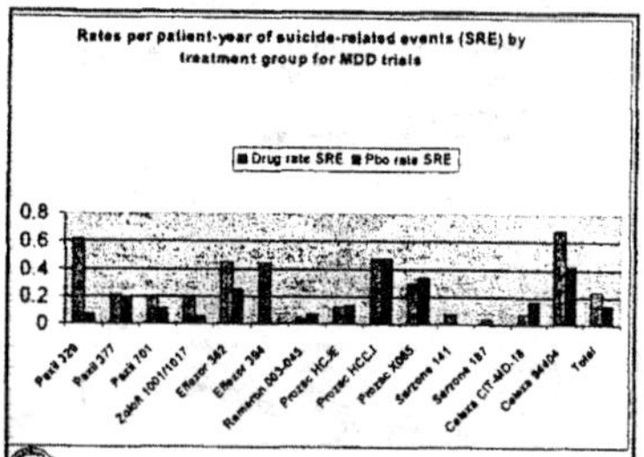

21 DRAFT

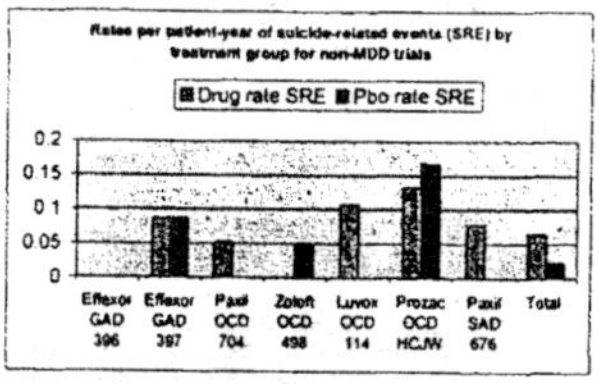

22 DRAFT

All suicide-related events by drug

Drug	Incidence rate ratios* (95% confidence interval), by drug: All suicide-related events
Paroxetine	2.65 (1.23-6.00)
Sertraline	2.07 (0.52-8.30)
Venlafaxine	2.31 (1.06-10.75)
Fluoxetine	0.87 (0.33-2.28)
Citalopram	1.36 (0.64-2.91)
Mirtazapine	0.53 (0.007-41.45)
Nefazodone	†
Fluvoxamine	†
MDD trials	1.80 (1.18-2.74)
Non-MDD trials	2.34 (0.67-8.22)
All trials	1.85 (1.24-2.76)

†Ratio undefined due to zero events in placebo group
*Mantel-Haenszel method

23 DRAFT

Analyses of serious adverse events related to suicidality

- Problems with case definition: difficulty distinguishing suicide attempt versus "gesture" versus non-suicidal self-harm
- Serious adverse drug experiences are fatal, are life-threatening, require or prolong inpatient hospitalization, are disabling, or involve a congenital defect. (21CFR 312.32). Determination of whether an adverse event in a clinical trial is serious is made by sponsor
- Focus on serious events provides a more specific, clinically meaningful case definition for analysis
- 72% of suicide-related events identified in these trials were designated serious by the sponsor

24 DRAFT

Serious suicide-related events by drug

Drug	Incidence rate ratios* (95% confidence interval), by drug: Serious suicide-related events
Paroxetine	2.19 (0.92-5.24)
Sertraline	2.58 (0.50-13.29)
Venlafaxine	1.79 (0.52-6.18)
Fluoxetine	0.87 (0.31-2.43)
Citalopram	2.45 (0.88-6.80)
Mirtazapine	†
Nefazodone	†
Fluvoxamine	†
MDD trials	1.94 (1.18-3.18)
Non-MDD trials	1.28 (0.25-6.57)
All trials	1.87 (1.17-3.01)

†Ratio undefined due to zero events in placebo group
*Mantel-Haenszel method

25 DRAFT

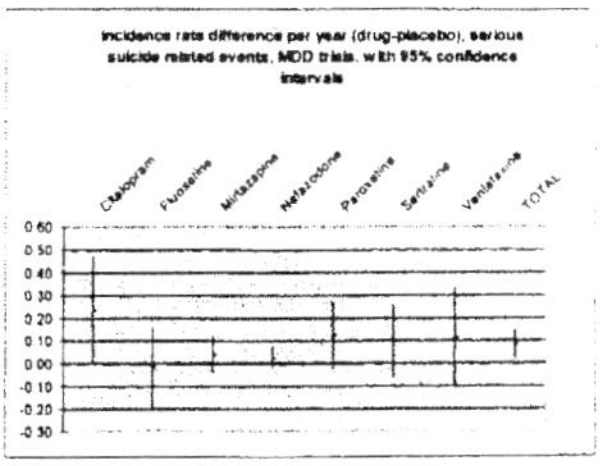

26 DRAFT

Estimating the attributable risk for suicide-related events

Category	Incidence rate difference per patient-year (drug minus placebo)	p-value
Suicide-related events		
All trials	0.084	0.002
Non-MDD trials	0.042	0.114
MDD trials	0.100	0.013
Serious suicide-related events		
All trials	0.064	0.006
Non-MDD trials	0.014	0.498
MDD trials	0.085	0.015

27 DRAFT

Limitations

- Case definition (previously noted): difficulty distinguishing suicide attempt versus "gesture" versus non-suicidal self-harm

28 DRAFT

Limitations

- Short-term trials only (only 2 trials longer than 12 weeks)
  - relevance to long-term treatment?
- Size of pediatric development programs varied considerably
  - This makes a balanced comparison between drugs difficult
- Difficult to know how findings from aggregated data apply to each specific drug

29 DRAFT

Limitations

- Limited size of clinical trial data set lessens reassurance obtained from observing no completed suicides
  - upper 95% confidence limit given 0 suicides in 407 patient-years is <1 completed suicide per 136 patient years
- Available data pertain to suicidal ideation and self-injurious behaviors, but outcome of most importance is completed suicide

30 DRAFT

Limitations

- Methodologic differences between sponsors
  - Fluoxetine: adverse events during 30-day follow-up time not reliably captured
  - Citalopram: blinded review of all adverse events: i.e.; not limited to serious events alone
  - Different methods of classifying post-study drug taper period
    - Venlafaxine: follow-up time
    - Paroxetine: on-treatment time

31 DRAFT

Conclusions

- This preliminary analysis indicates an association of suicide-related events with antidepressant drug treatment in short-term, placebo-controlled pediatric trials
  - Association most prominent in MDD trials
  - Degree to which this finding applies to specific individual drugs is unclear

32 DRAFT

Mosholder, Andrew D

From: Dubitsky, Gregory M
Sent: Friday, January 09, 2004 12:55 PM
To: Mosholder, Andrew D
Subject: RE: PDAC

Tab 20

Thanks, I'll send them to Glenn.

Yep, this gives one an uneasy feeling. We'll have to wait to see how it unfolds.

Greg

-----Original Message-----
From: Mosholder, Andrew D
Sent: Friday, January 09, 2004 12:40 PM
To: Dubitsky, Gregory M
Subject: RE: PDAC

Or, for that matter, please feel free to forward them to anyone else who's interested. Might as well get some use out of them.

And I agree, I'm not sure this is going to go over very well with the committee...

-Andy

-----Original Message-----
From: Mosholder, Andrew D
Sent: Friday, January 09, 2004 12:22 PM
To: Dubitsky, Gregory M
Subject: RE: PDAC

Sure, you can forward the slides to Glenn.
-Andy

-----Original Message-----
From: Dubitsky, Gregory M
Sent: Friday, January 09, 2004 12:04 PM
To: Mosholder, Andrew D
Subject: RE: PDAC

Wow - that's a bummer after all the work you put into it. Too bad they didn't think of that beforehand. But I would still think that your findings would be important to present. What are we going to say if the PDAC asks if the Agency has done their own analysis .... "Yes, we have, but it's not worth presenting??" It's very strange.

Anyway, sorry to hear that. Glenn Mannheim asked if he could get a copy of your slides. Do you mind if I forward them to him.

Greg

-----Original Message-----
From: Mosholder, Andrew D
Sent: Friday, January 09, 2004 10:58 AM
To: Dubitsky, Gregory M
Subject: RE: PDAC

Well, Greg, I guess you haven't heard the story...Rusty called me on Tuesday to say that he, Tom, RT, and John Jenkins decided to drop my talk from the agenda, because they don't agree with my view about the data. That is to say, my view is that although a more sophisticated analysis is desirable, one can't deny that the preliminary findings indicate there's a signal (and in fact I'll be skeptical if the new analysis makes it go away completely). Their point of view is that only the more sophisticated analysis being done by Columbia University is worth showing at all, and it's not ready yet--so no findings should be shown on Feb. 2. (Rusty did acknowledge that this is an ironic turn of events, considering that when he sent the consult to ODS he specifically asked for me to be assigned to the project, and now he's telling me to bow out.)

So, I won't be presenting any of my findings from the clinical trials, although they may still want me to present a very brief discussion of AERS reports of suicidal behaviors. I have prepared a consult which is an update to what I presented at the regulatory briefing in Sept., and you should be getting that as soon as Mark signs off on it.

In case you're interested, I'll attach the email with the slides I was planning to use on Feb. 2. But I don't think any of those slides will be shown.

Regards,
Andy

<< Message: Draft presentation RCT data for Feb. 2 AC mtg >>

-----Original Message-----
From: Dubitsky, Gregory M
Sent: Friday, January 09, 2004 10:21 AM
To: Mosholder, Andrew D
Subject: PDAC

Andy,

I got a copy of the PDAC package for the Feb 2 meeting but I didn't see anything there from you. Will you be presenting your findings at the meeting?

Greg

Mosholder, Andrew D

From: Trontell, Anne E
Sent: Tuesday, January 20, 2004 2:42 PM
To: Mosholder, Andrew D
Subject: Draft lanuage

Tab 21

Suggested alternative language;

In light of this preliminary analysis (by a single reviewer without access to blinded primary data), there appears to be an increased risk of suicidal behaviors in short-term studies of children being treated with paroxetine. Combined analyses with other RCTs of SSRI antidepressants in a variety of pediatric indications also show an increased risk of suicidal behaviors vs. placebo over all of the children enrolled in these trials; subanalyses of these trials by MDD versus nonMDD treatment show a statistically significant increase in risk within the MDD trials but not those for nonMDD endpoints (such as treatment of OCD, GAD, or other endpoints.)

Until definitive analyses are completed and expert input obtained, it seems prudent for clinicians to remain alert to the risk of suicide in pediatric patients being treated with SSRIs for MDD, particularly in the early months of therapy. Absent other information, clinicians contemplating starting pediatric patients with MDD on new antidepressant therapy with SSRIs would be well advised to give careful consideration to the following:

? FDA-approved product labeling indicating where efficacy in specific pediatric indications has been demonstrated and where excess risk of suicidal behaviors has been observed

? Assessing patient and environmental risks of suicidal behaviors

? Alerting patients, parents, and other caregivers of ways to prevent and detect suicidal behaviors before they are acted upon.

Clinicians with patients already taking SSRIs should monitor and educate their pediatric patients and family members concerning the risk of suicidal behaviors in light of their patients' duration on therapy, clinical response and stability, and other risk factors.

While FDA does not have regulatory authority to advise or otherwise direct physician behavior around therapeutic products other than through FDA-approved product labeling, clinical practice in the pharmacologic treatment of pediatric depressive disorders is consistent with the "prudent" advice above. Input and commentary from pediatric, psychiatric, and primary care professional organizations should be sought at the Advisory committee meeting being planned for February 2004.

Anne Trontell, M.D., M.P.H.
Deputy Director
Office of Drug Safety
Center for Drug Evaluation and Research
15B-33 Parklawn
HFD-400
5600 Fishers Lane
Rockville MD 20857
301-827-3219
301-443-5161 (fax)
trontella@cder.fda.gov

Mosholder, Andrew D

Tab 22

From: Willy, Mary E
Sent: Friday, January 23, 2004 8:55 AM
To: Trontell, Anne E
Cc: Mosholder, Andrew D; Avigan, Mark I
Subject: RE: Suggest we talk today

Anne, I am working at home today...give me a time and I will disconnect from my phone line so you can call in. (301) 493-8895

Mary Willy, PhD
Office of Drug Safety
(301) 827-3175

-----Original Message-----
From: Trontell, Anne E
Sent: Friday, January 23, 2004 8:51 AM
To: Willy, Mary E; Mosholder, Andrew D; Avigan, Mark I
Subject: Suggest we talk today

I spoke at length last night with Bob Temple and John Jenkins and I have encouraging news about some of our concerns. Let's talk today. We can call in Andy.

-----Original Message-----
From: Willy, Mary E
Sent: Friday, January 23, 2004 7:56 AM
To: Mosholder, Andrew D; Trontell, Anne E; Avigan, Mark I
Subject: RE: Press inquiry regarding pediatric antidepressant treatment

FYI, lucky me, I received a call from a reporter last night right in the middle of Friends!! Unfortunately, I thought he was a telemarketer and gave him my standard response (hang up) before I processed what he was saying to me!! Wish I could have been as articulate as Andy!

Mary Willy, PhD
Office of Drug Safety
(301) 827-3175

-----Original Message-----
From: Mosholder, Andrew D
Sent: Thursday, January 22, 2004 2:45 PM
To: Trontell, Anne E; Avigan, Mark I; Willy, Mary E
Cc: Cruzan, Susan M
Subject: Press inquiry regarding pediatric antidepressant treatment

Hello all,
Just to let you know: I received a phone call today from Rob Waters, the freelance reporter, seeking information about pediatric antidepressant drug treatment suicidality. He seemed to know that I am one of the people working on this issue, and asked if I was being pressured. I informed him of the upcoming advisory committee meeting (of which he said he was already well aware), and told him that for further inquiries he should contact Susan in Public Affairs.
Thanks,
Andy

Mosholder, Andrew D **Tab 23**

From: Mosholder, Andrew D
Sent: Wednesday, January 28, 2004 1:32 PM
To: Trontell, Anne E; Willy, Mary E
Cc: Avigan, Mark I; Seligman, Paul
Subject: RE: Feb 2 preparation for possible questions on RCT analyses by Andy

Hello all,
Here is my first crack at drafting answers to Anne's questions (see below).
Thanks,
Andy

Questions for which Andy should prepare a response:

What was the role of your analyses in this process? Why were they not included in the packet or presentations today? (Because they were only just completed?)
(Deferred.)

What did your analyses show? What is your conclusion? (Suggest giving exec summary version of results. No recommendations, just conclusions about what you think data indicate.

Results were as follows. Development programs for 8 antidepressant drugs included a total of 2227 pediatric patients treated with active drug and 1916 pediatric patients treated with placebo. There were 74 suicide related events with drug and 34 with placebo. Of these, the majority were serious; there were 54 serious events with drug and 24 with placebo. The combined relative risk for serious events was 1.9 (confidence limit 1.2-3.0) and the excess risk was equivalent to one additional serious suicide-related event per 12 patient-years of treatment with drug. These risks were principally observed in MDD trials. With respect to individual drugs, the strongest signal of risk was observed in the data for paroxetine and venlafaxine, while the most favorable risk estimate was seen for fluoxetine. (This mirrors the conclusions of the MHRA.) In addition, GSK's analysis of adult paroxetine trials showed no excess of suicidal events with paroxetine, in distinction to the findings from the pediatric trials.

Why is your conclusion different from the one being presented today? (Suggest you note here how your analyses are different, why you think they are unlikely to change. Would be a nice touch to acknowledge the limitations of your analyses relative to the definitive analyses being prepared.)

My analyses looked at the data sent by the sponsors in response to the July 22, 2003 requests that Dr. Laughren described to you.

To let you know how my approach to these data differed from that of the Neuropharm Division: First, in my analysis I included events that occurred within 30 days of treatment discontinuation. This made the biggest difference for paroxetine, with approximately ¼ of the suicide-related events occurring within 4 days of discontinuation of paroxetine. I based my calculations on patient-years of exposure rather than numbers of patients, to arrive at rates of events per patient-year of treatment. In addition to analyzing data from MDD trials, I also looked at data from trials with other indications. Finally, I combined data from different clinical trials, either by pooling or using the Mantel-Haenszel method, and applied statistical testing.

Because of the difficulties inherent in the case definition and concerns that clinically insignificant events were classified as "suicide attempts," I focused my analysis on events that met the regulatory definition of serious (as explained by Dr. Laughren).

With respect to the concerns about inconsistent case ascertainment by the sponsors: As a general principle, incomplete case ascertainment can be expected to bias an analysis towards the null; it would not be likely to generate a spurious signal. Consequently, while there were inconsistencies in methods from sponsor to sponsor (despite each sponsor having received the same instructions), in my view this would be more likely to introduce "noise" in the data and obscure a true signal than it would be to generate a false signal.

Regarding the concerns that the case definition is overly inclusive: A too-broad case definition would also be expected to obscure a signal with noise, while a more specific case definition would be more likely to reveal a statistical association.

Therefor, in my view, finding a statistical association *despite* these limitations and inconsistencies makes the finding difficult to dismiss, unless there was some unknown source of systematic bias.

Regarding the inconsistency of relative risk across individual studies: This is certainly an issue; however, the 95% confidence intervals for the relative risks overlap, and the data did not "fail" the Mantel-Haenszel test of homogeneity. Also, although there were a small number of studies indicating a high relative risk with active drug, there was an absence of studies showing a strong protective effect of active drug.

-----Original Message-----
From: Trontell, Anne E
Sent: Wednesday, January 28, 2004 10:43 AM
To: Mosholder, Andrew D; Willy, Mary E
Cc: Avigan, Mark I; Seligman, Paul; Trontell, Anne E
Subject: RE: Feb 2 preparation for possible questions on RCT analyses by Andy

Andy you are not at the table, but just behind it with the presenters. John Jenkins wanted you to be in a place you could address questions about the AERS and your RCT analysis should either come up.

To that end, I'm drafting some potential questions for you to prepare a response along with Mary & Mark's input. Once that's prepared, Paul and I would like to see what you plan to say and provide guidance on how to finesse the likelihood of a shouting match at the table.

Questions for which Andy should prepare a response:

What was the role of your analyses in this process? Why were they not included in the packet or presentations today? (Because they were only just completed?)

What did your analyses show? What is your conclusion? (Suggest giving exec summary version of results. No recommendations, just conclusions about what you think data indicate.

Why is your conclusion different from the one being presented today? (Suggest you note here how your analyses are different, why you think they are unlikely to change. Would be a nice touch to acknowledge the limitations of your analyses relative to the definitive analyses being prepared.)

FYI, concerning the Reporting rates absence; I will field this question and refer onto you only if necessary.

Anne

-----Original Message-----
From: Mosholder, Andrew D
Sent: Wednesday, January 28, 2004 8:48 AM
To: Trontell, Anne E; Willy, Mary E
Subject: RE: Feb 2

Thanks, but I really don't feel a need for a seat at the table. given the limited nature of my participation.
-Andy

-----Original Message-----
From: Trontell, Anne E
Sent: Tuesday, January 27, 2004 3:59 PM
To: Willy, Mary E
Cc: Mosholder, Andrew D
Subject: RE: Feb 2

Andy has been added per me, Temple, and Jenkins emails since Anuja's email was sent.

-----Original Message-----
From: Willy, Mary E

Sent: Tuesday, January 27, 2004 3:47 PM
To: Trontell, Anne E; Pamer, Carol; Avigan, Mark I; Mosholder, Andrew D
Subject: RE: Feb 2

I do not need to be near, but I would suggest that Andy should have a seat. Thanks

----

Mary Willy, PhD
Office of Drug Safety
(301) 827-3175

-----Original Message-----
From: Trontell, Anne E
Sent: Tuesday, January 27, 2004 3:44 PM
To: Pamer, Carol; Avigan, Mark I; Willy, Mary E
Cc: Patel, Anuja
Subject: FW: Feb 2

Pls email Anuja if you'd like to be near to help in answering questions. I hit the send key by mistake.

Anne

-----Original Message-----
From: Trontell, Anne E
Sent: Tuesday, January 27, 2004 3:43 PM
To: Patel, Anuja
Subject: RE: Feb 2

Anuja,
Will also reserve a seat behind the table for a nonpresenter but someone who may be called upon to answer questions on one of the presentations? That would be Carol Pamer, Pharm.D.. I'm copying Mark Avigan and Mary Willy to determine whether they would each also like a reserved seat to be able to help in fielding questions from the committeee.

Thanks.

Anne

-----Original Message-----
From: Patel, Anuja
Sent: Monday, January 26, 2004 8:39 AM
To: Murphy, Dianne; Trontell, Anne E; Galson, Steven; Temple, Robert; Jenkins, John K
Cc: Embrey, Jennifer; Seligman, Paul; Katz, Russell G; Cummins, Susan; Laughren, Thomas P; Somers, Karen M
Subject: RE: Feb 2
Importance: High

I'd like to check one last time to be sure that I have the most recent list of who will be at the table for the Feb 2 PDAC/Peds regarding SSRIs.

From sorting through the e-mails and conversations, my current list is

at the table:
Temple
Katz
Laughren
Murphy
Cummins
ODS??? (Trontell or Seligman) Please let me know!

in reserved seating behind the FDA at the table:
John Jenkins
Solomon Iyasu
Tarek Hammad
Judy Racoosin
Paul David

ANY ONE ELSE? - please let me know today!

This will be a very large table, 40 including six FDA at the table. The FDA section of seating will probably be fairly limited, so it will be a good idea to reserve seats for any critical people planning to attend. Because the table is large, there may not be room for all FDA who are "observing only" and some may have to sit in the audience.

Thanks
Anuja

-----Original Message-----
From: Murphy, Dianne
Sent: Friday, January 23, 2004 7:46 PM
To: Trontell, Anne E; Galson, Steven; Temple, Robert; Jenkins, John K
Cc: Patel, Anuja; Embrey, Jennifer; Seligman, Paul
Subject: RE: Feb 2

How about Temple, MurphyD, Katz, Laughren,Cummins, and ODS draft choice?

-----Original Message-----
From: Trontell, Anne E
Sent: Friday, January 23, 2004 5:13 PM
To: Galson, Steven; Temple, Robert; Jenkins, John K
Cc: Patel, Anuja; Embrey, Jennifer; Murphy, Dianne; Seligman, Paul
Subject: RE: Feb 2

I plan to attend the meeting, happy to sit wherever. Paul's attendance not clear from my looking at his calendar, will discuss his interests when he's back on Monday.

-----Original Message-----
From: Galson, Steven
Sent: Friday, January 23, 2004 4:57 PM
To: Temple, Robert; Jenkins, John K
Cc: Patel, Anuja; Embrey, Jennifer; Murphy, Dianne; PAUL J SELIGMAN .MD (seligmanp@CDER.FDA.gov); Trontell, Anne E
Subject: RE: Feb 2

I am not planning on attending. Would be good to have Anne or Paul up there too.

-----Original Message-----
From: Temple, Robert
Sent: Friday, January 23, 2004 4:52 PM
To: Galson, Steven; Jenkins, John K
Cc: Patel, Anuja
Subject: Feb 2

Do either of you intend to come to the antidepressant Ad Com. Anuja Patel is trying to figure who wants to be at the table. So far it seems like Dianne and me and I've urged Rusty and Tom.

Peds suicidality RCT consult.txt

From: Mosholder, Andrew D
Sent: Thursday, January 29, 2004 9:01 AM
To: Avigan, Mark I
Cc: Willy, Mary E
Subject: Peds suicidality RCT consult

Hi Mark, here is the consult, as we discussed. The new paragraph is highlighted in the exec summary and final portion.
Thanks,
Andy

Tab 24

-----Original Message-----
From: Mosholder, Andrew D
Sent: Tuesday, January 27, 2004 11:55 AM
To: Willy, Mary E
Subject: RCT consult

Hi Mary,
After several days of discussion and mulling it over, I find that I'm not apt to use Anne's proposed language for the recommendations.
I have slightly "wordsmithed" that paragraph, and I added a footnote referencing the MHRA's advisory (since it's similar). But it's not really different and I'm reasonably certain that Anne will want to write a dissenting memo.
I'll attach the document, with the changes (which appear where the placeholder for the recommendations was in the draft that was emailed).

How should I proceed at this point? I'm fine with Anne or anyone else adding a cover memo.
Thanks,
Andy

MEMORANDUM

DEPARTMENT OF HEALTH AND HUMAN SERVICES
PUBLIC HEALTH SERVICE
FOOD AND DRUG ADMINISTRATION
CENTER FOR DRUG EVALUATION AND RESEARCH

PID# D030341

DATE: January 23, 2004

FROM: Andrew D. Mosholder, M.D., M.P.H., Epidemiologist

THROUGH: Mark Avigan, M.D., Director
Division of Drug Risk Evaluation, HFD-430

TO: Russell Katz, M.D., Director
Division of Neuropharmacological Drug Products, HFD-120

SUBJECT: Suicidality in pediatric clinical trials with paroxetine and other antidepressant drugs: Follow-up to 9-4-03 consult

Drugs: paroxetine, sertraline, venlafaxine, fluoxetine, fluvoxamine, citalopram, nefazodone, mirtazapine, and bupropion

EXECUTIVE SUMMARY

This consult is a follow-up to the previous consult on this topic, dated 9-5-03. As described in that consult, GlaxoSmithKline (GSK) performed an analysis of suicidal behaviors in their paroxetine pediatric clinical trial database, and found that there was a statistically significant increase in suicide-related adverse events for paroxetine-treated subjects compared to placebo. The method GSK used for their analysis involved an electronic search of the adverse event data for certain events that might have represented suicidal behaviors, followed by a blinded review of these events to select those that appeared to be probably related to suicide. In July 2003, the Division of Neuropharmacological Drug Products (DNDP) requested the sponsors of the other antidepressant drugs to replicate GSK's analysis in their own pediatric clinical trial databases. This consult summarizes the results of these analyses for 22 short-term placebo-controlled trials involving 9 different antidepressant drugs.

These trials included a total of 4250 pediatric subjects, 2298 treated with active drug and 1952 treated with placebo. There were 108 patients with suicide-related events (74 on active drug and 34 on placebo); 78 of these adverse events were serious (54 on active drug and 24 on placebo).

Considering individual development programs separately, the data for venlafaxine and paroxetine showed a statistically significant increase in suicide-related events relative to placebo. Additionally, on one measure (the incidence rate difference for serious suicide-related events) the data for citalopram approached statistical significance (p-value = 0.063). The relative risks for suicide related events with two compounds, fluoxetine and mirtazapine, were below one, raising the possibility of a protective effect. However, the mirtazapine relative risk estimate of 0.5 was based on a very small number of events and had very broad confidence intervals. The relative risk of suicide-related events for fluoxetine was 0.9 (95% confidence limits 0.3-2.3). (For all the other drugs, the relative risk estimates were greater than one, or undefined because of no events on placebo.)

Overall, comparing active drug treatment to placebo, there was an association of suicide-related events (incidence rate difference 0.08/year, p-value = 0.002) and serious suicide-related events (incidence rate difference 0.06/year, p-value = 0.006) with active drug treatment. This association was observed principally in major depressive disorder (MDD) trials, where the relative risk was 1.8 (95% confidence limit 1.2—2.8) and the attributable risk was 0.24/patient year for drug minus 0.14/patient year for placebo, yielding a value of 0.10 per patient-year of exposure to drug (p-value = 0.013). For serious suicide-related events in MDD trials, the relative risk was 1.9 (95% confidence interval 1.2–3.2), and the attributable risk was was 0.19/patient year for drug minus 0.10/patient year for placebo, yielding a value of 0.085 events per patient-year of exposure to drug (p-value = 0.015), equivalent to approximately 1 excess serious suicide-related event per 12 years of drug treatment. For non-MDD trials, the data also showed a higher rate of events with active drug treatment, but the attributable risk for serious events was much smaller than for MDD trials (0.01/year), and the data were not statistically significant.

There are a number of limitations to this analysis, the chief among them being that the clinical trial data are limited to short-term use of these drugs. Unfortunately, there are not comparable data available regarding safety and efficacy of long-term use of these drugs in pediatric patients. Also, although there were attempts to standardize the methodology and case definitions among the various sponsors, in practice there may have been differences because each sponsor conducted their own separate analysis.

At the present time, a number of additional steps are under way to enhance the quality of the data for the assessment of this signal. These initiatives include arranging for a blinded review of the clinical trial cases by suicidology experts at Columbia University, requesting additional details on how each sponsor conducted their analysis, and obtaining electronic clinical trial datasets for each study to permit a more sophisticated statistical analysis.

However, while these efforts will yield valuable information, particularly at the level of the data for individual trials and drugs, in my view it is unlikely that the new information will alter the basic finding of an association of suicide-related events and serious suicide-related events with active treatment. This is because of the size of the effect and the statistical significance of the overall finding. Also, it seems less likely that misclassification or failure to identify relevant events would produce a false positive signal; rather, those types of errors tend to weaken a signal. Only systematic bias could be reasonably expected to yield a false positive signal of this magnitude, and that seems unlikely.

Recommendations: Given the strength of the association shown by the present data, the clinical importance of the apparent effect (i.e., an estimated excess of one additional serious suicide-related event per 12 patient-years of active treatment), and the fact that the additional analyses are likely to take several more months to complete while considerable numbers of pediatric patients are being exposed to these drugs, I favor an interim risk management plan regarding use of these drugs in the pediatric population. This might be of value to physicians, patients and families who are faced with the need to make a decision regarding pharmacotherapy at the present time. Specifically, I propose a risk management strategy directed at discouraging off-label pediatric use of antidepressant drugs, particularly the use of drugs other than fluoxetine in the treatment of pediatric MDD.[1] Conceivably, this might include discouraging the initiation of treatment of drug-naïve pediatric MDD patients with off-label drugs, in the absence of some over-riding clinical consideration. (Of course, all such warnings should be made in a manner that emphasizes the fact that the available data apply only to short-term, acute treatment, and that sudden discontinuation of antidepressant treatment, or discontinuation without medical supervision, are unwise.) I recommend this approach because fluoxetine is the only drug shown to be effective in pediatric MDD in two clinical studies (out of two MDD studies conducted), and although the confidence limits are broad, it is the drug for which the estimate of the relative risk of suicidal events appears most favorable.

BACKGROUND

This memorandum is in follow-up to our consult to DNDP dated 9-5-03. On May 22 of this year, GlaxoSmithKline submitted an analysis of adverse events related to suicidal behaviors in pediatric trials of paroxetine (Paxil, NDA 20-031). The sponsor performed this analysis by conducting an automated, electronic search of the safety database from their pediatric trials for adverse event terms that would suggest suicidal behaviors. This analysis showed a statistically significant increase in such behaviors with paroxetine treatment, compared to placebo. A previous consult reviewed these data, and also provided a preliminary analysis of data from seven other pediatric development programs for other antidepressant drugs.[2] Overall, there was a statistically significant increase in suicidal adverse events for active drug treatment compared to placebo, similar to the findings from the paroxetine trials. These findings were discussed at a CDER Regulatory Briefing.[3]

However, this preliminary review of pediatric trials with the other antidepressant drugs was limited to a manual search of the reports submitted to FDA. In order to provide a meaningful comparison to the paroxetine findings, the Division of Neuropharmacological Drug Products requested the sponsors of eight other drugs (sertraline, venlafaxine, fluoxetine, fluvoxamine, citalopram, nefazodone, mirtazapine, and bupropion) to conduct a search of their databases similar to the analysis performed by GlaxoSmithKline. All of the 8 sponsors responded to this request within the next few months. The purpose of this memorandum is to summarize the findings reported in those submissions.

With respect to pediatric indications for the antidepressant drugs, clomipramine, fluvoxamine, sertraline and fluoxetine are approved for pediatric obsessive compulsive disorder. (Clomipramine is an older tricyclic compound that was not part of this analysis.) For pediatric major depressive disorder (in children 8 years and up), the only drug approved is fluoxetine. Appendix table 5 presents a summary of the efficacy results from placebo-controlled trials with the aforementioned drugs, along with the regulatory status of the drugs for pediatric use.

METHODS

The sponsors of the aforementioned 8 drugs all received identical information request letters from DNDP dated 7-22-03. The letters asked for the following analyses for all randomized, placebo-

[1] The U.K.'s MHRA, after their recent evaluation of many of the same clinical trial results, concluded that only fluoxetine should be considered to have a favorable risk-benefit ratio for use in pediatric MDD (http://www.mhra.gov.uk/news/2003.htm#2003).
[2] PID# D030341, 9-4-03.
[3] CDER Regulatory Briefing 9-16-03

controlled trial involving pediatric subjects (the indented text below is reproduced from the letters):

> The identification of the following events should be done blinded to treatment to avoid bias. All adverse events occurring within 30 days of the last dose of drug should be included in the search.
>
> "Suicide-related events" should be identified using the following algorithm:
> • Any events coded to preferred terms that include the text strings "suic" or "overdos"
> • Exclude "accidental overdose" cases
> • Regardless of the preferred term to which the verbatim term is mapped, all verbatim terms should be searched for the following text strings: "attempt", "cut", "gas", "hang", "hung", "jump", "mutilat-", "overdos-", "self damag-", "self harm", "self inflict", "self injur-", "shoot", "slash", "suic-"
> • Any terms identified by this search because the text string was a substring of an unrelated word should be excluded (for example, the text string "cut" might identify the word "acute")
> • In addition to the algorithm above, narratives of all serious adverse events (SAEs) should be reviewed (in a blinded fashion) to identify any additional cases of suicidality or self- harm. In particular, SAEs related to mania and hostility should be examined closely for suicidality or self-harm.
> • Any death found to be due to suicide or overdose should be included (if not already identified by the previous search methods).
>
> We are also interested in an analysis of suicide attempts. "Suicide attempts" are a subset of the "suicide-related events" identified above; they should be identified using a blinded hands-on review of the records of all patients identified by the above algorithm as having a "suicide-related event". For the purposes of this analysis, any case in which the patient exhibited self-injurious behavior should be considered as a suicide attempt. Any case in which the patient's suicidal ideation did not lead to self-injurious behavior should be excluded from this subset.
>
> Separate analyses should be performed for the group of "suicide-related" events and the group of "suicide attempts". Both the risk (# of events/# of patients) and the rate (# of events/person-time exposure) should be presented by treatment group. All treatment groups should be presented, including active controls. If a study has a blinded extension phase, events identified while the patient is in that extension phase should be excluded.
>
> In addition to presenting the overall risks and rates across all indications and within each indication, the following stratified analyses should be performed:
> • Child (<12) vs. Adolescent (>= 12).
> • On-therapy vs. On-therapy + 30 days.
> • Within each indication, data from each trial should be presented separately.

Also requested were detailed clinical data about the patients identified as having suicidal events, in the form of narrative summaries and tabulations.

The analyses submitted by each sponsor are summarized herein. A brief description of the relevant pediatric clinical trials is presented for each drug. Also, Appendix table 3 lists each pediatric subject having a suicide-related event.

Although I reviewed all the narrative summaries of the identified adverse events, I have not reclassified any events myself; the sponsors maintained the blind on treatment when they categorized these events, and this is obviously not possible for me. Instead, I have simply noted the few cases where in my opinion a different classification of the event might reasonably have been made. For a few patients who experienced more than one event of interest, I have chosen to count each patient only once in the analysis, at the time of their first event; their subsequent events are described under "Comments" in appendix table 3. Also described under "Comments" are any other adverse events that were prominently associated with the suicidal events. For a few of the clinical development programs, there were a sufficient number of cases to warrant a discussion of possible contributing clinical factors such as dose and duration of treatment, and I have included those details where appropriate.

Also included is a summary analysis of the clinical trial data, both overall and by drug and indication, with statistical testing. This analysis examines the question of the association of these events with active drug treatment in two ways: by calculation of the attributable risk (more precisely, the incidence rate difference between drug and placebo), as well as the relative risk (i.e., incidence rate ratios for drug:placebo). All statistical calculations were performed with Stata version 7.0 software. (Grateful acknowledgement is made to Dr. Yi Tsong of OPSS for his comments on the statistical methods.)

RESULTS

Including the previously reviewed data on paroxetine, this analysis comprised a total of 22 randomized, placebo-controlled trials with 9 different antidepressant drugs in the pediatric population. A total of 2298 pediatric subjects were exposed to active drug, for a total of 406.9 patient-years; for placebo, there were 1952 subjects exposed for a total of 347.6 patient-years. (One trial, Study 329 for paroxetine, included an imipramine arm as an active control, in which the rate of suicide-related events was intermediate between paroxetine and placebo at 0.24 per patient-year, but I have omitted those data from this analysis. Also, patient-years of exposure were not available for the single trial with bupropion.)

The sponsors identified a total of 108 patients with suicide-related events in these trials, 74 on active drug and 34 on placebo. There were no completed suicides. All 83 patients with suicide-related events described in the previous consult were included among these 108 patients. Seventy-eight patients had events classified as serious (54 on drug and 24 on placebo), and 75 had events classified as "suicide attempts" under the method described above (with 49 suicide attempts on drug, and 26 on placebo). Appendix Table 1 presents the complete data on the numbers of these events from all 22 clinical trials, and Appendix Table 2 presents the derived rates of these events for each trial. Appendix Figures 1-4 depict graphically the rates enumerated in Appendix table 2, for MDD and non-MDD studies. Note that the placebo rates of events vary considerably from trial to trial, even within the subgroup of MDD studies. With respect to the classification of events, discussion at the 9-16-03 CDER Regulatory Briefing and subsequently has raised questions about the appropriateness of the "suicide attempts" classification, since this category actually includes all types of deliberate self-injury. Accordingly, in the following I have chosen to emphasize the category of serious suicide-related events, rather than the category of suicide attempts, as being perhaps more clinically meaningful. The data for the category "suicide attempt" are included in Appendix Tables 1 and 2 for completeness.

Overview of each sponsor's submission.

Bupropion (Wellbutrin, NDA 18-644, GlaxoSmithKline, submission dated 8-22-03)

There were no pediatric studies for the indications of major depressive disorder (MDD) or smoking cessation. There was one placebo-controlled pediatric study for the indication of attention deficit hyperactivity disorder (ADHD), as shown below. The requested electronic search of adverse event data revealed no suicide-related events in this study.

Indication	Protocol	No. of sites	Age range (yrs)	Duration (wks)	N	
					Bupropion	Placebo
ADHD	75	4	6-12	6	71	36

Thus, there are no available data on pediatric suicidality with bupropion in the relevant patient populations.

Mirtazapine (Remeron, NDA 20-415, Organon, submission dated 8-21-03 and email dated 11-24-03)

There was only one clinical protocol in the mirtazapine development program, described below; the sponsor conducted two identical studies under that protocol, which were combined for the analysis of safety information.

Indication	Protocol	No. of sites	Age range (yrs)	Duration (wks)	Dose (mg/day)	N	
						Mirtazapine	Placebo
MDD	003-045	34	7-17	8	15-45	170	88

The electronic search of the adverse events terms in study 003-045 yielded a total of 13 adverse events; these were listed in Organon's email submission dated 11-24-03. Of these 13 events, 10 were obviously not related to suicidal behaviors and were excluded, leaving 3 cases for further review; one of these cases ocurred pre-randomization and so was not part of the analysis. Additionally, a subject who was hospitalized for suicidal ideation was identified from the review of all serious adverse events (subject 0404), yielding a total of 3 cases, summarized in Appendix table 3. Note, however, that Organon excluded one of these events from the analysis: subject 0801, a 9 year old boy receiving mirtazapine treated in the emergency room for an overdose on 4 Depakote tablets. This was not considered a suicide attempt because the boy took the tablets "on a dare."

Fluoxetine (Prozac, NDA 18-936, Lilly)

N.B. The following summary is based primarily upon Lilly's submission to Health Canada dated 10-7-03, and not their submission to FDA dated 9-2-03, because Lilly discovered an additional fluoxetine-associated event while preparing their Canadian submission. For details, please refer to Lilly's correspondence dated 10-9-03.

There were four clinical trials relevant to this analysis, three in MDD and one in obsessive-compulsive disorder (OCD). Study HCCJ, a pilot study in adolescent depression, was excluded from the sponsor's Integrated Summary of Safety for the pediatric supplement, but is included in this analysis.

Indication	Study	No. of sites	Age range (yrs)	Duration (wks)	Dose (mg/day)	N	
						Fluoxetine	Pbo
OCD	HCJW	22	7-18	13	10-60	71	32
MDD	HCJE	22	8-18	19*	20	109	110
MDD	X065	1	8-18	8	20	48	48
MDD	HCCJ	1	12-17	6	20-60	21	19

*includes subacute phase (weeks 10-19), during which poorly responding patients could receive a higher dose of double-blind study medication

Lilly's search for adverse events of interest yielded a total of 220 possibly relevant events. Of these, 176 were considered obviously unrelated to the issue of suicidality and were not reviewed further (a list of these adverse events was provided by email 11-17-03, and I concur with the sponsor that none of the events involve self-harm). The remaining cases are summarized in the sponsor's table, reproduced below.

Number of patients in pediatric fluoxetine MDD and OCD trials, by search category (reproduced from sponsor's submission)

Patient Category	Number of Patients
1) Suicide-related events with suicide attempts (acute/subchronic phases[a])	10
2) Suicide-related events with no suicide attempts (acute/subchronic phases[a])	7
3) Accidental overdose/death	1
4) Could be suicide related, but insufficient information	3
5) Suicide-related event prior to treatment phase	14
6) Suicide-related event during extension phase	2
7) Suicide-related event that was not treatment emergent	7

[a] Defined as the acute treatment phases for Studies HCCJ, X065, and HCJW, and the acute and subchronic phases from Study Periods III through V of Study HCJE.

Lilly provided narratives on all the cases listed, in their aforementioned submission to Health Canada and also in their email submission 11-18-03. My own review of these narratives substantiated Lilly's categorization of them.

The 17 events in categories 1 and 2 above were included in the analysis; a listing of these patients appears in appendix table 3.

A few observations can be made regarding the clinical details of these cases. With respect to dose, among the 9 fluoxetine-treated subjects with suicide-related events, the daily dose at the time of event was 20 mg for 7 subjects, 30 mg for one, and 60 mg for one. Median duration of treatment for fluoxetine subjects at the time of their event was 38 days, and the corresponding median for placebo subjects was 33 days. The adolescent age category predominated; children under 12 years of age comprised 43% of the total sample of 458 clinical trial subjects, but only 3 (18%) of the 17 suicide-related events occurred in children, which is not surprising given the relative infrequency of suicidal behavior among children compared to adolescents. Of the 17 suicide-related events, 13 (76.5%) occurred in female subjects, although females comprised only 228 (49.8%) of the 458 subjects.

Regarding the relationship to drug discontinuation, only one of the events (a drug overdose by fluoxetine patient 001-6401 in study HCCJ) occurred during the 30-day follow-up period. This patient was regarded as having discontinued by virtue of being non-compliant with study medication. However, Lilly acknowledged that "events occurring after study completion were not systematically collected," and so some events in the 30-day follow-up period may have been missed.

Nefazodone (Serzone, NDA 20-152, Bristol Myers Squibb, submission dated 8-21-03)

The table below provides the details for the two randomized, placebo-controlled pediatric studies with nefazodone.

Indication	Protocol	No. of sites	Age range (yrs)	Duration (wks)	Dose (mg/day)	N	
						Nefazodone	Placebo
MDD	CN104141	15	12-18	8	100-600	95	95
MDD	CN104187	28	7-17	8	100-300 or 200-600	184 (both arms)	94

The sponsor performed the requested search and identified two suicide-related events in these trials, both occurring in nefazodone-treated patients (please refer to Appendix table 3). (In addition to these events, the sponsor reported a total of 5 suicide-related events that occurred during open label treatment with nefazodone in follow-up to study 187. However, only the two events during double-blind treatment are relevant for this analysis.)

Fluvoxamine (Luvox, NDA 21-519, Solvay, submission dated 8-22-03)

There was one randomized, placebo controlled pediatric trial with fluvoxamine, described in the table below.

Indication	Protocol	No. of sites	Age range (yrs)	Duration (wks)	Dose (mg/day)	N	
						Fluvoxamine	Placebo
OCD	114	20	8-17	10	50-200	57	63

Solvay's search of the safety dataset for this trial revealed a single suicide-related event in a fluvoxamine-treated patient.

Sertraline (Zoloft, NDA 19-839, Pfizer, submission dated 9-12-03)

There were three randomized, placebo-controlled trials in the pediatric population, summarized in the table below. In addition, Pfizer is conducting a pediatric trial in post-traumatic stress disorder, for which the treatment is still blinded. Note that there were two studies for MDD conducted under the same protocol, and these have been combined in this analysis.

Indication	Protocol	No. of sites	Age range (yrs)	Duration (wks)	Dose (mg/day)	N	
						Sertraline	Placebo
OCD	498	12	6-17	12	25-200	92	95
MDD	1001/1017	51	6-17	10	50-200	189	184

The electronic search of adverse event terms yielded 89 potential events from these trials. Pfizer's blinded review of the 89 cases identified 25 patients with possibly relevant events, and further review of these cases excluded 19 events (mostly associated with accidental injuries). This yielded a total of 9 events occurring among 8 subjects that were considered suicide-related. (My own review of the listing of these 89 events did not disclose any additional events that were obvious omissions.) In addition, Pfizer performed the requested review of all serious adverse events in these trials, yielding one additional case relevant to the analysis (subject 1001-29533-2006, who was hospitalized for suicidal ideation). Thus there were a total of 9 patients with suicide-related events. It should be noted, however, that in their submission Pfizer questioned the clinical relevance of events in two sertraline-treated patients (subject 30506-1076, with self-mutilation, and subject 6193-1022, who was hospitalized for suicidal threats), although they did not exclude these events from their analysis.

Although the number of events was probably too small for any meaningful characterizations, the median age among the 6 sertraline treated patients with events was 10 years, somewhat younger than seen in other development programs. These 6 subjects included 3 males and 3 females; their median dose was 100 mg/day, and all had MDD.

There were no events reported within the 30-day period after discontinuation of study medication, and no events in the OCD trial. Of the nine events, six occurred on drug and three on placebo. Six of the nine events occurred in female subjects. With respect to age, there was a somewhat different pattern from that seen in other clinical trial programs, since four events out of the nine occurred in children rather than adolescents (one event considered a suicide attempt occurred in a 6 year old boy). The duration of treatment among the six sertraline-associated events ranged from 21 to 50 days.

Citalopram (Celexa, NDA 20-822, Forest, submission dated 8-21-03)

There were two randomized, controlled clinical trials in the citalopram pediatric development program, summarized below.

Indication	Protocol	No. of sites	Age range (yrs)	Duration (wks)	Dose (mg/day)	N	
						Citalopram	Placebo
MDD	CIT-MD-18	21 in U.S.	7-17	8	20-40	89	85
MDD*	94404	31 in Europe	13-18	12	10-40	121	112

*subjects could be inpatients or outpatients

Note that in addition to these two completed trials, the sponsor is conducting study SCT-MD-15, a randomized, double blind, placebo controlled trial of escitalopram, the s-isomer of citalopram, in children and adolescents with MDD. This trial is still blinded; the total number of subjects planned is 264, and there have been two suicide-related events thus far.

Forest made a couple of departures from the requested methods for the adverse event search. They included an analysis of 8 patients who experienced worsening of depression, but not suicidal thoughts or behaviors; all these patients were treated with placebo. These events were not included in the analysis presented here; the interested reader should refer to their submission for details. Forest also reported that their search of all serious adverse events for events involving suicidality was not performed blind to treatment. (I reviewed the serious adverse events in these two trials myself, and although I was not blind to treatment group either, I did not find any cases that were obvious omissions. However, among the serious adverse events, there were 6 placebo-treated and 2 citalopram-treated patients in study 94404 with psychiatric hospitalizations. These events were not counted in the analysis, however, because suicidality was not specifically documented.)

In addition to the events selected for the analysis, Forest reported that the electronic search identified 11 patients with "false positives" who were excluded.[4] In addition to the electronic search, Forest conducted a manual search of all adverse events and patient narratives from the

[4] Email dated 11-17-03

two trials, yielding 6 patients with relevant events that were not disclosed in the electronic search. This made a total of 30 patients with events. In addition, one patient who took an extra dose of medication by mistake was considered to have taken an accidental overdose (patient 485 in study 94404); this event was not included in the analysis. Two events occurred prior to randomized treatment, yielding a total of 28 patients for the analysis (please refer to Appendix table 3 for a list of these patients). Note that 27 of the 28 events were classified as suicide attempts. However, Forest indicated in an email dated 11-17-03 that six of the study 94404 patients classified with "suicide attempts" (patients 664, 693, 867, 607, 152, and 713) were so categorized simply because the recorded preferred term was suicide attempt, and not because the event description documented self-injurious behavior.

Four placebo-treated patients and four citalopram-treated patients had events during the 30-day follow-up period after the end of randomized treatment. However, two of these 4 placebo patients also had events during double blind treatment, and so are counted as having events while on-treatment. Note that patient 007 in study 94404 was actually receiving fluoxetine, not citalopram, at the time of the event during the post-study period.

The median age of the 28 patients with events was 16 years; 19 were females and 9 males. Among the 13 patients receiving citalopram at the time of their event, the median dose was 20 mg/day, and the median duration on treatment was 27 days. Forest noted that 11 of the 16 citalopram-treated patients with suicide-related events in study 94404 had a past history of suicidality.

Forest also provided an analysis of scores on the suicidality item of the depression rating scales in the two trials; i.e., the CDRS-R in study CIT-MD-18, and the K-SADS in study 94404. There was a greater improvement on the suicidality item in study CIT-MD-18 with citalopram treatment compared to placebo, and this almost reached statistical significance. However, the mean change from baseline on item IX from the K-SADS in study 94404 was approximately equal between citalopram and placebo.[5]

Paroxetine (Paxil, NDA 20-031, GlaxoSmithKline)

Please refer to the consult dated 9-5-03 for details regarding the paroxetine pediatric clinical trial data. Subsequently, GSK provided the agency with a copy of their report to the Committee for Proprietary Medicinal Products of the European Agency for the Evaluation of Medicinal Products .[6] Included in this is an analysis of suicide-related events in adult trials with paroxetine that mirrors GSK's analysis of the pediatric clinical trials. The results of the adult trial analysis show essentially no difference in the rates of suicide-related events between paroxetine and placebo treatment groups, for all studies combined or for the subset of MDD trials. This is in contrast to the previously described pediatric trial data, which showed a statistically significant increase with paroxetine treatment. The sponsor's tables describing both the adult and the pediatric analyses are reproduced in Appendix Figure 5.

Venlafaxine (Effexor and Effexor XR, NDAs 20-151 and 20-699, Wyeth)

There were four randomized, double blind, placebo-controlled venlafaxine trials in pediatric patients, summarized in the following table. The sponsor also reported that two additional

---

[5] NDA 20-822 8-21-03 submission
[6] NDA 20-031 11-7-03 electronic submission

pediatric placebo-controlled trials, one in social anxiety disorder and one in panic disorder, have been completed but are not fully analyzed yet.

Indication	Protocol	No. of sites	Age range (yrs)	Duration (wks)	Dose* (mg/day)	N	
						Venlafaxine	Placebo
MDD	382	16	7-17	8 + taper	37.5-225	80	85
MDD	394	37	7-17	8 + taper	37.5-225	102	94
GAD**	396	39	6-17	8 + taper	37.5-225	80	84
GAD	397	35	6-17	8 + taper	37.5-225	77	79

*administered as Effexor XR in all trials; dosage based upon weight of subject, and tapered over ≤2 weeks following double-blind treatment
**Generalized Anxiety Disorder

Wyeth identified 16 randomized patients with suicide-related events, along with two MDD patients who had events before beginning the study and who were not counted in the analysis. Additionally, one more event was identified through review of adverse event narratives, yielding a total of 17 patients who experienced a total of 20 events of interest. Wyeth counted all 20 events, rather than simply enumerating the number of patients with events.[7] Note that two patients were considered to have had separate events a few days apart (patients 39402-0041 and 39428-1087); after review of the narrative summaries, I have elected to count these instead as single events. A third patient also had two events, patient 38211-012, but these were separated by approximately 3 weeks and I have elected to count only the first event in the analysis that follows. Thus, the analysis shown below is based upon the number of patients with events, rather than the number of events (as in Wyeth's analysis). The listing in the Appendix provides further details about the patients.

The patient-years of exposure were not provided in the response to the July 2003 letter, since only rates were displayed in that submission; however, the exposures were available from the original pediatric exclusivity supplement. Additionally, in Wyeth's analysis, the "on-therapy" period does not include the taper period, but only the period of randomized treatment during which patients received their full dose of study medication. Therefor, "on-therapy period + 30 days" does not include a full 30 days from the last dose of study medication, if the patient had a taper following the end of their study treatment. This is slightly different from GlaxoSmithKline's analysis of the paroxetine pediatric trials, in which the "on-therapy" period included the taper phase, through the last dose of study medication, and the "on-therapy + 30 days" period included a full 30 days from the last dose of study medication.

With respect to classification of events, there were some issues with the "suicide attempts" category. The reason that patient 38205-019 was not counted in the suicide attempt category for taking an overdose was unclear. Also, I was unable to verify Wyeth's count of 3 suicide attempts on venlafaxine and 2 on placebo in study 382.[8] Instead, I have used the counts from Wyeth's "Abbreviated Table of Patient Characteristics."[9]

The median age among the 17 patients with suicide-related events was 13 years. For the 13 venlafaxine-treated patients, at the time of the event the median dose was 112.5 mg/day, and the median duration of treatment was 24 days. Wyeth counted any events occurring within 1 day of

[7] NDA 20-151 submission 8-28-03
[8] Table 3A, NDA 20-151 submission 8-28-03
[9] Table 4A, NDA 20-151 submission 8-28-03

the last full dose of study medication as having occurred on-therapy. Five of the 17 events did not occur on-therapy, 3 with venlafaxine and 2 with placebo.

Risk estimates

Analysis of attributable risk

Pooling the exposure and event data by drug and by indication provides the results shown in tables 1 and 2. Appendix figure 6 displays these same results graphically. Here, an incidence rate difference greater than zero would indicate a risk associated with active drug versus placebo, while an incidence rate difference less than zero would indicate a protective effect of the drug.

Table 1.

Attributable risks (incidence rate differences) per patient-year for suicide-related events in pediatric trials

Trials	Incidence rate difference, drug minus placebo	95% confidence interval	p-value
Citalopram	0.14	-0.16-0.43	0.374
Fluoxetine	-0.03	-0.20-0.14	0.737
Fluvoxamine	0.11	-0.10-0.32	0.485
Mirtazapine	-0.04	-0.21-0.14	0.691
Nefazodone	0.05	-0.02-0.12	0.367
Paroxetine	0.12	0.04-0.20	0.005
Sertraline	0.06	-0.05-0.17	0.327
Venlafaxine	0.17	0.02-0.33	0.029
All MDD trials	0.10	0.02-0.18	0.013
All non-MDD trials	0.04	-0.01-0.09	0.114
All trials	0.08	0.03-0.14	0.002

Table 2

Attributable risks (incidence rate differences) per patient-year for serious suicide-related events in pediatric trials

Trials	Incidence rate difference, drug minus placebo	95% confidence interval	p-value
Citalopram	0.24	-0.01-0.48	0.063
Fluoxetine	-0.02	-0.18-0.14	0.775
Fluvoxamine	0	-	-
Mirtazapine	0.04	-0.04-0.12	0.654
Nefazodone	0.03	-0.02-0.08	0.606
Paroxetine	0.08	0.01-0.15	0.038
Sertraline	0.06	-0.04-0.16	0.276
Venlafaxine	0.06	-0.07-0.18	0.379
All MDD trials	0.09	0.02-0.15	0.015
All non-MDD trials	0.01	-0.02-0.05	0.498
All trials	0.06	0.02-0.11	0.006

The incidence rate differences by drug for MDD trials alone are shown in Appendix Tables 6 and 7. These data are displayed graphically in Appendix Figure 7.

It can be seen that overall the data are consistent with an increased risk of suicidal events with active drug treatment; the comparison between active treatment and placebo for all trials pooled together is statistically significant (p-value = 0.002 for all suicide-related events, and p-value = 0.006 for serious suicide-related events). For serious suicide-related events in MDD trials, the attributable risk was was 0.19/patient year for drug minus 0.10/patient year for placebo, yielding a value of 0.085 events per patient-year of exposure to drug (p-value = 0.015), equivalent to approximately 1 excess serious suicide-related event per 12 years of drug treatment. The observed serious event incidence rate differences are larger in MDD trials (0.085/year) than in trials with OCD, GAD and Social Anxiety Disorder (SAD) (0.014/year).
With respect to individual drugs, the incidence rate differences for all suicide-related events are largest for paroxetine, venlafaxine and citalopram, reaching statistical significance for paroxetine and venlafaxine. For serious suicide-related events, citalopram showed the largest incidence rate difference, which approached statistical significance (p-value = 0.063).

Analysis of relative risk

In addition to estimating the excess risk attributable to drug, the data can also be analyzed in terms of the relative risk, or more precisely, the ratio of the incidence rates for drug and placebo. Accordingly, Mantel-Haenszel combined incidence rate ratios were calculated, stratified by study. This approach has the advantage of providing stratification by study, while the analysis of excess risk shown above simply involved summing all the relevant data without regard for differences between trials. In addition to calculating the combined incidence rate ratio, the Stata software also tests for homogeneity of the individual study ratios.

The Stata output for the "All trials" category is shown in Appendix table 3. There were two studies by themselves that showed statistically significant rate ratios for suicide-related events, Paroxetine Study 329 and Venlafaxine Study 394. No individual study showed a statistically significant protective effect.

Table 3 below displays the relative risks (more precisely, the incidence rate ratios) for suicide-related events and serious suicide-related events for each of the antidepressant drugs, and for all 21 clinical trials combined. Here placebo is the reference, and thus a value less than one indicates a protective effect of the drug, and a value greater than one a risk associated with drug treatment. For each combined incidence rate ratio calculated, the Mantel-Haenszel chi-square test showed no lack of homogeneity (i.e., indicating that data from the individual studies can be combined statistically).

Table 3. Combined incidence rate ratios for suicide-related events and serious suicide-related events

Drug	Number of pediatric trials	Incidence rate ratios* (95% confidence interval), by drug	
		All suicide-related events	Serious suicide-related events
Paroxetine	5	2.69 (1.20-6.00)	2.19 (0.92-5.24)
Sertraline	2	2.03 (0.51-8.16)	2.52 (0.49-13.01)
Venlafaxine	4	3.33 (1.08-10.33)	1.80 (0.52-6.20)
Fluoxetine	4	0.88 (0.34-2.30)	0.88 (0.32-2.44)
Citalopram	2	1.41 (0.66-3.00)	2.54 (0.91-7.05)
Mirtazapine	1	0.53 (0.007-41.45)	†
Nefazodone	2	†	†
Fluvoxamine	1	†	†
MDD trials	14	1.81 (1.19-2.77)	1.95 (1.19-3.21)
Non-MDD trials	7	2.36 (0.67-8.33)	1.31 (0.26-6.72)
All trials	21	1.86 (1.25-2.78)	1.89 (1.18-3.04)

†Ratio undefined due to zero events in placebo group
*Mantel-Haenszel method

It will be seen that the suicide-related event incidence rate ratios for venlafaxine and paroxetine indicate an association with drug treatment, and that the corresponding confidence intervals exclude one. Overall, the incidence rate ratio of approximately 1.9 for both suicide-related events and the subcategory of serious suicide-related events indicate an association of these events with drug treatment. Put another way, compared to placebo, treatment with active drug increased the rate of suicide-related events by an estimated 85%, and by an estimated 87% for serious suicide-related events. For the subgroup of MDD trials, the incidence rate ratios were also statistically significant, while for non-MDD trials the incidence rate ratio estimates had very wide confidence intervals.

DISCUSSION AND CONCLUSIONS

In short-term pediatric trials, antidepressant drug treatment is associated with an increase in suicidal adverse events compared to placebo. This finding is seen for both the broad category of any suicide-related event, and the more specific category of serious suicide-related events. The association is more prominent in the MDD trial data, where the relative risk of serious suicide-related events is approximately 1.9. The rate of serious suicide-related events in MDD trials among drug-treated patients was 0.19/patient-year, and was 0.10/patient-year among placebo-treated patients. These rates represent one serious event per 5.4 patient-years for drug, and one serious event per 9.9 patient-years for placebo, yielding an attributable risk of one additional serious suicide-related event per 11.8 patient-years of drug treatment. The finding appears to be statistically robust, inasmuch as the p-value for the incidence rate difference for all suicide-related events across all trials is 0.002.

With respect to individual drugs, the data for paroxetine and venlafaxine show a statistically significant increase in suicide-related events with active treatment in their pediatric development programs. Also, the incidence rate difference for serious suicide-related events with citalopram was close to statistical significance (p-value = 0.063). For fluoxetine and mirtazapine, the point estimates were consistent with a protective effect, but the confidence intervals for mirtazapine were very broad, and even for fluoxetine the confidence interval on the incidence rate ratio includes a relative risk of greater than 2. Put another way, although an increase in suicide-related events reached statistical significance for two drugs (paroxetine and venlafaxine), for no drug was a protective effect demonstrated at a statistically significant level.

This analysis has several limitations. Most importantly, it is limited to short-term trials only. Conceivably, long-term treatment in patients who have responded positively to a drug might not produce an increased risk, or might even provide a protective effect. In other words, it may not be appropriate to extrapolate a finding of a risk in short-term trials to use of the drug for long-term maintenance treatment, especially if the patients have manifested a clinical response to the drug. Unfortunately, there is very little long-term controlled pediatric trial data for antidepressant drugs that is available for analysis.

Another limitation of this analysis is that although there is evidence of a class effect overall, it is difficult to know to what extent it applies to particular members of the class. Inspection of the confidence intervals for the risk estimates will show that the confidence limits for individual drugs overlap considerably. The existing clinical trial data, moreover, cannot provide a fair comparison between drugs, since the sizes of the clinical development programs and the specific indications studied vary from drug to drug, not to mention the fact that the intrinsic pharmacologic and pharmacokinetic properties of the drugs themselves are different.

A third limitation pertains to the difficulties in standardizing the methodology used by the nine different sponsors. Although all sponsors were given the same set of instructions in the letters issued 7-22-03, there were some discrepancies in how these instructions were applied. For example, Forest (sponsor of citalopram) performed not only the requested electronic search of all adverse event terms, but also a manual search, which yielded cases not found with the electronic search. Also, the 30-day follow-up period was interpreted differently by GSK (paroxetine) and Wyeth (venlafaxine). GSK counted followed-up time for 30 days after the last dose of study medication, and the taper phase was not part of that 30-day period. However, Wyeth began the 30-day period from the last full dose of study medication, so that the period of dosage taper was included in the 30-day follow-up time. Also, Lilly (sponsor of fluoxetine) reported that adverse event data was not consistently collected once patients discontinued their study treatment.

As Appendix figures 1-4 illustrate, there was considerable variability in the rates of these events from trial to trial, even within the same indication. This could be due to differences in the patient population (some trials included children, for example), or to differences in ascertainment of suicide-related events, or to both. This, of course, raises questions about whether it is appropriate to combine the data from different trials. The Mantel-Haenszel chi square test for homogeneity of the rate ratios, however, did not reveal any statistically significant lack of homogeneity.

The increase in suicidal events was most clearly demonstrated in MDD trials. However, events with active drug treatment were more frequent than events with placebo in non-MDD trials, although the numbers are small and the risk estimates are very uncertain. Nonetheless, this leaves open the possibility of a drug-associated risk of such behaviors for non-MDD patients, although at a much lower incidence rate difference than for MDD patients.

With respect to clinical factors that might be contributory, as described in the previous consult, the paroxetine data suggested a possible role for drug withdrawal, but this pattern was not as prominent in the data for other drugs. However, this observation might point to a lack of consistency across development programs with respect to ascertainment of adverse events following the end of double-blind treatment.

The absence of completed suicides in these data is only reassuring to a limited degree. The total drug exposure time in these trials was 407 patient-years. For assessing the rate of a rare event such as completed suicide with active drug treatment, this is a relatively small data set. To illustrate, the upper confidence limit (one sided, 95% level) for the actual rate in the population given an observation of no suicides in 407 patient-years is 1 completed suicide in approximately 136 patient years.

In contrast to the paroxetine pediatric data, the analysis of suicide-related events in adult paroxetine trials, employing methods identical to the corresponding analysis of pediatric trial data, failed to show an increase in the rate of such events with paroxetine treatment relative to placebo. This was despite the fact that the placebo rate for these events was similar between the adult MDD trials (0.10/year) and the pediatric MDD trials (0.13/year). This suggests that adults and pediatric patients may have different responses to paroxetine with respect to suicidality.

Several steps are being taken at the moment to evaluate this signal further. First, a joint meeting of the Psychopharmacologic Drugs Advisory Committee and the Pediatric Subcommittee of the Anti-Infective Drugs Advisory Committee will be held 2-2-04 to discuss this issue.[10] Secondly, DNDP has requested electronic data sets from the sponsors of these clinical trials that will permit a more sophisticated statistical analysis. This analysis will permit examination of a number of issues that were beyond the scope of this consult, such as adjustment for a number of relevant covariates and exploration of risk factors such as agitation and relevant family history. Thirdly, DNDP has arranged for a group of suicidology experts at Columbia University to review the clinical narrative summaries for all of the identified cases; this will permit a more sophisticated case classification, particularly with regards to whether the event was a serious suicide attempt, a gesture, or self-mutilation. Fourthly, on 11-24-03 DNDP sent a memo to all the sponsors requesting a more detailed description of the methods each sponsor used to generate the submissions reviewed in this consult, to ensure the highest possible quality of data for review by the Columbia University experts.

One suggestion can be made for the expert group involved in the review of the cases. Because the nature and quality of the case reports received from the sponsors (as listed in Appendix Table 3) vary considerably, it is likely that even experts in classifying suicidal behaviors will have some uncertainty about how to classify some of the case reports. Accordingly, it will be important to reserve a category of indeterminate cases with which to do a sensitivity analysis. The principle here would be to do an analysis including the doubtful cases, and another analysis excluding them, to see if the results are very dependent upon how uncertain cases are classified.

These initiatives should indeed provide higher-quality data for evaluation of this signal. However, in my view, the new analyses are more likely to change the findings for individual studies and drug compounds where the numbers are relatively small, than they are to alter the overall finding of an increase in suicide-related adverse events and serious suicide-related events with active drug treatment compared to placebo. There are, I believe, several reasons for this. First, the aggregate findings are statistically robust (e.g., p-value = 0.002). Secondly, the counts of serious suicide-related events are, in my view, less likely to be unstable, because of the methods routinely employed to account for serious adverse events in clinical trials, and the greater amount of clinical information that is often collected about serious adverse events compared to non-serious events. Additionally, to the extent that events have been misclassified or overlooked in the sponsor's searches, this would generally be expected to introduce "noise" that would weaken the signal and produce a false negative, not generate a false positive. Only a systematic bias that

[10] Federal Register Vol. 68, No. 211 Friday, October 31, 2003

caused events in the placebo group to be missed while events in the drug group were captured would be expected to produce a false positive, and it is difficult to conceive of what could produce such a bias.

As previously noted, fluoxetine is currently the only drug approved for pediatric MDD, although several drugs are approved for pediatric OCD (see Appendix table 5). As shown in that table, all of the four pediatric OCD trials were positive and provided evidence of efficacy for approval of the drugs for pediatric OCD. This is in contrast to the experience with pediatric MDD trials, for which only 3 of the 15 trials have been judged positive, two with fluoxetine and one with citalopram.

In sum, short-term pediatric clinical trials of antidepressant drugs demonstrate an increased rate of suicidal events with active drug compared to placebo.

Recommendations: Given the strength of the association shown by the present data, the clinical importance of the apparent effect (i.e., an estimated excess of one additional serious suicide-related event per 12 patient-years of active treatment), and the fact that the additional analyses are likely to take several more months to complete while considerable numbers of pediatric patients are being exposed to these drugs, I favor an interim risk management plan regarding use of these drugs in the pediatric population. This might be of value to physicians, patients and families who are faced with the need to make a decision regarding pharmacotherapy at the present time. Specifically, I propose a risk management strategy directed at discouraging off-label pediatric use of antidepressant drugs, particularly the use of drugs other than fluoxetine in the treatment of pediatric MDD. Conceivably, this might include discouraging the initiation of treatment of drug-naïve pediatric MDD patients with off-label drugs, in the absence of some over-riding clinical consideration. (Of course, all such warnings should be made in a manner that emphasizes the fact that the available data apply only to short-term, acute treatment, and that sudden discontinuation of antidepressant treatment, or discontinuation without medical supervision, are unwise.) I recommend this approach because fluoxetine is the only drug shown to be effective in pediatric MDD in two clinical studies (out of two MDD studies conducted), and although the confidence limits are broad, it is the drug for which the estimate of the relative risk of suicidal events appears most favorable.

Andrew D. Mosholder, M.D., M.P.H.
Epidemiologist

Mary Willy, Ph.D.
Epidemiology Team Leader

Appendix Table 1. Summary of pediatric clinical trial data on suicidal adverse events

Drug	Indication	Study	Drug					Placebo				
			N	Patient-years	Suicide-related events	Serious suicide-related Events	Suicide attempts	N	Patient-years	Suicide-related events	Serious suicide-related events	Suicide attempts
Paroxetine*	MDD	329†	93	13	8	7	5	88	13	1	1	0
	MDD	377	181	41	9	7	8	95	21	4	4	4
	MDD	701	104	16	3	3	2	102	17	2	1	1
	OCD	704	99	19	1	1	0	107	22	0	0	0
	SAD	676	165	51	4	0	1	157	47	0	0	0
	Paroxetine Total		*642*	*140*	*25*	*18*	*16*	*549*	*120*	*7*	*6*	*5*
Sertraline	MDD	1001/1017	189	32.2	6	5	3	184	32.5	2	2	2
	OCD	498	92	18.8	0	0	0	95	19.7	1	0	0
	Sertraline Total		*281*	*51*	*6*	*5*	*3*	*279*	*52.2*	*3*	*2*	*2*
Venlafaxine	MDD	382	80	11.01	5	3	1	85	11.73	3	3	3
	MDD	394	102	15.95	7	3	3	94	15.47	0	0	0
	GAD	396	80	13.08	0	0	0	84	13.56	0	0	0
	GAD	397	77	11.63	1	1	1	79	11.44	1	1	1
	Venlafaxine Total		*339*	*51.67*	*13*	*7*	*5*	*342*	*52.2*	*4*	*4*	*4*
Fluvoxamine	OCD	114	57	9.37	1	0	0	63	9.95	0	0	0
Mirtazapine	MDD	003-045	170	24.05	1	1	0	88	12.7	1	0	1
Fluoxetine	MDD	HCJE	109	31.57	4	3	1	110	27.96	4	3	2
	MDD	HCCJ	21	2.11	1	1	1	19	2.11	1	1	1
	MDD	X065	48	6.71	2	2	2	48	5.83	2	2	0
	OCD	HCJW	71	15.12	2	2	2	32	5.98	1	1	1
	Fluoxetine Total		*249*	*55.51*	*9*	*8*	*6*	*209*	*41.88*	*8*	*7*	*4*
Nefazodone	MDD	141	95	13.6	1	0	1	95	12.5	0	0	0
	MDD	187	184	25.4	1	1	1	94	12.9	0	0	0
	Nefazodone Total		*279*	*39*	*2*	*1*	*2*	*189*	*25.4*	*0*	*0*	*0*
Citalopram	MDD	CIT-MD-18	89	12.8	1	0	1	85	12	2	0	1
	MDD	94404	121	23.5	16	14	16	112	21.3	9	5	9
	Citalopram Total		*210*	*36.3*	*17*	*14*	*17*	*197*	*33.3*	*11*	*5*	*10*
Bupropion	ADHD	75	71	**	0	0	0	36	**	0	0	0
Grand Total			**2298**	**406.9**	**74**	**54**	**49**	**1952**	**347.63**	**34**	**24**	**26**

*Paroxetine patient-years of exposure were provided only to the nearest integer **Patient-years of exposure data were not provided †Imipramine arm omitted

Appendix Table 2. Rates of suicidal adverse events, per patient-year, in pediatric clinical trials

Drug	Indication	Study	Drug				Placebo			
			Patient-years	Rate of Suicide-related events	Rate of Serious suicide-related Events	Rate of Suicide attempts	Patient-years	Rate of Suicide-related events	Rate of Serious suicide-related events	Rate of Suicide attempts
Paroxetine	MDD	329	13	0.62	0.54	0.38	13	0.08	0.00	0.08
	MDD	377	41	0.22	0.17	0.20	21	0.19	0.19	0.19
	MDD	701	16	0.19	0.19	0.13	17	0.12	0.06	0.06
	OCD	704	19	0.05	0.05	0.00	22	0.00	0.00	0.00
	SAD	676	51	0.08	0.00	0.02	47	0.00	0.00	0.00
Sertraline	MDD	1001/1017	32.2	0.19	0.16	0.09	32.5	0.06	0.06	0.06
	OCD	498	18.8	0.00	0.00	0.00	19.7	0.05	0.00	0.00
Venlafaxine	MDD	382	11.01	0.45	0.27	0.09	11.73	0.26	0.26	0.26
	MDD	394	15.95	0.44	0.19	0.19	15.47	0.00	0.00	0.00
	GAD	396	13.08	0.00	0.00	0.00	13.56	0.00	0.00	0.00
	GAD	397	11.63	0.09	0.09	0.09	11.44	0.09	0.09	0.09
Fluvoxamine	OCD	114	9.37	0.11	0.00	0.00	9.95	0.00	0.00	0.00
Mirtazapine	MDD	003-045	24.05	0.04	0.04	0.00	12.7	0.08	0.08	0.00
Fluoxetine	MDD	HCJE	31.57	0.13	0.10	0.03	27.96	0.14	0.07	0.11
	MDD	HCCJ	2.11	0.47	0.47	0.47	2.11	0.47	0.47	0.47
	MDD	X065	6.71	0.30	0.30	0.30	5.83	0.34	0.34	0.00
	OCD	HCJW	15.12	0.13	0.13	0.13	5.98	0.17	0.17	0.17
Nefazodone	MDD	141	13.6	0.07	0.00	0.07	12.5	0.00	0.00	0.00
	MDD	187	25.4	0.04	0.04	0.04	12.9	0.00	0.00	0.00
Citalopram	MDD	CIT-MD-18	12.8	0.08	0.00	0.08	12	0.17	0.08	0.00
	MDD	94404	23.5	0.68	0.60	0.68	21.3	0.42	0.42	0.23
Total			406.9	0.18	0.13	0.12	347.63	0.10	0.07	0.07

Appendix Table 3. Listing of all patients with suicide-related events in pediatric antidepressant drug trials.

MIRTAZAPINE

Study	Indication	Patient ID	Age Sex	Treatment	Dose (mg/day) at time of event	Duration (days)	Event	Serious (y/n)	Comments
003-045	MDD	0404	15 M	Mirtazapine	15	7	Hospitalization for suicidal ideation	Y	
003-045	MDD	0801	9 M	Mirtazapine	45	52	Depakote overdose "on a dare"	Y	*Excluded by sponsor*
003-045	MDD	1603	12 F	Placebo	-	56	Self inflicted cuts	N	

FLUOXETINE

Study	Indication	Patient ID	Age Sex	Treatment	Dose (mg/day) at time of event	Duration (days)	Event	Serious (y/n)	Comments
HCCJ	MDD	001/6401	17 F	Fluoxetine	30	40	Overdose, details unknown; discontinued from trial	y	Patient poorly compliant with study drug
HCCJ	MDD	001-6408	13 M	Placebo	-	33	Overdose of aspirin	y	
HCJE	MDD	008-0806	15 M	Placebo	-	37	Hospitalized for suicidal ideation and self-mutilation	y	
HCJE	MDD	008/0804	15 F	Placebo	-	60	Overdose on study medication	y	
HCJE	MDD	009-0901	15 F	Fluoxetine	60	101	Self-mutilation	n	
HCJW	OCD	006-0609	15 F	Placebo	-	71	Self-injurious behavior	Y	No details provided
HCJW	OCD	013-1300	12 F	Fluoxetine	20	25	Tylenol overdose	Y	Hospitalized
HCJW	OCD	018-1811	7 F	Fluoxetine	20	60	Self-destructive cutting	y	
X065	MDD	001-2051	16 F	Fluoxetine	20	14	Multiple drug overdose	Y	Other adverse events included manic reaction
X065	MDD	001-2163	17 F	Fluoxetine	20	12	Overdose on unknown pills	Y	No psychiatric family history, no previous attempts
HCJE	MDD	004-0419	13 F	Fluoxetine	20	67	Hospitalized for suicidal ideation	Y	
HCJE	MDD	022-2216	15 F	Fluoxetine	20	38	Suicidal ideation	Y	
HCJE	MDD	003-0302	17 F	Fluoxetine	20	32	Suicidal thoughts	y	
HCJE	MDD	019-1901	11 F	Placebo	-	?	"wanting to die"	N	
HCJE	MDD	022-2203	9 M	Placebo	-	9	Suicidal ideation, intermittent	Y	Displayed self-injurious behavior during later extension phase of trial
X065	MDD	001-2052	16 M	Placebo	-	33	Suicidal ideation X 1 day (not hospitalized)	Y	Considered serious
X065	MDD	001-2087	14 F	Placebo	-	6	Hospitalized for suicidal ideation	y	

NEFAZODONE

Study	Indication	Patient ID	Age Sex	Treatment	Dose (mg/day) at time of event	Duration	Event	Serious (y/n)	Comments
141	MDD	3-1065	12 M	Nefazodone	600	38	Self mutilation (superficial cutting)	n	
187	MDD	18-322	13 F	Nefazodone	0	4 days post d/c	Overdose on 14 tablets of study medication	y	Hospitalized

FLUVOXAMINE

Study	Indication	Patient ID	Age Sex	Treatment	Dose (mg/day) at time of event	Duration (days)	Event	Serious (y/n)	Comments
RH1140201	OCD	65815	15 M	Fluvoxamine	200	36	Suicidal ideation	N	Self-mutilation during open label extension phase

SERTRALINE

Study	Indication	Patient ID	Age Sex	Treatment	Dose (mg/day) at time of event	Duration (days)	Event	Serious (y/n)	Comments
498	OCD	90N0242-19	12 F	Placebo	-	12	Suicidal ideation	N	
1001	MDD	29533-2006	12 M	Sertraline	100	49	Suicidal ideation	y	Hospitalized
1001	MDD	29534-1089	10 F	Sertraline	100	35	Suicidal ideation	Y	Hospitalized
1001	MDD	30506-1076	9 F	Sertraline	100	37	Self mutilation	n	Second episode of self mutilation on day 46
1001	MDD	6193-1022	10 M	Sertraline	100	21	Suicidal ideation	Y	Hospitalized. Also had mild agitation.
1017	MDD	29384-4022	16 F	Sertraline	150	50	Multidrug overdose	Y	Also noted to have restlessness
1017	MDD	30627-3095	6 M	Sertraline	100	34	Threatened to jump from vehicle, suicidal ideation	Y	Hospitalized; also experienced agitation
1017	MDD	31940-4329	17 F	Placebo	-	9	Attempted self-immolation	Y	Minor burn wounds. Subject later denied suicidality
1017	MDD	31942-4321	15 F	Placebo	-	63	Attempted suicide by hanging	Y	Second suicide attempt by overdose on day 66

CITALOPRAM

Study	Indication	Pt ID	Age Sex	Treatment	Dose (mg/day) at time of event	Duration (days)	Event	Serious (y/n)	Comments
CIT-MD-18	MDD	193	9 M	Citalopram	20	37	Cut self with knife	N	Agitation reported on previous day
CIT-MD-18	MDD	137	10 M	Placebo	-	31	Attempted to hang self (but not designated as a serious event)	N	Personality disorder; 24 days post-tx had another suicide-related event
CIT-MD-18	MDD	519	12 F	Placebo	-	41	Severe suicidal tendency (no details)	N	
94404	MDD	007	15 M	Citalopram	-	25 days post tx	Multiple drug overdose	Y	*Patient had received fluoxetine X 25 days since completing trial*
94404	MDD	009	17 F	Citalopram	20	15	Hospitalized for suicidality; overdose on naproxen on day 6 of hospitalization	Y	
94404	MDD	121	18 F	Citalopram	-	12 days post tx	Overdose of chlorxazone	Y	Patient had been discontinued from study on day 8 because of abnl clinical laboratories
94404	MDD	148	17 F	Citalopram	20	47	Overdose of 4-6 citalopram tablets	Y	Made a second overdose later in tria
94404	MDD	426	14 F	Citalopram	20	70	Overdose on 11 paracetamol tablets; denied suicidal intent	Y	Event coded as medication error
94404	MDD	573	14 F	Citalopram	20	88	Intentional ingestion of cigarettes	Y	Subject was an inpatient at screening
94404	MDD	575	14 F	Citalopram	20	55	Suicidal ideation, cut arm	Y	Subject was an inpatient at screening
94404	MDD	664	15 M	Citalopram	20	10	Re-hospitalized for suicidality	Y	Subject was an inpatient at screening
94404	MDD	713	16 M	Citalopram	30	27	Re-hospitalized for suicidality	N	Subject was an inpatient at screening. No explanation for why this was not designated a serious event.
94404	MDD	715	17 F	Citalopram	20	14	Hospitalized for suicidality, cut wrists, denied suicidal intent	Y	
94404	MDD	729	16 M	Citalopram	10	63	Ingested 15 caffeine pills plus alcohol	N	Event coded as medication error
94404	MDD	761	13 M	Citalopram	-	1 day post tx	Hospitalized for suicidality, event designated as a suicide attempt	Y	Also developed agitation, mood lability
94404	MDD	776	17 F	Citalopram	-	1 day post tx	Multiple drug overdose; only dose of study medication was the previous day	Y	Subject was an inpatient at screening. Also experienced anxiety
94404	MDD	867	17 F	Citalopram	30	20	Hospitalization due to suicidal thoughts	Y	Also experienced anxiety
94404	MDD	874	17 f	Citalopram	20	13	Overdose	Y	Patient cut her wrist 4 days after overdose
94404	MDD	884	16 F	Citalopram	20	16	Hospitalized after overdose on diazepam (9 tablets)	Y	On day 22, re-hospitalized for suicidality, and on day 81, another overdose
94404	MDD	071	16 F	Placebo	-	16	Hospitalized after self-inflicted wrist laceration	Y	Re-hospitalized for suicidality on day 36
94404	MDD	152	14 F	Placebo	-	8 days post tx	Hospitalized for suicidality	Y	Treated with citalopram after hospitalization
94404	MDD	412	18 F	Placebo	-	1 day post tx	Overdose on mother's medication	Y	Also receiving oxazepam for anxiety

Study	Indication	Pt ID	Age Sex	Treatment	Dose (mg/day) at time of event	Duration (days)	Event	Serious (y/n)	Comments
94404	MDD	605	13 M	Placebo	-	35	Self mutilation (forearm)	N	
94404	MDD	607	17 M	Placebo	-	62	Suicidal ideation and tension, treated with lorazepam	N	Inpatient at screening.
94404	MDD	691	17 F	Placebo	-	29	Self mutilation (palms)	N	
94404	MDD	693	16 F	Placebo	-	2	Hospitalized for suicidal ideation	Y	Later in trial had self-inflicted scratches on arm. After completing trial, started citalopram and was re-hospitalized for suicidal ideation 8 days later
94404	MDD	787	13 F	Placebo	-	29	Self-mutilation	N	
94404	MDD	871	17 F	Placebo	-	25	Overdose on 8 tablets of tolfenamic acid	Y	

PAROXETINE (Sources: 6-16-03 submission and Excel spreadsheet courtesy of Dr. Judith Racoosin, Division of Neuropharmacological Drug Products)

Study	Indication	Pt ID	AGe	SEx	Treatment	Dose (mg/day) at time of event	Duration (days)	Event	Serious (y/n)	Comments
329	MDD	32900300313	18	M	Paroxetine	20	11	Command hallucinations, self mutilation	Y	Hospitalized
329	MDD	32900400015	16	F	Paroxetine	20	31	Mild self mutilation	N	
329	MDD	32900600038	15	F	Paroxetine	20	57	Multiple drug overdose	Y	
329	MDD	32900200245	14	F	Paroxetine	20	13	Acetaminophen overdose (27-28 capsules)	Y	Treated in emergency room and released
329	MDD	32900500250	15	F	Paroxetine	30	28	Overcompliance (by 124%) with study medication	Y	Coded as "overdose intentional." (Same patient subsequently overdosed on 20 capsules of study medication during continuation treatment.)
329	MDD	32900100065	14	M	Paroxetine	20	13	Angry outburst (with destruction of property) followed by suicidal thoughts	Y	
329	MDD	32900500333	16	F	Paroxetine	20	+4 post study	Hospitalized for severe suicidal ideation	Y	
329	MDD	32900200106	15	F	Paroxetine	40	51	Combative with mother, threatened suicide	Y	Hospitalized
377	MDD	37701100061	17	F	Paroxetine	40	75	Overdose (28 tablets of study medication)	Y	Hospitalized
377	MDD	37702400158	14	F	Paroxetine	30	86	Slapping herself in the face (automutilation)	N	
377	MDD	37702300172	16	M	Paroxetine	30	38	Overdose on 5 gm paracetamol plus 600 mg aspirin	N	Considered a non-serious event by investigator
377	MDD	37703000181	18	F	Paroxetine	40	56	Hostility, depression, writing suicide notes; possible drug abuse (cannabis)	Y	Hospitalized
377	MDD	37700900225	17	F	Paroxetine	20	78	Overdose on study medication	Y	Hospitalized
377	MDD	37704200310	15	F	Paroxetine	20	23	Self-inflicted wrist lacerations, superficial	Y	

Study	Indication	Pt ID	AGe	SEx	Treatment	Dose (mg/day) at time of event	Duration (days)	Event	Serious (y/n)	Comments
377	MDD	37705300508	14	F	Paroxetine	20	54	Cut left wrist after arguing with mother	Y	
377	MDD	37704200315	15	F	Paroxetine	20	+4 post study	Overdose on 5 acetaminophen pills and two other pills, agitation, anxiety	Y	Hospitalized
377	MDD	37704900479	17	M	Paroxetine	40	+2 post study	Suicidal ideation, irritability	Y	Hospitalized
676	SAD	67601124283	15	M	Paroxetine	30	+1 post study	Vague suicidal ideation	N	
676	SAD	67601424376	13	F	Paroxetine	40	34	Worsening panic attacks, suicidal ideation	N	
676	SAD	67610024705	16	F	Paroxetine	20	43	Self-inflicted scratch on wrist	N	
676	SAD	67610124629	14	F	Paroxetine	40	99	Threatened suicide when brother hospitalized	N	
701	MDD	70116325718	16	F	Paroxetine	50	41	Patient reported taking an overdose of 100 paroxetine tablets	Y	Overdose not confirmed by urine drug screen
701	MDD	70118025639	15	F	Paroxetine	30	+2 post study	Cut arms, overdose on acetaminophen	Y	Required ICU admission
701	MDD	70118327620	11	F	Paroxetine	20	+4 post study	Threatened to hang self	Y	Hospitalized
704	OCD	70403325513	15	M	Paroxetine	40	25	Hospitalization due to suicidal thoughts	Y	
329	MDD	32900100123	16	F	Placebo	-	45	Worsening depression, suicidal thoughts	Y	
377	MDD	37700500231	14	F	Placebo	-	31	Overdose of study medication and chlorazepate	Y	
377	MDD	37701000068	14	F	Placebo	-	83	Overdose on 21 alprazolam tablets	Y	Hospitalized
377	MDD	37702900024	17	F	Placebo	-	29	Tried to kill herself with scissors	Y	Details not provided
377	MDD	37704100294	14	F	Placebo	-	84	Overdose on 10 gm of acetaminophen	Y	Hospitalized
701	MDD	70115425768	13	M	Placebo	-	5	Wrecked parent's car and became suicidal	Y	Hospitalized
701	MDD	70118327617	12	F	Placebo	-	3	Mild self-mutilation of arms	N	

VENLAFAXINE

Study	Indication	Pt ID	AGE	Sex	Treatment	Dose (mg/day)	Duration (days)	Event	Serious (y/n)	Comments
382	MDD	38202-036	13	F	Placebo	-	+18 post tx	Angry, kicked a cabinet	Y	Resulted in ER visit
382	MDD	38204-023	11	F	venlafaxine ER	112.5	21	Suicidal ideation	N	
382	MDD	38205-008	12	M	venlafaxine ER	75	29	Suicidal ideation, auditory hallucinations	Y	Hospitalized
382	MDD	38205-019	8	F	venlafaxine ER	NA	13	Overdose on venlafaxine 300 mg	Y	Hospitalized
382	MDD	38207-008	12	M	Placebo	-	+17 post tx	Suicidal ideation, scratching on arms	Y	Hospitalized
382	MDD	38207-023	14	F	Placebo	-	3	Overdose on study medication (~8 capsules)	Y	Treated at ER and released
382	MDD	38209-020	13	F	venlafaxine ER	37.5	13	Suicidal ideation with plan to overdose	Y	Hospitalized
382	MDD	38211-012	10	F	venlafaxine ER	112.5	23	Mild self-injurious behavior	N	On day 43 of trial, hospitalized for swallowing aftershave

394	MDD	39402-0041	7	M	venlafaxine ER	75	25 and 29	Suicidal ideation, plan to stab self	Y	Hospitalized (considered 2 events by sponsor)
394	MDD	39404-0126	14	M	venlafaxine ER	75	15	Suicidal and homicidal ideation	Y	Hospitalized
394	MDD	39411-0405	14	F	venlafaxine ER	150	51	Cut arm in context of family discord	N	Treated at ER and released
394	MDD	39420-0769	13	M	venlafaxine ER	225	36	Mild suicidal ideation	N	
394	MDD	39428-1087	16	M	venlafaxine ER	150	47 and 50	Rage attack, suicidal, homicidal	Y	Hospitalized; drug screen positive for PCP (considered 2 events by sponsor)
394	MDD	39435-1366	17	F	venlafaxine ER	37.5	5	Mild self-mutilation	N	
394	MDD	39440-1561	12	F	venlafaxine ER	-	+6 post tx	Overdose on study medication (17 capsules)	N	Treated at ER and released. Not considered a serious event
397	GAD	39701-0012	17	F	Placebo	-	15	Overdose of 18 Excedrin PM tablets following fight with boyfriend	Y	Hospitalized
397	GAD	39710-0361	10	M	venlafaxine ER	-	+3 post tx	Suicidal (wrapped cord around neck), agitated, and physically agressive	Y	Hospitalized

BUPROPION No cases

Appendix table 4. Stata outputs for calculation of combined incidence rate ratios

Category: **Suicide-related events**

Study	IRR	[95% Conf.	Interval]	M-H Weight	
003-045	.5281385	.0067291	41.45135	.6543909	(exact)
1001/1017	3.028078	.5414406	30.67137	.9953421	(exact)
114	.	.0272237	.	0	(exact)
141	.	.0235638	.	0	(exact)
187	.	.0130205	.	0	(exact)
329	8	1.072641	354.959	.5	(exact)
377	1.152439	.3216551	5.121634	2.645161	(exact)
382	1.775317	.3454063	11.43182	1.452651	(exact)
394	.	1.39804	.	0	(exact)
396	.	.	.	0	(exact)
397	.9837456	.0125341	77.21001	.5040969	(exact)
498	0	0	40.8801	.4882943	(exact)
676	.	.6083716	.	0	(exact)
701	1.59375	.1825649	19.08565	.969697	(exact)
704	.	.0296822	.	0	(exact)
94404	1.611357	.6704749	4.137106	4.720969	(exact)
CIT-MD-18	.46875	.0079441	9.004248	1.032258	(exact)
HCCJ	1	.0127412	78.48575	.5	(exact)
HCJE	.8856201	.1649537	4.754807	2.121318	(exact)
HCJW	.7910853	.0411829	46.67882	.7165671	(exact)
X065	.8689261	.0629945	11.98569	1.070133	(exact)
Crude	1.859448	1.223071	2.879198		(exact)
M-H combined	1.863115	1.246773	2.784147		

Test of homogeneity (M-H) chi2(13) = 7.67 Pr>chi2 = 0.8642

Category: **Serious suicide-related events**

Study	IRR	[95% Conf.	Interval]	M-H Weight	
003-045	.	.0135386	.	0	(exact)
1001/1017	2.523398	.4131554	26.50048	.9953421	(exact)
114	.	.	.	0	(exact)
141	.	.	.	0	(exact)
187	.	.0130205	.	0	(exact)
329	7	.8993189	315.599	.5	(exact)
377	.8963415	.2278526	4.175488	2.645161	(exact)
382	1.06519	.1426495	7.953972	1.452651	(exact)
394	.	.4008445	.	0	(exact)
396	.	.	.	0	(exact)
397	.9837456	.0125341	77.21001	.5040969	(exact)
498	.	.	.	0	(exact)
676	.	.	.	0	(exact)
701	3.1875	.2559633	167.3341	.4848485	(exact)
704	.	.0296822	.	0	(exact)
94404	2.537888	.8637632	9.002482	2.62276	(exact)
CIT-MD-18	.	.	.	0	(exact)
HCCJ	1	.0127412	78.48575	.5	(exact)
HCJE	.8856201	.1186016	6.613087	1.590989	(exact)
HCJW	.7910853	.0411829	46.67882	.7165671	(exact)
X065	.8689261	.0629945	11.98569	1.070133	(exact)
Crude	1.922267	1.168124	3.25143		(exact)
M-H combined	1.890265	1.175603	3.039376		

Test of homogeneity (M-H) chi2(10) = 6.44 Pr>chi2 = 0.7768

Appendix table 5. Summary of efficacy findings from eight pediatric antidepressant development programs

Drug	Indication	Approval status for pediatric use*	Study	N		
				Drug	Placebo	Efficacy results on primary variable
Paroxetine	MDD	NA	329	93	88	Failed (but + on secondary variables)
			377	181	95	Failed
			701	104	102	Failed
	OCD	AE	704	99	107	+
	SAD	Not submitted	676	165	157	? (not submitted)
Sertraline	MDD	NA	1001/1017	189	184	Two studies under same protocol, both failed (but + if data pooled)
	OCD	AP	498	92	95	+
Venlafaxine	MDD	NA	382	80	85	Failed
			394	102	94	Failed
	GAD	NA	396	80	84	Failed, by a small margin (p=0.09)
			397	77	79	+
Fluvoxamine	OCD	AP	114	57	63	+
Mirtazapine	MDD	NA	003-045	170	88	Two studies under this protocol, both failed
Fluoxetine	MDD	AP	HCJE	109	110	+
			X065	48	48	+
	OCD	AP	HCJW	71	32	+
Nefazodone	MDD	NA	141	102	99	Failed, by a small margin (p=0.08)
			187	184	94	Failed
Citalopram	MDD	NA	CIT-MD-18	89	85	+
			94404	121	112	Failed

* NA not approvable, AE approvable, AP approved

Appendix Table 6.

Attributable risks (incidence rate differences) per patient-year for suicide-related events in pediatric MDD trials			
Drug	Incidence rate difference, drug minus placebo	95% confidence interval	p-value
Citalopram	0.14	-0.16-0.43	0.374
Fluoxetine	-0.02	-0.21-0.17	0.829
Mirtazapine	-0.04	-0.21-0.14	0.691
Nefazodone	0.05	-0.02-0.12	0.367
Paroxetine	0.15	-0.01-0.31	0.088
Sertraline	0.12	-0.05-0.30	0.176
Venlafaxine	0.33	0.05-0.62	0.020
All MDD trials	0.10	0.02-0.18	0.013

Appendix Table 7.

Attributable risks (incidence rate differences) per patient-year for serious suicide-related events in pediatric MDD trials			
Drug	Incidence rate difference, drug minus placebo	95% confidence interval	p-value
Citalopram	0.24	-0.01-0.48	0.063
Fluoxetine	-0.02	-0.20-0.16	0.842
Mirtazapine	0.04	-0.04-0.12	0.654
Nefazodone	0.03	-0.02-0.08	0.606
Paroxetine	0.13	-0.02-0.27	0.121
Sertraline	0.09	-0.07-0.25	0.284
Venlafaxine	0.11	-0.11-0.33	0.337
All MDD trials	0.09	0.02-0.15	0.015

Appendix Figure 1.

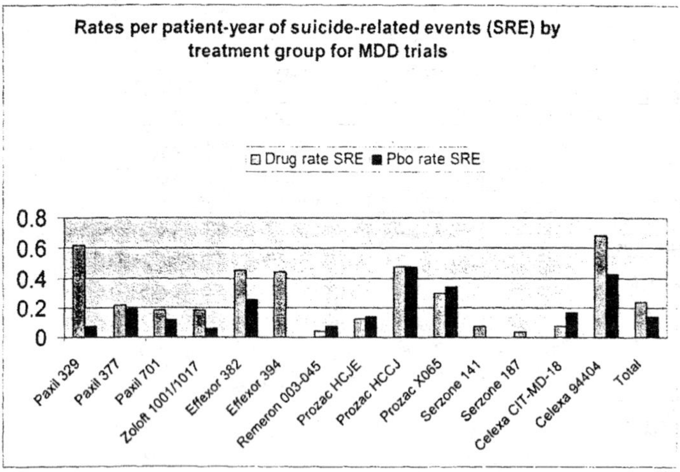

Appendix Figure 2.

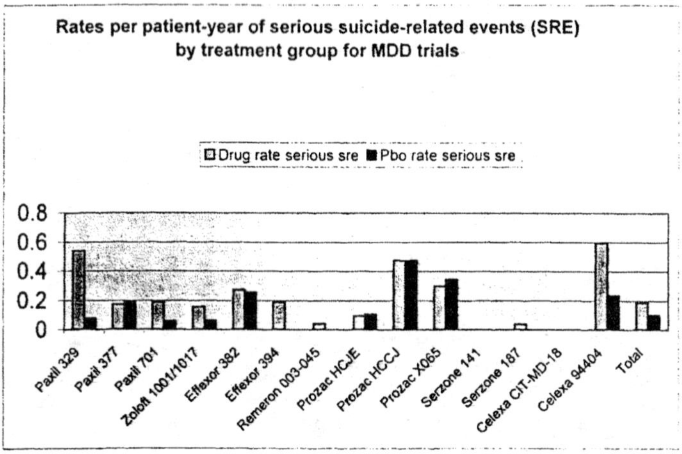

Appendix Figure 3.

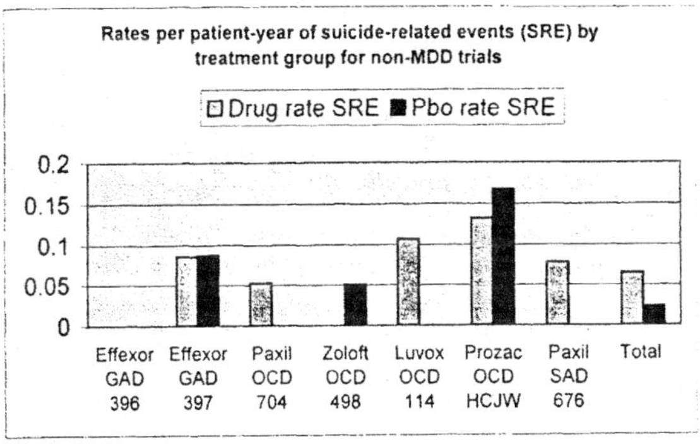

Appendix Figure 4.

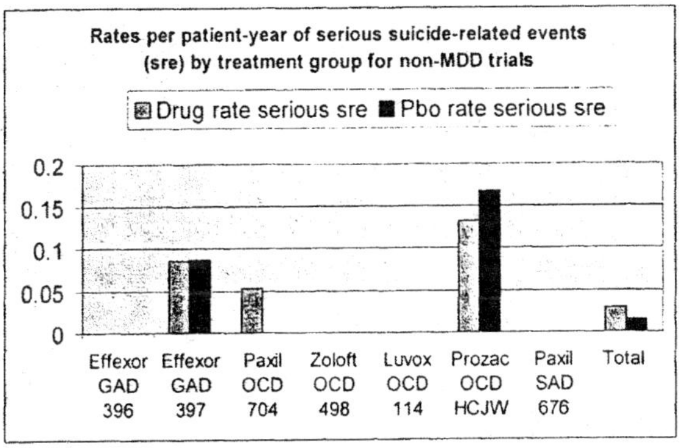

Appendix Figure 5 (reproduced from the sponsor's submission)

CONFIDENTIAL
Seroxat Article 31 - Consolidated Response Document

Table 2.9 **Incidence and Incidence Density for Possibly Suicide-Related Events by Treatment Group and Indication**
Paediatric Placebo Controlled Trials
On-Therapy (including Taper Phase) plus 30 days post-therapy

Indication		Paroxetine	Placebo	Odds Ratio (95% CI)	P value
Overall	n/N (%)	25/738 (3.4%)	8/647 (1.2%)	2.80 (1.25 , 6.25)	0.012
	PYE	176	149		
	n/PYE	0.14	0.05		0.017
Depression	n/N (%)	20/378 (5.3%)	8/285 (2.8%)	1.93 (0.84 , 4.46)	0.12
	PYE	85	61		
	n/PYE	0.24	0.13		0.16
OCD	n/N (%)	1/195 (0.5%)	0/205 (0.0%)		0.49
	PYE	41	41		
	n/PYE	0.02	0.00		
SAD	n/N (%)	4/165 (2.4%)	0/157 (0.0%)		0.12
	PYE	51	46		
	n/PYE	0.08	0.00		

Data Source: Appendix 2B, Table 2.56

CONFIDENTIAL
Seroxat Article 31 - Consolidated Response Document

Table 2.5 **Incidence and Incidence Density for Possibly Suicide-Related Events by Treatment Group and Indication**
Adult Placebo Controlled Trials
On-Therapy (including Taper Phase) plus 30 days post-therapy

Indication		Paroxetine	Placebo	Odds Ratio (95% CI)	P value
Overall	n/N (%)	92/8481 (1.1%)	63/5808 (1.1%)	1.00 (0.72 , 1.38)	1.00
	PYE	1916	1313		
	n/PYE	0.05	0.05		1.00
Depression	n/N (%)	74/3421 (2.2%)	44/2117 (2.1%)	1.04 (0.71 , 1.52)	0.92
	PYE	671	428		
	n/PYE	0.11	0.10		0.71
GAD	n/N (%)	2/1182 (0.2%)	2/985 (0.2%)	0.83 (0.12 , 5.92)	1.00
	PYE	259	211		
	n/PYE	0.01	0.01		0.84
OCD	n/N (%)	3/542 (0.6%)	4/265 (1.5%)	0.36 (0.08 , 1.63)	0.23
	PYE	141	61		
	n/PYE	0.02	0.07		0.14
PMDD	n/N (%)	0/760 (0.0%)	0/379 (0.0%)		
	PYE	208	102		
	n/PYE	0.00	0.00		
PTSD	n/N (%)	7/786 (0.9%)	6/598 (1.0%)	0.89 (0.30, 2.65)	1.00
	PYE	174	138		
	n/PYE	0.04	0.04		0.89
Panic	n/N (%)	3/920 (0.3%)	4/780 (0.5%)	0.63 (0.14, 2.84)	0.71
	PYE	237	186		
	n/PYE	0.01	0.02		0.48
SAD	n/N (%)	3/870 (0.3%)	3/684 (0.4%)	0.79 (0.16 , 3.90)	1.00
	PYE	225	187		
	n/PYE	0.01	0.02		0.82

Data Source: Appendix 2B, Table 2.02

Appendix Figure 6.

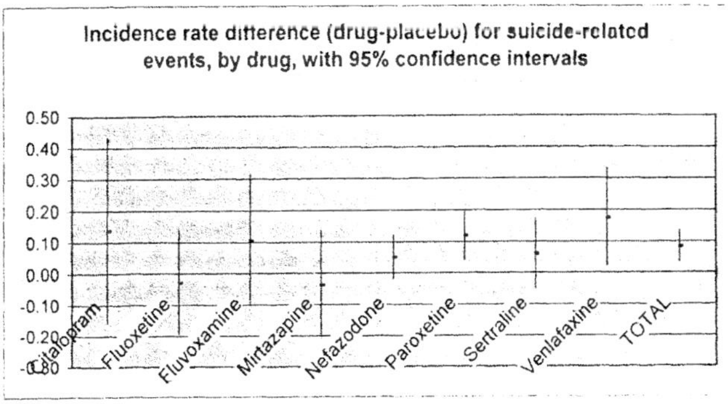

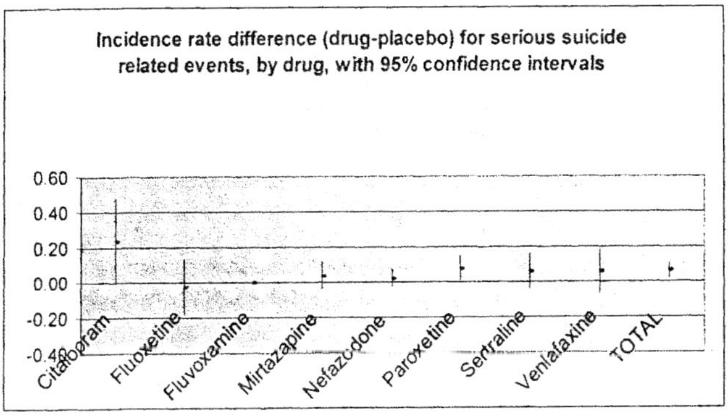

Appendix Figure 7.

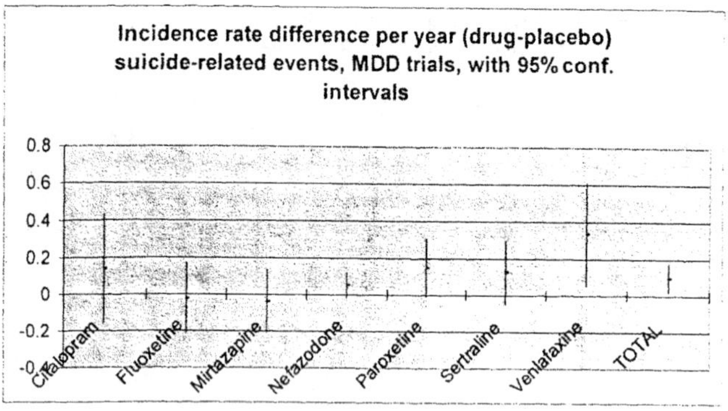

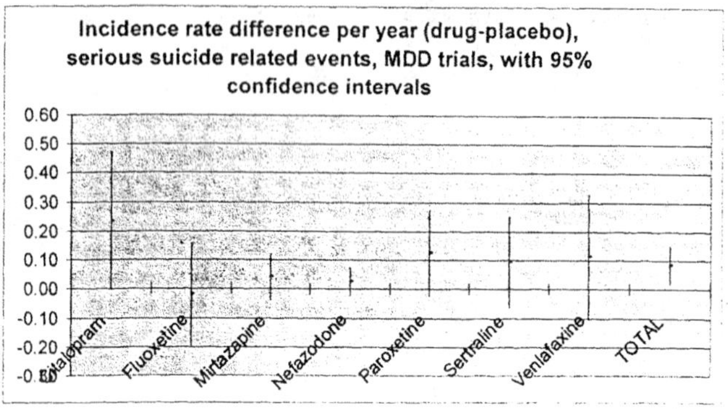

Tab 25

PROPOSED AGENDA FOR FEBRUARY 2
As Revised at the 12/9 Planning Meeting

TIME	TOPIC	PRESENTER
8:00	Welcome/Introductions	Russell Katz
8:10	Pediatric Drug Development Program	OCTAP
8:30	Epidemiology of Depression/Suicide and Suicide Attempts in Pediatrics	David Schaffer
8:50	Clinical Presentation of Depression in Children	Cynthia Pfeiffer
9:15	Break	
9:30	Open Public Hearing	
11:30	Lunch	
12:30	Limited Overview of Paxil Controlled Trials and Controlled Trials of Other Antidepressants	Andrew Mosholder
1:15	Presentation of AERS Data: Paxil/Celexa Obligatory 1-Year Reporting	Solomon Iyasu
1:30	AERS Data [scope to be determined]	ODS
	General Use Data	ODS/ David Schaffer?
	Specific Use Data	ODS
2:00	Open Public Hearing	
2:30	Break	
2:45	Overview of Proposed Analysis of All 8 Anti-Depressants - Reclassification and Patient Level Data Analysis	Thomas Laughren
3:15	Columbia Presentation	
3:30	Challenges of Analysis/Plans to Address Challenges - Patient Level Data Analysis	Tarek Hammad
3:45	Discussion	
5:45	Adjourn	

PROPOSED AGENDA FOR FEBRUARY 2
As Revised at the 12/9 Planning Meeting

TIME	TOPIC	PRESENTER
8:00	Welcome/Introductions	Russell Katz
8:10	Pediatric Drug Development Program	OCTAP
8:30	Epidemiology of Depression/Suicide and Suicide Attempts in Pediatrics	David Schaffer
8:50	Clinical Presentation of Depression in Children	Cynthia Pfeiffer
9:15	Break	
9:30	Open Public Hearing	
11:30	Lunch	
12:30	Limited Overview of Paxil Controlled Trials and Controlled Trials of Other Antidepressants	Andrew Mosholder
1:15	Presentation of AERS Data: Paxil/Celexa - Obligatory 1-Year Reporting	Solomon Iyasu
1:30	AERS Data [scope to be determined]	ODS
	General Use Data	ODS/ David Schaffer?
	Specific Use Data	ODS
2:00	Open Public Hearing	
2:30	Break	
2:45	Overview of Proposed Analysis of All 8 Anti-Depressants - Reclassification and Patient Level Data Analysis	Thomas Laughren
3:15	Columbia Presentation	
3:30	Challenges of Analysis/Plans to Address Challenges - Patient Level Data Analysis	Tarek Hammad
3:45	Discussion	
5:45	Adjourn	

PROPOSED AGENDA FOR FEBRUARY 2
As Revised by T. Laughren, 12/30/03

Tab 26

TIME	TOPIC	PRESENTER
8:00	Welcome/Introductions	Russell Katz
8:10	Pediatric Drug Development Program	OCTAP Dianne
8:30	Pediatric Depression and Its Treatment	Cynthia Pfeffer
8:50	Epidemiology of Depression and Suicide in Pediatrics	David Schaffer
9:15	Break	
9:30	Open Public Hearing	
11:30	Lunch	
12:30	Presentation of AERS Data: Paxil/Celexa Obligatory 1-Year Reporting	Solomon Iyasu - may need more than 15 min
~~12:45~~ 1:00	AERS Data - maybe epi studies	ODS
~~1:15~~ 1:30	Open Public Hearing	
2:00	Break	
2:15	Regulatory History on Antidepressants and Suicidality and Update on Current Plans for Analysis of Pediatric Suicidality Data	Thomas Laughren
3:00	Reclassification of Clinical Cases	Kelly Posner ✓ OK
3:15	Plans for Analysis of Patient Level Data for Pediatric Studies	Tarek Hammad
3:30	Commmittee Discussion	
5:45	Adjourn	

7 public speakers - 2-3 min apiece

Jan 24th - deadline for slides
web site posting tomorrow probably

PROPOSED AGENDA FOR FEBRUARY 2
As Revised by T. Laughren, 12/30/03

TIME	TOPIC	PRESENTER
8:00	Welcome/Introductions	Russell Katz
8:10	Pediatric Drug Development Program	OCTAP
8:30	Pediatric Depression and Its Treatment	Cynthia Pfeffer
8:50	Epidemiology of Depression and Suicide in Pediatrics	David Schaffer
9:15	Break	
9:30	Open Public Hearing	
11:30	Lunch	
12:30	Presentation of AERS Data: Paxil/Celexa Obligatory 1-Year Reporting	Solomon Iyasu
12:45	AERS Data	ODS
1:15	Open Public Hearing	
2:00	Break	
2:15	Regulatory History on Antidepressants and Suicidality and Update on Current Plans for Analysis of Pediatric Suicidality Data	Thomas Laughren
3:00	Reclassification of Clinical Cases	Kelly Posner ✓ ok
3:15	Plans for Analysis of Patient Level Data for Pediatric Studies	Tarek Hammad
3:30	Commmittee Discussion	
5:45	Adjourn	

AGENDA FOR FEBRUARY 2, 2004
As Revised at the 1/12/04 Planning Meeting

TIME	TOPIC	PRESENTER
8:00	Welcome/Introductions	Russell Katz
8:10	Pediatric Drug Development Program	Diane Murphy
8:30	Pediatric Depression and Its Treatment	Cynthia Pfeiffer
8:50	Epidemiology of Depression and Suicide in Pediatrics	David Schaffer
9:15	Break	
9:30	Open Public Hearing	
11:30	Lunch	
12:30	Presentation of AERS Data: Paxil/Celexa Obligatory 1-Year Reporting	Solomon Iyasu
12:50	AERS Data	ODS
1:30	Open Public Hearing	
2:00	Break	
2:15	Regulatory History on Antidepressants and Suicidality and Update on Current Plans for Analysis of Pediatric Suicidality Data	Thomas Laughren
3:00	Reclassification of Clinical Cases	Kelly Posner
3:15	Plans for Analysis of Patient Level Data for Pediatric Studies	Tarek Hammad
3:30	Committee Discussion	
5:45	Adjourn	

AGENDA FOR FEBRUARY 2, 2004
As Revised at the 1/12/04 Planning Meeting

Tab 27

TIME	TOPIC	PRESENTER
8:00	Welcome/Introductions	Chair
8:10	Overview of Issues	Russell Katz
8:15	Pediatric Drug Development Program	Diane Murphy
8:30	Pediatric Depression and Its Treatment	Cynthia Pfeffer
8:50	Epidemiology of Depression and Suicide in Pediatrics	David Shaffer
9:15	Break	
9:30	Open Public Hearing	
11:30	Lunch	
12:30	Presentation of AERS Data: Paxil/Celexa Obligatory 1-Year Reporting	Solomon Iyasu
12:50	Pediatric & Adolescent Antidepressant Drug Use in the U.S.	Gianna Rigoni
~~12:50~~1:10	~~AERS Data~~ Office of Drug Safety Data Resources for the Study of Suicidal Events Associated with Pediatric Use of Antidepressants	~~ODS~~Andrew Mosholder
1:30	Open Public Hearing	
2:00	Break	
2:15	Regulatory History on Antidepressants and Suicidality and Update on Current Plans for Analysis of Pediatric Suicidality Data	Thomas Laughren
3:00	Reclassification of Clinical Cases	Kelly Posner
3:15	Plans for Analysis of Patient Level Data for Pediatric Studies	Tarek Hammad
3:30	Committee Discussion	
5:45	Adjourn	

AGENDA FOR FEBRUARY 2, 2004
As Revised at the 1/12/04 Planning Meeting

TIME	TOPIC	PRESENTER
8:00	Welcome/Introductions	Russell Katz
8:10	Pediatric Drug Development Program	Diane Murphy
8:30	Pediatric Depression and Its Treatment	Cynthia Pfeiffer
8:50	Epidemiology of Depression and Suicide in Pediatrics	David Schaffer
9:15	Break	
9:30	Open Public Hearing	
11:30	Lunch	
12:30	Presentation of AERS Data: Paxil/Celexa Obligatory 1-Year Reporting	Solomon Iyasu
12:50	AERS Data	ODS
1:30	Open Public Hearing	
2:00	Break	
2:15	Regulatory History on Antidepressants and Suicidality and Update on Current Plans for Analysis of Pediatric Suicidality Data	Thomas Laughren
3:00	Reclassification of Clinical Cases	Kelly Posner
3:15	Plans for Analysis of Patient Level Data for Pediatric Studies	Tarek Hammad
3:30	Committee Discussion	
5:45	Adjourn	

RE Pediatric Suicide Labeling Changes.txt

Tab 28

From: Mosholder, Andrew D
Sent: Tuesday, February 10, 2004 11:07 PM
To: Willy, Mary E
Subject: RE: Pediatric Suicide Labeling Changes

I concur, Mary.

By the way, with the agency about to take some kind of action on this issue, is there any renewed interest on the part of Mark or Anne for finalizing my consult? If so, you can give me a call at home. I can put it in DFS from here if necessary. (Seems to me that if we wait until after the agency has acted, the consult will be moot.)

If there's still disagreement, we can always fall back on the Resolution of Disputes MaPP (attached).

Thanks,
Andy

-----Original Message-----
From: Willy, Mary E
Sent: Tuesday, February 10, 2004 9:18 AM
To: Pamer, Carol; Mosholder, Andrew D; Trontell, Anne E; Avigan, Mark I; Seligman, Paul
Subject: RE: Pediatric Suicide Labeling Changes

Mark, will you send these on to neuropharm or how will these thoughts be communicated?

Mary's comments (in italics): I think there should be more emphasis on the risk benefit -

"……….Although a causal link between antidepressant use and the emergence of such symptoms in association with suicidal impulses has not been definitely established, consideration should be given to the risk/benefit of treatment when initiating the medication and discontinuing the medication when such symptoms are severe, abrupt in onset, or were not part of the patient's presenting symptoms.

Carol's comment:

I only have one minor comment, since I did not review the clinical trials data or Andy's consult. I suggest adding to the 3rd paragraph "Families, caregivers, and educators of patients being treated...." since these are children who spend most of their days at school.

Andy's comments:

I think the proposed labeling offers sound advice to clinicians and patients. Its major weakness, in my opinion, is that it fails to distinguish between the current data for adults and pediatric patients. For adults, the evidence of drug-induced suicidality comes solely from case series and anecdotal reports; data from adult clinical trials have not shown an increase in these events relative to placebo controls. One interpretation is that if these events are truly adverse reactions to drug, they must be fairly rare and are thus invisible in the comparison between drug and placebo. For pediatric patients, on the other hand, the clinical trial data suggest that patients are actually more likely to have these events on drug than they are on placebo, with the possible exception of fluoxetine.

Of course, I realize that the folks in DNDP are not prepared to acknowledge a signal in the pediatric trials without confirmation by the Columbia University experts. Perhaps that is the reason for the statement, "...a causal link between antidepressant use and the emergence of such symptoms in association with suicidal impulses has not been established..." But it seems to me that for pediatric use, one would have to say that a causal link, if not established, is at least suspected.

It might be of interest to compare Wyeth's Dear Health Care Provider letter regarding Effexor (attached), though I'm told that DNDP has not accepted Wyeth's Changes Being Effected labeling.

I hope these comments are useful.

Andy

<< File: Dear HCP letter.pdf >>

-----Original Message-----
From: Trontell, Anne E
Sent: Monday, February 09, 2004 11:44 AM
To: Avigan, Mark I; Seligman, Paul; Willy, Mary E; Mosholder, Andrew D; Pamer, Carol
Subject: RE: Pediatric Suicide Labeling Changes
Importance: High

Mark,
Thanks for jumping on this one. Will you coordinate DDREs input with your own and run it past Paul or myself before sending it back to Paul David? Thanks.
Anne

-----Original Message-----
From: Avigan, Mark I
Sent: Monday, February 09, 2004 11:16 AM
To: Seligman, Paul; Trontell, Anne E; Willy, Mary E; Mosholder, Andrew D; Pamer, Carol
Subject: FW: Pediatric Suicide Labeling Changes
Importance: High

Folks in ODS,

I think that the general labeling changes that have been proposed are quite good. My only suggested edits are for some reordering and clarification of drug-related suicidality (as described by the AC).

Your thoughts before sending back to Paul David?

Mark A.

-----Original Message-----
From: David, Paul A
Sent: Monday, February 09, 2004 10:36 AM
To: Jenkins, John K; Galson, Steven; Kweder, Sandra L; Temple, Robert; Trontell, Anne E; Willy, Mary E; Mosholder, Andrew D; Seligman, Paul; Avigan, Mark I; Murphy, Dianne; Murphy, Shirley; Iyasu, Solomon; Addy, Rosemary; Cummins, Susan; Roberts, Rosemary
Cc: Katz, Russell G; Laughren, Thomas P; Andreason, Paul J; Stasko, Robert; Martin, Terry; Racoosin, Judith A; Hammad, Tarek
Subject: Pediatric Suicide Labeling Changes
Importance: High

As recommended by the advisory committee members at the 2-2-04 AC meeting, 120 has taken the lead in drafting revisions to labeling which will be sent out to all 9 drugs discussed at the AC meeting.

Once we have hammered out the labeling, 120 will issue CBE supplement request letters to the sponsors requesting that they implement these changes immediately. 120 also intends to draft a Public Health Advisory with the goal of this issuing in the next few weeks.

Another initiative, post labeling revisions and PHA, is to have the sponsors implement a MedGuide targeting this event as well as changing to unit of use packaging.

The Commissioner has been in contact with Dr. Steven Galson on this topic, and he would like the Agency to act quickly as a follow-up to our 2-2-04 meeting.

Therefore, we are requesting input on the proposed labeling revisions from the team by COB Wednesday 2/11.

Thanks,
Paul
<< File: Label 03.doc >>

MEMORANDUM

Tab 29

DEPARTMENT OF HEALTH AND HUMAN SERVICES
PUBLIC HEALTH SERVICE
FOOD AND DRUG ADMINISTRATION
CENTER FOR DRUG EVALUATION AND RESEARCH

PID#	D030341
DATE:	March 15, 2004
From:	Anne Trontell, M.D., M.P.H., Deputy Director Office of Drug Safety, HFD-400
TO:	Russell Katz, M.D., Director Division of Neuropharmacological Drug Products, HFD-120
SUBJECT:	Office of Drug Safety Cover Memorandum Follow-up Consult to 9-4-03 consult by Andrew Mosholder on Suicidality in pediatric clinical trials with paroxetine and other antidepressant drugs: Drugs: paroxetine, sertraline, venlafaxine, fluoxetine, fluvoxamine, citalopram, nefazodone, mirtazapine, and bupropion

Dr. Mosholder has concluded from his composite analysis of preliminary data from the randomized clinical trials (RCTs) of selective serotonin reuptake inhibitors (SSRIs) in pediatric psychiatric conditions, that short-term use of these drugs is associated with a statistically and clinically significant elevation in the risk of self-injurious events over placebo. He found the short-term excess risk of SSRIs relative to placebo to be statistically significant in trials of major depressive disorder (MDD), but not in those for nonMDD indications. Based on these findings and the limited number of SSRI trials showing efficacy in pediatric MDD, Dr. Mosholder advocates discouraging antidepressant drugs outside their labeled efficacy indications. Specifically, he notes that only fluoxetine has demonstrated efficacy in pediatric MDD, and that the point estimate of its relative risk for suicide-related events of 0.88 (95% CI 0.34-2.30) "appears most favorable."

Dr. Mosholder's conclusions are based upon thoughtful consideration of what are, at this point, preliminary data. Systematic data collection and coding have not been assured, and unblinded analyses by Dr. Mosholder were not possible. Dr. Mosholder notes these deficiencies, but expresses his belief that only systematic bias could explain away his findings, and so "interim risk management" around labeled efficacy should be done pending definitive analyses.

As Dr. Mosholder's supervisors, Dr. Avigan and I disagree with his proposed interim risk management which implies making treatment recommendations about off-label use for SSRIs in pediatric psychiatric illness. In particular, we disagree that the data are sufficiently robust to advocate preferential use of fluoxetine in pediatric MDD. We note that the point estimate suggesting a modest protective effect in serious suicide-related events was not statistically significant, and that the 95% confidence interval could not rule out a doubling of the risk. We share Dr. Mosholder's concern about the potential excess risk of self-injurious behavior in pediatric patients treated with SSRIs, and agree that these potential concerns should be transmitted widely to physicians, patients, and parents when these drugs are used. Such information-sharing should reinforce prudent use and close patient follow-up in initiating therapy with SSRIs, particularly among patients being treated for MDD. We support additional adjudicated analyses being done by Columbia University, and once they are complete, recommend their comparison to Dr.

Mosholder's preliminary findings with due consideration and appropriate sensitivity analyses around indeterminate cases of self-injury.

Like Dr. Avigan, I believe the current safety data from pediatric SSRI RCTs are insufficiently characterized to assure they are free from nonrandom sources of error that may lead to erroneous conclusions. In particular, I believe they do not warrant making treatment recommendations at this time addressing labeled or unlabeled uses, particularly to suggest relative safety for one product over another.

I agree with Dr. Avigan's comments that the studies as analyzed by Dr. Mosholder may not be sufficiently homogeneous to support their composite analysis. Additional examination of the clinical trial data, along with additional statistical testing for homogeneity should be done to determine if making conclusions based on the combined data is valid. Dr. Avigan notes that differences in the selection of patient populations among the different trials may have led to individual differences in the self-injury risk of patients. This concern is supported by the observation of differences among the placebo rates of suicide-related events among the different trials, as well as the differential rates and relative risk of self-injurious behaviors across individual drug trials. Dr. Mosholder himself notes that the post-hoc ascertainment methods for suicide-related events were different among the sponsors of different drug trials. He does not mention the possibility that ascertainment differences may also have influenced data collection during the RCTs themselves, since self-injurious behaviors were not elicited prospectively or systematically. Investigator practices in eliciting, recording, or coding these events were not likely to have been done in a consistent fashion.

In addition to inconsistent ascertainment of self-injurious adverse events, Dr. Mosholder's analyses do not describe imbalances in individual treatment times (e.g. time-adjusted survival analyses) that may have occurred due to differential dropout rates of placebo patients relative to treated patients. The common side-effect profile of SSRIs (including akathesia) may have led to the loss of true blinding by either the investigator, patient, or both, and so influenced decision-making about continuing participation in the trial. Such a scenario would allow for the possibility that more severely ill patients (perhaps at higher risk of self-injurious behavior) might have been preferentially retained in active treatment.

In conclusion, Division and Office management within the Office of Drug Safety support Dr. Mosholder's concerns that pediatric patients being treated for MDD with SSRIs may experience an increase in self-injurious behaviors that may in turn, place them at greater risk of suicidal behaviors. We disagree as to the conclusiveness of this finding for making of psychiatric treatment recommendations such as the preferential use of fluoxetine in pediatric MDD. We instead advocate widespread information-sharing with clinicians, patients, and parents addressing the potential emergence of self-injurious behavior in the initial treatment of pediatric psychiatric illness, and urge attentive patient follow-up by all parties. We support the timely completion of adjudicated data analyses by Columbia University, and a reexamination of the data and consideration of clinical treatment recommendations when the Joint FDA Pediatric and Neurological Advisory Committee is reconvened later in 2004.

MEMORANDUM

DEPARTMENT OF HEALTH AND HUMAN SERVICES
PUBLIC HEALTH SERVICE
FOOD AND DRUG ADMINISTRATION
CENTER FOR DRUG EVALUATION AND RESEARCH

PID# D030341

DATE: March 6, 2004

From: Mark Avigan, M.D., C.M., Director
Division of Drug Risk Evaluation, HFD-430

TO: Russell Katz, M.D., Director
Division of Neuropharmacological Drug Products, HFD-120

SUBJECT: Suicidality in pediatric clinical trials with paroxetine and other antidepressant drugs: Follow-up to 9-4-03 consult

Drugs: paroxetine, sertraline, venlafaxine, fluoxetine, fluvoxamine, citalopram, nefazodone, mirtazapine, and bupropion

The attached memorandum from Andrew D. Mosholder, M.D., M.P.H., an epidemiologist in the Division of Drug Risk Evaluation/Office of Drug Safety, contains an analysis of suicidality in pediatric clinical trials with paroxetine and other antidepressant drugs and recommendations for a plan of action. An emphasis has been placed in suicide-related outcomes in the *composite* of randomized controlled trials of each pediatric drug development program. In Dr. Mosholder's analysis, for most but not all drugs of this class, there is a trend towards an increased attributable risk of suicide-related events linked to randomization to active drug, compared to placebo. Moreover, a meta-analysis of Major Depressive Disorder(MDD) studies across all drug programs reveals that the active treatment arm is associated with an increased risk for these events.

This meta-analysis raises critical concerns that must be addressed to optimize pharmacotherapy of pediatric MDD and other psychiatric illness(es). As Director of the Division of Drug Risk Evaluation, I have reviewed this document and support the analyses and conclusions that it contains, with the following exceptions and/or additions:

- Based on limitations in the data-set that has been made available, the meta-analysis that has been performed does not justify a recommendation for a labeled contraindication for use in 'all pediatric patients' of any of the reviewed drugs, at this time.

- As pointed out in Dr. Laughren's review[1], between individual trials, for each drug, there are inconsistencies of results of suicidality. This observation beckons for a more rigorous analysis of similarities and differences between the trials in their design and implementation.

[1] Thomas P. Laughren; Background on Suicidality Associated with Antidepressant treatment; submitted January 5, 2004; presented at Psychopharmacologic Drugs Advisory Committee and Pediatric Subcommittee of the Anti-Infectives Advisory Committee, February 2, 2004

In reviewing the clinical trial database to understand differences in suicidality between trials the following elements should be elucidated:

- *enrollment criteria (patient characteristics)*
- *classification criteria for including/excuding suicidality events*
- *protocols for following and assessing patients before, during and after treatment*

- Reasons for absence of efficacy for different agents in pediatric trials remain unclear. Whether differences in trial results are related to inherent differences in pharmacological properties between agents, or in trial characteristics (enrollment, powering, efficacy measures, etc.) has not yet been elucidated. Thus, at this time, differential labeling of fluoxetine to imply more a more favorable benefit/risk profile should be approached with caution.

- Although the rates of severe agitation and completed suicides have been reported in pediatric patients treated with anti-depressants, other events, including 'possible' and even 'serious' suicide-related events, appear to be much more common. Further information to understand the predictive relationship between these outcomes is critical in the interpretation of safety events associated with clinical trials.

- Dr. Mosholder's recommendation to discourage initiation of 'off-label' treatment of pediatric patients is based on a justifiable concern that in this age group, with the exception of fluoxetine, efficacy to treat MDD has not been demonstrated. Although off-label treatment is not directly discourages, the FDA Public Health Advisory issued on October 27, 2003 states:

  ..*'FDA emphasizes that, for the 7 drugs evaluated in pediatric major depressive disorder (MDD), data reviewed by FDA were adequate to establish effectiveness in MDD for only one of these drugs, Prozac (fluoxetine). Failure to show effectiveness in any particular study in pediatric MDD, however, is not definitive evidence that the drug is not effective since trials may fail for many reasons, FDA recognizes that pediatric MDD is a serious condition for which there are few established options, and that clinicians often must make choices among treatments available for adult MDD.'*

  'FDA emphasizes that these drugs must be used with caution. ....'

  At this time, because of lack of information, I do not support an explicit labeled instruction to avoid all 'off-label' treatment. Rather, an interim plan should be implemented to comprehensively inform physicians, patients and their families of the possible serious risks attached to treatment (in addition to their underlying psychiatric condition) suggested by some spontaneous reports that the agency has received. As part of this effort, explicit labeling about the association of antidepressant treatment with an increase in agitation, akathisia, aggression, depression, etc., that has been observed in some cases should be adopted. In addition, strategies to effectively communicate this information, in order to enhance vigilance of patients and their families and promote appropriate physician follow-up, should be developed.

MEMORANDUM

DEPARTMENT OF HEALTH AND HUMAN SERVICES
PUBLIC HEALTH SERVICE
FOOD AND DRUG ADMINISTRATION
CENTER FOR DRUG EVALUATION AND RESEARCH

PID# D030341

DATE: February 18, 2004

FROM: Andrew D. Mosholder, M.D., M.P.H., Epidemiologist

THROUGH: Mark Avigan, M.D., Director
Division of Drug Risk Evaluation, HFD-430

TO: Russell Katz, M.D., Director
Division of Neuropharmacological Drug Products, HFD-120

SUBJECT: Suicidality in pediatric clinical trials with paroxetine and other antidepressant drugs: Follow-up to 9-4-03 consult

Drugs: paroxetine, sertraline, venlafaxine, fluoxetine, fluvoxamine, citalopram, nefazodone, mirtazapine, and bupropion

EXECUTIVE SUMMARY

This consult is a follow-up to the previous consult on this topic, dated 9-5-03. As described in that consult, GlaxoSmithKline (GSK) performed an analysis of suicidal behaviors in their paroxetine pediatric clinical trial database, and found that there was a statistically significant increase in suicide-related adverse events for paroxetine-treated subjects compared to placebo. The method GSK used for their analysis involved an electronic search of the adverse event data for certain events that might have represented suicidal behaviors, followed by a blinded review of these events to select those that appeared to be probably related to suicide. In July 2003, the Division of Neuropharmacological Drug Products (DNDP) requested the sponsors of the other antidepressant drugs to replicate GSK's analysis in their own pediatric clinical trial databases. This consult summarizes the results of these analyses for 22 short-term placebo-controlled trials involving 9 different antidepressant drugs.

These trials included a total of 4250 pediatric subjects, 2298 treated with active drug and 1952 treated with placebo. There were 108 patients with suicide-related events (74 on active drug and 34 on placebo); 78 of these adverse events were serious (54 on active drug and 24 on placebo).

Considering individual development programs separately, the data for venlafaxine and paroxetine showed a statistically significant increase in suicide-related events relative to placebo. Additionally, on one measure (the incidence rate difference for serious suicide-related events) the data for citalopram approached statistical significance (p-value = 0.063). The relative risks for suicide related events with two compounds, fluoxetine and mirtazapine, were below one, raising the possibility of a protective effect. However, the mirtazapine relative risk estimate of 0.5 was based on a very small number of events and had very broad confidence intervals. The relative risk of suicide-related events for fluoxetine was 0.9 (95% confidence limits 0.3-2.3). (For all the other drugs, the relative risk estimates were greater than one, or undefined because of no events on placebo.)

Overall, comparing active drug treatment to placebo, there was an association of suicide-related events (incidence rate difference 0.08/year, p-value = 0.002) and serious suicide-related events (incidence rate difference 0.06/year, p-value = 0.006) with active drug treatment. This association was observed principally in major depressive disorder (MDD) trials, where the relative risk was 1.8 (95% confidence limit 1.2—2.8) and the attributable risk was 0.24/patient year for drug minus 0.14/patient year for placebo, yielding a value of 0.10 per patient-year of exposure to drug (p-value = 0.013). For serious suicide-related events in MDD trials, the relative risk was 1.9 (95% confidence interval 1.2–3.2), and the attributable risk was was 0.19/patient year for drug minus 0.10/patient year for placebo, yielding a value of 0.085 events per patient-year of exposure to drug (p-value = 0.015), equivalent to approximately 1 excess serious suicide-related event per 12 years of drug treatment. For non-MDD trials, the data also showed a higher rate of events with active drug treatment, but the attributable risk for serious events was much smaller than for MDD trials (0.01/year), and the data were not statistically significant.

There are a number of limitations to this analysis, the chief among them being that the clinical trial data are limited to short-term use of these drugs. Unfortunately, there are not comparable data available regarding safety and efficacy of long-term use of these drugs in pediatric patients. Also, although there were attempts to standardize the methodology and case definitions among the various sponsors, in practice there may have been differences because each sponsor conducted their own separate analysis.

At the present time, a number of additional steps are under way to enhance the quality of the data for the assessment of this signal. These initiatives include arranging for a blinded review of the clinical trial cases by suicidology experts at Columbia University, requesting additional details on how each sponsor conducted their analysis, and obtaining electronic clinical trial datasets for each study to permit a more sophisticated statistical analysis.

However, while these efforts will yield valuable information, particularly at the level of the data for individual trials and drugs, in my view it is unlikely that the new information will alter the basic finding of an association of suicide-related events and serious suicide-related events with active treatment. This is because of the size of the effect and the statistical significance of the overall finding. Also, it seems less likely that misclassification or failure to identify relevant events would produce a false positive signal; rather, those types of errors tend to weaken a signal. Only systematic bias could be reasonably expected to yield a false positive signal of this magnitude, and that seems unlikely.

Recommendations: Given the strength of the association shown by the present data, the clinical importance of the apparent effect (i.e., an estimated excess of one additional serious suicide-related event per 12 patient-years of active treatment), and the fact that the additional analyses are likely to take several more months to complete while considerable numbers of pediatric patients are being exposed to these drugs, I favor an interim risk management plan regarding use of these drugs in the pediatric population. This might be of value to physicians, patients and families who are faced with the need to make a decision regarding pharmacotherapy at the present time. Specifically, I propose a risk management strategy directed at discouraging off-label pediatric use of antidepressant drugs, particularly the use of drugs other than fluoxetine in the treatment of pediatric MDD. Conceivably, this might include discouraging the initiation of treatment of drug-naïve pediatric MDD patients with off-label drugs, in the absence of some over-riding clinical consideration. (Of course, all such warnings should be made in a manner that emphasizes the fact that the available data apply only to short-term, acute treatment, and that sudden discontinuation of antidepressant treatment, or discontinuation without medical supervision, are unwise.)

I recommend this approach for two reasons. First, of all the drugs with pediatric MDD clinical trial programs, only fluoxetine is approved for pediatric MDD, on the basis of two positive clinical studies (out of two MDD studies conducted). Of course, the failure to demonstrate efficacy in pediatric MDD trials with other antidepressants does not necessarily mean that these other drugs are ineffective in pediatric MDD. Still, for drugs other than fluoxetine, judgement regarding their efficacy in pediatric MDD must remain a matter of speculation until further trials are conducted. Secondly, although the confidence limits are broad, fluoxetine is the drug for which the estimate of the relative risk of suicidal events appears most favorable.

BACKGROUND

This memorandum is in follow-up to our consult to DNDP dated 9-5-03. On May 22 of this year, GlaxoSmithKline submitted an analysis of adverse events related to suicidal behaviors in pediatric trials of paroxetine (Paxil, NDA 20-031). The sponsor performed this analysis by conducting an automated, electronic search of the safety database from their pediatric trials for adverse event terms that would suggest suicidal behaviors. This analysis showed a statistically significant increase in such behaviors with paroxetine treatment, compared to placebo. A previous consult reviewed these data, and also provided a preliminary analysis of data from seven other pediatric development programs for other antidepressant drugs.[2] Overall, there was a statistically significant increase in suicidal adverse events for active drug treatment compared to placebo, similar to the findings from the paroxetine trials. These findings were discussed at a CDER Regulatory Briefing.[3]

However, this preliminary review of pediatric trials with the other antidepressant drugs was limited to a manual search of the reports submitted to FDA. In order to provide a meaningful comparison to the paroxetine findings, the Division of Neuropharmacological Drug Products requested the sponsors of eight other drugs (sertraline, venlafaxine, fluoxetine, fluvoxamine, citalopram, nefazodone, mirtazapine, and bupropion) to conduct a search of their databases similar to the analysis performed by GlaxoSmithKline. All of the 8 sponsors responded to this request within the next few months. The purpose of this memorandum is to summarize the findings reported in those submissions.

With respect to pediatric indications for the antidepressant drugs, clomipramine, fluvoxamine, sertraline and fluoxetine are approved for pediatric obsessive compulsive disorder. (Clomipramine is an older tricyclic compound that was not part of this analysis.) For pediatric major depressive disorder (in children 8 years and up), the only drug approved is fluoxetine. Appendix table 5 presents a summary of the efficacy results from placebo-controlled trials with the aforementioned drugs, along with the regulatory status of the drugs for pediatric use.

METHODS

The sponsors of the aforementioned 8 drugs all received identical information request letters from DNDP dated 7-22-03. The letters asked for the following analyses for all randomized, placebo-

---

[2] PID# D030341, 9-4-03.
[3] CDER Regulatory Briefing 9-16-03

controlled trial involving pediatric subjects (the indented text below is reproduced from the letters):

> The identification of the following events should be done blinded to treatment to avoid bias. All adverse events occurring within 30 days of the last dose of drug should be included in the search.
>
> "Suicide-related events" should be identified using the following algorithm:
> • Any events coded to preferred terms that include the text strings "suic" or "overdos"
> • Exclude "accidental overdose" cases
> • Regardless of the preferred term to which the verbatim term is mapped, all verbatim terms should be searched for the following text strings: "attempt", "cut", "gas", "hang", "hung", "jump", "mutilat-", "overdos-", "self damag-", "self harm", "self inflict", "self injur-", "shoot", "slash", "suic-"
> • Any terms identified by this search because the text string was a substring of an unrelated word should be excluded (for example, the text string "cut" might identify the word "acute")
> • In addition to the algorithm above, narratives of all serious adverse events (SAEs) should be reviewed (in a blinded fashion) to identify any additional cases of suicidality or self- harm. In particular, SAEs related to mania and hostility should be examined closely for suicidality or self-harm.
> • Any death found to be due to suicide or overdose should be included (if not already identified by the previous search methods).
>
> We are also interested in an analysis of suicide attempts. "Suicide attempts" are a subset of the "suicide-related events" identified above; they should be identified using a blinded hands-on review of the records of all patients identified by the above algorithm as having a "suicide-related event". For the purposes of this analysis, any case in which the patient exhibited self-injurious behavior should be considered as a suicide attempt. Any case in which the patient's suicidal ideation did not lead to self-injurious behavior should be excluded from this subset.
>
> Separate analyses should be performed for the group of "suicide-related" events and the group of "suicide attempts". Both the risk (# of events/# of patients) and the rate (# of events/person-time exposure) should be presented by treatment group. All treatment groups should be presented, including active controls. If a study has a blinded extension phase, events identified while the patient is in that extension phase should be excluded.
>
> In addition to presenting the overall risks and rates across all indications and within each indication, the following stratified analyses should be performed:
> • Child (<12) vs. Adolescent (>= 12).
> • On-therapy vs. On-therapy + 30 days.
> • Within each indication, data from each trial should be presented separately.

Also requested were detailed clinical data about the patients identified as having suicidal events, in the form of narrative summaries and tabulations.

The analyses submitted by each sponsor are summarized herein. A brief description of the relevant pediatric clinical trials is presented for each drug. Also, Appendix table 3 lists each pediatric subject having a suicide-related event.

Although I reviewed all the narrative summaries of the identified adverse events, I have not reclassified any events myself; the sponsors maintained the blind on treatment when they categorized these events, and this is obviously not possible for me. Instead, I have simply noted the few cases where in my opinion a different classification of the event might reasonably have been made. For a few patients who experienced more than one event of interest, I have chosen to count each patient only once in the analysis, at the time of their first event; their subsequent events are described under "Comments" in appendix table 3. Also described under "Comments" are any other adverse events that were prominently associated with the suicidal events. For a few of the clinical development programs, there were a sufficient number of cases to warrant a discussion of possible contributing clinical factors such as dose and duration of treatment, and I have included those details where appropriate.

Also included is a summary analysis of the clinical trial data, both overall and by drug and indication, with statistical testing. This analysis examines the question of the association of these events with active drug treatment in two ways: by calculation of the attributable risk (more precisely, the incidence rate difference between drug and placebo), as well as the relative risk (i.e., incidence rate ratios for drug:placebo). All statistical calculations were performed with Stata version 7.0 software. (Grateful acknowledgement is made to Dr. Yi Tsong of OPSS for his comments on the statistical methods.)

RESULTS

Including the previously reviewed data on paroxetine, this analysis comprised a total of 22 randomized, placebo-controlled trials with 9 different antidepressant drugs in the pediatric population. A total of 2298 pediatric subjects were exposed to active drug, for a total of 406.9 patient-years; for placebo, there were 1952 subjects exposed for a total of 347.6 patient-years. (One trial, Study 329 for paroxetine, included an imipramine arm as an active control, in which the rate of suicide-related events was intermediate between paroxetine and placebo at 0.24 per patient-year, but I have omitted those data from this analysis. Also, patient-years of exposure were not available for the single trial with bupropion.)

The sponsors identified a total of 108 patients with suicide-related events in these trials, 74 on active drug and 34 on placebo. There were no completed suicides. All 83 patients with suicide-related events described in the previous consult were included among these 108 patients. Seventy-eight patients had events classified as serious (54 on drug and 24 on placebo), and 75 had events classified as "suicide attempts" under the method described above (with 49 suicide attempts on drug, and 26 on placebo). Appendix Table 1 presents the complete data on the numbers of these events from all 22 clinical trials, and Appendix Table 2 presents the derived rates of these events for each trial. Appendix Figures 1-4 depict graphically the rates enumerated in Appendix table 2, for MDD and non-MDD studies. Note that the placebo rates of events vary considerably from trial to trial, even within the subgroup of MDD studies. With respect to the classification of events, discussion at the 9-16-03 CDER Regulatory Briefing and subsequently has raised questions about the appropriateness of the "suicide attempts" classification, since this category actually includes all types of deliberate self-injury. Accordingly, in the following I have chosen to emphasize the category of serious suicide-related events, rather than the category of suicide attempts, as being perhaps more clinically meaningful. The data for the category "suicide attempt" are included in Appendix Tables 1 and 2 for completeness.

Overview of each sponsor's submission.

Bupropion (Wellbutrin, NDA 18-644, GlaxoSmithKline, submission dated 8-22-03)

There were no pediatric studies for the indications of major depressive disorder (MDD) or smoking cessation. There was one placebo-controlled pediatric study for the indication of attention deficit hyperactivity disorder (ADHD), as shown below. The requested electronic search of adverse event data revealed no suicide-related events in this study.

Indication	Protocol	No. of sites	Age range (yrs)	Duration (wks)	N	
					Bupropion	Placebo
ADHD	75	4	6-12	6	71	36

Thus, there are no available data on pediatric suicidality with bupropion in the relevant patient populations.

Mirtazapine (Remeron, NDA 20-415, Organon, submission dated 8-21-03 and email dated 11-24-03)

There was only one clinical protocol in the mirtazapine development program, described below; the sponsor conducted two identical studies under that protocol, which were combined for the analysis of safety information.

Indication	Protocol	No. of sites	Age range (yrs)	Duration (wks)	Dose (mg/day)	N	
						Mirtazapine	Placebo
MDD	003-045	34	7-17	8	15-45	170	88

The electronic search of the adverse events terms in study 003-045 yielded a total of 13 adverse events; these were listed in Organon's email submission dated 11-24-03. Of these 13 events, 10 were obviously not related to suicidal behaviors and were excluded, leaving 3 cases for further review; one of these cases ocurred pre-randomization and so was not part of the analysis. Additionally, a subject who was hospitalized for suicidal ideation was identified from the review of all serious adverse events (subject 0404), yielding a total of 3 cases, summarized in Appendix table 3. Note, however, that Organon excluded one of these events from the analysis: subject 0801, a 9 year old boy receiving mirtazapine treated in the emergency room for an overdose on 4 Depakote tablets. This was not considered a suicide attempt because the boy took the tablets "on a dare."

Fluoxetine (Prozac, NDA 18-936, Lilly)

N.B. The following summary is based primarily upon Lilly's submission to Health Canada dated 10-7-03, and not their submission to FDA dated 9-2-03, because Lilly discovered an additional fluoxetine-associated event while preparing their Canadian submission. For details, please refer to Lilly's correspondence dated 10-9-03.

There were four clinical trials relevant to this analysis, three in MDD and one in obsessive-compulsive disorder (OCD). Study HCCJ, a pilot study in adolescent depression, was excluded from the sponsor's Integrated Summary of Safety for the pediatric supplement, but is included in this analysis.

Indication	Study	No. of sites	Age range (yrs)	Duration (wks)	Dose (mg/day)	N	
						Fluoxetine	Pbo
OCD	HCJW	22	7-18	13	10-60	71	32
MDD	HCJE	22	8-18	19*	20	109	110
MDD	X065	1	8-18	8	20	48	48
MDD	HCCJ	1	12-17	6	20-60	21	19

*includes subacute phase (weeks 10-19), during which poorly responding patients could receive a higher dose of double-blind study medication

Lilly's search for adverse events of interest yielded a total of 220 possibly relevant events. Of these, 176 were considered obviously unrelated to the issue of suicidality and were not reviewed further (a list of these adverse events was provided by email 11-17-03, and I concur with the sponsor that none of the events involve self-harm). The remaining cases are summarized in the sponsor's table, reproduced below.

Number of patients in pediatric fluoxetine MDD and OCD trials, by search category (reproduced from sponsor's submission)

Patient Category	Number of Patients
1) Suicide-related events with suicide attempts (acute/subchronic phases[a])	10
2) Suicide-related events with no suicide attempts (acute/subchronic phases[a])	7
3) Accidental overdose/death	1
4) Could be suicide related, but insufficient information	3
5) Suicide-related event prior to treatment phase	14
6) Suicide-related event during extension phase	2
7) Suicide-related event that was not treatment emergent	7

a Defined as the acute treatment phases for Studies HCCJ, X065, and HCJW, and the acute and subchronic phases from Study Periods III through V of Study HCJE.

Lilly provided narratives on all the cases listed, in their aforementioned submission to Health Canada and also in their email submission 11-18-03. My own review of these narratives substantiated Lilly's categorization of them.

The 17 events in categories 1 and 2 above were included in the analysis; a listing of these patients appears in appendix table 3.

A few observations can be made regarding the clinical details of these cases. With respect to dose, among the 9 fluoxetine-treated subjects with suicide-related events, the daily dose at the time of event was 20 mg for 7 subjects, 30 mg for one, and 60 mg for one. Median duration of treatment for fluoxetine subjects at the time of their event was 38 days, and the corresponding median for placebo subjects was 33 days. The adolescent age category predominated; children under 12 years of age comprised 43% of the total sample of 458 clinical trial subjects, but only 3 (18%) of the 17 suicide-related events occurred in children, which is not surprising given the relative infrequency of suicidal behavior among children compared to adolescents. Of the 17 suicide-related events, 13 (76.5%) occurred in female subjects, although females comprised only 228 (49.8%) of the 458 subjects.

Regarding the relationship to drug discontinuation, only one of the events (a drug overdose by fluoxetine patient 001-6401 in study HCCJ) occurred during the 30-day follow-up period. This patient was regarded as having discontinued by virtue of being non-compliant with study medication. However, Lilly acknowledged that "events occurring after study completion were not systematically collected," and so some events in the 30-day follow-up period may have been missed.

Nefazodone (Serzone, NDA 20-152, Bristol Myers Squibb, submission dated 8-21-03)

The table below provides the details for the two randomized, placebo-controlled pediatric studies with nefazodone.

Indication	Protocol	No. of sites	Age range (yrs)	Duration (wks)	Dose (mg/day)	N	
						Nefazodone	Placebo
MDD	CN104141	15	12-18	8	100-600	95	95
MDD	CN104187	28	7-17	8	100-300 or 200-600	184 (both arms)	94

The sponsor performed the requested search and identified two suicide-related events in these trials, both occurring in nefazodone-treated patients (please refer to Appendix table 3). (In addition to these events, the sponsor reported a total of 5 suicide-related events that occurred during open label treatment with nefazodone in follow-up to study 187. However, only the two events during double-blind treatment are relevant for this analysis.)

Fluvoxamine (Luvox, NDA 21-519, Solvay, submission dated 8-22-03)

There was one randomized, placebo controlled pediatric trial with fluvoxamine, described in the table below.

Indication	Protocol	No. of sites	Age range (yrs)	Duration (wks)	Dose (mg/day)	N	
						Fluvoxamine	Placebo
OCD	114	20	8-17	10	50-200	57	63

Solvay's search of the safety dataset for this trial revealed a single suicide-related event in a fluvoxamine-treated patient.

Sertraline (Zoloft, NDA 19-839, Pfizer, submission dated 9-12-03)

There were three randomized, placebo-controlled trials in the pediatric population, summarized in the table below. In addition, Pfizer is conducting a pediatric trial in post-traumatic stress disorder, for which the treatment is still blinded. Note that there were two studies for MDD conducted under the same protocol, and these have been combined in this analysis.

Indication	Protocol	No. of sites	Age range (yrs)	Duration (wks)	Dose (mg/day)	N	
						Sertraline	Placebo
OCD	498	12	6-17	12	25-200	92	95
MDD	1001/1017	51	6-17	10	50-200	189	184

The electronic search of adverse event terms yielded 89 potential events from these trials. Pfizer's blinded review of the 89 cases identified 25 patients with possibly relevant events, and further review of these cases excluded 19 events (mostly associated with accidental injuries). This yielded a total of 9 events occurring among 8 subjects that were considered suicide-related. (My own review of the listing of these 89 events did not disclose any additional events that were obvious omissions.) In addition, Pfizer performed the requested review of all serious adverse events in these trials, yielding one additional case relevant to the analysis (subject 1001-29533-2006, who was hospitalized for suicidal ideation). Thus there were a total of 9 patients with suicide-related events. It should be noted, however, that in their submission Pfizer questioned the clinical relevance of events in two sertraline-treated patients (subject 30506-1076, with self-mutilation, and subject 6193-1022, who was hospitalized for suicidal threats), although they did not exclude these events from their analysis.

Although the number of events was probably too small for any meaningful characterizations, the median age among the 6 sertraline treated patients with events was 10 years, somewhat younger than seen in other development programs. These 6 subjects included 3 males and 3 females; their median dose was 100 mg/day, and all had MDD.

There were no events reported within the 30-day period after discontinuation of study medication, and no events in the OCD trial. Of the nine events, six occurred on drug and three on placebo. Six of the nine events occurred in female subjects. With respect to age, there was a somewhat different pattern from that seen in other clinical trial programs, since four events out of the nine occurred in children rather than adolescents (one event considered a suicide attempt occurred in a 6 year old boy). The duration of treatment among the six sertraline-associated events ranged from 21 to 50 days.

Citalopram (Celexa, NDA 20-822, Forest, submission dated 8-21-03)

There were two randomized, controlled clinical trials in the citalopram pediatric development program, summarized below.

Indication	Protocol	No. of sites	Age range (yrs)	Duration (wks)	Dose (mg/day)	N	
						Citalopram	Placebo
MDD	CIT-MD-18	21 in U.S.	7-17	8	20-40	89	85
MDD*	94404	31 in Europe	13-18	12	10-40	121	112

*subjects could be inpatients or outpatients

Note that in addition to these two completed trials, the sponsor is conducting study SCT-MD-15, a randomized, double blind, placebo controlled trial of escitalopram, the s-isomer of citalopram, in children and adolescents with MDD. This trial is still blinded; the total number of subjects planned is 264, and there have been two suicide-related events thus far.

Forest made a couple of departures from the requested methods for the adverse event search. They included an analysis of 8 patients who experienced worsening of depression, but not suicidal thoughts or behaviors; all these patients were treated with placebo. These events were not included in the analysis presented here; the interested reader should refer to their submission for details. Forest also reported that their search of all serious adverse events for events involving suicidality was not performed blind to treatment. (I reviewed the serious adverse events in these two trials myself, and although I was not blind to treatment group either, I did not find any cases that were obvious omissions. However, among the serious adverse events, there were 6 placebo-treated and 2 citalopram-treated patients in study 94404 with psychiatric hospitalizations. These events were not counted in the analysis, however, because suicidality was not specifically documented.)

In addition to the events selected for the analysis, Forest reported that the electronic search identified 11 patients with "false positives" who were excluded.[4] In addition to the electronic search, Forest conducted a manual search of all adverse events and patient narratives from the

[4] Email dated 11-17-03

two trials, yielding 6 patients with relevant events that were not disclosed in the electronic search. This made a total of 30 patients with events. In addition, one patient who took an extra dose of medication by mistake was considered to have taken an accidental overdose (patient 485 in study 94404); this event was not included in the analysis. Two events occurred prior to randomized treatment, yielding a total of 28 patients for the analysis (please refer to Appendix table 3 for a list of these patients). Note that 27 of the 28 events were classified as suicide attempts. However, Forest indicated in an email dated 11-17-03 that six of the study 94404 patients classified with "suicide attempts" (patients 664, 693, 867, 607, 152, and 713) were so categorized simply because the recorded preferred term was suicide attempt, and not because the event description documented self-injurious behavior.

Four placebo-treated patients and four citalopram-treated patients had events during the 30-day follow-up period after the end of randomized treatment. However, two of these 4 placebo patients also had events during double blind treatment, and so are counted as having events while on-treatment. Note that patient 007 in study 94404 was actually receiving fluoxetine, not citalopram, at the time of the event during the post-study period.

The median age of the 28 patients with events was 16 years; 19 were females and 9 males. Among the 13 patients receiving citalopram at the time of their event, the median dose was 20 mg/day, and the median duration on treatment was 27 days. Forest noted that 11 of the 16 citalopram-treated patients with suicide-related events in study 94404 had a past history of suicidality.

Forest also provided an analysis of scores on the suicidality item of the depression rating scales in the two trials; i.e., the CDRS-R in study CIT-MD-18, and the K-SADS in study 94404. There was a greater improvement on the suicidality item in study CIT-MD-18 with citalopram treatment compared to placebo, and this almost reached statistical significance. However, the mean change from baseline on item IX from the K-SADS in study 94404 was approximately equal between citalopram and placebo.[5]

Paroxetine (Paxil, NDA 20-031, GlaxoSmithKline)

Please refer to the consult dated 9-5-03 for details regarding the paroxetine pediatric clinical trial data. Subsequently, GSK provided the agency with a copy of their report to the Committee for Proprietary Medicinal Products of the European Agency for the Evaluation of Medicinal Products .[6] Included in this is an analysis of suicide-related events in adult trials with paroxetine that mirrors GSK's analysis of the pediatric clinical trials. The results of the adult trial analysis show essentially no difference in the rates of suicide-related events between paroxetine and placebo treatment groups, for all studies combined or for the subset of MDD trials. This is in contrast to the previously described pediatric trial data, which showed a statistically significant increase with paroxetine treatment. The sponsor's tables describing both the adult and the pediatric analyses are reproduced in Appendix Figure 5.

Venlafaxine (Effexor and Effexor XR, NDAs 20-151 and 20-699, Wyeth)

There were four randomized, double blind, placebo-controlled venlafaxine trials in pediatric patients, summarized in the following table. The sponsor also reported that two additional

---

[5] NDA 20-822 8-21-03 submission

[6] NDA 20-031 11-7-03 electronic submission

pediatric placebo-controlled trials, one in social anxiety disorder and one in panic disorder, have been completed but are not fully analyzed yet.

Indication	Protocol	No. of sites	Age range (yrs)	Duration (wks)	Dose* (mg/day)	N	
						Venlafaxine	Placebo
MDD	382	16	7-17	8 + taper	37.5-225	80	85
MDD	394	37	7-17	8 + taper	37.5-225	102	94
GAD**	396	39	6-17	8 + taper	37.5-225	80	84
GAD	397	35	6-17	8 + taper	37.5-225	77	79

*administered as Effexor XR in all trials; dosage based upon weight of subject, and tapered over ≤2 weeks following double-blind treatment

**Generalized Anxiety Disorder

Wyeth identified 16 randomized patients with suicide-related events, along with two MDD patients who had events before beginning the study and who were not counted in the analysis. Additionally, one more event was identified through review of adverse event narratives, yielding a total of 17 patients who experienced a total of 20 events of interest. Wyeth counted all 20 events, rather than simply enumerating the number of patients with events.[7] Note that two patients were considered to have had separate events a few days apart (patients 39402-0041 and 39428-1087); after review of the narrative summaries, I have elected to count these instead as single events. A third patient also had two events, patient 38211-012, but these were separated by approximately 3 weeks and I have elected to count only the first event in the analysis that follows. Thus, the analysis shown below is based upon the number of patients with events, rather than the number of events (as in Wyeth's analysis). The listing in the Appendix provides further details about the patients.

The patient-years of exposure were not provided in the response to the July 2003 letter, since only rates were displayed in that submission; however, the exposures were available from the original pediatric exclusivity supplement. Additionally, in Wyeth's analysis, the "on-therapy" period does not include the taper period, but only the period of randomized treatment during which patients received their full dose of study medication. Therefor, "on-therapy period + 30 days" does not include a full 30 days from the last dose of study medication, if the patient had a taper following the end of their study treatment. This is slightly different from GlaxoSmithKline's analysis of the paroxetine pediatric trials, in which the "on-therapy" period included the taper phase, through the last dose of study medication, and the "on-therapy + 30 days" period included a full 30 days from the last dose of study medication.

With respect to classification of events, there were some issues with the "suicide attempts" category. The reason that patient 38205-019 was not counted in the suicide attempt category for taking an overdose was unclear. Also, I was unable to verify Wyeth's count of 3 suicide attempts on venlafaxine and 2 on placebo in study 382.[8] Instead, I have used the counts from Wyeth's "Abbreviated Table of Patient Characteristics."[9]

The median age among the 17 patients with suicide-related events was 13 years. For the 13 venlafaxine-treated patients, at the time of the event the median dose was 112.5 mg/day, and the median duration of treatment was 24 days. Wyeth counted any events occurring within 1 day of

[7] NDA 20-151 submission 8-28-03

[8] Table 3A, NDA 20-151 submission 8-28-03

[9] Table 4A, NDA 20-151 submission 8-28-03

the last full dose of study medication as having occurred on-therapy. Five of the 17 events did not occur on-therapy, 3 with venlafaxine and 2 with placebo.

Risk estimates

Analysis of attributable risk

Pooling the exposure and event data by drug and by indication provides the results shown in tables 1 and 2. Appendix figure 6 displays these same results graphically. Here, an incidence rate difference greater than zero would indicate a risk associated with active drug versus placebo, while an incidence rate difference less than zero would indicate a protective effect of the drug.

Table 1.

Attributable risks (incidence rate differences) per patient-year for suicide-related events in pediatric trials

Trials	Incidence rate difference, drug minus placebo	95% confidence interval	p-value
Citalopram	0.14	-0.16-0.43	0.374
Fluoxetine	-0.03	-0.20-0.14	0.737
Fluvoxamine	0.11	-0.10-0.32	0.485
Mirtazapine	-0.04	-0.21-0.14	0.691
Nefazodone	0.05	-0.02-0.12	0.367
Paroxetine	0.12	0.04-0.20	0.005
Sertraline	0.06	-0.05-0.17	0.327
Venlafaxine	0.17	0.02-0.33	0.029
All MDD trials	0.10	0.02-0.18	0.013
All non-MDD trials	0.04	-0.01-0.09	0.114
All trials	0.08	0.03-0.14	0.002

Table 2

Attributable risks (incidence rate differences) per patient-year for serious suicide-related events in pediatric trials

Trials	Incidence rate difference, drug minus placebo	95% confidence interval	p-value
Citalopram	0.24	-0.01-0.48	0.063
Fluoxetine	-0.02	-0.18-0.14	0.775
Fluvoxamine	0	-	-
Mirtazapine	0.04	-0.04-0.12	0.654
Nefazodone	0.03	-0.02-0.08	0.606
Paroxetine	0.08	0.01-0.15	0.038
Sertraline	0.06	-0.04-0.16	0.276
Venlafaxine	0.06	-0.07-0.18	0.379
All MDD trials	0.09	0.02-0.15	0.015
All non-MDD trials	0.01	-0.02-0.05	0.498
All trials	0.06	0.02-0.11	0.006

The incidence rate differences by drug for MDD trials alone are shown in Appendix Tables 6 and 7. These data are displayed graphically in Appendix Figure 7.

It can be seen that overall the data are consistent with an increased risk of suicidal events with active drug treatment; the comparison between active treatment and placebo for all trials pooled together is statistically significant (p-value = 0.002 for all suicide-related events, and p-value = 0.006 for serious suicide-related events). For serious suicide-related events in MDD trials, the attributable risk was was 0.19/patient year for drug minus 0.10/patient year for placebo, yielding a value of 0.085 events per patient-year of exposure to drug (p-value = 0.015), equivalent to approximately 1 excess serious suicide-related event per 12 years of drug treatment. The observed serious event incidence rate differences are larger in MDD trials (0.085/year) than in trials with OCD, GAD and Social Anxiety Disorder (SAD) (0.014/year).
With respect to individual drugs, the incidence rate differences for all suicide-related events are largest for paroxetine, venlafaxine and citalopram, reaching statistical significance for paroxetine and venlafaxine. For serious suicide-related events, citalopram showed the largest incidence rate difference, which approached statistical significance (p-value = 0.063).

Analysis of relative risk

In addition to estimating the excess risk attributable to drug, the data can also be analyzed in terms of the relative risk, or more precisely, the ratio of the incidence rates for drug and placebo. Accordingly, Mantel-Haenszel combined incidence rate ratios were calculated, stratified by study. This approach has the advantage of providing stratification by study, while the analysis of excess risk shown above simply involved summing all the relevant data without regard for differences between trials. In addition to calculating the combined incidence rate ratio, the Stata software also tests for homogeneity of the individual study ratios.

The Stata output for the "All trials" category is shown in Appendix table 3. There were two studies by themselves that showed statistically significant rate ratios for suicide-related events, Paroxetine Study 329 and Venlafaxine Study 394. No individual study showed a statistically significant protective effect.

Table 3 below displays the relative risks (more precisely, the incidence rate ratios) for suicide-related events and serious suicide-related events for each of the antidepressant drugs, and for all 21 clinical trials combined. Here placebo is the reference, and thus a value less than one indicates a protective effect of the drug, and a value greater than one a risk associated with drug treatment. For each combined incidence rate ratio calculated, the Mantel-Haenszel chi-square test showed no lack of homogeneity (i.e., indicating that data from the individual studies can be combined statistically).

Table 3. Combined incidence rate ratios for suicide-related events and serious suicide-related events

Drug	Number of pediatric trials	Incidence rate ratios* (95% confidence interval), by drug	
		All suicide-related events	Serious suicide-related events
Paroxetine	5	2.69 (1.20-6.00)	2.19 (0.92-5.24)
Sertraline	2	2.03 (0.51-8.16)	2.52 (0.49-13.01)
Venlafaxine	4	3.33 (1.08-10.33)	1.80 (0.52-6.20)
Fluoxetine	4	0.88 (0.34-2.30)	0.88 (0.32-2.44)
Citalopram	2	1.41 (0.66-3.00)	2.54 (0.91-7.05)
Mirtazapine	1	0.53 (0.007-41.45)	†
Nefazodone	2	†	†
Fluvoxamine	1	†	†
MDD trials	14	1.82 (1.19-2.77)	1.95 (1.19-3.21)
Non-MDD trials	7	2.36 (0.67-8.33)	1.31 (0.26-6.72)
All trials	21	1.86 (1.25-2.78)	1.89 (1.18-3.04)

†Ratio undefined due to zero events in placebo group
*Mantel-Haenszel method

It will be seen that the suicide-related event incidence rate ratios for venlafaxine and paroxetine indicate an association with drug treatment, and that the corresponding confidence intervals exclude one. Overall, the incidence rate ratio of approximately 1.9 for both suicide-related events and the subcategory of serious suicide-related events indicate an association of these events with drug treatment. Put another way, compared to placebo, treatment with active drug increased the rate of suicide-related events by an estimated 85%, and by an estimated 87% for serious suicide-related events. For the subgroup of MDD trials, the incidence rate ratios were also statistically significant, while for non-MDD trials the incidence rate ratio estimates had very wide confidence intervals.

DISCUSSION AND CONCLUSIONS

In short-term pediatric trials, antidepressant drug treatment is associated with an increase in suicidal adverse events compared to placebo. This finding is seen for both the broad category of any suicide-related event, and the more specific category of serious suicide-related events. The association is more prominent in the MDD trial data, where the relative risk of serious suicide-related events is approximately 1.9. The rate of serious suicide-related events in MDD trials among drug-treated patients was 0.19/patient-year, and was 0.10/patient-year among placebo-treated patients. These rates represent one serious event per 5.4 patient-years for drug, and one serious event per 9.9 patient-years for placebo, yielding an attributable risk of one additional serious suicide-related event per 11.8 patient-years of drug treatment. The finding appears to be statistically robust, inasmuch as the p-value for the incidence rate difference for all suicide-related events across all trials is 0.002.

With respect to individual drugs, the data for paroxetine and venlafaxine show a statistically significant increase in suicide-related events with active treatment in their pediatric development programs. Also, the incidence rate difference for serious suicide-related events with citalopram was close to statistical significance (p-value = 0.063). For fluoxetine and mirtazapine, the point estimates were consistent with a protective effect, but the confidence intervals for mirtazapine were very broad, and even for fluoxetine the confidence interval on the incidence rate ratio includes a relative risk of greater than 2. Put another way, although an increase in suicide-related events reached statistical significance for two drugs (paroxetine and venlafaxine). for no drug was a protective effect demonstrated at a statistically significant level.

This analysis has several limitations. Most importantly, it is limited to short-term trials only. Conceivably, long-term treatment in patients who have responded positively to a drug might not produce an increased risk, or might even provide a protective effect. In other words, it may not be appropriate to extrapolate a finding of a risk in short-term trials to use of the drug for long-term maintenance treatment, especially if the patients have manifested a clinical response to the drug. Unfortunately, there is very little long-term controlled pediatric trial data for antidepressant drugs that is available for analysis.

Another limitation of this analysis is that although there is evidence of a class effect overall, it is difficult to know to what extent it applies to particular members of the class. Inspection of the confidence intervals for the risk estimates will show that the confidence limits for individual drugs overlap considerably. The existing clinical trial data, moreover, cannot provide a fair comparison between drugs, since the sizes of the clinical development programs and the specific indications studied vary from drug to drug, not to mention the fact that the intrinsic pharmacologic and pharmacokinetic properties of the drugs themselves are different.

A third limitation pertains to the difficulties in standardizing the methodology used by the nine different sponsors. Although all sponsors were given the same set of instructions in the letters issued 7-22-03, there were some discrepancies in how these instructions were applied. For example, Forest (sponsor of citalopram) performed not only the requested electronic search of all adverse event terms, but also a manual search, which yielded cases not found with the electronic search. Also, the 30-day follow-up period was interpreted differently by GSK (paroxetine) and Wyeth (venlafaxine). GSK counted followed-up time for 30 days after the last dose of study medication, and the taper phase was not part of that 30-day period. However, Wyeth began the 30-day period from the last full dose of study medication, so that the period of dosage taper was included in the 30-day follow-up time. Also, Lilly (sponsor of fluoxetine) reported that adverse event data was not consistently collected once patients discontinued their study treatment.

As Appendix figures 1-4 illustrate, there was considerable variability in the rates of these events from trial to trial, even within the same indication. This could be due to differences in the patient population (some trials included children, for example), or to differences in ascertainment of suicide-related events, or to both. This, of course, raises questions about whether it is appropriate to combine the data from different trials. The Mantel-Haenszel chi square test for homogeneity of the rate ratios, however, did not reveal any statistically significant lack of homogeneity.

The increase in suicidal events was most clearly demonstrated in MDD trials. However, events with active drug treatment were more frequent than events with placebo in non-MDD trials, although the numbers are small and the risk estimates are very uncertain. Nonetheless, this leaves open the possibility of a drug-associated risk of such behaviors for non-MDD patients, although at a much lower incidence rate difference than for MDD patients.

With respect to clinical factors that might be contributory, as described in the previous consult, the paroxetine data suggested a possible role for drug withdrawal, but this pattern was not as prominent in the data for other drugs. However, this observation might point to a lack of consistency across development programs with respect to ascertainment of adverse events following the end of double-blind treatment.

The absence of completed suicides in these data is only reassuring to a limited degree. The total drug exposure time in these trials was 407 patient-years. For assessing the rate of a rare event such as completed suicide with active drug treatment, this is a relatively small data set. To illustrate, the upper confidence limit (one sided, 95% level) for the actual rate in the population given an observation of no suicides in 407 patient-years is 1 completed suicide in approximately 136 patient years.

In contrast to the paroxetine pediatric data, the analysis of suicide-related events in adult paroxetine trials, employing methods identical to the corresponding analysis of pediatric trial data, failed to show an increase in the rate of such events with paroxetine treatment relative to placebo. This was despite the fact that the placebo rate for these events was similar between the adult MDD trials (0.10/year) and the pediatric MDD trials (0.13/year). This suggests that adults and pediatric patients may have different responses to paroxetine with respect to suicidality.

Several steps are being taken at the moment to evaluate this signal further. First, a joint meeting of the Psychopharmacologic Drugs Advisory Committee and the Pediatric Subcommittee of the Anti-Infective Drugs Advisory Committee will be held 2-2-04 to discuss this issue.[10] Secondly, DNDP has requested electronic data sets from the sponsors of these clinical trials that will permit a more sophisticated statistical analysis. This analysis will permit examination of a number of issues that were beyond the scope of this consult, such as adjustment for a number of relevant covariates and exploration of risk factors such as agitation and relevant family history. Thirdly, DNDP has arranged for a group of suicidology experts at Columbia University to review the clinical narrative summaries for all of the identified cases; this will permit a more sophisticated case classification, particularly with regards to whether the event was a serious suicide attempt, a gesture, or self-mutilation. Fourthly, on 11-24-03 DNDP sent a memo to all the sponsors requesting a more detailed description of the methods each sponsor used to generate the submissions reviewed in this consult, to ensure the highest possible quality of data for review by the Columbia University experts.

One suggestion can be made for the expert group involved in the review of the cases. Because the nature and quality of the case reports received from the sponsors (as listed in Appendix Table 3) vary considerably, it is likely that even experts in classifying suicidal behaviors will have some uncertainty about how to classify some of the case reports. Accordingly, it will be important to reserve a category of indeterminate cases with which to do a sensitivity analysis. The principle here would be to do an analysis including the doubtful cases, and another analysis excluding them, to see if the results are very dependent upon how uncertain cases are classified.

These initiatives should indeed provide higher-quality data for evaluation of this signal. However, in my view, the new analyses are more likely to change the findings for individual studies and drug compounds where the numbers are relatively small, than they are to alter the overall finding of an increase in suicide-related adverse events and serious suicide-related events with active drug treatment compared to placebo. There are, I believe, several reasons for this. First, the aggregate findings are statistically robust (e.g., p-value = 0.002). Secondly, the counts of serious suicide-related events are, in my view, less likely to be unstable, because of the methods routinely employed to account for serious adverse events in clinical trials, and the greater amount of clinical information that is often collected about serious adverse events compared to non-serious events. Additionally, to the extent that events have been misclassified or overlooked in the sponsor's searches, this would generally be expected to introduce "noise" that would weaken the signal and produce a false negative, not generate a false positive. Only a systematic bias that

---

[10] Federal Register Vol. 68, No. 211 Friday, October 31, 2003

caused events in the placebo group to be missed while events in the drug group were captured would be expected to produce a false positive, and it is difficult to conceive of what could produce such a bias.

As previously noted, fluoxetine is currently the only drug approved for pediatric MDD, although several drugs are approved for pediatric OCD (see Appendix table 5). As shown in that table, all of the four pediatric OCD trials were positive and provided evidence of efficacy for approval of the drugs for pediatric OCD. This is in contrast to the experience with pediatric MDD trials, for which only 3 of the 15 trials have been judged positive, two with fluoxetine and one with citalopram.

In sum, short-term pediatric clinical trials of antidepressant drugs demonstrate an increased rate of suicidal events with active drug compared to placebo.

Recommendations: Given the strength of the association shown by the present data, the clinical importance of the apparent effect (i.e., an estimated excess of one additional serious suicide-related event per 12 patient-years of active treatment), and the fact that the additional analyses are likely to take several more months to complete while considerable numbers of pediatric patients are being exposed to these drugs, I favor an interim risk management plan regarding use of these drugs in the pediatric population. This might be of value to physicians, patients and families who are faced with the need to make a decision regarding pharmacotherapy at the present time. Specifically, I propose a risk management strategy directed at discouraging off-label pediatric use of antidepressant drugs, particularly the use of drugs other than fluoxetine in the treatment of pediatric MDD. Conceivably, this might include discouraging the initiation of treatment of drug-naïve pediatric MDD patients with off-label drugs, in the absence of some over-riding clinical consideration. (Of course, all such warnings should be made in a manner that emphasizes the fact that the available data apply only to short-term, acute treatment, and that sudden discontinuation of antidepressant treatment, or discontinuation without medical supervision, are unwise.)

I recommend this approach for two reasons. First, of all the drugs with pediatric MDD clinical trial programs, only fluoxetine is approved for pediatric MDD, on the basis of two positive clinical studies (out of two MDD studies conducted). Of course, the failure to demonstrate efficacy in pediatric MDD trials with other antidepressants does not necessarily mean that these other drugs are ineffective in pediatric MDD. Still, for drugs other than fluoxetine, judgement regarding their efficacy in pediatric MDD must remain a matter of speculation until further trials are conducted. Secondly, although the confidence limits are broad, fluoxetine is the drug for which the estimate of the relative risk of suicidal events appears most favorable.

Andrew D. Mosholder, M.D., M.P.H.
Epidemiologist

Mary Willy, Ph.D.
Epidemiology Team Leader

Appendix Table 1. Summary of pediatric clinical trial data on suicidal adverse events

Drug	Indication	Study	Drug: N	Drug: Patient-years	Drug: Suicide-related events	Drug: Serious suicide-related Events	Drug: Suicide attempts	Placebo: N	Placebo: Patient-years	Placebo: Suicide-related events	Placebo: Serious suicide-related events	Placebo: Suicide attempts
Paroxetine*	MDD	329†	93	13	8	7	5	88	13	1	1	0
	MDD	377	181	41	9	7	8	95	21	4	4	4
	MDD	701	104	16	3	3	2	102	17	2	1	1
	OCD	704	99	19	1	1	0	107	22	0	0	0
	SAD	676	165	51	4	0	1	157	47	0	0	0
	Paroxetine Total		*642*	*140*	*25*	*18*	*16*	*549*	*120*	*7*	*6*	*5*
Sertraline	MDD	1001/1017	189	32.2	6	5	3	184	32.5	2	2	2
	OCD	498	92	18.8	0	0	0	95	19.7	1	0	0
	Sertraline Total		*281*	*51*	*6*	*5*	*3*	*279*	*52.2*	*3*	*2*	*2*
Venlafaxine	MDD	382	80	11.01	5	3	1	85	11.73	3	3	3
	MDD	394	102	15.95	7	3	3	94	15.47	0	0	0
	GAD	396	80	13.08	0	0	0	84	13.56	0	0	0
	GAD	397	77	11.63	1	1	1	79	11.44	1	1	1
	Venlafaxine Total		*339*	*51.67*	*13*	*7*	*5*	*342*	*52.2*	*4*	*4*	*4*
Fluvoxamine	OCD	114	57	9.37	1	0	0	63	9.95	0	0	0
Mirtazapine	MDD	003-045	170	24.05	1	1	0	88	12.7	1	0	1
Fluoxetine	MDD	HCJE	109	31.57	4	3	1	110	27.96	4	3	2
	MDD	HCCJ	21	2.11	1	1	1	19	2.11	1	1	1
	MDD	X065	48	6.71	2	2	2	48	5.83	2	2	0
	OCD	HCJW	71	15.12	2	2	2	32	5.98	1	1	1
	Fluoxetine Total		*249*	*55.51*	*9*	*8*	*6*	*209*	*41.88*	*8*	*7*	*4*
Nefazodone	MDD	141	95	13.6	1	0	1	95	12.5	0	0	0
	MDD	187	184	25.4	1	1	1	94	12.9	0	0	0
	Nefazodone Total		*279*	*39*	*2*	*1*	*2*	*189*	*25.4*	*0*	*0*	*0*
Citalopram	MDD	CIT-MD-18	89	12.8	1	0	1	85	12	2	0	1
	MDD	94404	121	23.5	16	14	16	112	21.3	9	5	9
	Citalopram Total		*210*	*36.3*	*17*	*14*	*17*	*197*	*33.3*	*11*	*5*	*10*
Bupropion	ADHD	75	71	**	0	0	0	36	**	0	0	0
Grand Total			**2298**	**406.9**	**74**	**54**	**49**	**1952**	**347.63**	**34**	**24**	**26**

*Paroxetine patient-years of exposure were provided only to the nearest integer **Patient-years of exposure data were not provided †Imipramine arm omitted

Appendix Table 2. Rates of suicidal adverse events, per patient-year, in pediatric clinical trials

Drug	Indication	Study	Drug				Placebo			
			Patient-years	Rate of Suicide-related events	Rate of Serious suicide-related Events	Rate of Suicide attempts	Patient-years	Rate of Suicide-related events	Rate of Serious suicide-related events	Rate of Suicide attempts
Paroxetine	MDD	329	13	0.62	0.54	0.38	13	0.08	0.00	0.08
	MDD	377	41	0.22	0.17	0.20	21	0.19	0.19	0.19
	MDD	701	16	0.19	0.19	0.13	17	0.12	0.06	0.06
	OCD	704	19	0.05	0.05	0.00	22	0.00	0.00	0.00
	SAD	676	51	0.08	0.00	0.02	47	0.00	0.00	0.00
Sertraline	MDD	1001/1017	32.2	0.19	0.16	0.09	32.5	0.06	0.06	0.06
	OCD	498	18.8	0.00	0.00	0.00	19.7	0.05	0.00	0.00
Venlafaxine	MDD	382	11.01	0.45	0.27	0.09	11.73	0.26	0.26	0.26
	MDD	394	15.95	0.44	0.19	0.19	15.47	0.00	0.00	0.00
	GAD	396	13.08	0.00	0.00	0.00	13.56	0.00	0.00	0.00
	GAD	397	11.63	0.09	0.09	0.09	11.44	0.09	0.09	0.09
Fluvoxamine	OCD	114	9.37	0.11	0.00	0.00	9.95	0.00	0.00	0.00
Mirtazapine	MDD	003-045	24.05	0.04	0.04	0.00	12.7	0.08	0.08	0.00
Fluoxetine	MDD	HCJE	31.57	0.13	0.10	0.03	27.96	0.14	0.07	0.11
	MDD	HCCJ	2.11	0.47	0.47	0.47	2.11	0.47	0.47	0.47
	MDD	X065	6.71	0.30	0.30	0.30	5.83	0.34	0.34	0.00
	OCD	HCJW	15.12	0.13	0.13	0.13	5.98	0.17	0.17	0.17
Nefazodone	MDD	141	13.6	0.07	0.00	0.07	12.5	0.00	0.00	0.00
	MDD	187	25.4	0.04	0.04	0.04	12.9	0.00	0.00	0.00
Citalopram	MDD	CIT-MD-18	12.8	0.08	0.00	0.08	12	0.17	0.08	0.00
	MDD	94404	23.5	0.68	0.60	0.68	21.3	0.42	0.42	0.23
Total			406.9	0.18	0.13	0.12	347.63	0.10	0.07	0.07

Appendix Table 3. Listing of all patients with suicide-related events in pediatric antidepressant drug trials.

MIRTAZAPINE

Study	Indication	Patient ID	Age Sex	Treatment	Dose (mg/day) at time of event	Duration (days)	Event	Serious (y/n)	Comments
003-045	MDD	0404	15 M	Mirtazapine	15	7	Hospitalization for suicidal ideation	Y	
003-045	MDD	0801	9 M	Mirtazapine	45	52	Depakote overdose "on a dare"	Y	*Excluded by sponsor*
003-045	MDD	1603	12 F	Placebo	-	56	Self inflicted cuts	N	

FLUOXETINE

Study	Indication	Patient ID	Age Sex	Treatment	Dose (mg/day) at time of event	Duration (days)	Event	Serious (y/n)	Comments
HCCJ	MDD	001/6401	17 F	Fluoxetine	30	40	Overdose, details unknown, discontinued from trial	y	Patient poorly compliant with study drug
HCCJ	MDD	001-6408	13 M	Placebo	-	33	Overdose of aspirin	y	
HCJE	MDD	008-0806	15 M	Placebo	-	37	Hospitalized for suicidal ideation and self-mutilation	y	
HCJE	MDD	008/0804	15 F	Placebo	-	60	Overdose on study medication	y	
HCJE	MDD	009-0901	15 F	Fluoxetine	60	101	Self-mutilation	n	
HCJW	OCD	006-0609	15 F	Placebo	-	71	Self-injurious behavior	Y	No details provided
HCJW	OCD	013-1300	12 F	Fluoxetine	20	25	Tylenol overdose	Y	Hospitalized
HCJW	OCD	018-1811	7 F	Fluoxetine	20	60	Self-destructive cutting	y	
X065	MDD	001-2051	16 F	Fluoxetine	20	14	Multiple drug overdose	Y	Other adverse events included manic reaction
X065	MDD	001-2163	17 F	Fluoxetine	20	12	Overdose on unknown pills	Y	No psychiatric family history, no previous attempts
HCJE	MDD	004-0419	13 F	Fluoxetine	20	67	Hospitalized for suicidal ideation	Y	
HCJE	MDD	022-2216	15 F	Fluoxetine	20	38	Suicidal ideation	Y	
HCJE	MDD	003-0302	17 F	Fluoxetine	20	32	Suicidal thoughts	y	
HCJE	MDD	019-1901	11 F	Placebo	-	?	"wanting to die"	N	
HCJE	MDD	022-2203	9 M	Placebo	-	9	Suicidal ideation, intermittent	Y	Displayed self-injurious behavior during later extension phase of trial
X065	MDD	001-2052	16 M	Placebo	-	33	Suicidal ideation X 1 day (not hospitalized)	Y	Considered serious
X065	MDD	001-2087	14 F	Placebo	-	6	Hospitalized for suicidal ideation	y	

NEFAZODONE

Study	Indication	Patient ID	Age Sex	Treatment	Dose (mg/day) at time of event	Duration	Event	Serious (y/n)	Comments
141	MDD	3-1065	12 M	Nefazodone	600	38	Self mutilation (superficial cutting)	n	
187	MDD	18-322	13 F	Nefazodone	0	4 days post d/c	Overdose on 14 tablets of study medication	y	Hospitalized

FLUVOXAMINE

Study	Indication	Patient ID	Age Sex	Treatment	Dose (mg/day) at time of event	Duration (days)	Event	Serious (y/n)	Comments
RH1140201	OCD	65815	15 M	Fluvoxamine	200	36	Suicidal ideation	N	Self-mutilation during open label extension phase

SERTRALINE

Study	Indication	Patient ID	Age Sex	Treatment	Dose (mg/day) at time of event	Duration (days)	Event	Serious (y/n)	Comments
498	OCD	90N0242-19	12 F	Placebo	-	12	Suicidal ideation	N	
1001	MDD	29533-2006	12 M	Sertraline	100	49	Suicidal ideation	y	Hospitalized
1001	MDD	29534-1089	10 F	Sertraline	100	35	Suicidal ideation	Y	Hospitalized
1001	MDD	30506-1076	9 F	Sertraline	100	37	Self mutilation	n	Second episode of self mutilation on day 46
1001	MDD	6193-1022	10 M	Sertraline	100	21	Suicidal ideation	Y	Hospitalized. Also had mild agitation.
1017	MDD	29384-4022	16 F	Sertraline	150	50	Multidrug overdose	Y	Also noted to have restlessness
1017	MDD	30627-3095	6 M	Sertraline	100	34	Threatened to jump from vehicle, suicidal ideation	Y	Hospitalized; also experienced agitation
1017	MDD	31940-4329	17 F	Placebo	-	9	Attempted self-immolation	Y	Minor burn wounds. Subject later denied suicidality
1017	MDD	31942-4321	15 F	Placebo	-	63	Attempted suicide by hanging	Y	Second suicide attempt by overdose on day 66

CITALOPRAM

Study	Indication	Pt ID	Age Sex	Treatment	Dose (mg/day) at time of event	Duration (days)	Event	Serious (y/n)	Comments
CIT-MD-18	MDD	193	9 M	Citalopram	20	37	Cut self with knife	N	Agitation reported on previous day
CIT-MD-18	MDD	137	10 M	Placebo	-	31	Attempted to hang self (but not designated as a serious event)	N	Personality disorder; 24 days post-tx had another suicide-related event
CIT-MD-18	MDD	519	12 F	Placebo	-	41	Severe suicidal tendency (no details)	N	
94404	MDD	007	15 M	Citalopram	-	25 days post tx	Multiple drug overdose	Y	*Patient had received fluoxetine X 25 days since completing trial*
94404	MDD	009	17 F	Citalopram	20	15	Hospitalized for suicidality; overdose on naproxen on day 6 of hospitalization	Y	
94404	MDD	121	18 F	Citalopram	-	12 days post tx	Overdose of chlorxazone	Y	Patient had been discontinued from study on day 8 because of abnl clinical laboratories
94404	MDD	148	17 F	Citalopram	20	47	Overdose of 4-6 citalopram tablets	Y	Made a second overdose later in trial
94404	MDD	426	14 F	Citalopram	20	70	Overdose on 11 paracetamol tablets; denied suicidal intent	Y	Event coded as medication error
94404	MDD	573	14 F	Citalopram	20	88	Intentional ingestion of cigarettes	Y	Subject was an inpatient at screening
94404	MDD	575	14 F	Citalopram	20	55	Suicidal ideation, cut arm	Y	Subject was an inpatient at screening
94404	MDD	664	15 M	Citalopram	20	10	Re-hospitalized for suicidality	Y	Subject was an inpatient at screening
94404	MDD	713	16 M	Citalopram	30	27	Re-hospitalized for suicidality	N	Subject was an inpatient at screening. No explanation for why this was not designated a serious event.
94404	MDD	715	17 F	Citalopram	20	14	Hospitalized for suicidality, cut wrists, denied suicidal intent	Y	
94404	MDD	729	16 M	Citalopram	10	63	Ingested 15 caffeine pills plus alcohol	N	Event coded as medication error
94404	MDD	761	13 M	Citalopram	-	1 day post tx	Hospitalized for suicidality, event designated as a suicide attempt	Y	Also developed agitation, mood lability
94404	MDD	776	17 F	Citalopram	-	1 day post tx	Multiple drug overdose; only dose of study medication was the previous day	Y	Subject was an inpatient at screening. Also experienced anxiety
94404	MDD	867	17 F	Citalopram	30	20	Hospitalization due to suicidal thoughts	Y	Also experienced anxiety
94404	MDD	874	17 f	Citalopram	20	13	Overdose	Y	Patient cut her wrist 4 days after overdose
94404	MDD	884	16 F	Citalopram	20	16	Hospitalized after overdose on diazepam (9 tablets)	Y	On day 22, re-hospitalized for suicidality, and on day 81, another overdose
94404	MDD	071	16 F	Placebo	-	16	Hospitalized after self-inflicted wrist laceration	Y	Re-hospitalized for suicidality on day 36
94404	MDD	152	14 F	Placebo	-	8 days post tx	Hospitalized for suicidality	Y	Treated with citalopram after hospitalization
94404	MDD	412	18 F	Placebo	-	1 day post tx	Overdose on mother's medication	Y	Also receiving oxazepam for anxiety

Study	Indication	Pt ID	Age Sex	Treatment	Dose (mg/day) at time of event	Duration (days)	Event	Serious (y/n)	Comments
94404	MDD	605	13 M	Placebo	-	35	Self mutilation (forearm)	N	
94404	MDD	607	17 M	Placebo	-	62	Suicidal ideation and tension, treated with lorazepam	N	Inpatient at screening.
94404	MDD	691	17 F	Placebo	-	29	Self mutilation (palms)	N	
94404	MDD	693	16 F	Placebo	-	2	Hospitalized for suicidal ideation	Y	Later in trial had self-inflicted scratches on arm. After completing trial, started citalopram and was re-hospitalized for suicidal ideation 8 days later
94404	MDD	787	13 F	Placebo	-	29	Self-mutilation	N	
94404	MDD	871	17 F	Placebo	-	25	Overdose on 8 tablets of tolfenamic acid	Y	

PAROXETINE (Sources: 6-16-03 submission and Excel spreadsheet courtesy of Dr. Judith Racoosin, Division of Neuropharmacological Drug Products)

Study	Indication	Pt ID	Age	Sex	Treatment	Dose (mg/day) at time of event	Duration (days)	Event	Serious (y/n)	Comments
329	MDD	32900300313	18	M	Paroxetine	20	11	Command hallucinations, self mutilation	Y	Hospitalized
329	MDD	32900400015	16	F	Paroxetine	20	31	Mild self mutilation	N	
329	MDD	32900600038	15	F	Paroxetine	20	57	Multiple drug overdose	Y	
329	MDD	32900200245	14	F	Paroxetine	20	13	Acetaminophen overdose (27-28 capsules)	Y	Treated in emergency room and released
329	MDD	32900500250	15	F	Paroxetine	30	28	Overcompliance (by 124%) with study medication	Y	Coded as "overdose intentional" (Same patient subsequently overdosed on 20 capsules of study medication during continuation treatment.)
329	MDD	32900100065	14	M	Paroxetine	20	13	Angry outburst (with destruction of property) followed by suicidal thoughts	Y	
329	MDD	32900500333	16	F	Paroxetine	20	+4 post study	Hospitalized for severe suicidal ideation	Y	
329	MDD	32900200106	15	F	Paroxetine	40	51	Combative with mother, threatened suicide	Y	Hospitalized
377	MDD	37701100061	17	F	Paroxetine	40	75	Overdose (28 tablets of study medication)	Y	Hospitalized
377	MDD	37702400158	14	F	Paroxetine	30	86	Slapping herself in the face (automutilation)	N	
377	MDD	37702300172	16	M	Paroxetine	30	38	Overdose on 5 gm paracetamol plus 600 mg aspirin	N	Considered a non-serious event by investigator
377	MDD	37703000181	18	F	Paroxetine	40	56	Hostility, depression, writing suicide notes; possible drug abuse (cannabis)	Y	Hospitalized
377	MDD	37700900225	17	F	Paroxetine	20	78	Overdose on study medication	Y	Hospitalized
377	MDD	37704200310	15	F	Paroxetine	20	23	Self-inflicted wrist lacerations, superficial	Y	

Study	Indication	Pt ID	AGe	SEx	Treatment	Dose (mg/day) at time of event	Duration (days)	Event	Serious (y/n)	Comments
377	MDD	37705300508	14	F	Paroxetine	20	54	Cut left wrist after arguing with mother	Y	
377	MDD	37704200315	15	F	Paroxetine	20	+4 post study	Overdose on 5 acetaminophen pills and two other pills, agitation, anxiety	Y	Hospitalized
377	MDD	37704900479	17	M	Paroxetine	40	+2 post study	Suicidal ideation, irritability	Y	Hospitalized
676	SAD	67601124283	15	M	Paroxetine	30	+1 post study	Vague suicidal ideation	N	
676	SAD	67601424376	13	F	Paroxetine	40	34	Worsening panic attacks, suicidal ideation	N	
676	SAD	67610024705	16	F	Paroxetine	20	43	Self-inflicted scratch on wrist	N	
676	SAD	67610124629	14	F	Paroxetine	40	99	Threatened suicide when brother hospitalized	N	
701	MDD	70116325718	16	F	Paroxetine	50	41	Patient reported taking an overdose of 100 paroxetine tablets	Y	Overdose not confirmed by urine drug screen
701	MDD	70118025639	15	F	Paroxetine	30	+2 post study	Cut arms, overdose on acetaminophen	Y	Required ICU admission
701	MDD	70118327620	11	F	Paroxetine	20	+4 post study	Threatened to hang self	Y	Hospitalized
704	OCD	70403325513	15	M	Paroxetine	40	25	Hospitalization due to suicidal thoughts	Y	
329	MDD	32900100123	16	F	Placebo	-	45	Worsening depression, suicidal thoughts	Y	
377	MDD	37700500231	14	F	Placebo	-	31	Overdose of study medication and chlorazepate	Y	
377	MDD	37701000068	14	F	Placebo	-	83	Overdose on 21 alprazolam tablets	Y	Hospitalized
377	MDD	37702900024	17	F	Placebo	-	29	Tried to kill herself with scissors	Y	Details not provided
377	MDD	37704100294	14	F	Placebo	-	84	Overdose on 10 gm of acetaminophen	Y	Hospitalized
701	MDD	70115425768	13	M	Placebo	-	5	Wrecked parent's car and became suicidal	Y	Hospitalized
701	MDD	70118327617	12	F	Placebo	-	3	Mild self-mutilation of arms	N	

VENLAFAXINE

Study	Indication	Pt ID	AGE	Sex	Treatment	Dose (mg/day)	Duration (days)	Event	Serious (y/n)	Comments
382	MDD	38202-036	13	F	Placebo	-	+18 post tx	Angry, kicked a cabinet	Y	Resulted in ER visit
382	MDD	38204-023	11	F	venlafaxine ER	112.5	21	Suicidal ideation	N	
382	MDD	38205-008	12	M	venlafaxine ER	75	29	Suicidal ideation, auditory hallucinations	Y	Hospitalized
382	MDD	38205-019	8	F	venlafaxine ER	NA	13	Overdose on venlafaxine 300 mg	Y	Hospitalized
382	MDD	38207-008	12	M	Placebo	-	+17 post tx	Suicidal ideation, scratching on arms	Y	Hospitalized
382	MDD	38207-023	14	F	Placebo	-	3	Overdose on study medication (~8 capsules)	Y	Treated at ER and released
382	MDD	38209-020	13	F	venlafaxine ER	37.5	13	Suicidal ideation with plan to overdose	Y	Hospitalized
382	MDD	38211-012	10	F	venlafaxine ER	112.5	23	Mild self-injurious behavior	N	On day 43 of trial, hospitalized for swallowing aftershave

394	MDD	39402-0041	7	M	venlafaxine ER	'75	25 and 29	Suicidal ideation, plan to stab self	Y	Hospitalized (considered 2 events by sponsor)
394	MDD	39404-0126	14	M	venlafaxine ER	75	15	Suicidal and homicidal ideation	Y	Hospitalized
394	MDD	39411-0405	14	F	venlafaxine ER	150	51	Cut arm in context of family discord	N	Treated at ER and released
394	MDD	39420-0769	13	M	venlafaxine ER	225	36	Mild suicidal ideation	N	
394	MDD	39428-1087	16	M	venlafaxine ER	150	47 and 50	Rage attack, suicidal, homicidal	Y	Hospitalized; drug screen positive for PCP (considered 2 events by sponsor)
394	MDD	39435-1366	17	F	venlafaxine ER	37.5	5	Mild self-mutilation	N	
394	MDD	39440-1561	12	F	venlafaxine ER	-	+6 post tx	Overdose on study medication (17 capsules)	N	Treated at ER and released. Not considered a serious event
397	GAD	39701-0012	17	F	Placebo	-	15	Overdose of 18 Excedrin PM tablets following fight with boyfriend	Y	Hospitalized
397	GAD	39710-0361	10	M	venlafaxine ER	-	+3 post tx	Suicidal (wrapped cord around neck), agitated, and physically agressive	Y	Hospitalized

BUPROPION No cases

Appendix table 4. Stata outputs for calculation of combined incidence rate ratios

Category: Suicide-related events

Study	IRR	[95% Conf.	Interval]	M-H Weight	
003-045	.5281385	.0067291	41.45135	.6543909	(exact)
1001/1017	3.028078	.5414406	30.67137	.9953421	(exact)
114	.	.0272237	.	0	(exact)
141	.	.0235638	.	0	(exact)
187	.	.0130205	.	0	(exact)
329	8	1.072641	354.959	.5	(exact)
377	1.152439	.3216551	5.121634	2.645161	(exact)
382	1.775317	.3454063	11.43182	1.452651	(exact)
394	.	1.39804	.	0	(exact)
396	.	.	.	0	(exact)
397	.9837456	.0125341	77.21001	.5040969	(exact)
498	0	0	40.8801	.4882943	(exact)
676	.	.6083716	.	0	(exact)
701	1.59375	.1825649	19.08565	.969697	(exact)
704	.	.0296822	.	0	(exact)
94404	1.611357	.6704749	4.137106	4.720969	(exact)
CIT-MD-18	.46875	.0079441	9.004248	1.032258	(exact)
HCCJ	1	.0127412	78.48575	.5	(exact)
HCJE	.8856201	.1649537	4.754807	2.121318	(exact)
HCJW	.7910853	.0411829	46.67882	.7165671	(exact)
X065	.8689261	.0629945	11.98569	1.070133	(exact)
Crude	1.859448	1.223071	2.879198		(exact)
M-H combined	1.863115	1.246773	2.784147		

Test of homogeneity (M-H) chi2(13) = 7.67 Pr>chi2 = 0.8642

Category: Serious suicide-related events

Study	IRR	[95% Conf.	Interval]	M-H Weight	
003-045	.	.0135386	.	0	(exact)
1001/1017	2.523398	.4131554	26.50048	.9953421	(exact)
114	.	.	.	0	(exact)
141	.	.	.	0	(exact)
187	.	.0130205	.	0	(exact)
329	7	.8993189	315.599	.5	(exact)
377	.8963415	.2278526	4.175488	2.645161	(exact)
382	1.06519	.1426495	7.953972	1.452651	(exact)
394	.	.4008445	.	0	(exact)
396	.	.	.	0	(exact)
397	.9837456	.0125341	77.21001	.5040969	(exact)
498	.	.	.	0	(exact)
676	.	.	.	0	(exact)
701	3.1875	.2559633	167.3341	.4848485	(exact)
704	.	.0296822	.	0	(exact)
94404	2.537888	.8637632	9.002482	2.62276	(exact)
CIT-MD-18	.	.	.	0	(exact)
HCCJ	1	.0127412	78.48575	.5	(exact)
HCJE	.8856201	.1186016	6.613087	1.590989	(exact)
HCJW	.7910853	.0411829	46.67882	.7165671	(exact)
X065	.8689261	.0629945	11.98569	1.070133	(exact)
Crude	1.922267	1.168124	3.25143		(exact)
M-H combined	1.890265	1.175603	3.039376		

Test of homogeneity (M-H) chi2(10) = 6.44 Pr>chi2 = 0.7768

Appendix table 5. Summary of efficacy findings from eight pediatric antidepressant development programs

Drug	Indication	Approval status for pediatric use*	Study	N		
				Drug	Placebo	Efficacy results on primary variable
Paroxetine	MDD	NA	329	93	88	Failed (but + on secondary variables)
			377	181	95	Failed
			701	104	102	Failed
	OCD	AE	704	99	107	+
	SAD	Not submitted	676	165	157	? (not submitted)
Sertraline	MDD	NA	1001/1017	189	184	Two studies under same protocol, both failed (but + if data pooled)
	OCD	AP	498	92	95	+
Venlafaxine	MDD	NA	382	80	85	Failed
			394	102	94	Failed
	GAD	NA	396	80	84	Failed, by a small margin (p=0.09)
			397	77	79	+
Fluvoxamine	OCD	AP	114	57	63	+
Mirtazapine	MDD	NA	003-045	170	88	Two studies under this protocol, both failed
Fluoxetine	MDD	AP	HCJE	109	110	+
			X065	48	48	+
	OCD	AP	HCJW	71	32	+
Nefazodone	MDD	NA	141	102	99	Failed, by a small margin (p=0.08)
			187	184	94	Failed
Citalopram	MDD	NA	CIT-MD-18	89	85	+
			94404	121	112	Failed

* NA not approvable, AE approvable, AP approved

Appendix Table 6.

Attributable risks (incidence rate differences) per patient-year for suicide-related events in pediatric MDD trials			
Drug	Incidence rate difference, drug minus placebo	95% confidence interval	p-value
Citalopram	0.14	-0.16-0.43	0.374
Fluoxetine	-0.02	-0.21-0.17	0.829
Mirtazapine	-0.04	-0.21-0.14	0.691
Nefazodone	0.05	-0.02-0.12	0.367
Paroxetine	0.15	-0.01-0.31	0.088
Sertraline	0.12	-0.05-0.30	0.176
Venlafaxine	0.33	0.05-0.62	0.020
All MDD trials	0.10	0.02-0.18	0.013

Appendix Table 7.

Attributable risks (incidence rate differences) per patient-year for serious suicide-related events in pediatric MDD trials			
Drug	Incidence rate difference, drug minus placebo	95% confidence interval	p-value
Citalopram	0.24	-0.01-0.48	0.063
Fluoxetine	-0.02	-0.20-0.16	0.842
Mirtazapine	0.04	-0.04-0.12	0.654
Nefazodone	0.03	-0.02-0.08	0.606
Paroxetine	0.13	-0.02-0.27	0.121
Sertraline	0.09	-0.07-0.25	0.284
Venlafaxine	0.11	-0.11-0.33	0.337
All MDD trials	0.09	0.02-0.15	0.015

Appendix Figure 1.

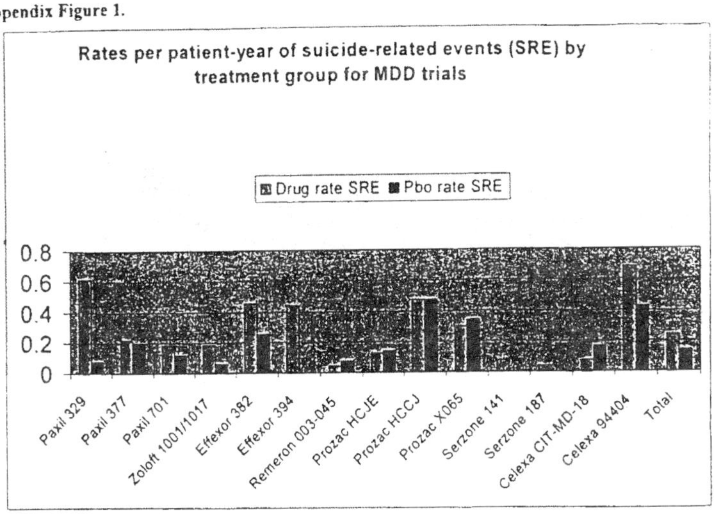

Appendix Figure 2.

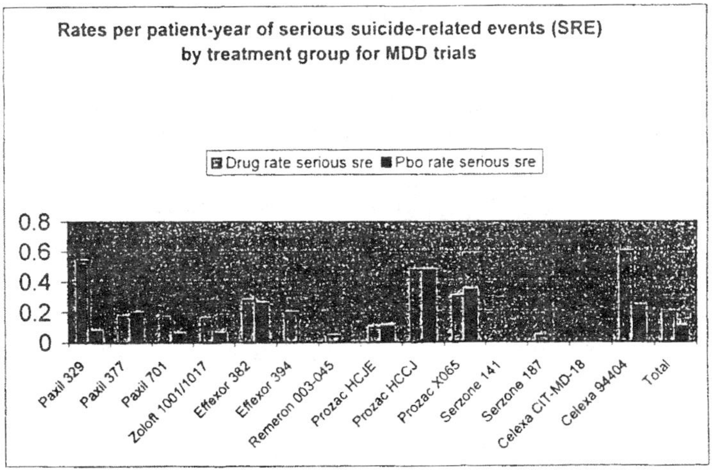

Appendix Figure 3.

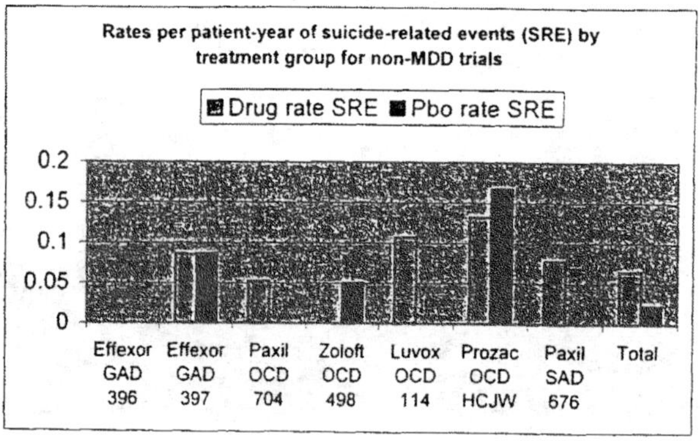

Appendix Figure 4.

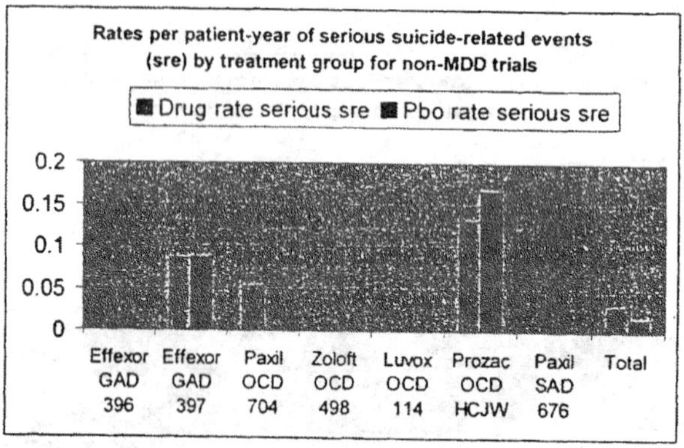

Appendix Figure 5 (reproduced from the sponsor's submission)

CONFIDENTIAL
Seroxat Article 31 - Consolidated Response Document

Table 2.9 **Incidence and Incidence Density for Possibly Suicide-Related Events by Treatment Group and Indication Paediatric Placebo Controlled Trials On-Therapy (including Taper Phase) plus 30 days post-therapy**

Indication		Paroxetine	Placebo	Odds Ratio (95% CI)	P value
Overall	n/N (%)	25/738 (3.4%)	8/647 (1.2%)	2.80 (1.25 , 6.25)	0.012
	PYE	176	149		
	n/PYE	0.14	0.05		0.017
Depression	n/N (%)	20/378 (5.3%)	8/285 (2.8%)	1.93 (0.84 , 4.46)	0.12
	PYE	85	61		
	n/PYE	0.24	0.13		0.16
OCD	n/N (%)	1/195 (0.5%)	0/205 (0.0%)		0.49
	PYE	41	41		
	n/PYE	0.02	0.00		
SAD	n/N (%)	4/165 (2.4%)	0/157 (0.0%)		0.12
	PYE	51	46		
	n/PYE	0.08	0.00		

Data Source: Appendix 28, Table 2.56

CONFIDENTIAL
Seroxat Article 31 - Consolidated Response Document

Table 2.5 **Incidence and Incidence Density for Possibly Suicide-Related Events by Treatment Group and Indication Adult Placebo Controlled Trials On-Therapy (including Taper Phase) plus 30 days post-therapy**

Indication		Paroxetine	Placebo	Odds Ratio (95% CI)	P value
Overall	n/N (%)	92/8481 (1.1%)	63/5808 (1.1%)	1.00 (0.72 , 1.38)	1.00
	PYE	1916	1313		
	n/PYE	0.05	0.05		1.00
Depression	n/N (%)	74/3421 (2.2%)	44/2117 (2.1%)	1.04 (0.71 , 1.52)	0.92
	PYE	671	428		
	n/PYE	0.11	0.10		0.71
GAD	n/N (%)	2/1182 (0.2%)	2/985 (0.2%)	0.83 (0.12 , 5.92)	1.00
	PYE	259	211		
	n/PYE	0.01	0.01		0.84
OCD	n/N (%)	3/542 (0.6%)	4/265 (1.5%)	0.36 (0.08 , 1.63)	0.23
	PYE	141	61		
	n/PYE	0.02	0.07		0.14
PMDD	n/N (%)	0/760 (0.0%)	0/379 (0.0%)		
	PYE	208	102		
	n/PYE	0.00	0.00		
PTSD	n/N (%)	7/786 (0.9%)	6/598 (1.0%)	0.89 (0.30, 2.65)	1.00
	PYE	174	138		
	n/PYE	0.04	0.04		0.89
Panic	n/N (%)	3/920 (0.3%)	4/780 (0.5%)	0.63 (0.14, 2.84)	0.71
	PYE	237	186		
	n/PYE	0.01	0.02		0.48
SAD	n/N (%)	3/870 (0.3%)	3/684 (0.4%)	0.79 (0.16 , 3.90)	1.00
	PYE	225	187		
	n/PYE	0.01	0.02		0.82

Data Source: Appendix 28, Table 2.02

Appendix Figure 6.

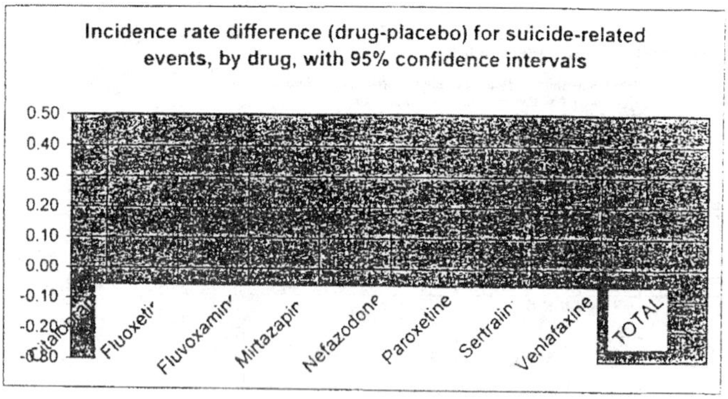

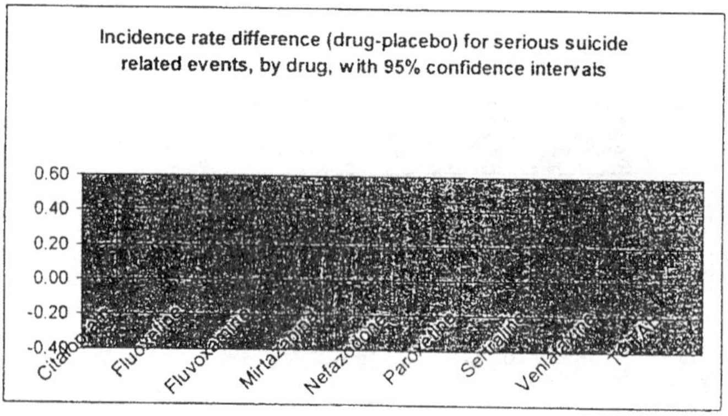

Appendix Figure 7.

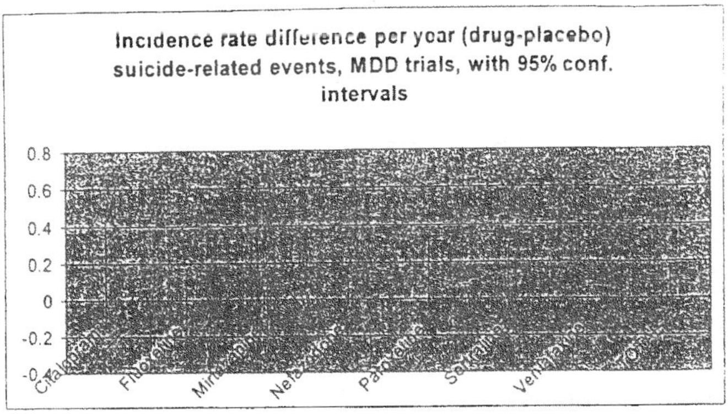

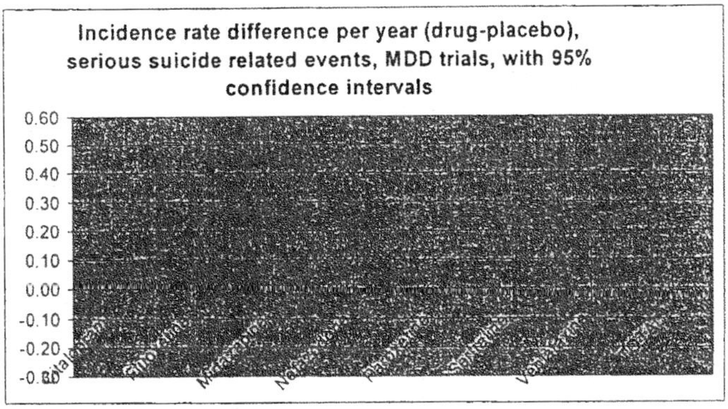

This is a representation of an electronic record that was signed electronically and this page is the manifestation of the electronic signature.

/s/

Andy Mosholder
3/19/04 01:31:42 PM
DRUG SAFETY OFFICE REVIEWER

Mary Willy
3/19/04 01:36:03 PM
DRUG SAFETY OFFICE REVIEWER

Mark Avigan
3/19/04 02:53:51 PM
DRUG SAFETY OFFICE REVIEWER

Anne Trontell
3/19/04 05:17:16 PM
DRUG SAFETY OFFICE REVIEWER

Tab 30

Subject:	Adult MDD Suicide Data Discussion
Location:	CDER WOC2 4FL-E Conf Room
Start:	Fri 5/28/2004 8:30 AM
End:	Fri 5/28/2004 9:30 AM
Show Time As:	Tentative
Recurrence:	(none)
Meeting Status:	Not yet responded
Required Attendees:	Temple, Robert; Katz, Russell G; Laughren, Thomas P; Racoosin, Judith A; Hammad, Tarek

Tab 31

Interim Results of the Analysis of Pediatric Trials

7/19/04

Tarek A. Hammad, MD, PhD, MSc, MS

Medical Reviewer

Division of Neuropharmacological Drug Products
Center for Drug Evaluation and Research, FDA

Objectives

- To investigate the relationship between psychotropic drugs and pediatric suicidality reported as AEs
  - AEs included in the analysis were blindly adjudicated and classified by a group of suicidology experts assembled by Columbia University
- To investigate the relationship between psychotropic drugs and pediatric suicidality as suggested by scores of the suicidality item(s) reported in pertinent depression questionnaires
- To understand the source(s) of inconsistency in any of the outcomes listed in the first two objectives by investigating possible source(s) of variation or imbalance in the data e.g. trial design, duration of exposure, patient population, and other potential confounders

FDA

Data Domain

- **25 controlled trials conducted in pediatric patients in nine drug development programs**

- Drugs - number of trials:
  - SSRIs group
    - Fluoxetine (Prozac) - 4
    - Sertraline (Zoloft) - 3
    - Paroxetine (Paxil) - 6
    - Fluvoxamine (Luvox) - 1
    - Citalopram (Celexa) - 2
  - Atypical antidepressants group
    - Bupropion (Wellbutrin) - 2
    - Venlafaxine (Effexor) - 4
    - Nefazodone (Serzone) - 2
    - Mirtazapine (Remeron) - 1

FDA

Data Domain, continued ...

- Indications - number of trials
  - Major Depressive Disorder - 15
  - Anxiety Disorders
    - Obsessive Compulsive Disorder - 5
    - Generalized Anxiety Disorder - 2
    - Social anxiety Disorder/Social Phobia - 1
  - Attention Deficit Hyperactivity Disorder – 2

- **Two trials excluded (Paxil 453-relapse prevention, Wellbutrin 41-uncontrolled)**

- **Trial year: 1983 to 2001**

- **Duration: 4 to 19 weeks**

FDA

Codes for Columbia University Classification

- 1: suicide attempt
- 2: preparatory actions towards imminent suicidal behavior
- 3: self-injurious behavior, intent unknown
- 4: self-injurious behavior, no intent, primarily to affect circumstance
- 5: self-injurious behavior, no intent, primarily to affect internal state
- 6: suicidal ideation
  - 6a: suicidal ideation, passive
  - 6b: suicidal ideation, active
  - 6c: suicidal ideation, active with plan
  - 6d: suicidal ideation, type unknown
- 7: other: accident
- 8: other: psychiatric
- 9: other: medical
- 10: not enough information
- 11: self-injurious behavior, no suicidal intent (unspecified type, i.e. rater not sure if it is 4 or 5)
- 12: "other"

FDA

Outcomes Based on AEs

- Included events that occurred in double-blind acute treatment phase or within one day of the end of this phase

FDA

Disposition of Events

[redacted]

[redacted]

[redacted]

[redacted]

[redacted]

[redacted]

Relationship Between Sponsor's and Columbia's Classifications

Columbia	Sponsor		Total
	No	Yes	
No event	4418	[redacted]	4435
Definitive suicidal behavior (codes 1 & 2) (1)	[redacted]	32	33
Suicidal ideation (code 6) (10)	[redacted]	35	45
Definitive suicidal behavior /ideation (codes 1,2, & 6) (11)	[redacted]	67	78
Possible suicidal behavior/ideation (codes 1, 2, 3, 6, & 10) (22)	[redacted]	87	109
Self-injurious behavior, non-suicidal (codes 4, 5, & 11) (2)	[redacted]	[redacted]	11

[redacted]

Outcomes Based on Suicidality Scores

Worsening of suicidality score

- Patient reached the threshold for "worsening of suicidal ideation" at any time during the controlled portion of the trial based on an increase of **one point or more** on the HAM-D item 3 or **two points or more** on the suicidality item 13 in CDRS-R or on the suicidality item 10 in MADRS, regardless of subsequent change.

- The definition of this variable is intended to capture only patients that exhibit the listed changes in their suicidality items in relation to their respective **baseline values**.

FDA

Emergence of suicidal ideation

(a subset of the previous one)

Definition of patient reaching the threshold of "emergence of suicidal ideation" depends on the scale used to rate suicidality:

- HAM-D
  - The patient is assigned a value of "1" if there is a change in rating of "suicide" item (item number 3) from 0 at baseline to 1 or more, or from 1 at baseline to 2 or more, at any time during the controlled phase of the trial. The variable should reflect the first time such a change occurs regardless of subsequent changes.
- CDRS-R
  - The patient is assigned a value of "1" if there is a change in rating of "suicidal ideation" item (item number 13) from 1 or 2 at baseline to 3 or more at any time during the controlled phase of the trial. The variable should reflect the first time such a change occurs regardless of subsequent changes.
- MADRS
  - The patient is assigned a value of "1" if there is a change in rating of "suicidal thoughts" item (item number 10) from 0 or 1 at baseline to 2 or more at any time during the controlled phase of the trial. The variable should reflect the first time such a change occurs regardless of subsequent changes.

Outcomes Used in the Analysis

Outcomes	Description	Number of events
Outcome1	Definitive suicidal behavior (1,2)	n=33
Outcome2	Suicidal ideation (6)	n=45
Outcome3	Definitive suicidal behavior/ideation (1,2,6)	n=78
Outcome4	Possible suicidal behavior/ideation (1,2,3,6,10)	n=109
Outcome5	Self-injurious behavior, non-suicidal (4,5,11)	n=11
Outcome6	Worsening of suicidality score	n=434
Outcome7	Emergence of suicidal ideation (a subset of outcome6)	n=349

All trials, all indications
(Fixed effect model)

Study	Risk ratio (95% CI)	% Weight
[redacted]	[redacted]	[redacted]
EFFEX(GAD, 397)	1.03 (0.07,16.11)	7.3
EFFEX(MDD,394)	2.77 (0.11,67.10)	3.9
[redacted]	[redacted]	[redacted]
PROZ(MDD,HCCJ)	0.30 (0.01,7.02)	11.7
PROZ(MDD,X065)	5.00 (0.25,101.48)	3.7
PROZ(OCD,HCJW)	1.38 (0.06,32.87)	5.1
[redacted]	[redacted]	[redacted]
Overall (95% CI)	1.78 (0.92,3.47)	

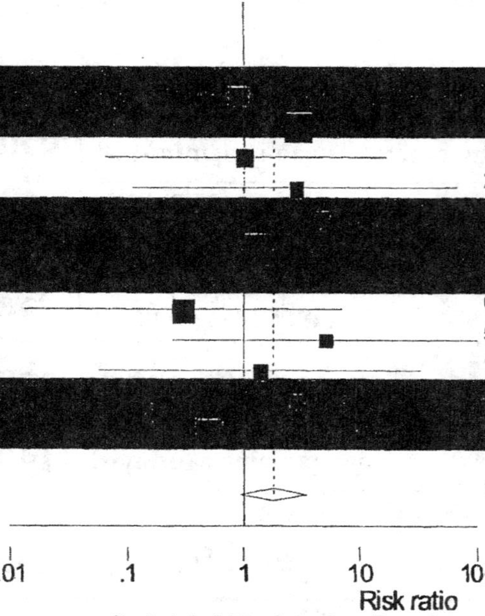

Suicidal Behavior [codes 1 & 2]

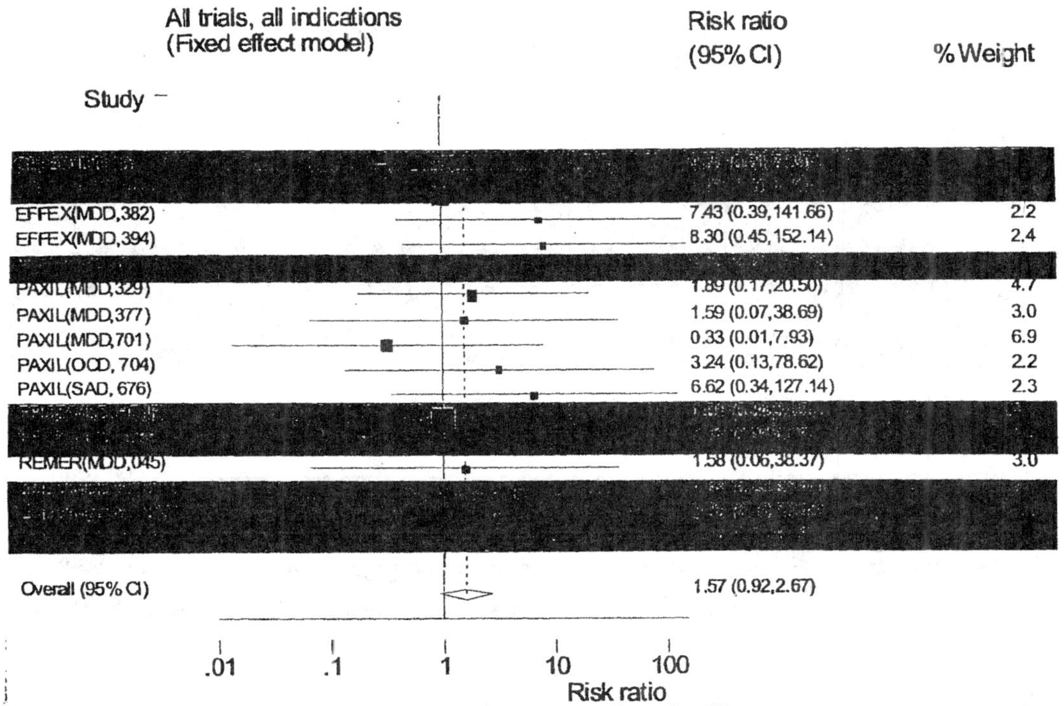

Suicidal Ideation [code 6]

14

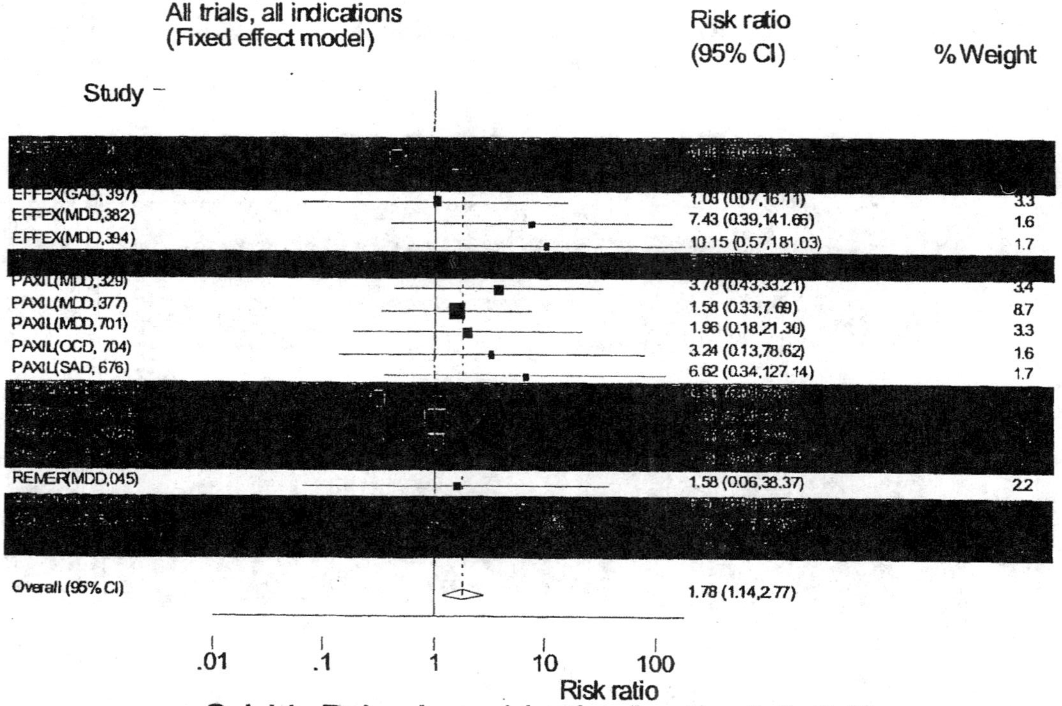

Suicide Behavior or Ideation [codes 1, 2, & 6]

15

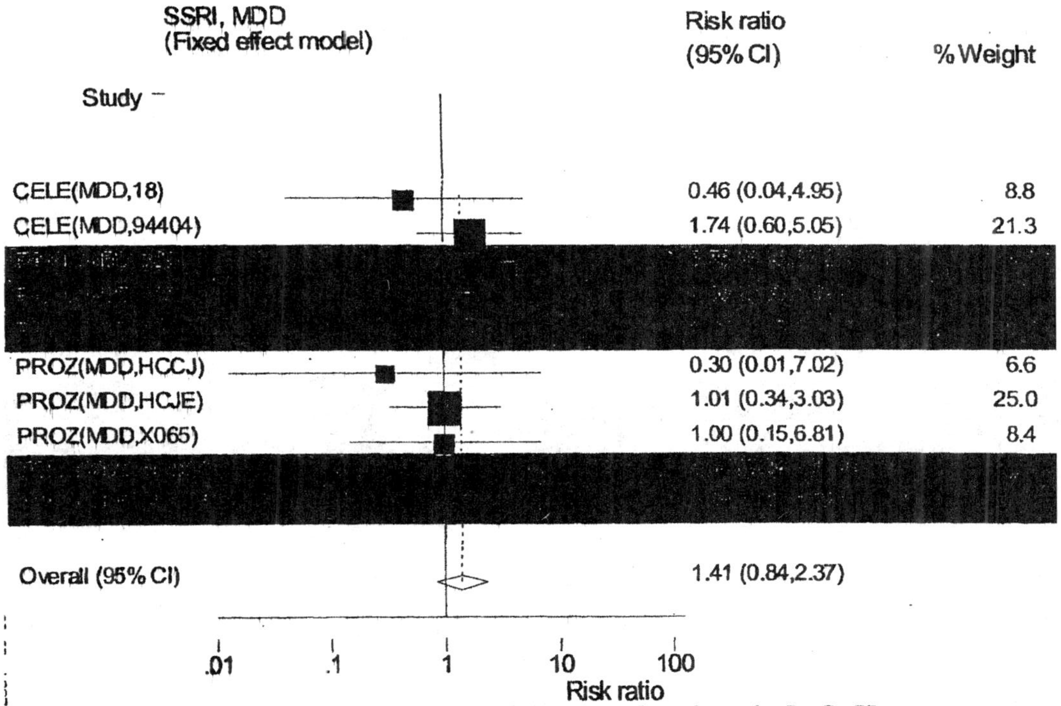

Suicide Behavior or Ideation [codes 1, 2, & 6]

16

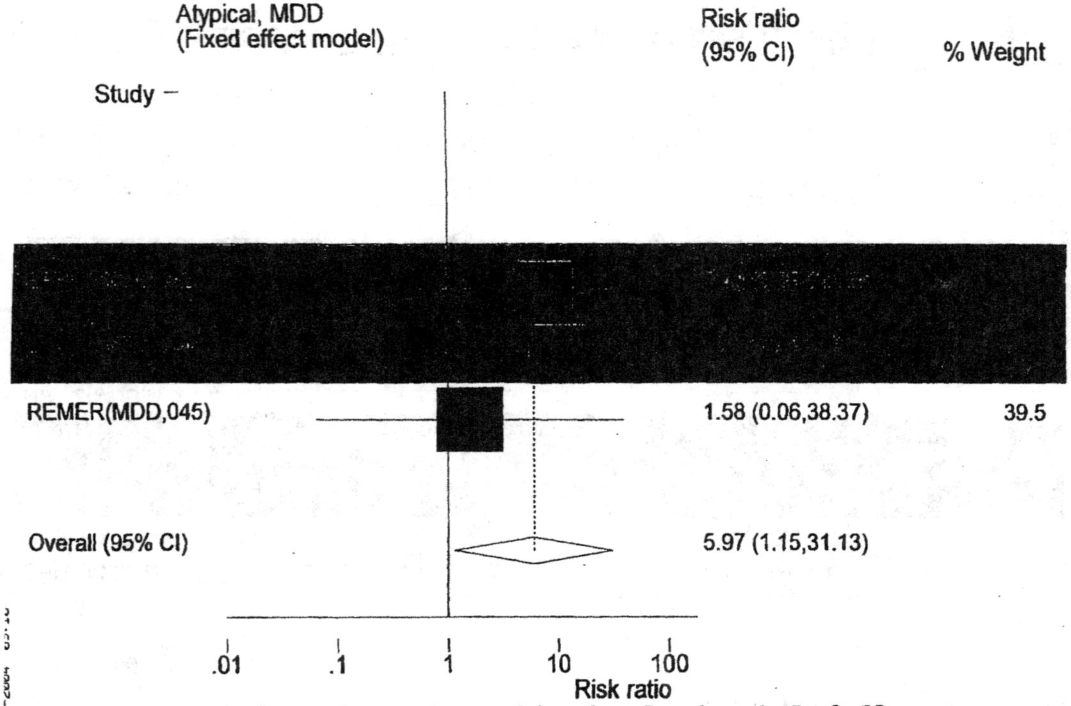

Suicide Behavior or Ideation [codes 1, 2, & 6]

17

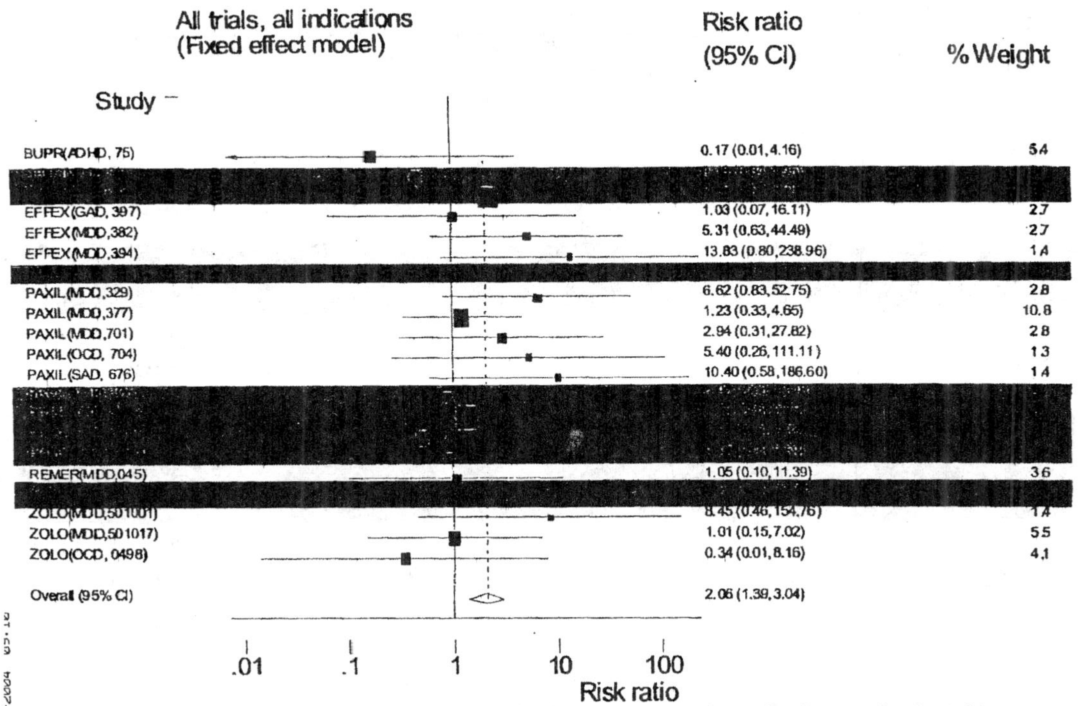

Possible suicidal behavior/Ideation [codes 1, 2, 3, 6, & 10] **18**

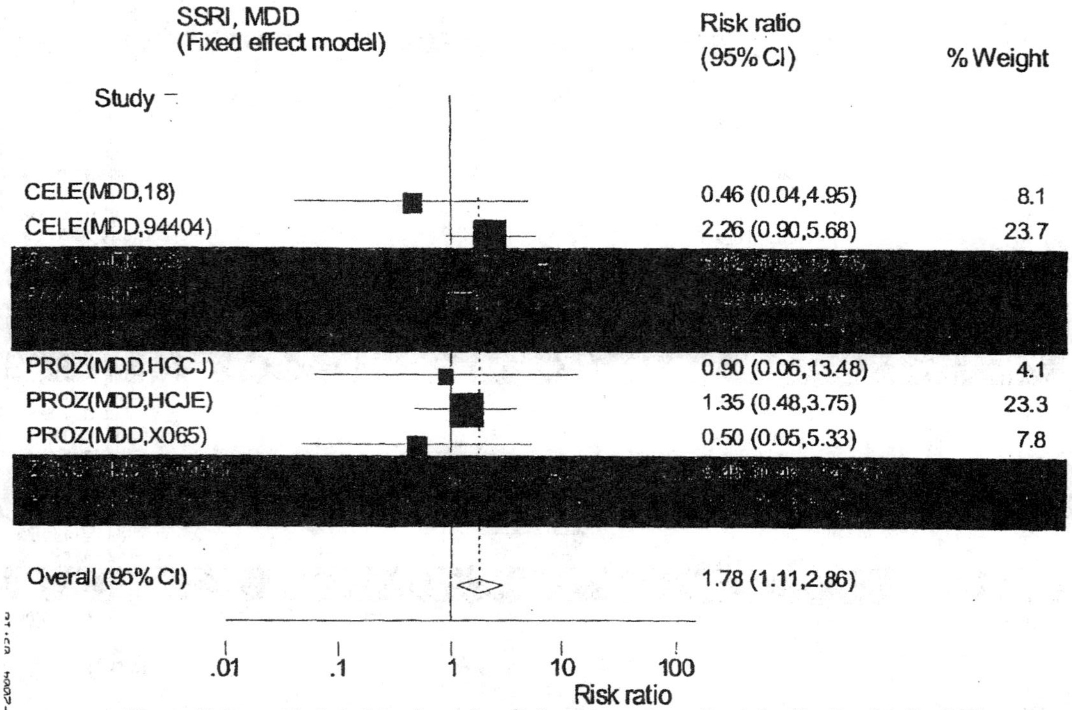

Possible suicidal behavior/Ideation [codes 1, 2, 3, 6, & 10] **19**

AUG-05-2004 09:18

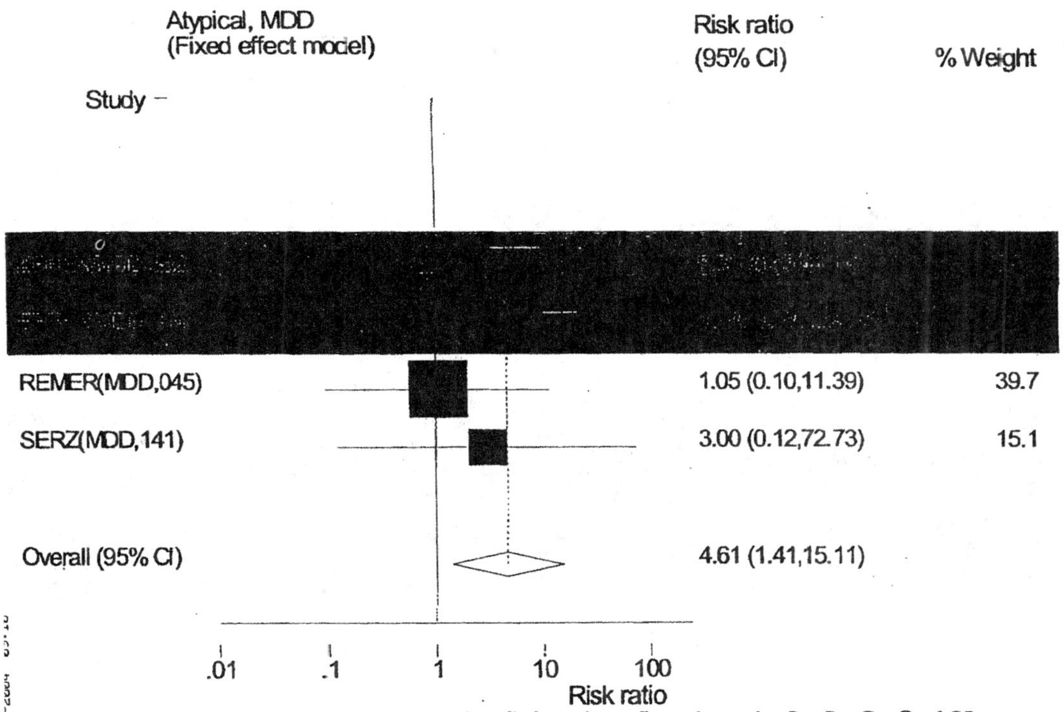

Possible suicidal behavior/Ideation [codes 1, 2, 3, 6, & 10] **20**

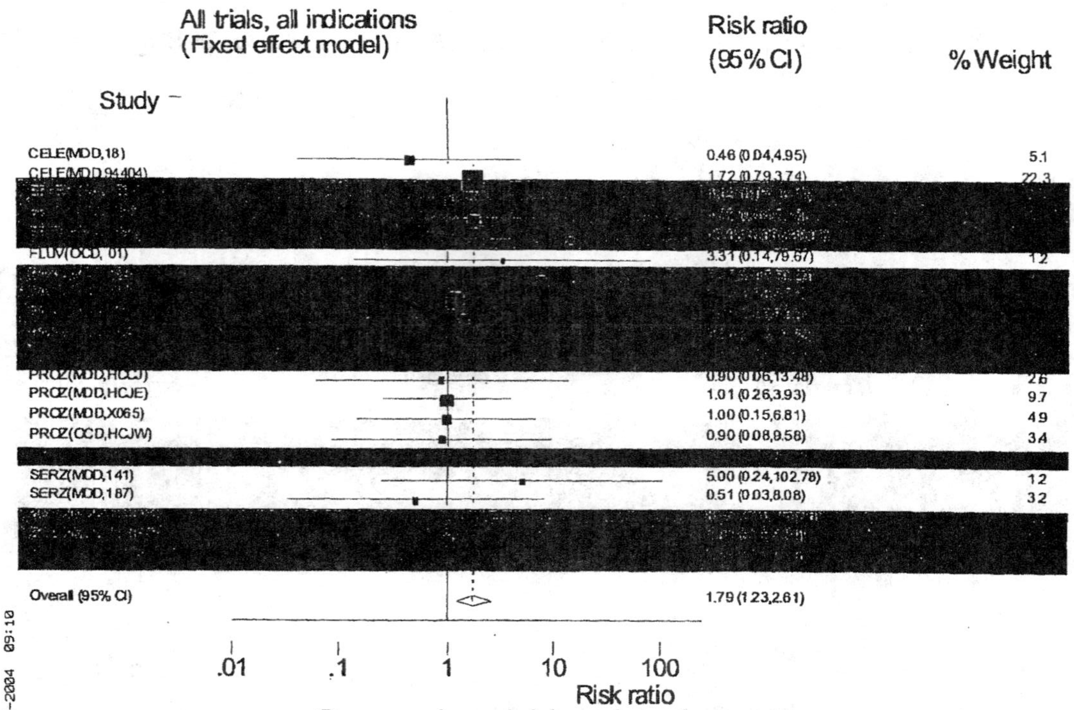

Sponsor's suicide-related events

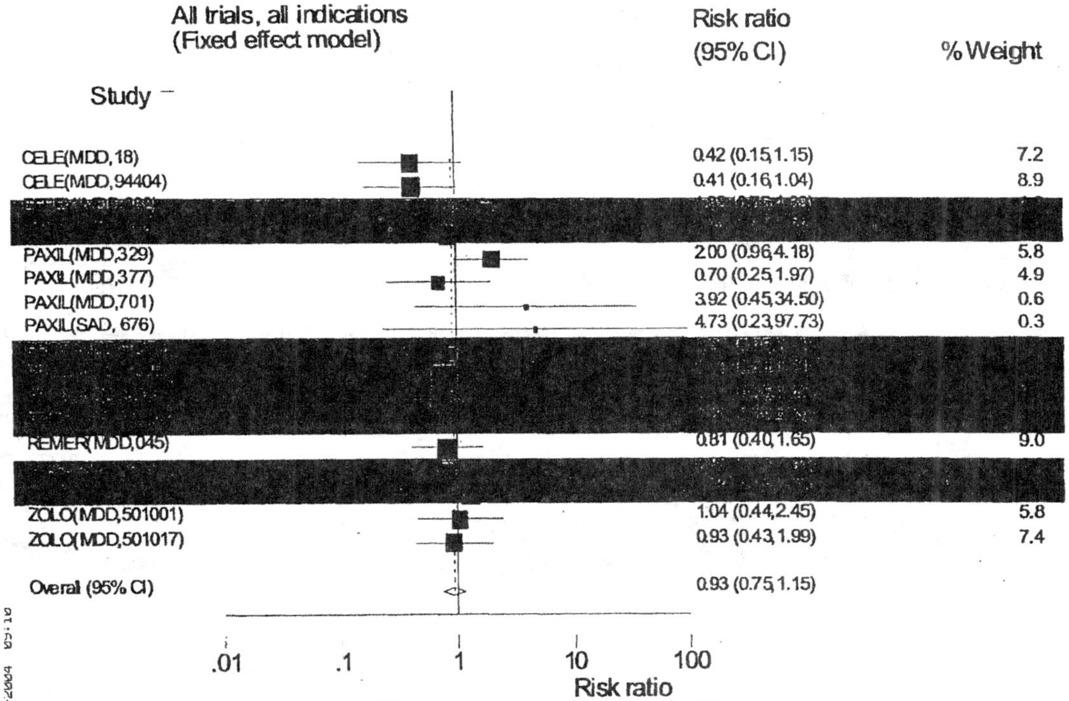

Emergence of Suicidality

22

All trials, all indications
(Fixed effect model)

Study	Risk ratio (95% CI)	% Weight
CELE(MDD,18)	0.38 (0.14,1.04)	6.3
CELE(MDD,94404)	0.54 (0.26,1.12)	9.2
[redacted]	[redacted]	[redacted]
PAXIL(MDD,329)	1.14 (0.68,1.90)	10.4
PAXIL(MDD,377)	0.66 (0.32,1.35)	7.9
PAXIL(MDD,701)	1.84 (0.82,4.15)	4.1
PAXIL(SAD, 676)	1.42 (0.24,8.37)	1.0
[redacted]	[redacted]	[redacted]
REMER(MDD,045)	0.86 (0.42,1.73)	7.3
[redacted]	[redacted]	[redacted]
ZOLO(MDD,501001)	1.04 (0.44,2.45)	4.7
ZOLO(MDD,501017)	0.93 (0.45,1.94)	6.5
Overal (95% CI)	0.92 (0.76,1.11)	

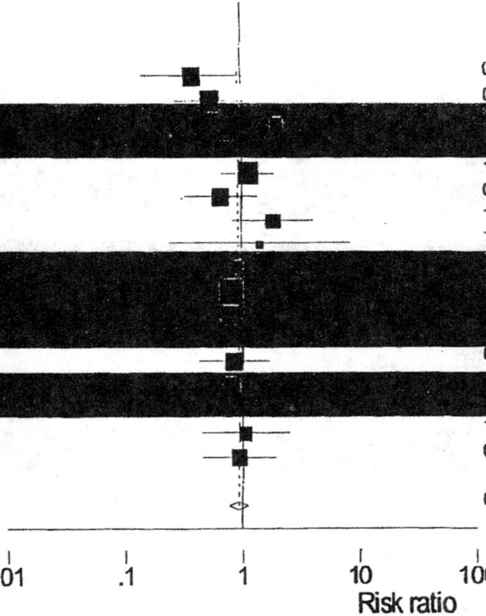

Worsening/Emergence of Suicidality

MEMORANDUM

Tab 32

DEPARTMENT OF HEALTH AND HUMAN SERVICES
PUBLIC HEALTH SERVICE
FOOD AND DRUG ADMINISTRATION
CENTER FOR DRUG EVALUATION AND RESEARCH

PID# D040495

DATE: August 16, 2004

From: Paul Seligman, M.D., M.P.H.
Acting Director, Office of Drug Safety, HFD-400
(hard copy signed 8-16-04)

Anne Trontell, M.D., M.P.H., Deputy Director
Office of Drug Safety, HFD-400
(hard copy signed 8-16-04)

TO: Russell Katz, M.D., Director
Division of Neuropharmacological Drug Products, HFD-120

SUBJECT: Office of Drug Safety Cover Memorandum
Follow-up Consult of August 16, 2004 by Andrew Mosholder on Suicidality in pediatric clinical trials with paroxetine and other antidepressant drugs:

Drugs: paroxetine, sertraline, venlafaxine, fluoxetine, fluvoxamine, citalopram, nefazodone, mirtazapine, and bupropion

The results of Dr. Mosholder's analyses (dated February 18, 2004) are very similar to those obtained using other statistical methods and a reclassification of suicidality events by Columbia University. Remaining questions to be addressed are whether the overall finding of increased risk applies to all or selected drug products among the nine products studied, and what additional regulatory actions are merited. On those topics, we reference the Office of Drug Safety memorandum written by Anne Trontell and dated March 15, 2004.

M E M O R A N D U M

DEPARTMENT OF HEALTH AND HUMAN SERVICES
PUBLIC HEALTH SERVICE
FOOD AND DRUG ADMINISTRATION
CENTER FOR DRUG EVALUATION AND RESEARCH

PID#	D040495
DATE:	August 16, 2004
FROM:	Andrew D. Mosholder, M.D., M.P.H., Epidemiologist Division of Drug Risk Evaluation, HFD-430
THROUGH:	Mark Avigan, M.D., C.M., Director Division of Drug Risk Evaluation, HFD-430 *(hard copy signed 8-16-04)*
TO:	Paul J. Seligman, M.D., M.P.H., Acting Director Office of Drug Safety, HFD-400 Anne Trontell, M.D., M.P.H., Deputy Director Office of Drug Safety, HFD-400
SUBJECT:	Suicidality in pediatric clinical trials of antidepressant drugs: Comparison between previous analyses and Colombia University classification Drugs: paroxetine, sertraline, venlafaxine, fluoxetine, fluvoxamine, citalopram, nefazodone, and mirtazapine

BACKGROUND

Please refer to the 3-19-04 consult[1] regarding suicidal adverse events in pediatric clinical trials of antidepressant drugs. That consult described a meta-analysis by the undersigned of suicidal adverse events in short-term placebo-controlled pediatric clinical trials, showing a statistically significant association of suicidal adverse events with antidepressant drug treatment. However, because of concerns regarding misclassification of cases, FDA expanded the case finding algorithm, and arranged to have expert consultants jury the cases prior to any definitive analyses. Please refer to the materials from the February 2, 2004 Advisory Committee Meeting on this topic for additional details.

The aforementioned case reclassification has recently been completed by an expert panel convened by Columbia University. Dr. Tarek Hammad of FDA's Division of Neuropharmacological Drug Products (DNDP) has performed a new meta-analysis, based on the reclassification that was performed by Columbia University, which I will refer to herein as the DNDP analysis. I was asked to examine the impact of the Columbia University reclassification of cases on my analysis performed prior to the Columbia University reclassification, as described in

[1] PID# D030341

the 3-19-04 consult, which I will refer to in this memorandum as the ODS analysis. I have also compared my results, that were obtained using different analytic methods, with those of Dr. Hammad. For these purposes, Dr. Hammad has kindly provided me with his results, which are included below.

METHODS

A full description of the methodology is beyond the scope of this memorandum, so the interested reader should refer to the reviews by Dr. Hammad and myself for details on the analytic methods and clinical trial data. It should be noted that the two analyses used different case ascertainment strategies and different case criteria; the ODS analysis used only cases identified by the sponsors through an electronic search of their adverse event databases, while the DNDP analysis supplemented this approach with additional search methods. Some salient differences between the two analyses are the following: (1) the ODS analysis did not employ a correction for zero cells, whereas the DNDP analysis does; (2) the ODS analysis used rate ratios, with person-time for denominators, while the DNDP analysis uses risk ratios, with numbers of patients for denominators; (3) the ODS analysis included events occurring up to 30 days after discontinuation of treatment, while the DNDP analysis uses a 1-day post-treatment window; and (4) the ODS analysis included taper phase events, which are excluded from the DNDP analysis.

This memorandum will present the following three modes of comparing the DNDP and ODS analyses.

Comparison of risk ratios obtained with ODS and DNDP statistical methods

In order to determine how the two different statistical methods affect the values for the relative risks, we compare the relative risks obtained with identical patient populations and classifications of cases. For this purpose, all possibly suicide-related events were included regardless of whether they were serious or not; this outcome variable was common to both sets of data, thereby allowing a comparison. While this outcome may be accorded relatively little inferential value because of the concerns about case misclassification, it does permit a direct comparison between results from the two statistical methods.

Comparison of case classifications

In order to assess the degree of agreement or lack thereof between the Columbia University and ODS case classifications, the "primary" outcome for the respective analyses must be defined. For the DNDP analysis, this is "Outcome 3," definitive suicidal behavior/ideation, a composite of Columbia University codes 1 (suicide attempt), 2 (preparatory actions towards imminent suicidal behavior), and 6 (suicidal ideation). In contrast, for the ODS analysis, performed using the classification prior to the Columbia University reclassification, the primary outcome was serious suicide-related events, comprising events selected as possibly suicide-related by each sponsor under the search strategy requested by FDA in July 2003, and also designated as serious adverse events by the sponsors under the standard regulatory criteria for "serious." By focusing on these primary outcomes, a comparison of the impact of the two systems of case classification is presented.

Comparison of risk estimates obtained with the two analyses

Finally, the risk estimates obtained from the two analyses are directly compared.

RESULTS

Comparison of statistical methods

Table 1 below displays the relative risks obtained by the two analytic methods when identical patient populations and classification of cases are used in the respective analyses.

Table 1: Comparison of results from two methods for sponsor's classification of suicide related events

Category of trials	All sponsor-defined suicide-related events	
	ODS analysis: Combined incidence rate ratios*	DNDP analysis: Risk ratios*
Paroxetine	2.69 (1.20-6.00)	2.47 (1.16-5.27)
Sertraline	2.03 (0.51-8.16)	1.72 (0.50-5.89)
Venlafaxine	3.33 (1.08-10.33)	3.03 (1.04-8.80)
Fluoxetine	0.88 (0.34-2.30)	0.98 (0.38-2.50)
Citalopram	1.41 (0.66-3.00)	1.49 (0.72-3.06)
Mirtazapine	0.53 (0.007-41.45)	0.52 (0.003-8.27)
Nefazodone	†	2.17 (0.23-20.08)
Fluvoxamine	†	3.31 (0.14-79.67)
MDD trials	1.81 (1.19-2.77)	Not done
SSRI** MDD trials	1.58 (0.99-2.52)	1.62 (1.03-2.54)
Non-MDD trials	2.36 (0.67-8.33)	1.93 (0.68-5.45)
All trials	1.86 (1.25-2.78)	1.81 (1.24-2.64)

†Ratio undefined due to zero events in placebo group
*Mantel-Haenszel method, fixed effects model
**includes paroxetine, sertraline, fluoxetine, citalopram, fluvoxamine

There is generally good agreement between the two methods, suggesting that the findings are not sensitive to changes in statistical computing methodology.

Comparison of case classifications

The ODS analysis included a total of 78 serious, suicide-related events, as defined above. Of these 78 cases, 61 (78.2%) were classified by the Columbia University group as Outcome 3 (definitive suicidal behavior). Of the remaining 17 cases, an additional 13 (16.7%) were classified as self-injurious behavior with unknown intent (Code 3), and the remaining 4 cases were classified in other outcomes.

Conversely, the Columbia University group identified a total of 95 cases as definitive suicidal behavior (Outcome 3). Of these 95 cases, 61 (64.2%) were serious, suicide-related events in the ODS analysis; sixteen (16.8%) of the 95 cases were sponsor-defined suicide-related but nonserious events, and thus were excluded from the ODS primary analysis; and 18 cases were new, i.e., were identified through the expanded search for cases that was not part of the ODS analysis.

On a net basis, the DNDP analyses considered 17 more cases than the ODS analysis.

Comparison of risk estimates

Table 2 below compares the risk estimates derived from the two analyses, using the above-mentioned case definitions.

Table 2: Comparison of Columbia University Outcome 3 with Serious suicide-related events

Category of Trials	Total N Drug	Total N Pbo	Incidence rate ratios, serious suicide-related events (ODS analysis)*	Risk ratios, Columbia University Outcome 3, (DNDP analysis)*
Paroxetine	642	549	2.19 (0.92-5.24)	2.65 (1.00-7.02)
Sertraline	281	279	2.52 (0.49-13.01)	1.48 (0.42-5.24)
Venlafaxine	339	342	1.80 (0.52-6.20)	4.97 (1.09-22.72)
Fluoxetine	249	209	0.88 (0.32-2.44)	0.92 (0.39-2.19)
Citalopram	210	197	2.54 (0.91-7.05)	1.37 (0.53-3.50)
Mirtazapine	170	88	†	1.58 (0.06-38.37)
Nefazodone	279	189	†	**
Fluvoxamine	57	63	†	5.52 (0.27-112.55)
Bupropion	71	36	**	**
All MDD trials	1586	1299	1.95 (1.19-3.21)	1.71 (1.05-2.77)
SSRI†† MDD trials	955	843	1.87 (1.10-3.18)	1.41 (0.84-2.37)
Non-MDD trials	712	653	1.31 (0.26-6.72)	2.17 (0.72-6.48)
All trials	2298	1952	1.89 (1.18-3.04)	1.78 (1.14-2.77)

*Mantel-Haenszel method, fixed effects model

**No events in either arm

†Ratio undefined due to zero events in placebo group

††includes paroxetine, sertraline, fluoxetine, citalopram, fluvoxamine

The overall risk estimate for the primary outcome for the "all trials" analysis decreased with the Columbia University reclassification analysis from 1.89 to 1.78; the confidence intervals for both risk estimates exclude one. For the category of SSRI MDD trials, the risk estimate decreased and lost statistical significance with the Columbia University reclassification analysis. In terms of results for individual drugs, the risk estimates for paroxetine and venlafaxine increased.

CONCLUSIONS

Consistent with the analysis described in the 3-19-04 consult, the DNDP meta-analysis also indicates a statistically significant association of suicidal events with antidepressant drug treatment in short-term pediatric clinical trials for all indications. In terms of subgroups of trials, the major differences were that the risk estimate for the category of SSRI MDD trials was lower and not statistically significant with the DNDP analysis, while the risk estimates for two drugs (paroxetine and venlafaxine) increased. In all three cases, however, the new point estimate falls within the confidence limits of the previous result.

RECOMMENDATIONS

With respect to what further analyses might be undertaken with the Columbia University dataset, I propose an analysis that examines events occurring after treatment discontinuation, since there appears to be a signal for at least paroxetine in this regard (please refer to the previous consults by the undersigned for details).

Beyond what else may be done with the current dataset, I also propose an analysis with psychiatric inpatient hospitalization as the outcome. While not specific for suicidal behavior, this might give insight into more general behavioral toxicities, and would have the advantage of being easily determined from the existing case reports. In addition, I agree with the plans to analyze the new data from the NIMH Treatment of Adolescent Depression Study (TADS), which will provide additional data for fluoxetine. With respect to possible regulatory actions, please refer to my recommendations in the 3-19-04 consult; the results from the DNDP meta-analysis using the Columbia University reclassification do not materially affect the recommendations I made previously.

(hard copy signed 8-16-04)
Andrew D. Mosholder, M.D., M.P.H.
Epidemiologist

(hard copy signed 8-16-04)
Mary Willy, Ph.D.
Epidemiology Team Leader

Tab 33

MISSION

The Center for Drug Evaluation and Research promotes and protects public health by assuring that safe and effective drugs are available to Americans. The Food and Drug Administration Modernization Act of 1997 affirmed the center's public health protection role, clarified the FDA's mission and called for the FDA to:

1. Promote the public health by promptly and efficiently reviewing clinical research and taking appropriate action on the marketing of human drugs in a timely manner.
2. Protect the public health by ensuring that human drugs are safe and effective.
3. Participate through appropriate processes with representatives of other countries to reduce the burden of regulation, harmonize regulatory requirements and achieve appropriate reciprocal arrangements.
4. Carry out its mission in consultation with experts in science, medicine and public health and in cooperation with consumers, users, manufacturers, importers, packers, distributors and retailers of human drugs.

This report is available on the Internet in Adobe Acrobat Portable Document Format and in hypertext markup language. The charts and graphs are available as Microsoft PowerPoint slides. The locations are:

PDF: http://www.fda.gov/cder/reports/rtn/2002/rtn2002.pdf

HTML: http://www.fda.gov/cder/reports/rtn/2002/rtn2002.htm

Slides: http://www.fda.gov/cder/reports/rtn/2002/rtn2002.ppt

Suggested citation: Food and Drug Administration. *CDER 2002 Report to the Nation: Improving Public Health Through Human Drugs*. Rockville, Maryland, 20857.

DAVID

APR 28 1999

NDA 20-031
NDA 20-710

Tab 34

SmithKline Beecham Pharmaceuticals
Attention: Thomas F. Kline
Manager, U.S. Regulatory Affairs
1250 South Collegeville Road, P.O. Box 5089
Collegeville, Pennsylvania 19426-0989

Three Years From the APR 28 2002
Date of This Letter ____________

Dear Mr. Kline:

Reference is made to your Proposed Pediatric Study Request submitted on August 27, 1998 and October 15, 1998 to your New Drug Applications for Paxil (paroxetine hydrochloride) 10 mg, 20 mg, 30 mg, and 40 mg tablets (NDA 20-031) and 10 mg/5 ml oral suspension (NDA 20-710).

We have completed our review of your submission and concluded that your proposed pediatric study request is incomplete.

To obtain needed pediatric information on paroxetine, the Food and Drug Administration (FDA) is hereby making a formal Written Request, pursuant to Section 505A of the Federal Food, Drug, and Cosmetic Act (the Act), that you submit information from the trials in pediatric patients with depression and Obsessive Compulsive Disorder (OCD) described below.

PEDIATRIC DEPRESSION

Background Comments on Pediatric Depression
Under current regulations [21 CFR 201.57(f)(9)(iv)], a new claim in a pediatric population could be established by extrapolating the effectiveness results of adequate and well controlled studies in adults for the same entity if it were believed that depression was essentially the same disease in adults and children. Under FDAMA (1997), a claim might be based on a single study in pediatric patients along with confirmatory evidence from another source, perhaps adult data for that disorder, an approach considered in the draft guidance document entitled "Guidance for Industry - Providing Clinical Evidence of Effectiveness for Human Drug and Biological Products". This approach too requires some degree of belief that the course of the disease and the effects of the drug are sufficiently similar in the pediatric and adult populations to make data from the adult efficacy studies pertinent to pediatric patients. Unfortunately, in our view there is little reason to assume continuity between adult and pediatric depression and our concern about the extrapolability of adult depression data to pediatric depression is more than theoretical. While we, of course, acknowledge the one published positive report of fluoxetine in pediatric depression (Emslie, et al. 1997), we are concerned about the preponderance of negative studies

of antidepressants in pediatric populations. We recognize that all of these negative studies utilized tricyclic antidepressants, and that, in addition, there are other possible explanations for the negative outcomes, e.g., sample size, entry criteria, outcome measures, etc. Nevertheless, these negative trials (at least 12 in number) lead to a substantial concern about the ability to extrapolate positive antidepressant findings from adult to pediatric patients. Consequently, we believe that a pediatric depression claim for any antidepressant already approved in adult depression would need to be supported by two independent, adequate and well controlled clinical trials in pediatric depression. In addition, a pediatric depression program would need to include pharmacokinetic information and safety information in the relevant pediatric age groups. For pediatric depression, we consider the relevant age groups to include children (ages 7 through 11) and adolescents (ages 12 through 17).

Specific Study Requirements for Development Program in Pediatric Depression

Types of Studies
Pediatric Efficacy and Safety Studies
Pediatric Pharmacokinetic Study
Pediatric Safety Study

Objective/Rationale
The overall goal of the development program is to establish the safety and efficacy of the study drug in the treatment of pediatric depression, and to develop other information, e.g., pharmacokinetic, pertinent to using the drug in the pediatric population.

Study Design
Pediatric Efficacy and Safety Studies

- For the controlled efficacy studies, conduct two randomized, double-blind, parallel group, placebo-controlled acute treatment trial, with a recommended duration of at least 6 to 8 weeks. We recommend that at least one of the two studies should be a fixed dose study including two or more fixed doses of the study drug. You may consider dosing patients on the basis of patient weight. Randomization must be stratified by the two age groups studied. Ideally, a relapse prevention trial would follow from the acute treatment trials, involving the randomization of responders from the acute treatment trials to continuation on either study drug or placebo, with follow-up observation for relapse for a period of 6 months or more. Please note that a relapse prevention trial is not required under this written request.

Pediatric Pharmacokinetic Study

- A pharmacokinetic study to provide information pertinent to dosing of the study drug in the relevant pediatric population. These data could come from traditional pharmacokinetic studies, or alternatively, from population kinetic approaches applied to controlled efficacy trials or to other safety trials. You should be aware that a guidance document on population pharmacokinetic studies is available under [www.fda.gov/cder/guidance/1852fnl.pdf].

Pediatric Safety Study

- Safety data should be collected in the controlled efficacy trials. Longer-term safety data should be generated in longer-term open extensions from these trials and/or in separate longer-term open safety studies.

Age Group in Which Study(ies) will be Performed – All Studies

Both children (ages 7 to 11) and adolescents (ages 12 to 17) should be equally represented in the samples, and there should be a reasonable distribution of both sexes in these strata.

Number of Patients to be Studied or Power of Study to be Achieved

Pediatric Efficacy and Safety Studies

- While it is difficult to specify the sample size needed to show a difference between drug and placebo in this population, it should be noted that, in the only published positive antidepressant trial in pediatric depression (Emslie, et al, 1997), there were 48 patients in each of the two treatment arms.

Pediatric Pharmacokinetic Study

- A sufficient number of subjects to adequately characterize the pharmacokinetics in the above age groups.

Pediatric Safety Study

- A sufficient number of pediatric patients to adequately characterize the safety of paroxetine at clinically effective doses for a sufficient duration.

Entry Criteria

The protocols should include a valid and reliable diagnostic method for recruiting children and adolescents with major depressive disorder.

Study Endpoints

Pediatric Efficacy and Safety Studies

- It is essential to identify a single primary outcome for the controlled efficacy trials, and ordinarily this should be change from baseline to endpoint on whatever symptom rating scale you have chosen for your trials.

Pediatric Pharmacokinetic Study

- Pharmacokinetic measurements as appropriate.

Pediatric Safety Study

- Appropriately frequent standard measures of safety (clinical - including signs and symptoms and laboratory).

Statistical Information

Pediatric Efficacy and Safety Studies

- These trials should have a detailed statistical plan. Ordinarily these trials should be designed with at least 80% statistical power to detect a treatment effect of conventional ($p=0.05$) statistical significance.

Pediatric Pharmacokinetic Study
- Descriptive analysis of the pharmacokinetic parameters.

Pediatric Safety Study
- Descriptive analysis of the safety data.

Study Evaluations
Pediatric Efficacy and Safety Studies
- A scale specific to pediatric depression and sensitive to the effects of drug treatment of pediatric depression, e.g., the Children's Depression Rating Scale—Revised, and a global measure, e.g., the Clinical Global Impression (CGI).

Pediatric Pharmacokinetic Study
- The pharmacokinetic assessments should be made with respect to the study drug and any metabolites that make substantial contributions to its efficacy and/or toxicity. For the parent and each metabolite followed, the data collected should provide estimates of the pharmacokinetic parameters including AUC, half-life, C_{max}, t_{max}, and apparent oral clearance in pediatric subjects in the relevant age range. You should be aware that a draft guidance document on pediatric pharmacokinetic studies is available under [www.fda.gov/cder/guidance/index.htm, under Clinical/Pharmacological (Draft)].

Pediatric Safety Study
- Routine safety assessments should include vital signs, weight, clinical laboratory, ECGs, and monitoring for adverse events. Although not a part of this Written Request, we remind you that it may be important to determine the effect of the study drug on the growth and development of pediatric patients, and we encourage you to consider longer-term studies of a year or more to address this question if the acute studies demonstrate antidepressant activity.

Drug Information
Use age appropriate formulations in the studies described above. Since the pediatric patient population consists of both children (ages 7 to 11) and adolescents (ages 12 to 17), your marketed solid dosage formulation should be adequate for these studies.

Drug Concerns
No specific concerns related to administration to pediatric patients were identified while studying paroxetine in adults, nor have specific concerns been identified during the postmarketing experience.

PEDIATRIC OBSESSIVE COMPULSIVE DISORDER (OCD)

Background Comments on Pediatric OCD
Under current regulations [21 CFR 201.57(f)(9)(iv)], a new claim in a pediatric population could be established by extrapolating the effectiveness results of adequate and well controlled studies in adults for the same entity if it were believed that OCD was essentially the same disease in adults and children. Under FDAMA (1997), a claim might be based on a single study in pediatric patients along with confirmatory evidence from another source, perhaps adult data for that disorder, and approach considered in the draft guidance document entitled "Guidance for Industry - Providing Clinical Evidence of Effectiveness for Human Drug and Biological Products". This approach too requires some degree of belief that the course of the disease and the effects of the drug are sufficiently similar in the pediatric and adult populations to make data from the adult efficacy studies pertinent to pediatric patients. In the case of OCD, we believe a sufficiently strong case has been made for continuity between adult and pediatric OCD to permit a pediatric claim for a drug already approved in adults to be supported by a single independent, adequate and well controlled clinical trial in pediatric OCD. In addition, a pediatric OCD program would need to include pharmacokinetic information and safety information in the relevant pediatric age groups. For pediatric OCD, we consider the relevant age groups to include children (ages 7 through 11) and adolescents (ages 12 through 17). In keeping with the overall objective of a pediatric OCD development program, there would need to be a minimum of one adequate and well-controlled trial (to be defined under design below) to determine the effectiveness of the study drug in the treatment of pediatric OCD.

Specific Study Requirements for Development Program in OCD

Types of Studies
Pediatric Efficacy and Safety Studies
Pediatric Pharmacokinetic Study
Pediatric Safety Study

Objective/Rationale
The overall goal of the development program would be to establish the safety and efficacy of the study drug in the treatment of pediatric OCD, and to develop other information, e.g., pharmacokinetic, pertinent to using the drug in the pediatric population.

Study Design
Pediatric Efficacy and Safety Studies

- For the controlled efficacy study, the design must be a randomized, double-blind, parallel group, placebo-controlled acute treatment trial, with a recommended duration of at least 10 to 12 weeks. Ideally the study would be a fixed dose study including two or more fixed doses of the study drug. You may consider dosing patients on the basis of patient weight. Randomization should be stratified by the two age groups studied. Ideally, a relapse prevention trial would follow from the acute treatment trial, involving the randomization of responders from the acute treatment trials to continuation on either study drug or placebo, with follow-up observation for relapse for a period of 6 months or more. Please note that a relapse prevention trial is not required under this written request.

Pediatric Pharmacokinetic Study

- In addition, there would need to be pharmacokinetic data to provide information pertinent to dosing of the study drug in the relevant pediatric population. These data could come from traditional pharmacokinetic studies, or alternatively, from population kinetic approaches applied to controlled efficacy trials or from other safety trials. Please refer to the previous paragraph under "Specific Study Requirements for Development Program in Pediatric Depression".

Pediatric Safety Study

- Safety data could come from controlled efficacy trials. Longer-term safety data should be generated in longer-term open extensions from these trials and/or in separate longer-term open safety studies. Safety data will also be available, of course, from the pediatric depression studies.

Age Group in Which Study(ies) will be Performed – All Studies
Both children (ages 7 to 11) and adolescents (ages 12 to 17) should be equally represented in the samples, and there should be a reasonable distribution of both sexes in these strata.

Number of Patients to be Studied or Power of Study to be Achieved
Pediatric Efficacy and Safety Studies

- While it is difficult to specify the sample size needed to show a difference between drug and placebo in this population, it should be noted that other positive trials in pediatric OCD have utilized samples of roughly 45-95 patients in each treatment arm.

Pediatric Pharmacokinetic Study

- A sufficient number of subjects to adequately characterize the pharmacokinetics in the above age groups.

Pediatric Safety Study

- A sufficient number of pediatric patients to adequately characterize the safety of paroxetine at clinically effective doses for a sufficient duration.

Entry Criteria
The protocols should include a valid and reliable diagnostic method for recruiting children and adolescents with OCD.

Study Endpoints
Pediatric Efficacy and Safety Studies

- It is essential to identify a single primary outcome for the controlled efficacy trials, and ordinarily this should be change from baseline to endpoint on whatever symptom rating scale you have chosen for your trial.

Pediatric Pharmacokinetic Study

- **Pharmacokinetic measurements as appropriate.**

Pediatric Safety Study

- Appropriately frequent standard measures of safety (clinical - including signs and symptoms and laboratory).

Statistical Information

Pediatric Efficacy and Safety Studies

- This trial should have a detailed statistical plan. Ordinarily this trial should be designed with at least 80% statistical power to detect a treatment effect of conventional ($p=0.05$) statistical significance.

Pediatric Pharmacokinetic Study

- Descriptive analysis of the pharmacokinetic parameters.

Pediatric Safety Study

- Descriptive analysis of the safety data.

Study Evaluations

Pediatric Efficacy and Safety Studies

- The efficacy assessments should include a validated symptom rating scale specific to pediatric OCD and expected to be sensitive to the effects of drug treatment of pediatric OCD, e.g., the Children's Yale-Brown Obsessive Compulsive Scale (CYBOCS), and a global measure, e.g., the Clinical Global Impression (CGI).

Pediatric Pharmacokinetic Study

- The pharmacokinetic assessments should be made with respect to the study drug and any metabolites that make substantial contributions to its efficacy and/or toxicity. For the parent and each metabolite followed, the data collected should provide estimates of the pharmacokinetic parameters including AUC, half-life, C_{max}, t_{max}, and apparent oral clearance in pediatric subjects in the relevant age range. You should be aware that a draft guidance document on pediatric pharmacokinetic studies is available under [www.fda.gov/cder/guidance/index.htm, under Clinical/Pharmacological (Draft)].

Pediatric Safety Study

- Routine safety assessments should include vital signs, weight, clinical laboratory, ECGs, and monitoring for adverse events. Although not a part of this Written Request, we remind you that it may be important to determine the effect of the study drug on the growth and development of pediatric patients, and we encourage you to consider longer-term studies of a year or more to address this question if the acute studies demonstrate efficacy.

Drug Information

Use age appropriate formulations in the studies described above. Since the pediatric patient population consists of both children (ages 7 to 11) and adolescents (ages 12 to 17), your marketed solid dosage formulation should be adequate for these studies.

Drug Concerns
No specific concerns related to administration to pediatric patients were identified while studying paroxetine in adults, nor have specific concerns been identified during the postmarketing experience.

Labeling That May Result from the Studies
The pediatric depression efficacy, safety, and pharmacokinetic studies described in this request could result in the addition to labeling of information pertinent to these studies. Similarly, the data generated from the OCD efficacy, safety, and pharmacokinetic studies described in this request could result in the addition to labeling of information pertinent to these studies.

Format of Reports to be Submitted
Full study reports or analyses, not previously submitted to the Agency, addressing the issues outlined in this request, with full analysis, assessment, and interpretation.

Timeframe for Submitting Reports of the Study(ies)
Reports of the above studies must be submitted to the Agency within 3 years from the date of this letter to be eligible to qualify for pediatric exclusivity extension under Section 505A of the Act. Please remember that pediatric exclusivity extends only existing patent protection or exclusivity that has not expired at the time you submit your reports of studies in response to this Written Request.

Please submit protocols for the above studies to an investigational new drug application (IND) and clearly mark your submission **"PEDIATRIC PROTOCOL SUBMITTED FOR PEDIATRIC EXCLUSIVITY STUDY"** in large font, bolded type at the beginning of the cover letter of the submission. We recommend you seek a written agreement with FDA before developing pediatric studies. Please notify us as soon as possible if you wish to enter into a written agreement by submitting a proposed written agreement. Clearly mark your submission **"PROPOSED WRITTEN AGREEMENT FOR PEDIATRIC STUDIES"** in large font, bolded type at the beginning of the cover letter of the submission.

Reports of the studies should be submitted as a supplement to your approved NDA with the proposed labeling changes you believe would be warranted based on the data derived from these studies. When submitting the reports, please clearly mark your submission **"SUBMISSION OF PEDIATRIC STUDY REPORTS – PEDIATRIC EXCLUSIVITY DETERMINATION REQUESTED"** in large font, bolded type at the beginning of the cover letter of the submission and include a copy of this letter. Please also send a copy of the cover letter of your submission, via fax (301-594-0183) or messenger to the Director, Office of Generic Drugs, HFD-600, Metro Park North II, 7500 Standish Place, Rockville, MD 20855-2773.

If you wish to discuss any amendments to this Written Request, please submit proposed changes and the reasons for the proposed changes to your application. Submissions of proposed changes to this request should be clearly marked **"PROPOSED CHANGES IN WRITTEN REQUEST FOR PEDIATRIC STUDIES"** in large font, bolded type at the beginning of the cover letter of the submission. You will be notified in writing if any changes to this Written Request are agreed upon by the Agency.

We hope you will fulfill this pediatric study request. We look forward to working with you on this matter in order to develop additional pediatric information that may produce health benefits to the pediatric population.

If you have any questions, contact Paul A. David, Regulatory Project Manager, at (301) 594-5530.

Sincerely yours,

Robert Temple 4/28/99

Robert Temple, M.D.
Director
Office of Drug Evaluation I
Center for Drug Evaluation and Research

cc:
Archival NDA 20-031 and 20-710
HFD-120/division file
HFD-120/PDavid
HFD-120/RKatz/TLaughren/Amosholder/Rglass/GDubitsky
HFD-100/RTemple
HFD-600/Office of Generic Drugs
HFD-2/MLumpkin
HFD-104/DMurphy
HFD-6/KRoberts
Drafted by:03/22/99am;rg
Rev:03/29/99tl; 04/02/99rt;04/12/99tl;4/21/99pdit
Final:04/22/99pd
filename: DAVID\PEDIATRICS\PAXILPEDS02.DOC

PEDIATRIC WRITTEN REQUEST LETTER
INFORMATION REQUEST (IR)

RECEIVED
MAY 2 7 2003
HFD-120/CDER

May 22, 2003

GlaxoSmithKline

GlaxoSmithKline
U.S. Regulatory Affairs
One Franklin Plaza
P.O. Box 7929
Philadelphia, PA
19101-7929
USA

Telephone: 215 751 3868
Fax: 215 751 4926
www.gsk.com

Russell G. Katz, M.D., Director
Division of Neuropharmacological Drug Products
Center for Drug Evaluation and Research
Office of Drug Evaluation I
Food and Drug Administration
HFD-120, WOC2, Room 4049
1451 Rockville Pike
Rockville, MD 20852

Tab 35

DUPLICATE

SE5-037(BZ)

Re: NDA 20-031; PAXIL® (paroxetine hydrochloride) Tablets
Response to FDA Request/Comment: Clinical, Statistical

SUPPLEMENT AMENDMENT

Dear Dr. Katz:

Reference is made to our approved New Drug Application for Paxil® (paroxetine hydrochloride) Tablets, NDA 20-031. Additional reference is made to our pediatric supplemental application NDA 20-031/S-037 and its associated "approvable letter," dated October 10, 2002.

Because pediatric applications will soon be submitted to various foreign regulatory authorities, and because it may be several more weeks before a complete response to the approvable letter is available, GSK wanted to ensure that FDA received two additional analyses we have conducted in connection with the term "emotional lability," which was the subject of Questions 7 and 8 of the approvable letter.

Subsequent to the analyses submitted to FDA on May 2, 2002, and February 6, 2003, concerning the overall clinical trial population (adult and pediatric), we conducted analyses of the reports of suicide attempts and "possibly suicide-related" events (as this term was defined) from the pediatric-only clinical trials (Attachments 1 and 2). Each analysis looked at two treatment periods from the placebo-controlled trials: (1) on-therapy (including taper phase); and (2) on-therapy plus 30 days post-therapy. The analyses also broke down the events by indication.

The analysis of suicide attempts demonstrated that there was no statistically significant difference between paroxetine and placebo during the "on-therapy" period. Similarly, with respect to "possibly suicide-related" events, there was no statistically significant difference between paroxetine and placebo during the "on-

① GSK needs to send us the data that they sent to UK.
② They need to look at the scale to see if there was a change.
③ / Call GSK
④ [illegible]
⑤ Get [illegible] to look at Paxil & the other SSRIs.

(226)

Russell G. Katz, M.D.
May 22, 2003
Page 2

therapy" period. By contrast, there was a statistically significant difference between paroxetine and placebo in terms of events occurring during the "on-therapy plus 30 days post-therapy period," with respect to both suicide attempts and "possibly suicide-related" events, when data from all pediatric studies/indications was pooled. For all analyses, there was no statistically significant difference between paroxetine and placebo for any of the specific individual pediatric indications.

Please note that we are including with this submission an internal report that provides greater detail concerning the events that were the subject of the two analyses (Attachment 3). As always, we will continue to evaluate whether any additional analyses are required. If they are, we will provide such analyses, as appropriate.

Finally, we are planning to submit revised labeling to the Division in the upcoming complete response to the October 10, 2002 letter.

Please do not hesitate to contact me at (215) 751-4054 if you have any questions or require additional information.

Sincerely,

Thomas F. Kline
Director
Regulatory Affairs

Paroxetine

Clinical Evaluation of "Possibly Suicide-Related" Adverse Events in Paroxetine Hydrochloride Pediatric Clinical Trials

Philip Perera M.D.*

*Director - Clinical Development and Medical Affairs North America, Psychiatry

Tab 36

TABLE OF CONTENTS

I. Background

In response to an FDA inquiry about the constituent symptoms included in the preferred term "emotional lability" a post-hoc analysis of adverse events, possibly related to suicidality, was conducted. Thirty three subjects in the pediatric placebo controlled trials of paroxetine for any indication were identified in a post-hoc statistical analysis of "possibly suicide–related" Adverse Events (AEs). As with any statistical analysis confined to a narrow categorical limit, especially when it is not prospectively defined, the analysis of "possibly suicide–related" Adverse Events (AEs) did not take into account relevant and potentially contributing clinical factors. This report focuses on a clinical review of these 33 cases.

Only the controlled sections of these pediatric placebo controlled trials were utilized in the statistical analysis, i.e. uncontrolled extension phases and run-in periods were not included. Subjects were included in the "possibly suicide-related" category if they met the "broad analysis" definition criteria under the preferred term "emotional lability" and verbatim terms containing a number of text strings related to suicidal ideation, suicide attempts, and self inflicted harm. Subjects who met criteria under the preferred term of "overdose" and "intentional overdose" were also included. Essentially, all subjects with a post-randomization suicide attempt and subjects with new or worsening suicidal ideation occurring after randomization, including those in the taper and post discontinuation phases, were included in the clinical analysis. It should be noted that the post discontinuation phase was uncontrolled, and the data from this phase are difficult to interpret since new medications may have been started; patients were aware that the study was ending; follow-up was variable and less systematic; no accounting is made for the possible return of symptoms, and discontinuation symptoms may have resulted in inadvertent unblinding.

The thirty three cases with " possibly suicide–related " AEs were identified out of 1385 subjects in pediatric clinical trials 329, 377, 701, 676, 704 and 453. Studies 329, 377 and 701 were pediatric depression studies and twenty eight of the thirty three suicidal subjects assigned to either paroxetine or placebo were identified in these trials. Sufficient efficacy was not demonstrated in these pediatric depression trials to warrant submission to regulatory authorities requesting a claim of efficacy. Four patients with suicidality were identified in the Social Anxiety Disorder trial 676, and one suicidal patient was identified in study 704 in Obsessive Compulsive Disorder (OCD). Efficacy was demonstrated in these pediatric Social Anxiety Disorder and Obsessive Compulsive Disorder trials. Study 453 in pediatric OCD had no reported suicide-related AEs in the double-blind phase. Therefore, all 33 cases were identified in studies 329, 377, 701, 676, and 704. No deaths were reported in any of these pediatric studies (Tables 1 and 2).

Serious adverse event narratives and case report forms were used as reference materials for the clinical review which included an overview of verbatim descriptions of the suicidal events and an analysis of several key clinical factors including the treatment phase during which these events occurred, investigator reported relatedness to study drug, demographics, comorbidity, study drug dosage before and during the events, duration of treatment, concomitant medications, depression scale suicidality scores before, during, and after the event when available, comorbid psychiatric and medical history and the presence of proximate psychosocial stressors.

II. Study Phase

The incidence of events of suicidality were analyzed in two ways. These included an analysis of all events occurring post randomization (Table 1) and a second analysis of events occurring only on study drug, including taper phase events (Table 2). Most events of suicidality occurred during the treatment phase for both the paroxetine and placebo groups.

Paroxetine events - 17/25 occurred during the treatment phase, 1/25 occurred during the taper phase, and 7/25 events occurred during the 30 day post last dose period.

Placebo events - 6/8 occurred during the treatment phase and 1/8 occurred one day after the initiation of the taper phase and 1/8 occurred during the 30 day post last dose period.

As noted there were seven paroxetine and one 30 day post last dose events. All eight 30 day post last dose events occurred within 4 days of stopping either paroxetine or placebo.

III. Relatedness

Most reports of post-randomisation suicidality were judged by the clinical investigator to be unrelated to either paroxetine or placebo. Only "unrelated" and "probably unrelated" events required an explanation on the SAE form if the event was considered serious. Non-serious AEs did not require any explanation. In these trials the explanation as to why these events were unrelated and probably unrelated were under reported as only 7/16 investigators completed this information.

Paroxetine Events - Related 1, Possibly Related 3, Probably Unrelated 5, Unrelated 16

Placebo Events - Related 1, Possibly Related 2, Probably Unrelated 1, Unrelated 4

The one related event for the subject on placebo was reported by the investigator as related to "lack of efficacy".

The one paroxetine patient with a "related" SAE of suicidality, which occurred during the taper phase, was a 16 year old white female who reported that she ingested 100 tablets of paroxetine following a fight with her mother one day after being withdrawn from the study due to lack of efficacy and approximately 6 weeks after the initiation of study medication. She was on 50 mg paroxetine/day the day before the event. The patient was brought to the emergency room approximately 7 to 8 hours after the time she reportedly ingested the overdose of medication and approximately 32 hours after her last per protocol scheduled dose of paroxetine. A urine drug screen conducted by the emergency room physician was found to be negative for approximately 700 compounds including paroxetine and other antidepressants. The drug screen was only positive for caffeine, opening up the possibility that the patient did not actually ingest 100 tablets of paroxetine and that she was not taking her study medication as required per protocol.

With respect to ratings on the CDRS this patient had shown slight improvement in her depressed mood on the day prior to the event (CDRS; Item 11= 4 compared to baseline CDRS; Item 11= 6). The patient did not endorse significant depressed mood on the KADS at baseline (score = 0 "hardly ever") nor on the day prior to the event (score = 0). Ratings of irritability on both the CDRS and the KADS were improved on the day prior to the event, when the patient indicated she "hardly ever" felt irritable, compared to baseline when she felt irritable "most of the time".

There was no evidence of suicidal ideation on either the CDRS or the KADS the day prior to the event.

The patient did not display any signs of worsening mood or irritability at the early withdrawal visit, nor were there signs of suicidal ideation. In fact. the patient's condition was considered by the investigator to be "minimally improved". The patient was not taking any concomitant medications. The only adverse event that she experienced during the trial was insomnia which lasted for approximately 8 days and did not overlap with the event. Given this patient's negative urine drug screen for the presence of paroxetine, possible lack of compliance with study medication improved CDRS and KADS rating scale scores just prior to the event, and the presence of a proximate psychosocial stressor. relatedness of the SAE of suicidality to paroxetine in this case cannot be accounted for in the record.

IV. Dose Range

Fixed dose studies to determine dose response and dose related adverse events were not included in the pediatric program. All suicidal events occurred while subjects were enrolled in flexible dose studies, and all events occurred while subjects were on paroxetine across a range of doses from 20 mg to 50 mg daily with most events taking place while subjects were on between 20 mg to 40 mg daily. One event occurred at 50 mg daily. Four subjects on paroxetine had an escalation of 10 mg in their daily dose within one week prior to the event. Four patients assigned to paroxetine were on no medication at the time of the event (stopped prior to event). None of the 8 placebo patients had a dose escalation within one week prior to the suicidal event. No determination of a dose dependent effect on the emergence or worsening of suicidality can be ascertained from these data.

V. Duration of Treatment

Subjects with new or worsening post-randomisation suicidality were on paroxetine for an average of 54 days prior to their suicidal event and on placebo for an average of 61 days prior to the event with a range of 11-156 days for paroxetine and 5-108 days for placebo. The median number of days exposure prior to the event was 42 days for the paroxetine group and 63.5 days for those on placebo. No clear relationship between time on study drug and the development of suicidality is apparent.

VI. Concomitant Medications and Substances

Subjects were on a variety of concomitant medications for multiple different medical indications. Only one patient on paroxetine was on a concomitant medication, "Benzocaine for weight loss," with a possible contributing psychoactive component; one other patient overdosed on tranxene which may also have been taken concomitantly at other times; one admitted to smoking marijuana several days prior to the event, and one was found to have cannanaboids on a drug screen. Subjects on placebo were on no concomitant medication with a significant contributing psychoactive component.

VII. Demographics

In the all patients (children and adolescents combined) all studies population (329, 377, 701, 704, 676) there were more females randomized to paroxetine compared to placebo (57.6% [370/642] female paroxetine patients versus 50.1% [275/549] female placebo patients). For adolescents (ages 12-18 years) in the all studies population, there was also a higher proportion of females randomized to paroxetine compared to placebo (61.0% [296/485] female adolescent paroxetine patients compared to 53.4% [213/399] female adolescent placebo patients). Gender characteristics for the child age subgroup (ages 7-11 years) are not presented here since all but one of the suicidal subjects were adolescents. Unlike the higher proportion of females randomized to paroxetine in the all studies population (total and adolescent subgroups), there were similar proportions of females between groups in MDD studies 329, 701 and 377 in the adolescent age subgroup (63.0% [206/327] female paroxetine patients compared to 62.6% [149/238] female placebo patients).

In the "broad analysis" of suicidality there were a total of 645/1191 (54.1%) female and 546/1191 (45.8%) male pediatric subjects ages 7-18 years of age in studies 329, 377,701, 676 and 704. Adolescent females ages 12-18 years accounted for 509/884 (57.6%) of total subjects and adolescent males ages 12-18 years accounted for 375/884 (42.4%) of total subjects.

Of the 33 subjects with post-randomisation new or worsening suicidality there was a preponderance of females. Twenty-six out of 33 (79%) of suicidal subjects were female and 7/33 (21%) were male. There were 20/25 (80%) female subjects in the paroxetine group with suicidality and 5/25 (20%) male subjects. There were 6/8 (75%) female and 2/8 (25%) male subjects included in the placebo group with suicidality.

Most paroxetine and placebo patients with suicidality characterized themselves as white (18/25 on paroxetine 5/8 on placebo).

Study 704 in OCD and 701 in Major Depressive Disorder included children ages 7-11 and adolescents ages 12-18. Study 701 had one child age 11 with suicidality. No children under the age of 11 years were reported as suicidal. The age range for adolescents who reported suicidality was 12 to 18 years. The average age for the paroxetine group reporting suicidality in all pediatric studies was 15.4 years and 14.3 years for the placebo group.

VIII. Cormorbidity

Seven out of 25 paroxetine subjects had at least one ongoing comorbid DSM-IV psychiatric diagnosis at the time of entry into the study and 3/25 paroxetine subjects had a history of past psychiatric diagnosis at the time of entry into the study. Five out of 8 subjects on placebo had either a past or concurrent comorbid psychiatric disorder. No pattern of comorbid concurrent or past psychiatric history emerged as contributing to suicidality. However, the presence of comorbid concurrent and past psychiatric disorders such as Substance Abuse, ADHD, Borderline Personality (traits), Conduct Disorder and Anxiety Disorders cannot be ruled out as possibly contributing to a worsening in the patient's condition or at least rendering the patient less prone to treatment response. One patient developed what was reported as new onset auditory hallucinations. Evidence of a thorough evaluation of previous psychotic symptomatology was not apparent in the records available for review, and incipient bipolar or psychotic disorder cannot be ruled out for this subject.

IX. Nature and History of Suicidality

Post Randomization Suicide Attempts vs Suicidal Ideation:
Twenty-five out of 33 (76%) of the total reports of "possibly suicide–related" adverse events were in the paroxetine group and 8/33 (24%) were in the placebo group. Seventeen out of 25 (68%) of patients reported as suicidal on paroxetine had suicide attempts vs. 6/8 (75%) patients on placebo. The remaining 8/25 (32%) subjects on paroxetine had suicidal ideation only vs. 2/8 (25%) on placebo with suicidal ideation only. No clear relationship between drug and suicidal attempt vs. ideation is apparent. Subject PID: 377.024.00158 is described as experiencing an episode of "automutilation" in the form of face slapping. There is no mention of suicidal ideation or suicidal intent, and although this subject is counted as a

suicide attempt in the paroxetine group it is the clinical reviewer's opinion that this subject should not be included as suicidal.

Method of Suicidality:
The most common method of suicide attempt for both the paroxetine and placebo groups was overdose. Several subjects in both groups made "suicide gestures" in particular wrist scratching and superficial cutting are noted by the investigators. No clear relationship between drug and method of suicidal attempt is apparent..

History of Past Suicide Attempts and/or Past Suicidal Ideation:
Sixteen out of 25 subjects randomized to paroxetine and 6/8 subjects randomized to placebo who were identified with worsening or new suicidality after randomization had a history of one or more suicide attempts and/or suicidal ideation prior to their entry into the study as reported on the suicidal ideation/suicidal acts questions of their KSADS-L (used in MDD studies 329 and 377) or by the investigator's report of the subjects' past psychiatric history. Of these 16 subjects on paroxetine, 10 subjects had past suicidal ideation alone. 3 subjects had both past suicidal ideation and one or more suicide attempts and 3 subject had a past suicide attempt. Of the 6 subjects on placebo, 3 subjects had past suicidal ideation alone, one subject had both past suicidal ideation and one or more past suicide attempts, 2 subjects had a past suicide attempt. No clear relationship between drug and history of suicidal attempt and/or ideation is apparent.

Presence of Suicidality at Randomization:
Eight out of 25 (32%) of the subjects in the paroxetine group and 4/8 (50%) of the placebo group had suicidality already present at randomization prior to taking study medication as measured by a HAM-D Item 3 score ≥ 3 in study 329, MADRS Item 10 ≥ 3 in study 377, or CDRS item 13 ≥ 3 in studies 701 and 676. Study 704 in OCD had no depression scale or suicide item measurement. Five out of 25 (20%) of these subjects on paroxetine and 2/8 (25%) of these subjects on placebo scored 4 on the MADRS Item 10 indicating the presence of serious suicidality at the time of randomization and before starting study medication. No clear relationship between drug and suicidality at randomization is apparent.

Presence of Suicidality at Randomization and Subsequent Suicide Attempts vs. Suicidal Ideation:
Six out of 17 (35%) of patients on paroxetine identified as attempting suicide subsequent to randomization had suicidal ideation already present at the time of randomization as did 3/6 (50%) of the placebo group who had a post

randomization suicide attempt. Two out of 8 (25%) of patients on paroxetine who were identified with suicidal ideation subsequent to randomization had suicidal ideation already present at the time of randomization as did 1/2 (50%) of the placebo group with post randomization suicidal ideation.

Presence of Suicidality at Randomization and Overlapping History of Suicide Attempts, Suicidality, and Psychosocial Stressors: Six out of 25 subjects on paroxetine and 3/8 subjects on placebo had overlapping suicidality reported at randomization, a past history of suicide attempts and/or suicidality, and/or psychosocial stressors.

X. Proximate Psychosocial Events

Psychosocial factors were prominent prior to the suicidal event in 10/25 of the paroxetine cases with post-randomization suicidality and 1/8 subjects on placebo.

XI. Summary

Thirty three cases of "possibly suicide-related" adverse events were identified in the treatment, taper, and post discontinuation phases of pediatric clinical trials 329, 377,701, 676 and 704, with most events occurring in depression trials 329, 377 and 701. Sufficient efficacy was not demonstrated in these pediatric depression trials to warrant submission to regulatory authorities requesting a claim of efficacy. The disorder specific statistical analyses of the incidence of "possibly suicide-related" adverse events for subjects in the treatment, taper, and post discontinuation phases showed no statistically significant differences between the paroxetine and placebo groups (Table 1). An overall statistical analysis of "possibly suicide-related" adverse events that included subjects in the treatment, taper, and post discontinuation phases for all indications combined showed that the paroxetine group had a numerically and statistically greater number "possibly suicide-related" AE compared to the placebo group (Table 1). However, when "possibly suicide-related" AEs for subjects who discontinued paroxetine were excluded from this analysis, i.e. when only treatment and taper events were included, there was no statistically significant difference in "possibly suicide-related" AEs between the paroxetine and placebo groups in both the individual disorders analysis as well as the overall combined disorders analysis (Table 2).

The analyses for "on-drug" subjects is seen to be the more relevant and scientifically defensible analysis as this is limited to a more controlled drug-placebo comparison, i.e. during the randomized, placebo-controlled portions of the study. The analysis which includes subjects in the 30-day "off-drug" period (Table 1) is confounded by a number of different factors. New medications may have been started; patients were aware that the study was ending; follow-up was variable and less systematic; no accounting is made for the possible return of symptoms, and discontinuation symptoms may have resulted in unintended unblinding. It should also be noted that the "on therapy plus 30-days" analyses, include, in the numerator, all events occurring during the double-blind phase as well as any events in the 30 days after stopping treatment. The denominator however, (exposure and PYE) includes only those days during the double-blind phase, and not the 30 day period after stopping treatment.

A further clinical review of these 33 cases confirms that paroxetine was not associated with any completed suicide. Also, the method of suicide attempt did not appear to be any more impulsive or serious for the suicidal subjects in the paroxetine group compared to the placebo group. Among the events identified in subjects on paroxetine with a post-randomisation "possibly suicide–related" serious adverse event, 21/25 (84%) events were judged by the clinical investigators to be unrelated or probably unrelated to paroxetine.

No determination of a dose dependent effect on the emergence or worsening of suicidality related to paroxetine can be ascertained from the data. No clear relationship between the number of days on paroxetine or placebo and the development of suicidality was apparent..

Concomitant medications and substances with a psychoactive component may have played a role in complicating the clinical course of at least 4 subjects with suicidality assigned to the paroxetine group and none in the placebo group. However, concomitant medications and cannabis abuse or its presence as part of a drug screen were not reported by any investigator as directly leading to suicidality in any subject.

Several subjects on paroxetine and placebo had one or more past or concurrent comorbid psychiatric disorder. Proportionally more subjects on placebo had such disorders. The presence of comorbid concurrent and/or past psychiatric disorders such as Substance Abuse, ADHD, Borderline Personality (traits), Conduct Disorder and Anxiety Disorders seen in subjects with suicidality in these trials cannot be ruled out as possibly contributing to treatment resistance or a worsening clinical course for both paroxetine and placebo treated subjects with suicidality

The all patients all pediatric studies and "broad analysis" calculation of gender distribution showed a greater total number of female adolescents randomized to either paroxetine or placebo compared to males. In both analyses there was a greater number of female adolescents randomized to paroxetine compared to placebo and there was between 3 to 4 times as many females than males among the 33 post-randomisation suicidality cases. The imbalance of females with suicidality compared to males suggests that females were at greater risk for post randomisation emergence of suicide attempts or new or worsening suicidal ideation in these studies. This is consistent with what has been reported in the adolescent literature. When unequal gender distribution between paroxetine and placebo groups is not a factor, which was the case in depression studies 329, 377 and 701, a statistical analysis of post-randomisation suicidality in these studies shows no statistical difference in "possibly suicide-related" adverse events between the paroxetine and placebo groups.

A history of suicide attempts and/or suicidal ideation as well as the presence of suicidality at randomization measured by the suicide item of the HAM-D, MADRS, or CDRS was likely to have complicated the clinical course of a significant number of subjects who reported suicidality after randomization in both the paroxetine and placebo groups. Subject PID: 377.024.00158 with the face slapping related AE should not be counted as having a "possibly suicide-related" event. Also, post-randomisation psychosocial factors were pointed to by investigators as contributing to post-randomisation suicidality in both groups.

XII. Discussion

A statistical analysis confined to categorical limits such as "possibly suicide-related" AEs or new and worsening post randomisation suicidality may obscure important contributing clinical findings and should prompt us to impose limits on how we interpret such data. Further caution should be taken when interpreting the clinical meaning of the relative incidence of suicidal ideation and suicide attempts between the paroxetine and placebo groups in these pediatric studies when we consider that there were no completed suicides while subjects were on paroxetine and that 21/25 (84%) of the reported suicidal events occurring while subjects were on paroxetine were judged by the clinical investigators to be unrelated and probably unrelated to paroxetine.

In addition, seriously suicidal subjects are generally excluded from clinical drug trials. e.g. subjects with MADRS scores of 4. This was not the case in our pediatric trials. Instead, as is sometimes allowed, it was left up to the investigator's clinical judgement to determine suicide risk and then include or exclude suicidal subjects accordingly. Since past suicidal ideation and suicide attempts in adolescents are among the strongest predictors of future suicidal behaviours, this same positive correlation seen in our pediatric trials cannot be discounted and may have contributed to the reported incidence of suicidality seen in these studies, especially considering that some of these suicidal subjects were included with potentially confounding comorbid psychiatric disorders and psychosocial stressors.

Also, the total number of adolescents randomised to the paroxetine group contained a greater proportion of female adolescents compared to the placebo group. Female adolescents are reported to be at 2 to 4 times higher risk for suicidal ideation and attempts compared to their male counterparts who complete suicide more frequently. This higher proportion of females in the total paroxetine group may have contributed to the higher incidence of suicidality seen with paroxetine.

During the course of a psychiatric clinical drug trial in a pediatric population there are many factors that can account for adverse event reports of aggression, emotional lability, impulsivity, agitation, suicidal ideation and suicide attempts. Emotional regulation, in general, is a developmentally acquired process that requires a child and adolescent to experience a variety of situations from which they learn coping skills. This process is complex, not well understood, and is impacted by biological/neurological and environmental factors. By virtue of their age and inexperience children and adolescents have less developed coping skills than adults which may place them at greater risk for emotional dysregulation. especially when they are experiencing the stress of a mental disorder. In part, this may account for why completed suicide is the third leading cause of death among young people and why adverse events related to emotional dysregulation are likely to be reported in pediatric trials and in clinical settings (NIMH 1999, King RA et al 1991, Keller MB et al 2001, Emslie GJ 2002)

In summary, confounding clinical, demographic, psychosocial and developmental factors were present in subjects enrolled in our pediatric clinical trials. From a clinical perspective these should be viewed as contributing to the incidence and cause of adverse events such as aggression, emotional lability, impulsivity.

agitation, suicidal ideation and suicide attempts and not attributed solely to paroxetine or placebo.

XIII. TABLES

Table 1: Incidence, person year exposure, and incidence density for "possibly suicide-related" events, by treatment group and indication (On Therapy plus 30 days post-therapy)

Indication		Paroxetine	Placebo	P-value
Depression	n/N (%)	20/378 (5.3%)	8/285 (2.8%)	0.12
	PYE	85	51	
	n/PYE (rate relative to exposure)	0.24	0.13	0.16
OCD	n/N (%)	1/195 (0.5%)	0/205 (0.0%)	0.49
	PYE	41	41	
	n/PYE (rate relative to exposure)	0.02	0.00	n/a
Social Anxiety	n/N (%)	4/165 (2.4%)	0/157 (0.0%)	0.12
	PYE	51	47	
	n/PYE (rate relative to exposure)	0.08	0.00	n/a
Overall	n/N (%)	25/738 (3.4%)	8/647 (1.2%)	0.01
	PYE	176	149	
	n/PYE (rate relative to exposure)	0.14	0.05	0.02

Footnotes to Table 1

1. Exposure for one placebo patient (676.015.24401) could not be calculated due to missing start and stop dates of medication.
2. No early onset attempted suicides occurred for patients tapering from single blind / open label paroxetine prior to receiving randomized placebo.

Table 2: Incidence, person year exposure, and incidence density for "possibly suicide-related" events, by treatment group and indication (On Therapy)				
Indication		Paroxetine	Placebo	P-value
Depression	n/N (%)	14/378 (3.7%)	7/285 (2.5%)	0.50
	PYE	85	61	
	n/PYE (rate relative to exposure)	0.16	0.11	0.43
OCD	n/N (%)	1/195 (0.5%)	0/205 (0.0%)	0.49
	PYE	41	41	
	n/PYE (rate relative to exposure)	0.02	0.00	n/a
Social Anxiety	n/N (%)	3/165 (1.8%)	0/157 (0.0%)	0.25
	PYE	51	47	
	n/PYE (rate relative to exposure)	0.06	0.00	n/a
Overall	n/N (%)	18/738 (2.4%)	7/647 (1.1%)	0.07
	PYE	176	149	
	n/PYE (rate relative to exposure)	0.10	0.05	0.08

Footnotes to Table 2

1. Exposure for one placebo patient (676.015.24401) could not be calculated due to missing start and stop dates of medication.
2. No early onset attempted suicides occurred for patients tapering from single blind / open label paroxetine prior to receiving randomized placebo.

The following eight patients experienced possibly suicide-related events during the 30 day window post therapy and therefore do not contribute to the event counts: (329.002.00058, 329.005.00333, 377.042.00315, 377.049.00479, 701.154.25768, 701.180.25639, 701.183.27620 (Depression) and 676.011.24283 (Social Anxiety).

XIV. References

Emslie GJ, Heiligenstein JH, Wagner KD, Hoog SL, Ernest DE, Brown E, Nilsson M, Jacobson JG. Fluoxetine for acute treatment of depression in children and adolescents: a placebo-controlled, randomized clinical trial. J Am Acad Child Adolesc Psychiatry 2002 Oct;41(10):1205-15

Keller MB, Ryan ND, Strober M. Klein RG, Kutcher SP, Birmaher B, Hagino OR, Koplewicz H, Carlson GA, Clarke GN, Emslie GJ, Feinberg D, Geller B, Kusumakar V, Papatheodorou G. Sack WH, Sweeney M, Wagner KD, Weller EB, Winters NC, Oakes R, McCafferty JP. Efficacy of paroxetine in the treatment of adolescent major depression: a randomized, controlled trial. J Am Acad Child Adolesc Psychiatry 2001 Jul;40(7):762-72

King RA, Riddle MA, Chappell PB, Hardin MT, Anderson GM, Lombroso P, Scahill L. Emergence of self-destructive phenomena in children and adolescents during fluoxetine treatment. J Am Acad Child Adolesc Psychiatry 1991 Mar;30(2):179-86

National Institute of Mental Health Suicide Facts, Completed Suicides, U.S. 1999 http://www.nimh.nih.gov/research/suifact.htm

Tab 37

FDA Talk Paper

T03-43
June 19, 2003

Media Inquiries: 301-827-6242
Consumer Inquiries: 888-INFO-FDA

FDA Statement Regarding the Anti-Depressant Paxil for Pediatric Population

ADVISORY: DESPITE THE NEW POSSIBLE SAFETY CONCERNS ABOUT USE OF PAXIL IN CHILDREN, IT IS ESSENTIAL THAT PATIENTS TAKING PAXIL (paroxetine hydrochloride) DO NOT SUDDENLY DISCONTINUE USE OF THE DRUG. ANY CHANGES MUST TAKE PLACE UNDER MEDICAL SUPERVISION.

The Food and Drug Administration (FDA) said today it is reviewing reports of a possible increased risk of suicidal thinking and suicide attempts in children and adolescents under the age of 18 treated with the drug Paxil for major depressive disorder (MDD). Although the FDA has not completed its evaluation of the new safety data, FDA is recommending that Paxil not be used in children and adolescents for the treatment of MDD. There is currently no evidence that Paxil is effective in children or adolescents with MDD, and Paxil is not currently approved for use in children and adolescents. Other approved treatment options are available for depression in children.

Paxil is approved for use in adults for the treatment of Obsessive Compulsive Disorder (OCD), MDD, Panic Disorder, Social Anxiety Disorder (SAD), Generalized Anxiety Disorder, and Post-traumatic Stress Disorder. There is no evidence that Paxil is associated with an increased risk of suicidal thinking in adults.

Three well-controlled trials in pediatric patients with MDD failed to show that the drug was more effective than placebo. The new safety information that is currently under review was derived from trials of Paxil in pediatric patients.
Following its review of the same data, the UK Department of Health issued a Press Release on June 10 stating that paroxetine (brand name Seroxat in the UK) must not be used to treat children and teenagers under the age of 18 years for depressive illness because UK authorities have concluded that there is an increase in the rate of self harm and potentially suicidal behavior in this age group, when paroxetine is used for depressive illness.

FDA advises that caretakers of pediatric patients already receiving treatment with Paxil for MDD talk to their doctor before stopping use of the drug. Patients should not discontinue use of Paxil without first consulting their physicians, and it is important that Paxil not be abruptly discontinued.

More information about today's statement is available at http://www.fda.gov/cder/drug/infopage/paxil/default.htm

####

MEETING MINUTES
NDA 20-031/SE5-037

Date: September 16, 2003
Location: CDER WOC2 6FL-G Conf Room
Time: 2:00 – 4:00 PM EST
Firm: GlaxoSmithKline
Meeting Type: Internal Meeting
Drug: Paxil (paroxetine HCl) Tablets
Indication: Pediatric Major Depressive Disorder (MDD) & Obsessive Compulsive Disorder
Meeting Chair: John Jenkins, M.D., Director, OND
Meeting Recorder: Paul David, R.Ph., Senior Regulatory Project Manager, DNDP, HFD-120

Tab 38

Participants
See attached list (Attachment 1).

Meeting Objective
1. Discussion of suicidality data in pediatric patients treated with the modern drugs approved for MDD.
2. Discussion of suicidality data in adult patients treated with the modern drugs approved for MDD.

Background
1. 4-11-02: GSK submits pediatric exclusivity supplement for paroxetine, NDA 20-031 supplement 37, for which exclusivity is granted.
2. 10-10-02: Approvable letter for this supplement requests additional data on behavioral adverse events in clinical trials.
3. 5-22-03: GSK submits analyses of suicidal adverse events showing a higher incidence with paroxetine treatment than with placebo.
4. 6-18-03: FDA Talk Paper recommends against use of paroxetine for pediatric major depressive disorder (MDD)

Purpose:
1. The meeting was requested at the Office Level in order for the Division to apprise upper management on what work has been completed as well as in progress to address the pediatric suicidality issue.

2. Dr. Mosholder presented a PowerPoint presentation (Attachment 2) on the pediatric suicidality data.

3. Dr. Hammad presented a PowerPoint presentation (Attachment 3) on the adult suicidality data.

Discussion:
1. We need to get a better sense of what the events from these studies really are, i.e., are they legitimate, suicide-associated thoughts/actions or self-mutilation acts that are becoming increasingly common in the adolescent population today and are not generally associated with a sincere intent to die.

2. Dr. Temple believes randomized, controlled withdrawal studies are needed to answer the question of whether these drugs are effective in the treatment of pediatric depression.

3. It was not clear whether the majority thought narratives or a study or both would be needed to address the question. However, there was general agreement that more studies would be desirable.

4. With respect to obtaining additional studies, this class of drugs might prove to be a good candidate for the off-patent WR process.

5. Dr. Andreason noted that there should be better screening in future studies for patients with borderline personality disorder, as antidepressant drugs may not be effective in these patients (they may even exacerbate their underlying emotional lability), and so their inclusion in these studies may confound the outcome.

6. There was agreement that if the suicidal ideation/behavior finding is real, labeling will need to be revised to include this finding. It will be essential to accurately and fully characterize the finding in labeling.

7. The Division is taking this issue to the February Psychopharmacologic Drugs AC meeting. Because many non-psychiatrists (e.g., family practitioners, pediatricians) prescribe these drugs to children and adolescents, there was a suggestion to include on the committee several internists, GPs, etc. It was noted that the Division may want to solicit the committee's feedback on the design of a study that would be adequate to address the issue.

8. Dr. O'Neill suggested that better information on the use of antidepressants in the pediatric population could be obtained from health care databases available to FDA through the existing cooperative agreements.

Conclusions:

?? The Division will keep upper management apprised on its continuing efforts to address the pediatric suicidality issue.

Minutes Preparer

Concurrence, Chair (or designated authority)

Attachments (3)

MEETING MINUTES
NDA 20-031/SE5-037

Date: September 16, 2003
Location: CDER WOC2 6FL-G Conf Room
Time: 2:00 – 4:00 PM EST
Firm: GlaxoSmithKline
Meeting Type: Internal Meeting
Drug: Paxil (paroxetine HCl) Tablets
Indication: Pediatric Major Depressive Disorder (MDD) & Obsessive Compulsive Disorder
Meeting Chair: John Jenkins, M.D., Director, OND
Meeting Recorder: Paul David, R.Ph., Senior Regulatory Project Manager, DNDP, HFD-120

Participants
See attached list (Attachment 1).

Meeting Objective
1. Discussion of suicidality data in pediatric patients treated with the modern drugs approved for MDD.
2. Discussion of ~~suicidality~~ data on completed suicides in adult patients treated with the modern drugs approved for MDD.

Background
1. 4-11-02: GSK submits pediatric exclusivity supplement for paroxetine, NDA 20-031 supplement 37, for which exclusivity is granted.
   10-10-02: Approvable letter for this supplement requests additional data on behavioral adverse events in clinical trials.
3. 5-22-03: GSK submits analyses of suicidal adverse events showing a higher incidence with paroxetine treatment than with placebo.
4. 6-18-03: FDA Talk Paper recommends against use of paroxetine for pediatric major depressive disorder (MDD)

Purpose:
1. The meeting was requested at the Office Level in order for the Division to apprise upper management on what work has been completed as well as in progress to address the pediatric suicidality issue.

2. Dr. Mosholder presented a PowerPoint presentation (Attachment 2) on the pediatric suicidality data.

3. Dr. Hammad presented a PowerPoint presentation (Attachment 3) on a study of completed suicides in the adult MDD short term randomized controlled trials ~~suicidality data~~.

Discussion:
1. We need to get a better sense of what the events from these studies really are, i.e., are they legitimate, suicide-associated thoughts/actions or self-mutilation acts that are becoming increasingly common in the adolescent population today and are not generally associated with a sincere intent to die.

2. Dr. Temple believes randomized, controlled withdrawal studies are needed to answer the question of whether these drugs are effective in the treatment of pediatric depression. He also noted that fluoxetine, because of its long half-life can not be "discontinued" easily. Hence if the behavioral toxicity is related to withdrawal, that might explain why the signal for fluoxetine is not substantial.

3. It was not clear whether the majority thought narratives or a study or both would be needed to address the question. However, there was general agreement that more studies would be desirable.

4. Dr. Woodcock suggested that a trial was needed to examine the emergence of behavioral toxicity in children and adolescents treated with antidepressants. She added that the focus of the trial should not be efficacy.

4.

4.5. With respect to obtaining additional studies, this class of drugs might prove to be a good candidate for the off-patent WR process.

5.6. Dr. Andreason noted that there should be better screening in future studies for patients with borderline personality disorder, as antidepressant drugs may not be effective in these patients (they may even exacerbate their underlying emotional lability), and so their inclusion in these studies may confound the outcome.

6.7. There was agreement that if the suicidal ideation/behavior finding is real, labeling will need to be revised to include this finding. It will be essential to accurately and fully characterize the finding in labeling.

7.8. The Division is taking this issue to the February Psychopharmacologic Drugs AC meeting. Because many non-psychiatrists (e.g., family practitioners, pediatricians) prescribe these drugs to children and adolescents, there was a suggestion to include on the committee several internists, GPs, etc. It was noted that the Division may want to solicit the committee's feedback on the design of a study that would be adequate to address the issue. The discussion should also focus on unanswered questions about the treatment of MDD in the pediatric population.

8.9. Dr. O'Neill suggested that better information on the use of antidepressants in the pediatric population could be obtained from health care databases available to FDA through the existing cooperative agreements.

Conclusions:

?? The Division will keep upper management apprised on its continuing efforts to address the pediatric suicidality issue.

Minutes Preparer

Concurrence, Chair (or designated authority)

Attachments (3)

Tab 39 *FDA Talk Paper*

T03-70
October 27, 2003

Media Inquiries: 301-827-6242
Consumer Inquiries: 888-INFO-FDA

FDA Issues Public Health Advisory Entitled: Reports Of Suicidality in Pediatric Patients Being Treated with Antidepressant Medications for Major Depressive Disorder (MDD)

The Food and Drug Administration (FDA) is issuing a Public Health Advisory to alert physicians to reports of suicidal thinking (and suicide attempts) in clinical studies of various antidepressant drugs in pediatric patients with major depressive disorder (MDD).

FDA recognizes that pediatric MDD is a serious condition for which there are few established treatment options. In addition to use of non-medication approaches to treatment, clinicians must often make choices among drug treatments available for adult MDD. Currently, Prozac (fluoxetine) is the only drug labeled for use in Pediatric MDD, and was approved recently under the Pediatric Exclusivity provision.

FDA has completed a preliminary review of reports for eight antidepressant drugs -- citalopram, fluoxetine, fluvoxamine, mirtazapine, nefazodone, paroxetine, sertraline, and venlafaxine -- all studied under the pediatric exclusivity provision of the FDA Modernization Act (FDAMA, 1997). (Although fluvoxamine data were reviewed along with the other antidepressant drugs, it should be noted that it is not approved as an antidepressant in the United States.)

FDA notes, to date, that the data do not clearly establish an association between the use of these drugs and increased suicidal thoughts or actions by pediatric patients. Nevertheless, it is not possible at this point to rule out an increased risk of these adverse events for any of these drugs, including Paxil (paroxetine), which was the subject of a FDA Talk Paper on June 19, 2003. That talk paper advised that FDA is reviewing the safety concerns related to off-label use of Paxil in children based on recent trials of this drug.

FDA emphasizes that, for the seven drugs evaluated in pediatric major depressive disorder (MDD), data FDA reviewed were adequate to establish effectiveness in MDD only for Prozac (fluoxetine). Failure to show effectiveness in any particular study in pediatric MDD, however, is not definitive evidence that the drug is not effective because trials may fail for many reasons.

FDA is aware of press and medical journal reports of suicide attempts and completed suicides in pediatric patients receiving antidepressants, and many such reports have also been submitted to FDA as spontaneous reports. Such reports are very difficult to interpret, however, in the absence of a control group, as these events also occur in untreated patients with depression.

FDA emphasized the need for additional data, analyses and a public discussion of available data. As we recognize that this is a serious illness, we need a better understanding of how to use the products we have.

In order to promote a public discussion of data and pertinent regulatory actions, FDA has scheduled a meeting on February 2, 2004, before the Psychopharmacologic Drugs Advisory committee and the Pediatric Subcommittee of the Anti-Infective Drugs Advisory Committee.

The agency also reminds physicians and patients that these drugs must be used with caution, both in adults and children. The labeling of antidepressant drugs already carries precautionary language that the possibility of a suicide attempt is inherent in MDD and may persist until significant remission occurs. Close supervision of high-risk patients should accompany initial drug therapy.

In its Public Health Advisory, FDA recommends that caretakers of pediatric patients receiving treatments with any of these antidepressants talk to their doctors before stopping the use of these drugs. Patients should not discontinue use of any of these drugs without first consulting with their physicians, and for certain of these drugs it is important that they not be abruptly discontinued.

FDA sent the advisory through its Medwatch partners, which includes doctors and organizations. FDA provides more information on the clinical study data in its Public Health Advisory, which is available on the FDA website at http://www.fda.gov/cder/drug/advisory/mdd.htm.

####

Tab 40

Food and Drug Administration

Center for Drug Evaluation and Research

SUMMARY MINUTES OF THE

Psychopharmacologic Drugs Advisory Committee Meeting and the Pediatric Subcommittee of the anti-infective drugs advisory committee

February 2, 2004

Members Present (Voting)
Matthew Rudorfer, M.D. (Chair)
Tana Grady-Weliky, M.D.
Irene Ortiz, M.D.
Richard Malone, M.D.
Andrew Leon, Ph.D.
Philip Wang, M.D., M.P.H., Dr. PH
Wayne Goodman, M.D.
James McGough, M.D.
Jean Bronstein, R.N., M.S. (Consumer Representative)

FDA Participants
Robert Temple, M.D.
Russell Katz, M.D.
Thomas Laughren, M.D.
M. Dianne Murphy, M.D.,
Susan Cummins, M.D., M.P.H.,
Anne Trontell, M.D., M.P.H.

Executive Secretary
Anuja M. Patel, M.P.H.

Consultants to the Psychopharmocologic Drugs Advisory Committee (Voting)
Gail Griffith, B.A., M.A. (Patient Representative)
Cynthia Pfeffer, M.D.

Psychopharmacologic Drugs Advisory Committee Consultant (non-voting):
Daniel Pine, M.D.
David Shaffer, M.D.

Psychopharmacologic Drugs Advisory Committee Industry Representative (Non-voting):
Dilip Mehta, M.D., Ph.D.

Pediatric Subcommittee Consultant Members of the Anti-Infective Advisory Committee (voting):
Joan Chesney, M.D.
Robert Nelson, M.D. Ph.D.
Victor Santana, M.D.
David Danford, M.D.
Robert Fink, M.D.
Mark Hudak, M.D.
Susan Fuchs, M.D.
Richard Gorman, M.D., FAAP
Norman Fost, M.D., M.P.H. (CBER Consultant)

AIDAC Members of the Pediatric Subcommittee of the Anti-Infective Advisory Committee (voting):
Mary Glode, M.D.
Judith O'Fallon, Ph.D.
Steven Ebert, Pharm.D. (Consumer Representative)

Pediatric Subcommittee of the Anti-Infective Advisory Committee Consultants (voting):
Charles Irwin, Jr., M.D.
James Perrin, M.D.
Laurel Leslie, M.D., FAAP
Elizabeth Andrews, Ph.D.

Pediatric Subcommittee of the Anti-Infective Advisory Committee Acting Industry Representative (non-voting):
Samuel Maldonado, M.D., M.P.H.

Cardio-Renal AC Members Absent:
None

Guest Speaker (non-voting):
Kelly Posner, Ph.D

These summary minutes for the February 2, 2004, meeting of the Psychopharmacologic Drugs Advisory Committee and the Pediatric Subcommittee of the Anti-Infective Drugs Advisory Committee were approved on March 4, 2004.

I certify that I attended the February 2, 2004, meeting of the Psychopharmacologic Drugs Advisory Committee and the Pediatric Subcommittee of the Anti-Infective Drugs Advisory Committee meeting and that these minutes accurately reflect what transpired.

//S//	//S//
Anuja M. Patel, M.P.H.	Matthew Rudorfer, M.D.
Executive Secretary	Chair

On February 2, 2004, the Psychopharmacologic Drugs Advisory Committee and the Pediatric Subcommittee of the Anti-Infective Drugs Advisory Committee met in open session at the Holiday Inn, at 8120 Wisconsin Avenue, in Bethesda, Maryland. The Committees discussed reports of the occurrence of suicidality (both suicidal ideation and suicide attempts) in clinical trials for various anti-depressant drugs in pediatric patients with major depressive disorder (MDD). The Committees also considered optimal approach to the analysis of data from these trials, as well as further research needs to address these issues.

Prior to the meeting, the members and the invited consultants had been provided the background material from the FDA and written statements submitted by the public. The meeting was called to order by Matthew Rudorfer, M.D. (Committee Chair); the Conflict of Interest Statement was read into the record by Anuja M. Patel, M.P.H. (Executive Secretary). There were approximately 450 persons in attendance. There were approximately 54 speakers for the Open Public Hearing session.

Open Public Hearing Speakers:

- David Antonuccio, Ph.D. and Irving Kirsch, Ph.D.
- Lisa VanSyckel
- Anne Blake Tracy, Ph.D.
- Mark Miller
- Jay and Corey Baadsgaard
- Joyce Storey
- Jennifer and Jame Tierney
- Donna Taylor
- Shannon Baker
- Dawn Rider and Vincent Boehm , A.S.P.I.R.E
- Sara Bostock
- Vera Sharav, The Alliance for Human Research Protection
- Cynthia Brockman
- Rosie Meysenburg
- Rachel Adler and Sheila McDonald, Child and Adolescent Bipolar Foundation
- Andy Vickery
- Pepper Draper
- Donald Marks, M.D., Ph.D.
- Leah Harris M.A.
- Donald Farber, Esq., Law Office of Donald J. Farber
- Lorraine, Robert, and Jonathan Slater
- Paul Domb and Matthew Piepenburg
- Terri Williams
- Glenn McIntoch
- Delnora Duprey
- Joe Pittman
- Richard Mack
- Gloria and Noah Wright
- Tod and Eileen Shivak
- Suzanne Vogel-Scibilia, M.D., The National Alliance of the Mentally Ill
- Dennis Winter
- Steve Cole
- Allan Routhier
- Daniel Safer, M.D.
- Julie Magno Zito, Ph.D., UMD School of Pharmacy
- Joseph Glenmullen, M.D.
- Linda Cheslek
- Jeff Avery
- Harry Skigis
- Sharon McBride
- David Fassler, M.D. American Psychiatric Association
- Lawrence Diller, M.D.
- Thomas Moore, M.D.
- Pamela Wild
- Karen Menzies
- Amy Coburn
- Gary Cheslek, M.D.

- Marion Goff
- Sherri Walton, Mental Health Association of Arizona
- Peter Breggin, M.D.
- Robert Fritz
- Lawrence Greenhill, M.D., American Academy of Child & Adolescent Psychiatry
- Tom Woodward

FDA Presentations:

Overview of Issues — Russell Katz, M.D., Director, Division of Neuropharmacological Drug Products, FDA

Pediatric Drug Development — Dianne Murphy, M.D., Director, Office of Counter-Terrorism and Drug Development, FDA

Pediatric Depression and Its Treatment — Cynthia Pfeffer, M.D., Weill Medical College of Cornell University

Suicide and Related Problems in Adolescents — David Shaffer, F.R.C.P. (Lond), F.R.C. Psych, Columbia University

Pediatric and adolescent Antidepressant Drug Use in the U.S. — Gianna C. Rigoni, Pharm.D., M.S., Epidemiologist, Office of Drug Safety, FDA

One Year Post-Exclusivity Mandated Adverse Event Review for Paroxetine and Citalopram — Solomon Iyasu, M.D., M.P.H, Lead Medical Officer, Division of Pediatrics Drug Development, FDA

Office of Drug Safety Data Resources for the Study of Suicidal Events — Andrew Mosholder, M.D., M.P.H., Epidemiologist, Office of Drug Safety, FDA

Regulatory History on Antidepressants and Suicidality and Update on Current Plans for Analysis of Pediatric Suicidality Data — Thomas Laughren, M.D., Team Leader, Division of Neuropharmacological Drug Products, FDA

Suicidality Classification Project — Kelly Posner, Ph.D., Columbia University

Plans for Analysis of Patient Level Data for Pediatric Studies — Tarek Hammad, M.D., Ph.D., M.Sc., M.S., Safety Reviewer, Division of Neuropharmacological Drug Products, FDA

Questions to the Committee:

Topics Directly Pertinent to Continuing Evaluation of Data from Pediatric Controlled Trials:

1. Possible Failure to Fully Capture All Events of Potential Interest with Regard to Suicidality

The first step in the process of evaluation for suicidality was to find events of potential interest. GSK (Glaxo Smith Kline) had developed an algorithm for searching for events possibly representing suicidality in their database, and FDA proposed a variation of this to other sponsors. However, this was admittedly a compromise. It is conceivable that certain cases of interest might have been missed by the search methods employed. The only fail safe approach to identifying all possible events of interest would be to have experts blindly evaluate every case report form for the more than 4000 patients who participated in these trials. Since that is not feasible, FDA welcomes advice from the committee on possible modifications to the search strategies used for identifying cases that might have been missed. Additional searches at this point would further delay the analyses of these data, and this needs to be taken into consideration. However, if the committees feel there are serious deficiencies in the search methods employed, it would be helpful to hear about alternative approaches.

The overall consensus of the Committees was that the FDA should proceed with the planned re-analysis of the data once a team of mental health experts at Columbia University and elsewhere have reclassified the cases. The re-analysis, however, may not yield accurate results. The Committees' concern in this respect reflected impressions that the data had been collected during the medication trials in a fashion that would not easily allow the generation of an accurate estimate of adverse behavioral reactions associated with suicidal behavior or ideation. Despite these concerns, the statisticians on the Committees felt that the methodological concepts learned from the re-analyses will be valuable. The Committees encouraged the Agency to go back and examine data on adverse effects in individual study participants for signs of what has been labeled the "stimulation" or "activation" syndrome. These terms have been used to refer to a constellation of behaviors, including agitation, restlessness, hyperactivity, and disinhibition. In severe cases, probably representing a very small percentage of treated patients, the clinical picture may resemble frank akathisia, accompanied by considerable subjective distress. Treatment-emergent mood lability, irritability, or hostility should also be noted. The Committees encouraged study of these and related phenomena. In particular, the Committees inquired about whether the presence of these behaviors may be associated with drug levels or with suicidal ideation, suicidal behavior, or impulsive acts, and the response of such behaviors to drug discontinuation or dosage change (either decrease or increase). Although not necessarily available in the planned data re-analysis, the Committees recommended the use of clearer inclusion/exclusion criteria, the collection of additional data including drug concentrations for pharmacokinetic analysis, and more established endpoints in future antidepressant clinical trials in children and adolescents. With respect to study entry criteria and endpoints, the Committees encouraged an evaluation of study quality. This could be accomplished partially by examining the degree to which cross-site reliability was established in each individual study for the rating of criteria and endpoints. In addition, the Committee felt that off-label prescription including dispensing of antidepressant medication samples, by non-psychiatrists is problematic. Therefore, improved labeling information, highlighting potential side effects of greatest concern, was suggested by the Committee.

In conceptualizing future plans for re-analysis of data on adverse behavioral reactions, some discussion focused on defining the boundaries of events that should be considered indicative of suicidal behavior. Committee members recognized the need to define these boundaries more precisely than in the reviewed studies and offered some guidelines. In particular, some Committee members recommended that "cutting" should not be considered a symptom of suicidal behavior.

The Chair summarized the consensus of the committee stating that although individual members had reservations about the limitations of the existing database, the Committee endorses the continuation of the re-classification of data with some additional measures as mentioned above. The Committee advised the FDA to attempt to recreate the process of identifying cases of suicide-related events and look for multiple different types of definitions that may be subsumed under "stimulation (or activation) syndrome." This would necessarily require keeping definition(s) as broad as possible.

2. Approaches to Classifying Events into Meaningful Categories for the Purpose of Further Analysis

As noted, an important next step is to decide on categories into which events of interest might be classified, along with operational definitions for such classifications. The approach used by sponsors thus far has been to classify cases first into a crude category of "possibly suicide-related," and then a further sub-grouping of that broader group into a "suicide attempt" class. Since we are just now

beginning to address this question with our outside experts, we would welcome any advice the committees might have on how to classify these events for the purpose of further analysis.

The consensus of the Committees was that a level of certainty and variability in analysis be included in the reclassification of data. The Committees were concerned that the general quality of the data, as they were originally collected, was relatively low. This complicates any effort of reclassification. Efforts at re-creating the methodology used at various sites of the different trials are important for understanding the specific information that was actually gathered in each data set. The Committees encouraged the identification of treatment-emergent agitation and related behaviors as potentially relevant mediators of self-harm ideation or actions.

3. Patient Level Data Analysis

Since we are in the preliminary stages of designing an appropriate analysis of patient level data, this would be an opportune time to get feedback on how to approach this analysis. In addition, you have seen our list of potential covariates for inclusion in this analysis, and we would welcome any thoughts you might have on this list. If we have left out important covariates, please let us know, since this would be the time to try to gather any additional information that you feel might be helpful in trying to understand these data.

As noted, the Committees did have suggestions for additional covariates that might be collected from these databases to assist in designing an appropriate analysis plan. Individual committee members provided multiple suggestions to approaches to identifying covariates, and mentioned the potential value of evaluating observed events in relation to time of dosing or other intervention changes. Committee members expressed an interest in seeing data from various patient-level variables. These included a broader array of adverse effect variables, related to the broader "stimulation/activation" syndrome described above, as well as potential patient-level data that may have moderated therapeutic or adverse effects delineated in the available studies. Committee members inquired specifically about data on co-morbid psychopathology, such as anxiety or disruptive behavior disorders, adverse environmental events, and family history or other variables that may relate to the risk for bipolar disorder. In sum, the Committee felt that extending the analysis of patient level data beyond the focus specifically on suicidality related or mediating variables would be of value. These would include family history of mood and other mental disorders, pretreatment pre-morbid conditions such as hypomanic/manic symptoms or akathisia, careful delineation of the diagnosis where possible, e.g. unipolar vs. bipolar depression vs. schizophrenia spectrum, comorbidities (other mental and physical disorders, substance use), administration of other medications. As noted, particular attention to the presence of signs and symptoms of treatment-emergent agitation and activation is recommended, to include time to development and severity of such behaviors both pre- and post-treatment in both patients on medication and control group members.

Topics of Future Interest

4. Ascertainment for Suicidality

As we reviewed the descriptive information for the events identified by sponsors as possibly suggestive of suicidality, it became apparent that ascertainment for emergence of suicidality was not optimal. The case descriptions were frequently sparse and lacking the kind of detail that would ordinarily be useful in assessing whether or not the events might legitimately be considered to represent suicidality. Of course, these studies were not designed with that goal in mind. Indeed, patients who were judged to be suicidal at screening were excluded. Nor did we emphasize such assessment for suicidality in our Written Requests for these pediatric programs. Furthermore, there is, of course, no fix for this problem with regard to these studies. However, one of our outside experts

will address the issue of how one might develop guidance for more adequate assessment for emergent suicidality in future studies. We would welcome any advice from the committees on the development of such guidance.

The Committee's consensus was that the review of the available data pointed to the pressing need for more research on this topic in new samples of children and adolescents studied in randomized controlled trials. In such future studies, the Committee noted the importance of including children on various other medications while gathering high-quality data on adverse events. The Committee also recognized the importance of including placebos in such trials, in order to sort out the disease from the treatment and to evaluate the data accurately. Particular focus on behavioral toxicity early in treatment, including various forms of dysphoric activation, as noted above, is recommended for more definitive assessment in future clinical trials to try to capture instances of treatment-emergent difficulties that might precede or occur in association with frank suicidality. Pressing methodological issues for future clinical trials include the desirability of standardizing assessment instruments to capture suicidality or antecedent adverse effects of interest and permit better analysis across sites and across trials. Such measures should include self-assessment instruments for use by patients and their parents/guardians.

5. Future Approaches to Trying to Address the Question of What Benefits These Drugs Might Have in Pediatric MDD

Due to time constraints the Committee did not discuss this item completely. The Committee was mixed on the idea of drug-discontinuation designs. Some Committee members clearly recognized the potential superior statistical power in this design, given results from studies using this design in adults. Other Committee members noted that this design does not address key questions concerning the safety and efficacy of delivering antidepressants as opposed to other treatments for a child or adolescent presenting for the first time with symptoms of an untreated major depressive disorder. To the extent that this question remains central, it may be important to utilize various research designs beyond a randomized withdrawal design.

In answering these questions please keep in mind that the FDA does not regulate the practice of medicine, but is responsible for providing information on the safety and efficacy of the products it regulates. As a reminder, the FDA issued a Public Health Advisory on October 27, 2003, which stated:

"FDA emphasizes that these drugs must be used with caution. Prescribers are reminded of the following statement present in all antidepressant labeling:

Suicide: The possibility of a suicide attempt is inherent in major depressive disorder and may persist until significant remission occurs. Close supervision of high-risk patients should accompany initial drug therapy. Prescriptions for Drug X should be written for the smallest quantity of tablets consistent with good patient management, in order to reduce the risk of overdose".

The Committee discussed the need to consider revising this statement, in light of recent data. As noted, there was a consensus of the Committee that labeling include a more prominent warning of the risk of behavioral toxicity, particularly dysphoric agitation/activation, early in the course of antidepressant treatment. It was also noted that the last statement in the existing warning cited above, emphasizing the risk of medication overdose, is a legacy of the tricyclic antidepressant era, and is no longer appropriate, as drug overdose per se as a means of suicide is not a concern with the SSRIs and other newer antidepressants. Similarly, a bolded warning in all current Selective Serotonin Reuptake Inhibitor (SSRI) labeling regarding the necessity to avoid a potentially fatal drug-drug interaction with monoamine oxidase (MAO) inhibitor antidepressants, while true, may well not reflect current medical practice, which entails only rare use of MAO inhibitors. Consideration to replacement of these outdated warnings with labeling more representative of modern medical practice and concern is recommended.

6. A public meeting is planned in late summer to discuss the results of further analyses of the controlled trials. Until that time, should the FDA provide additional advice to practicing physicians regarding the use of these drugs?

- **If your answer is yes, please provide specific information on what that advice should be.**

The Committee advised the FDA to issue a warning in the interim to the physicians and the public on the potential side effects of the SSRIs and other newer antidepressants. The Committee advised the FDA to inform the public and health care workers including pediatricians and family practitioners of the level of concern regarding possible harm to a minority of children on antidepressants and the signs associated with the side effects. Specifically, the Committee felt that the necessity of close follow-up, with monitoring for emergent adverse effects, during the first weeks of treatment of children and adolescents with antidepressants should be stated explicitly. Parents or other responsible adults should be informed of the signs and symptoms of the "activation syndrome" and of the urgency of having the child seen by physician should such behaviors emerge, especially early in the treatment course.

The Committee advised the FDA to inform the public and health care workers, including pediatricians and family practitioners, that the data on the efficacy of SSRIs for pediatric major depression is less compelling than Committee members had recognized prior to recent events discussed by the Committee. The Committee is concerned that health care workers are unaware of the fact that the strong majority of randomized controlled trials of SSRIs do not demonstrate superiority over placebo in the treatment of major depression in children and adolescents. The Committee felt that it was important for the FDA to communicate this fact as it bears on the risk-benefit ratio for the use of SSRIs in pediatric major depression.

7. **Should FDA involve other professional organizations in the community? If so, how should FDA involve these organizations? What messages should these organizations provide?**

The Committee felt that the Agency should involve all health care organizations whose membership includes physicians and other medical personnel who might prescribe or be asked questions about antidepressant use in children and adolescents. Such health care professionals would include pediatricians, child and adult psychiatrists and psychologists, internists, family practitioners, emergency room, intensive care, and rehabilitation physicians, nurse practitioners, pharmacists, and physicians' assistants. Other professionals who work with young people, including teachers and social workers, should also be included. Examples of such professional organizations cited by Committee members include medical organizations such as the American Academy of Pediatrics (AAP) and the American Association of Family Practitioners (AAFP), and similar organizations representing the other health care professions. Professional publications, e.g. Pediatric News, while heightening awareness of the prevalence of depression and risk of suicide, may play a role in informing health care workers and family members of the relative benefits and risks, including possible side effects, of antidepressant drugs.

These organizations and the Agency should provide information to health care providers through a variety of sources, including newsletters and the Internet, as well as face-to-face meetings and panel discussions.

In addition, the organizations should also inform and educate parents so that when they make collaborative decisions with their child's physician they are fully informed and understand completely the serious potential risks of the drug. The adults responsible for the young person being treated with antidepressants should be aware of the small but real risk of an "activation syndrome" developing in their children and informed of the need to be vigilant about this concern and to immediately contact the prescribing health care professional should any behavioral toxicity emerge during treatment.

Following the discussion session, the meeting adjourned at approximately 6:15 PM.

3/19/04

DEPARTMENT OF HEALTH & HUMAN SERVICES

Public Health Service

Food and Drug Administration
Rockville MD 20857

032/00990081R

NDA 20-151/S-028/S-030
NDA 20-699/S-041/S-048

Tab 41

Wyeth Pharmaceuticals, Inc.
Attention: Kenneth R. Bonk
Director, Worldwide Regulatory Affairs
P.O. Box 8299
Philadelphia, PA 19101-1245

Dear Mr. Bonk:

We acknowledge receipt of your supplemental New Drug Applications (NDAs) dated August 8, 2003 (NDAs 20-151/S-028 & 20-699/S-041), and December 10, 2003 (NDAs 20-151/S-030 & 20-699/S-048), submitted under section 505(b) of the Federal Food, Drug, and Cosmetic Act for Effexor (venlafaxine hydrochloride) Immediate Release (NDA 20-151) and Effexor XR (venlafaxine hydrochloride) Extended Release Capsules (NDA 20-699).

We additionally acknowledge receipt of your amendments to NDAs 20-151/S-028 & 20-699/S-041 dated August 25, and 29, 2003.

Reference is also made to the February 2, 2004 meeting of the Psychopharmacologic Drugs Advisory Committee and the Pediatric Subcommittee of the Anti-Infective Advisory Committee to discuss reports of the occurrence of suicidality in clinical trials for various antidepressant drugs in pediatric patients with major depressive disorder.

Supplemental applications 20-151/S-028 & 20-699/S-041 submitted under "Changes Being Effected in 30 days" provide for the following revisions to product labeling:

1. Revisions to the **PRECAUTIONS-Usage in Children** section to denote hostility and suicide related adverse events in pediatric clinical trials.
2. The addition of the term "tinnitus" to the **DOSAGE AND ADMINISTRATION-Discontinuing Effexor** or **Effexor XR** sections.
3. Revisions to the Patient Brief Summary.

Supplemental applications 20-151/S-030 & 20-699/S-048 submitted as "Prior Approval" applications provide for revisions to the **DOSAGE and ADMINISTRATION/Discontinuing Effexor** or **Effexor XR** sections of product labeling.

We completed our review of these applications, as amended, and they are approvable. Before these applications may be approved, however, you must submit final printed labeling revised as follows:

1. Based upon the recommendations made by the committee members, we believe that labeling changes are warranted in order to caution practitioners and patients about the need for close observation of patients being treated with antidepressants for clinical worsening, for the emergence of suicidality, and for the emergence of a variety of other symptoms that may represent a precursor to suicidality. The committees felt that it would be important to warn prescribers and families of the need to be vigilant for such behaviors, regardless of the role antidepressants may have in the emergence of suicidal ideation/attempts in patients taking antidepressants

   Because we do not believe that a causal association between children taking venlafaxine and the emergence of suicidality has as yet been definitively established, we do not agree with the labeling changes proposed in your August 8, 2003 submission. We feel that, both for the terms "suicide-related adverse events" and "hostility," there is a need for more clinically meaningful classification of the events subsumed under these very broad terms in order to interpret the findings from these trials in a meaningful way.

   As stated, later in this letter, we are requesting all sponsors of modern drugs to treat major depressive disorder to submit revisions to labeling, as a "Changes Being Effected in 30 days" supplemental new drug application, to incorporate this information.

2. The addition of the term "tinnitus" to the list of adverse experiences possibly related to venlafaxine dose reduction or discontinuation is acceptable. However, we do not concur with the addition of the phrase "and spontaneous postmarketing reports" to the **DOSAGE and ADMINISTRATION/Discontinuing Effexor or Effexor XR** sections of product labeling since we are revising labeling, as stated later in this letter, in regard to discontinuation as part of a class labeling initiative.

   Additionally, since there are a number of cases of tinnitus which emerge during venlafaxine treatment, we request that tinnitus be added to the subsection **ADVERSE REACTIONS/Postmarketing Reports** section immediately following the mention of shock-like electrical sensations as follows: "shock-like electrical sensations or tinnitus (in some cases, subsequent to the discontinuation of venlafaxine or tapering of dose)."

3. The revisions to the Patient Brief Summary are acceptable.

As stated previously, and based upon our February 2, 2004 meeting, we are requesting revisions to your labeling in order to incorporate the committee's recommendations. Specifically, we are requesting the following revisions to product labeling.

1. Under **WARNINGS**, we are requesting the addition of a new subsection entitled **Clinical Worsening and Suicide.** Please note that the title of this new section should be bolded, as well as two statements embedded in this labeling language.

   WARNINGS-Clinical Worsening and Suicide

   Patients with major depressive disorder, both adult and pediatric, can experience worsening of their depression and/or the emergence of suicidal ideation and behavior (suicidality), whether or not they are taking antidepressant medications, and this risk may persist until significant remission occurs. Although there has been a long-standing concern that antidepressants may have a role in inducing worsening of depression and the emergence of suicidality in certain patients, a causal role for antidepressants in inducing such behaviors has not been established. **Nevertheless, patients being treated with antidepressants should be observed closely for clinical worsening and suicidality, especially at the beginning of a course of drug therapy, or at the time of dose changes, either increases or decreases.** Consideration should be given to discontinuing the medication in patients whose depression is persistently worse or whose emergent suicidality is severe, abrupt in onset, or was not part of the patient's presenting symptoms.

Antidepressants have been shown to cause, in some patients, anxiety, agitation, panic attacks, insomnia, irritability, hostility, impulsivity, akathisia, hypomania, and mania. These symptoms have been reported in adult and pediatric patients being treated with antidepressants for major depressive disorder as well as for other indications, both psychiatric and nonpsychiatric. Although a causal link between the emergence of such symptoms and either the worsening of depression and/or the emergence of suicidal impulses has not been established, consideration should be given to discontinuing the medication in patients for whom such symptoms are severe, abrupt in onset, or were not part of the patient's presenting symptoms.

Families and caregivers of patients being treated with antidepressants for major depressive disorder or other indications should be alerted about the need to monitor patients for the emergence of agitation, irritability, and the other symptoms described above, as well as the emergence of suicidality, and to report such symptoms immediately to health care providers. Prescriptions for [Insert EFFEXOR or EFFEXOR XR] should be written for the smallest quantity of capsules consistent with good patient management, in order to reduce the risk of overdose.

If the decision has been made to discontinue treatment, medication should be tapered, as rapidly as is feasible, but with recognition that abrupt discontinuation can be associated with certain symptoms (see Precautions and Dosage and Administration, Discontinuation of Treatment with [Insert EFFEXOR or EFFEXOR XR], for a description of the risks of discontinuation of [Insert EFFEXOR or EFFEXOR XR]).

It should be noted that [Insert EFFEXOR or EFFEXOR XR] is not approved for use in treating any indications in the pediatric population.

A major depressive episode may be the initial presentation of bipolar disorder. It is generally believed (though not established in controlled trials) that treating such an episode with an antidepressant alone can increase the likelihood of precipitation of a mixed/manic episode in patients at risk for bipolar disorder. Whether any of the symptoms described above represent such a conversion is unknown. However, prior to initiating treatment with an antidepressant, patients should be adequately screened to determine if they are at risk for bipolar disorder; such screening should include a detailed psychiatric history, including a family history of suicide, bipolar disorder, and depression. It should be noted that [Insert EFFEXOR or EFFEXOR XR] is not approved for use in treating bipolar depression.

2. Under **PRECAUTIONS-Information for Patients,** the following language should be added:

Patients and their families should be encouraged to be alert to the emergence of anxiety, agitation, panic attacks, insomnia, irritability, hostility, impulsivity, akathisia, hypomania, mania, worsening of depression, and suicidal ideation, especially early during antidepressant treatment. Such symptoms should be reported to the patient's physician if they are severe, abrupt in onset, or were not part of the patient's presenting symptoms.

3. Delete the section in **PRECAUTIONS-General** entitled "Suicide".

Additionally, we are taking this opportunity, in a class labeling initiative for all of the selective serotonin reuptake inhibitors (SSRIs) and serotonin and norepinephrine reuptake inhibitors (SNRIs), to change labeling in regards to discontinuation symptoms and to adverse events occurring in neonates exposed to any of the SSRIs or SNRIs late in the third trimester.

Therefore, we are requesting the following revisions to labeling (double underline font denotes additions to labeling and strike through font denotes deletions to labeling):

4. Under **PRECAUTIONS-General**, please add the new subsection below:

Discontinuation of Treatment with [insert EFFEXOR or EFFEXOR XR]

Discontinuation symptoms have been systematically evaluated in patients taking venlafaxine, to include prospective analyses of clinical trials in Generalized Anxiety Disorder and retrospective surveys of trials in depression. Abrupt discontinuation or dose reduction of venlafaxine at various doses has been found to be associated with the appearance of new symptoms, the frequency of which increased with increased dose level and with longer duration of treatment. Reported symptoms include agitation, anorexia, anxiety, confusion, coordination impaired, diarrhea, dizziness, dry mouth, dysphoric mood, fasciculation, fatigue, headaches, hypomania, insomnia, nausea, nervousness, nightmares, sensory disturbances (including shock-like electrical sensations), somnolence, sweating, tremor, vertigo, and vomiting.

During marketing of [insert EFFEXOR or EFFEXOR XR] and other SSRIs and SNRIs (Serotonin and Norepinephrine Reuptake Inhibitors), there have been spontaneous reports of adverse events occurring upon discontinuation of these drugs, particularly when abrupt, including the following: dysphoric mood, irritability, agitation, dizziness, sensory disturbances (e.g. paresthesias such as electric shock sensations), anxiety, confusion, headache, lethargy, emotional lability, insomnia, hypomania, tinnitus, and seizures. While these events are generally self-limiting, there have been reports of serious discontinuation symptoms.

Patients should be monitored for these symptoms when discontinuing treatment with [insert EFFEXOR or EFFEXOR XR]. A gradual reduction in the dose rather than abrupt cessation is recommended whenever possible. If intolerable symptoms occur following a decrease in the dose or upon discontinuation of treatment, then resuming the previously prescribed dose may be considered. Subsequently, the physician may continue decreasing the dose but at a more gradual rate (see DOSAGE AND ADMINISTRATION).

5. Under **PRECAUTIONS-PREGNANCY**, the following new class labeling subsection should be added (double underline font denotes class labeling):

PREGNANCY-Pregnancy-Nonteratogenic Effects

Neonates exposed to [insert EFFEXOR or EFFEXOR XR] and other SSRIs or serotonin and norepinephrine reuptake inhibitors (SNRIs), late in the third trimester have developed complications requiring prolonged hospitalization, respiratory support, and tube feeding. Such complications can arise immediately upon delivery. Reported clinical findings have included respiratory distress, cyanosis, apnea, seizures, temperature instability, feeding difficulty, vomiting, hypoglycemia, hypotonia, hypertonia, hyperreflexia, tremor, jitteriness, irritability, and constant crying. These features are consistent with either a direct toxic effect of SSRIs and SNRIs or, possibly, a drug discontinuation syndrome. It should be noted that, in some cases, the clinical picture is consistent with serotonin syndrome (see WARNINGS). When treating a pregnant woman with [insert EFFEXOR or EFFEXOR XR] during the third trimester, the physician should carefully consider the potential risks and benefits of treatment (see DOSAGE AND ADMINISTRATION).

6. Under **DOSAGE AND ADMINISTRATION**, please add a new section entitled **Special Populations**. Your current sections entitled **Patients with Hepatic Impairment, Patients with Renal Impairment**, and **Elderly Patients** may be placed in this section as well as the following new section entitled **Treatment of Pregnant Women During the Third Trimester** (double underline font denotes class labeling):

Treatment of Pregnant Women During the Third Trimester
Neonates exposed to [insert EFFEXOR or EFFEXOR XR] and other SSRIs or SNRIs, late in the third trimester have developed complications requiring prolonged hospitalization, respiratory support, and tube feeding (see PRECAUTIONS). When treating pregnant women with [insert EFFEXOR or EFFEXOR XR] during the third trimester, the physician should carefully consider the potential risks and benefits of treatment. The physician may consider tapering [insert EFFEXOR or EFFEXOR XR] in the third trimester.

7. Under **DOSAGE AND ADMINISTRATION**, please revise the section entitled **Discontinuing EFFEXOR [EFFEXOR XR]** as follows:

EFFEXOR LABELING
Discontinuing Effexor (venlafaxine hydrochloride)
Symptoms associated with discontinuation of Effexor and other SSRIs and SNRIs, have been reported (see PRECAUTIONS). Patients should be monitored for these symptoms when discontinuing treatment. A gradual reduction in the dose rather than abrupt cessation is recommended whenever possible. If intolerable symptoms occur following a decrease in the dose or upon discontinuation of treatment, then resuming the previously prescribed dose may be considered. Subsequently, the physician may continue decreasing the dose but at a more gradual rate.

~~When discontinuing Effexor after more than 1 week of therapy, it is generally recommended that the dose be tapered to minimize the risk of discontinuation symptoms. Patients who have received Effexor for 6 weeks or more should have their dose tapered gradually over at least a 2-week period.~~

~~Discontinuation symptoms have been systematically evaluated in patients taking venlafaxine, to include prospective analyses of clinical trials in Generalized Anxiety Disorder and retrospective surveys of trials in depression. Abrupt discontinuation or dose reduction of venlafaxine at various doses has been found to be associated with the appearance of new symptoms, the frequency of which increased with increased dose level and with longer duration of treatment. Reported symptoms include agitation, anorexia, anxiety, confusion, coordination impaired, diarrhea, dizziness, dry mouth, dysphoric mood, fasciculation, fatigue, headaches, hypomania, insomnia, nausea, nervousness, nightmares, seizures, sensory disturbances (including shock-like electrical sensations), somnolence.~~

~~sweating, tinnitus, tremor, vertigo, and vomiting. It is therefore recommended that the dosage of Effexor be tapered gradually and the patient monitored. The period required for tapering may depend on the dose, duration of therapy and the individual patient. Discontinuation effects are well known to occur with antidepressants.~~

EFFEXOR XR LABELING

Discontinuing Effexor XR
Symptoms associated with discontinuation of Effexor XR and other SSRIs and SNRIs, have been reported (see PRECAUTIONS). Patients should be monitored for these symptoms when discontinuing treatment. A gradual reduction in the dose rather than abrupt cessation is recommended whenever possible. If intolerable symptoms occur following a decrease in the dose or upon discontinuation of treatment, then resuming the previously prescribed dose may be considered. Subsequently, the physician may continue decreasing the dose but at a more gradual rate. ~~When discontinuing Effexor XR after more than 1 week of therapy, it is generally recommended that the dose be tapered to minimize the risk of discontinuation symptoms. Patients who have received Effexor XR for 6 weeks or more should have their dose tapered over at least a 2 week period.~~ In clinical trials with Effexor XR, tapering was achieved by reducing the daily dose by 75 mg at 1 week intervals. Individualization of tapering may be necessary.

~~Discontinuation symptoms have been systematically evaluated in patients taking venlafaxine, to include prospective analyses of clinical trials in Generalized Anxiety Disorder and retrospective surveys of trials of major depressive disorder. Abrupt discontinuation or dose reduction of venlafaxine at various doses has been found to be associated with the appearance of new symptoms, the frequency of which increased with increased dose level and with longer duration of treatment. Reported symptoms include agitation, anorexia, anxiety, confusion, coordination impaired, diarrhea, dizziness, dry mouth, dysphoric mood, fasciculation, fatigue, headaches, hypomania, insomnia, nausea, nervousness, nightmares, seizures, sensory disturbances (including shock-like electrical sensations), somnolence, sweating, tinnitus, tremor, vertigo, and vomiting. It is therefore recommended that the dosage of Effexor XR be tapered gradually and the patient monitored. The period required for tapering may depend on the dose, duration of therapy and the individual patient. Discontinuation effects are well known to occur with antidepressants.~~

Within 10 days after the date of this letter, you are required to amend the supplemental applications, notify us of your intent to file an amendment, or follow one of your other options under 21 CFR 314.120. In the absence of any such action, FDA may proceed to withdraw these supplemental applications. Any amendment should respond to all the deficiencies listed. We will not process a partial reply as a major amendment nor will the review clock be reactivated until all deficiencies have been addressed.

Please submit twenty copies of final printed labeling, ten of which are individually mounted on heavyweight paper or similar material, exactly as specified above as a "**Supplement - Changes Being Effected**". Incorporate all previous revisions as reflected in the most recently approved package insert. To facilitate review of your submission, provide a highlighted or marked-up copy that shows the changes that are being made.

These supplements should be submitted within 30 days from the date of this letter.

If you have any questions, call Paul David, R.Ph., Senior Regulatory Project Manager, at (301) 594-5530.

Sincerely,

{See appended electronic signature page}

Russell Katz, M.D.
Director
Division of Neuropharmacological Drug Products
Office of Drug Evaluation I
Center for Drug Evaluation and Research

RECEIVED
MAR 2 9 2004
KEN BONK
REGULATORY AFFAIRS

This is a representation of an electronic record that was signed electronically and this page is the manifestation of the electronic signature.

/s/

Russell Katz
3/19/04 04:06:47 PM

DEPARTMENT OF HEALTH & HUMAN SERVICES

Public Health Service

Food and Drug Administration
Rockville, MD 20857

CERTIFIED MAIL
RETURN RECEIPT REQUESTED

NDA 18-644
NDA 20-358
NDA 20-711

Tab 42

Glaxo Wellcome Inc.
Attention: James E. Murray
Director, Regulatory Affairs
P.O. Box 13398
Research Triangle Park, North Carolina 27709

Dear Mr. Murray:

Please refer to the Written Request, originally issued on July 21, 2000, that you received from the Center for Drug Evaluation and Research. This Written Request was issued under Section 505A of the Federal Food, Drug, and Cosmetic Act to conduct pediatric studies using bupropion hydrochloride. As you know, on January 4, 2002, the President signed into law the "Best Pharmaceuticals for Children Act," (BPCA) which both extended the pediatric exclusivity program established in the 1997 FDA Modernization Act (FDAMA) and provided new mechanisms for studying pediatric uses for drugs. The BPCA also contains new provisions of which you should be aware related to user fees, priority review, drug labeling, and disclosure of pediatric study results. FDA is revising its Guidance for Industry: Qualifying for Pediatric Exclusivity Under Section 505A of the Federal Food, Drug, and Cosmetic Act to provide additional information on the pediatric drugs study provisions of the BPCA.

FDA has received questions about whether sponsors who were issued Written Requests to conduct pediatric studies prior to passage of the BPCA, but who had not as yet submitted the reports of the studies as of January 4, 2002, would be governed by the provisions of FDAMA or the BPCA. In order to maximize the benefit to be derived from the BPCA and to minimize uncertainty and delay in implementing the pediatric exclusivity program, FDA has decided to reissue those Written Requests originally issued prior to passage of the BPCA for which studies have not already been submitted.

This letter is your notification that the Written Request (and any subsequent amendments) described above is considered to be reissued as of the date of this letter. The terms of the Written Request are not otherwise altered by this letter. If you believe that the Written Request should be amended, please contact the division directly.

Please note that if the original Written Request was issued under Section 505A(a), it will now be considered to be issued under Section 505A(b), due to the reordering of the sections, as described in Section 19 of the BPCA. If the original Written Request was issued under Section 505A(c), it will still be considered to be issued under Section 505A(c).

An important change to note is that, if the drug for which FDA issued the Written Request under 505A(c) has listed patent or exclusivity protection, new section 505(d)(4)(A) states that within 180 days of receipt of this "reissued" Written Request, you must notify FDA when the pediatric studies will be initiated, or that you do not agree to conduct the requested studies. New provisions at Section 505(d)(4)(B)-(F) describe alternative methods for obtaining these pediatric studies.

NDA 18-644
NDA 20-358
NDA 20-711
Page 2

If you have questions regarding the BPCA, please contact the Division of Pediatric Drug Development at (301) 594-7337. As noted above, requests to amend your Written Request should be directed to the review division.

Sincerely,

{See appended electronic signature page}

M. Dianne Murphy, M.D.
Director
Office of Counter-terrorism and Pediatric Drug Development
Center for Drug Evaluation and Research

This is a representation of an electronic record that was signed electronically and this page is the manifestation of the electronic signature.

/s/

Dianne Murphy
7/2/02 07:21:25 PM

DEPARTMENT OF HEALTH & HUMAN SERVICES

Public Health Service

Food and Drug Administration
Rockville MD 20857

Tab 43

NDA 20-031/S-037

Glaxo SmithKline
Attention: Thomas Kline
Director, U.S. Regulatory Affairs
1250 S. Collegeville Road, P.O. Box 5089
Collegeville, PA 19426-0989

Dear Mr. Kline:

Please refer to your supplemental new drug application dated and received April 11, 2002, submitted under section 505(b) of the Federal Food, Drug, and Cosmetic Act for Paxil (paroxetine hydrochloride) Immediate Release Tablets.

We acknowledge receipt of your amendments dated July 3, and August 8, 2002.

This supplemental new drug application proposes the use of Paxil in the treatment of major depressive disorder (MDD) and obsessive compulsive disorder (OCD) in the pediatric population.

We have completed the review of this application, as amended, and it is approvable. Before the application may be approved, however, it will be necessary for you to submit the following information and respond to the following issues:

Labeling

We agree that the results from Study 704 demonstrate the short-term efficacy of Paxil in pediatric patients with OCD, and that the results from Studies 329, 377, and 701 failed to demonstrate the efficacy of Paxil in pediatric patients with MDD. Given the fact that negative trials are frequently seen, even for antidepressant drugs that we know are effective, we agree that it would not be useful to describe these negative trials in labeling.

Accompanying this letter (Attachment) is the Agency's proposal for the labeling of Paxil in the treatment of pediatric OCD. We have used, as our base labeling, the most recently acceptable paroxetine labeling (see Agency letter dated October 2, 2002). Double underline font denotes additions to the labeling, and strikeout font denotes deletions to the labeling. Brackets [] embedded within the text that follows include comments and explanations concerning our proposed labeling. The Agency's revisions are based on the labeling changes proposed in your April 11, 2002 submission. For some sections, few changes were proposed, while others required extensive modification

Request for Additional Information

1. As conveyed in an electronic communication to you dated August 30, 2002, we are requesting that you submit additional ECG analyses. The ECG QT interval data which you included for study 715 (pharmacokinetic study) was only summary data.
   The following raw data is requested:

   a) QTc interval and heart rate data for the studies in children and adolescents.
   b) Any complete (i.e., collected for an entire dosing interval) adult PK, QTc interval and heart rate data.

2. As conveyed in an electronic communication to you dated July 15, 2002, we noted that you did not provide any analysis of ECG interval data for the controlled studies. The results provided for studies 701 and 704 consisted of a count of the numbers of patients with ECG abnormalities. In study 329, ECG abnormalities were considered adverse events but were not otherwise analyzed.

   In order to complete our review of this application, we are requesting that you submit the typical kind of analyses conducted for these type of data; i.e., an analysis of mean change from baseline for measured ECG intervals, and a count of the numbers of patients on drug or placebo exceeding potentially clinically significant thresholds. We request that you use the ECG data from the placebo-controlled, parallel group trials that included pre-treatment and on-treatment ECGs (studies 329, 701 and 715).

3. Please provide the exposure (total number of patients and person-years) for placebo in all studies combined.

4. Please prepare a table showing the duration of exposure and mean daily dose for all paroxetine patients. In this table, the columns should represent mean daily dose and the rows should represent duration of exposure. Patients should be enumerated within each cell, and each patient should be counted in only one cell, according to the patient's duration of exposure and mean daily dose. We can provide an example of such a table if it would be helpful.

5. ISS tables 18.43 through 18.47 provide a listing of paroxetine patients with serious adverse events. Please provide a similar listing for placebo patients. It would also be helpful to provide a summary tabulation of these serious adverse events, similar to ISS table 4.1.2.

6. Please provide further information on the serious adverse events that occurred in study 676; at the time of this submission, the treatment assignments were still blinded.

7. Table 6.14 in the ISS listed paroxetine treated patients who experienced adverse events coded under the terms hostility, emotional lability or agitation. However, the table did not include placebo patients, nor did it include psychiatric adverse events that were coded under other terms. Please prepare an expanded version of this table, including all psychiatric and behavioral adverse events, and also those that occurred among placebo patients. In addition, it would be helpful if you could attach the narrative case summaries for those events that were either serious or resulted in premature discontinuation.

8. Please provide your rationale for coding suicide attempts and other forms of self-injurious behavior under the

WHOART term "emotional lability."

9. ISS table 4.2.6 provides a comparison of weight gain velocity between paroxetine and placebo in study 329; however, the comparison is shown only by age subgroups. Please provide a comparison pooling all paroxetine and placebo patients across ages.

10. Weight corrected clearance was shown to be significantly higher in male children than in female children. Although section 16 of the ISS described analyses of adverse events according to age and gender subgroups, you did not explore the effect of gender on adverse event incidences within age subgroups. Please conduct an appropriate analysis to address this issue.

11. Tables 11.14, 11.15, and 11.16 in the ISS present the mean change from baseline for vital signs (including height and weight), for all subjects combined, children alone, and adolescents alone. Please perform an appropriate statistical test for the differences between treatment groups on these parameters.

12. We note that your application did not contain any information on environmental impact as required under 21 CFR 25.15. Please submit either a claim for environmental exclusion under 21 CFR 25.30 or 21 CFR 25.31 or an environmental assessment under 21 CFR 25.40.

Safety Update

Our assessment of the safety of Paxil in the pediatric population is based on our review of all safety information provided in your original submission. Please provide a final serious events update to include serious adverse events up to a more recent cutoff date.

Regulatory Status Update

Please provide any new information on the regulatory status of Paxil in the pediatric population worldwide.

Worldwide Literature Update

Please provide an updated worldwide literature search for paroxetine.

Phase 4 Commitments

As requested in an Agency letter dated January 10, 2001 and as part of the Agency's pediatric initiative, we believe that additional studies in young animals will be needed to support a complete pediatric assessment. Therefore, we are requesting that you commit, as a Phase 4 commitment, to conduct juvenile animal studies.

Since there are no standard protocols in this area, we suggest that you design a study that would address drug effects in animals of an age range which is analogous to that of the proposed patient population. In addition to the usual toxicological parameters, such a study would presumably evaluate effects on growth and neurological, behavioral, and reproductive development.

If additional information relating to the safety or effectiveness of this drug becomes available, revision of the labeling may be required.

Within 10 days after the date of this letter, you are required to amend the supplemental applications, notify us of your intent to file amendments, or follow one of your other options under 21 CFR 314.110. In the absence of any such action FDA may proceed to withdraw the applications. Any amendment should respond to all the deficiencies listed. We will not process a partial reply as a major amendment nor will the review clock be reactivated until all deficiencies have been addressed.

This product may be considered to be misbranded under the Federal Food, Drug, and Cosmetic Act if it is marketed with these changes prior to approval of this supplemental application.

If you have any questions, call Paul David, R.Ph., Senior Regulatory Project Manager, at (301) 594-5530.

Sincerely,

{See appended electronic signature page}

Russell Katz, M.D.
Director
Division of Neuropharmacological Drug Products
Office of Drug Evaluation I
Center for Drug Evaluation and Research

Attachment

FDA Public Health Advisory

FDA Public Health Advisory **Tab 44**

March 22, 2004

Subject: WORSENING DEPRESSION AND SUICIDALITY IN PATIENTS BEING TREATED WITH ANTIDEPRESSANT MEDICATIONS

Today the Food and Drug Administration (FDA) asked manufacturers of the following antidepressant drugs to include in their labeling a Warning statement that recommends close observation of adult and pediatric patients treated with these agents for worsening depression or the emergence of suicidality. The drugs that are the focus of this new Warning are: Prozac (fluoxetine); Zoloft (sertraline); Paxil (paroxetine); Luvox (fluvoxamine); Celexa (citalopram); Lexapro (escitalopram); Wellbutrin (bupropion); Effexor (venlafaxine); Serzone (nefazodone); and Remeron (mirtazapine).

Warning Information

- Health care providers should carefully monitor patients receiving antidepressants for possible worsening of depression or suicidality, especially at the beginning of therapy or when the dose either increases or decreases. Although FDA has not concluded that these drugs cause worsening depression or suicidality, health care providers should be aware that worsening of symptoms could be due to the underlying disease or might be a result of drug therapy.

- Heath care providers should carefully evaluate patients in whom depression persistently worsens, or emergent suicidality is severe, abrupt in onset, or was not part of the presenting symptoms, to determine what intervention, including discontinuing or modifying the current drug therapy, is indicated.

- Anxiety, agitation, panic attacks, insomnia, irritability, hostility, impulsivity, akathisia (severe restlessness), hypomania, and mania have been reported in adult and pediatric patients being treated with antidepressants for major depressive disorder as well as for other indications, both psychiatric and nonpsychiatric. Although FDA has not concluded that these symptoms are a precursor to either worsening of depression or the emergence of suicidal impulses, there is concern that patients who experience one or more of these symptoms may be at increased risk for worsening depression or suicidality. Therefore, therapy should be evaluated, and medications may need to be discontinued, when symptoms are severe, abrupt in onset, or were not part of the patient's presenting symptoms.

- If a decision is made to discontinue treatment, certain of these medications should be tapered rather than stopped abruptly (see labeling for individual drug products for details).

- Because antidepressants are believed to have the potential for inducing manic episodes in patients with bipolar disorder, there is a concern about using antidepressants alone in this population. Therefore, patients should be adequately screened to determine if they are at risk for bipolar disorder before initiating antidepressant treatment so that they can be appropriately monitored during treatment. Such screening should include a detailed psychiatric history, including a family history of suicide, bipolar disorder, and depression.

- Health care providers should instruct patients, their families and their caregivers to be alert for the emergence of agitation, irritability, and the other symptoms described above, as well as the emergence of suicidality and worsening depression, and to report such symptoms immediately to their health care provider.

Background

Among antidepressants, only Prozac (fluoxetine) is approved for the treatment of pediatric major depressive disorder. Prozac (fluoxetine), Zoloft (sertraline), and Luvox (fluvoxamine) are approved for pediatric obsessive compulsive disorder. None of these drugs is approved as monotherapy for use in treating bipolar depression, either in adults or children.

The requested labeling changes are consistent with recommendations made to the Agency at a meeting of the Psychopharmacological Drugs Advisory Committee (PDAC) and the Pediatric Subcommittee of the Anti-Infective Drugs Advisory Committee (Peds AC), held on February 2, 2004. The possibility of suicidality associated with the use of antidepressant drug products in the pediatric population was also the subject of two previous FDA communications (FDA Talk Paper on June 19, 2003, and FDA Public Health Advisory on October 27, 2003).

FDA is continuing to review available clinical trial data for pediatric patients with depression and other psychiatric disorders to try to determine whether there is evidence that some or all antidepressants increase the risk of suicidality. Later this summer, the FDA plans to update the PDAC and Peds AC about the results of this review.

FDA plans to work closely with each of the nine manufacturers of the antidepressants that are the subject of today's request to continue investigating how to optimize the safe use of these drugs and implement the proposed labeling changes and other safety communications in a timely manner.

Back to Top Back to Antidepressant Info

Date created: March 22, 2004

Wyeth Pharmaceuticals Inc.
P.O. Box 8299
Philadelphia, PA 19101-8299

Worldwide Regulatory Affairs

Wyeth

Tab 45

April 2, 2004

Effexor (venlafaxine HCl) Tablets
NDA No. 20-151/S-028

Response to March 31, 2004 Teleconference

Russell Katz, M.D., Director
Food and Drug Administration
Center for Drug Evaluation and Research
Division of Neuropharmacological Drug Products (HFD-120)
Attn.: Document Room 4008
1451 Rockville Pike
Rockville, MD 20852

Dear Dr. Katz,

Reference is made to our "Changes Being Effected" (CBE) supplement for Effexor (venlafaxine HCl) Tablets (NDA No. 20-151/S-028) submitted on August 8, 2003. In that CBE supplement, Wyeth inserted the following wording into the Effexor package insert:

> "In pediatric clinical trials, there were increased reports of hostility and, especially in Major Depressive Disorder, suicide-related adverse events such as suicidal ideation and self-harm."

Reference is further made to the March 19, 2004 FDA approvable letter, in which the Agency stated they do not agree with the changes to the package insert in our August 8, 2003 submission.

Additionally, reference is also made to the March 30, 2004 e-mail sent by me to Mr. Paul David, Senior Regulatory Project Manager, in which Wyeth informed FDA of our position to retain this wording in our package insert and to provide a cross-reference to the new class labeling subsection ("**WARNINGS-Clinical Worsening and Suicide**") presented in FDA's March 19, 2004 letter.

Response to March 31, 2004 Teleconference
Page No. 2

In a March 31, 2004 conversation, Mr. David reiterated FDA's stance that no causality had been established yet between the pediatric population taking venlafaxine and the emergence of suicidality. However, Mr. David also indicated that the current proposed wording might be acceptable if text was added that conveyed the lack of a definitive causality. Therefore, Wyeth is proposing the following text for your consideration:

> **"PRECAUTIONS**
> **Pediatric Use**
> Safety and effectiveness in pediatric patients have not been established.
>
> In pediatric clinical trials, there were increased reports of hostility and, especially in Major Depressive Disorder, suicide-related adverse events such as suicidal ideation and self-harm. However, a causal association between children and adolescents taking venlafaxine and the emergence of suicidality has not been definitively established (see **WARNINGS-Clinical Worsening and Suicide**)."

Wyeth also agrees to add "tinnitus" to the subsection **ADVERSE REACTIONS/Postmarketing Reports** as requested by FDA in the March 19, 2004 approvable letter:

If there are any questions regarding this submission, please contact me at (484) 865-3103.

Sincerely,
Wyeth Pharmaceuticals, Inc.

Kenneth R. Bonk

Kenneth R. Bonk, Director
Worldwide Regulatory Affairs

S:\CNS\FDA\Effexor\NDA\S052.doc

CONFIDENTIAL & PROPRIETARY

DEPARTMENT OF HEALTH & HUMAN SERVICES

Food and Drug Administration
Rockville MD 20857

Tab 46

The Honorable Joe Barton
Chairman
Committee on Energy and Commerce
U.S. House of Representatives
Washington, D.C. 20515-6115

APR 14 2004

Dear Mr. Chairman:

Thank you for your letter of March 24, 2004, concerning the Food and Drug Administration's (FDA or the Agency) decision to issue its March 22, 2004, *Talk Paper* entitled, "FDA Issues Public Health Advisory on Cautions for Use of Antidepressants in Adults and Children" and events surrounding an FDA internal consult prepared by Andrew D. Mosholder, M.D., M.P.H. on this issue.

Certain of the enclosed documents contain trade secret, commercial confidential, or other privileged information protected from disclosure to the public under the Freedom of Information Act (Title 5, United States Code [U.S.C.] section 552), the Trade Secrets Act (18, U.S.C. section 1905), and FDA regulations. The Committee should not publish or otherwise make public any such information. We would be glad to discuss with the Committee staff the protected status of any specific information. IMS Health and ADVANCEPCS utilization data is contained in a memo prepared by Dr. Mosholder. FDA obtained this data under contracts with IMS Health and ADVANCEPCS. The terms of the contracts stipulate that the utilization data cannot be released to the public. We request that the Committee not publish or otherwise make public this information. Finally, as discussed with Committee staff, we have redacted personal privacy information from the enclosed documents.

Your letter expressed a concern about evidence or reports developed or obtained by FDA staff regarding possible suicide-related adverse events associated with the use of specific drugs and also a concern that information relating to using these drugs safely in pediatric populations may not have been made public in a timely way. We want to assure you that at this time, based on our review, we do not believe that to have been the case.

FDA fully recognizes the critical public health importance of a possible link between use of antidepressant drugs in children and suicidal thoughts or behavior. Our goal has been, and remains, to carefully evaluate all the available data in a scientifically rigorous manner before reaching a conclusion. Our judgments in this matter will strongly influence how antidepressants are prescribed in children in the future. What we must do is give parents and physicians the very best information, because the health risks of incorrect conclusions are potentially great. In conducting its evaluation, FDA has followed its usual practice of engaging the expertise of experienced reviewers from different parts of the Agency and from outside sources to ensure that these issues are rigorously examined. The collective input from the various expert sources has been the basis for developing the Agency's current position on this issue.

Background on FDA's Review of Antidepressant Drugs

To place FDA's recent public announcements on this issue in proper perspective, it is important to briefly review the history of our examination of the issue of a possible link between the use of antidepressants in children and suicidal thoughts or behavior. Under the pediatric exclusivity provisions of the Food and Drug Administration Modernization Act, FDA issued requests to manufacturers of antidepressants for studies of these drugs in children. During our review of a supplemental new drug application submitted by GlaxoSmithKline (GSK) that contained the requested studies of the use of Paxil (paroxetine) in children, reviewers in the Division of Neuropharmacological Drug Products (DNDP) of FDA's Center for Drug Evaluation and Research (CDER or the Center) noted a greater number of adverse events that were coded under the term "emotional liability" in the group of patients treated with Paxil compared to placebo in some, but not all, of the studies. The reviewers noted that the actual events that were coded under this term included suicide thoughts and attempts as well as other forms of non-suicidal self-injurious behavior. In an effort to better understand these events and to further explore the extent of episodes of suicidal thoughts or behavior in children treated with Paxil, DNDP requested that GSK reanalyze their data and better characterize the adverse events that were identified under the term emotional liability.

GSK submitted their report to the Center on May 22, 2003, and on June 6, 2003, Dr. Russ Katz, the director of DNDP, requested that the Office of Drug Safety (ODS) perform a consultative review of the newly submitted safety data. Dr. Katz requested that Dr. Andy Mosholder be assigned as the primary reviewer for the consult since Dr. Mosholder had previously been involved in reviewing data on the safety of antidepressants when he worked as a reviewer in DNDP.

Following its initial review of these new data for Paxil, FDA issued a *Talk Paper* on June 19, 2003, that stated: "Although the FDA has not completed its evaluation of the new safety data, FDA is recommending that Paxil not be used in children or adolescents for the treatment of major depressive disorder (MDD)." FDA also expanded its investigation of a possible link between use of antidepressants in children and suicidal thoughts or behavior by requesting data similar to that submitted by GSK from the manufacturers of eight other antidepressant drugs that had been studied in children. On July 22, 2003, requests for data were sent to the manufacturers of the following drugs: Prozac (fluoxetine), Zoloft (setraline), Luvox (fluvoxamine), Celexa (citalopram), Wellbutrin (bupropion), Effexor (venlafaxine), Serzone (nefazodone), and Remeron (mirtazapine). These data requests from the Center, and the submissions from the manufacturers in response to them, have provided the core data on which the Agency has developed its scientific review of this issue.

As the reviewers in DNDP and ODS began conducting their more detailed reviews of these new safety data and carefully evaluated the narrative descriptions of the reported adverse events, the reviewers identified several new issues for further evaluation. These additional issues included the following matters:

1. A number of the adverse events classified under the category "possibly suicide related." For example, one child had hit her head with her hand, a number of children had engaged in superficial cutting behavior, and a number of children had ingested small numbers of pills in sight of parents, which while potentially of concern, taken alone, would not necessarily be an indication of suicidal behavior.
2. Although there were more adverse events that were characterized as "possibly suicide related" in patients taking the antidepressant drug compared to those taking placebo in some of the trials in children, this pattern was not consistently observed across all of the trials, even within individual drug programs.
3. There was a concern that due to the methods used by the manufacturers in searching their database, the possibility existed that not all adverse events of possible interest in addressing the potential risk of suicidality had in fact been captured.

To more fully evaluate these new issues, the DNDP determined that additional data searches and analyses were necessary. To further address issue 1, whether the reported adverse events represented suicidal behavior, Agency staff determined that an independent panel of experts in suicidology should be convened to carefully evaluate and reclassify the reported adverse events. DNDP arranged for this work to be performed under a contract with Columbia University and this review is ongoing. Once the reclassification of the adverse events is completed, the Center believes that it may be able to conduct more definitive analyses of the data. To further address issues 2 and 3, on November 24, 2003, DNDP requested additional data from the manufacturers of the other antidepressants that had been studied in children. The division specifically requested individual patient data for all the studies. The availability of these more detailed data would permit a more refined analysis, taking into consideration possible imbalances across study groups in these trials, and a more complete accounting of the search methods employed by these companies to ensure that possible cases of suicidality had not been overlooked. We expect these additional analyses to be completed this summer, and we will present these new analyses to the Advisory Committee for discussion. We expect this second Advisory Committee meeting to occur in late summer.

While the Center was conducting its more in-depth review of the data from the pediatric clinical trials, planning was also under way to hold an Advisory Committee meeting February 2, 2004, to review the post-marketing safety reporting for a number of products that had been granted pediatric exclusivity. A review of the post-marketing safety data is mandated for such products under the Best Pharmaceuticals for Children Act. One of the drugs scheduled for review at the February 2, 2004 Advisory Committee meeting was Paxil. In planning for the discussion of the safety of the use of Paxil in children at the Advisory Committee meeting, the Agency initially intended to broaden the meeting to include a discussion of the Agency's review of the safety concerns that arose from the data from studies of the use of antidepressants in children. However, as the reviews and meeting planning progressed, it became clear that the additional analyses of the data from the clinical trials of antidepressants in children would not be complete in time to present the Agency's final assessment of these data at that meeting. Therefore, the Agency decided to proceed with the plans to discuss the post-marketing safety data for Paxil at the meeting, to brief the Advisory Committee on the Agency's progress in evaluating the data from the clinical trials of antidepressants in children, and to solicit advice and comment regarding the Agency's plans for further analyses. The plan included returning to the Advisory Committee for another meeting after the Agency's more definitive analyses of the clinical trial data were complete to solicit Advisory Committee input prior to further regulatory action.

While CDER was moving ahead with plans for the February 2, 2004, Advisory Committee meeting, Dr. Mosholder was nearing completion of his review of the data from the clinical trials. Based on his review, he believed that the available data were sufficient to reach a conclusion about an association between the use of antidepressants and suicidality in children and to recommend that additional regulatory action would be appropriate without the need for the more in-depth case classification or analyses that had already been initiated by DNDP. Dr. Mosholder shared his conclusions with his supervisors and with the rest of the team involved in reviewing this issue. However, the other members of the review team, including his direct supervisors, did not agree with his regulatory conclusion that no further analyses were needed and continued to believe that additional analyses should be conducted before the Agency could reach a conclusion on these data. There was a discussion within the review team as to whether Dr. Mosholder's regulatory conclusions on the data should be presented in some form at the February 2, 2004, meeting. After considering the issue carefully, CDER staff decided that the data from which Dr. Mosholder reached his conclusions would be presented to the Advisory Committee meeting and that they would acknowledge as part of their presentation to the Committee that some reviewers had reached a conclusion that the data at this time were sufficient to conclude that there was a link between antidepressant use and suicidality in children. However, given the Agency's concerns regarding the limitations of the data and the plans to pursue case reclassification and more in-depth analyses, CDER decided that having Dr. Mosholder present his conclusion to the Advisory Committee, with the appearance that it was an Agency determination, would be potentially harmful to public health as it might lead patients who were actually benefiting from the use of these drugs to inappropriately discontinue therapy. CDER believed that disclosure of the available data to the Advisory Committee at the meeting along with a description of the limitations of those data in supporting a definitive conclusion, as well as a description of the Agency's plans to further evaluate the data was the best way to serve the public health on this very complex and important issue. The Agency takes very seriously its responsibility to the public to find the right answer to this question, and a premature conclusion that the drugs are harmful that does not hold up to more careful review would be a disservice to the public health given the serious, and potentially life-threatening nature of severe depression.

At the Advisory Committee meeting, Dr. Katz made an opening presentation of the issues and questions and made clear that some within the Agency believed that the data were conclusive. Dr. Tom Laughren from DNDP gave a more extensive presentation in which he carefully reviewed the available data and its strengths and weaknesses. Dr. Laughren also described to the Committee the Agency's plans to further evaluate the data and to return to the Committee for a more definitive review once those analyses were complete. Dr. Laughren specifically presented the same data from which Dr. Mosholder had reached his conclusions and the same data from which the Medicines and Healthcare Products Regulatory Agency (MHRA) in the UK reached its conclusions.

Although Dr. Mosholder did not present the clinical trial data or his conclusions at the Advisory Committee meeting, he is a member of the review team for this project and did make a presentation to the Committee regarding his evaluation of the postmarketing safety data for Paxil. The presentation of the clinical trial data by the staff in DNDP and the postmarketing safety data by the staff in ODS is fully consistent with CDER's normal, approach to the division of these review responsibilities.

In summary, the Center's review process involves a multidisciplinary approach to ensure that expertise from various areas of the Agency and from outside groups is brought to bear on an issue to ensure that a comprehensive and rigorous scientific analysis is completed that serves as the basis for the Agency's conclusions and actions. The review process honors and explicitly encourages individual reviewers to share their conclusions and recommendations with the review team to help inform the Center's decisions and actions. In some cases, the opinion of an individual reviewer may not be consistent with the Center's position on an issue. This occurs regularly and is to be expected in a large scientific organization that values open discussion of issues. In such cases the Center has procedures in place to ensure that the reviewer's position is documented, fully considered, and addressed by managers as part of the process.

Those procedures were followed in this case and, in the interest of full disclosure and open debate, the Agency ensured that the data were presented for public review. We specifically acknowledged at the public meeting that some within the Agency had reached different conclusions. The Advisory Committee fully discussed the available data regarding the safety of the use of antidepressants in children and concurred with the Agency's plans for further analyses prior to reaching more definitive conclusions. At the meeting, based on the presentations, the Advisory Committee recommended that FDA take interim steps to warn physicians, patients, and parents of the potential safety concern and the need to carefully monitor patients for evidence of suicidal thoughts or behavior while taking antidepressant drugs. The Agency concurred with the Advisory Committee's recommendations and issued a Public Health Advisory on this issue on March 22, 2004, along with a request to each of the manufacturers that they update the labeling for their product to reflect this information. The Agency is continuing its review of this important issue and plans to return to the Advisory Committee for further discussion when the additional analyses are complete later this summer.

FDA raised serious questions about the antidepressants, took the initiative in acquiring the relevant data, and has proceeded with careful analyses of the data from different perspectives inside and outside the Agency. The assessment of whether the antidepressant drugs under review increase the risk of suicidal thinking or behavior is critically important to patient safety. FDA's assessment on this issue is designed to achieve the most scientifically rigorous review possible.

In the meantime, we recognize the important role of Congress and the Committee, and share the objective of assuring an open and transparent process for evaluating these potential safety concerns. In response to your March 24, 2004, letter requesting a large voluume of materials, information and data, the Agency has been working closely with Committee staff to produce the necessary information. On April 1 and April 13, and April 14, 2004, in conversations between Patrick McGarey of FDA's Office of Legislation and Kelli Andrews and Alan Slobodin of the

Committee staff, we agreed to partially respond by providing responses to questions numbered 11 and 12 and a partial response to questions 1, 2, and 4. We have restated your questions followed by our answer. We sill continue to work with Committee staff on this document request, and may provide additional responsive materials to these questions if they are identified.

1. **All records provided by or to the FDA in connection with the February 2, 2004 FDA Advisory Committee meeting involving the Psychopharmacological Drugs Advisory Committee (PDAC) and the Pediatric SubCommittee of the Anti-Infective Drugs Advisory Committee (Peds AC), including, but not limited to, records relating to the planning of this meeting and its agenda.**

Based on conversations with Committee staff, we are providing records provided by or to the Advisory Committee Staff from outside parties related to the February 2, 2004, FDA Advisory Committee Meeting. The documents are enclosed at Tab A. As we discussed with Committee staff, due to the very large volume of documents that are responsive to this question, and in light of the difficulty we had reviewing and redacting personal privacy information and producing these documents by the time we issued this letter, we are providing a partial response at this time. We will discuss with Committee staff the timetable and need to produce further documents in response to this question.

As part of the meeting process, we published a transcript and documents. These documents also may be relevant to your inquiry and can be found at:
http://www.fda.gov/cder/drug/antidepressants/default.htm

2. **All records of Dr. Andrew Mosholder, Dr. Mary Willy, Dr. Russell Katz, Ms. Anne Trontell and Dr. Thomas Laughren, relating to efficacy and safety of anti-depressants in the pediatric and/or adolescent population, including, but not limited to, all draft or final reports, internal correspondence, e-mails and notes concerning pediatric or adolescent anti-depressant clinical trials and any records relating to spontaneous reports (AERS system) on the same issue.**

Based on conversations with Committee staff, we are providing the records compiled by Dr. Andrew Mosholder beginning with records created on January 1, 2003. The documents are enclosed at Tab B.

4. **All records relating to GlaxoSmithKline's submission of data analyses in pediatric/adolescent clinical trials involving Paxil, including, but not limited to, all submissions contained as attachments to their May 22, 2003 letter to the FDA.**

Based on conversations with Committee staff, we are providing records from the NDA file beginning with records created on October 10, 2002. The documents are enclosed at Tab C. In particular, please note that these materials contain or are reasonably likely to contain trade secret, commercial confidential, or otherwise privileged information that would not be subject to public disclosure under the Agency's FOI regulations.

11. A listing of all the pediatric/adolescent clinical trials involving anti-depressants that the FDA received data for which there was an obligation for the company to submit the data to the FDA. For each such trial, include the following information:

a. Name of the company;
b. Name of the anti-depressant;
c. Date when pediatric clinical trial data was submitted to the FDA;
d. Date when pediatric clinical trial was completed by company;
e. Summary of FDA's "response" to the clinical trial and what, if any, regulatory action FDA took with respect to approving the particular drug for an indication in the pediatric population.

We have provided this information in chart form at Tab D.

12. State the person(s) at FDA responsible for evaluating and providing a written analysis of the data that was requested by FDA, in the summer and fall of 2003, from various manufacturers of anti-depressants who performed clinical trials in children.

Dr. Andrew Mosholder of the Office of Drug Safety was responsible for evaluating the summary data from the pediatric clinical trials on antidepressants that was submitted in response to the Agency's July, 2003 letters. Drs. Tarek Hammad and Judy Racoosin from the Safety Group within the Division of Neuropharmacological Drug Products have responsibility for analyzing the patient-level data submitted by sponsors in response to the Agency's October, 2003 request for these electronic data sets. The analysis of these patient-level data are tied to the reclassification of clinical cases is accomplished by the expert panel that has been assembled by our consultants at Columbia University.

Thank you for your interest in this matter. A similar letter is being sent to Chairman Greenwood without the enclosure. If we can be of further assistance, please let us know.

Sincerely,

Robert C. McEwen, Acting

Amit K. Sachdev
Associate Commissioner
for Legislation

Enclosures

M E M O R A N D U M **DEPARTMENT OF HEALTH AND HUMAN SERVICES**
PUBLIC HEALTH SERVICE
FOOD AND DRUG ADMINISTRATION
CENTER FOR DRUG EVALUATION AND RESEARCH

DATE: August 16, 2004

Tab 47

FROM: Thomas P. Laughren, M.D.
Team Leader, Psychiatric Drug Products
Division of Neuropharmacological Drug Products
HFD-120

SUBJECT: Overview for September 13 & 14, 2004 Meeting of Psychopharmacological Drugs Advisory Committee (PDAC) and Pediatric Drugs Advisory Committee (Peds AC)

TO: Members of PDAC and Peds AC

On September 13th and 14th, the PDAC and Peds AC will meet to consider the occurrence of suicidality in the course of treatment of pediatric patients with various antidepressants. This September meeting is followup to a meeting on this same topic held on February 2, 2004. At the February meeting, the committees were presented with preliminary data on suicidality occurring in clinical trials involving pediatric patients being treated with various antidepressants. The major focus of that meeting was on FDA's plans for a more definitive evaluation and analysis of these data. The two key aspects of FDA's plans for evaluation of these data were the following: (1) the classification of suicidality events captured under the broad category of "possibly suicide-related" into more specific and meaningful categories by experts in pediatric suicidality; and, (2) an analysis of patient-level data from these trials that would permit adjustment for potential confounders. The committees generally endorsed FDA's proposed plan for further evaluation of these data. This additional work has now been completed, and the committees will be presented the results of these analyses.

The committees recommended at the February meeting that, while we were completing our analyses of the pediatric suicidality data, FDA should strengthen the labeling for these products. In particular, there was concern that some patients being treated with these drugs may not be closely monitored for suicidality. There was a consensus of the committees that, whether or not any of these drugs could be shown more definitively to have a role in the induction of suicidality, it would be important to remind clinicians treating patients with any of these drugs to be alert to the emergence of suicidality and to various other symptoms that might represent precursors to suicidality. FDA issued a Public Health Advisory on March 22, 2004, announcing an initiative to ask companies to add Warning statements to address this concern. This new Warning language has been accepted by the sponsors for all of these products.

The new language warns clinicians to observe closely patients who are being treated with antidepressants, for clinical worsening and suicidality, especially at the beginning of a course of therapy, or at times of dose changes. Clinicians are advised to consider changing the therapeutic regimen in patients whose depression is persistently worse or whose emergent suicidality is severe, abrupt in onset, or was not part of the patient's presenting symptoms. The new language notes that a causal role for antidepressants in inducing such behaviors has not been established. The new warning applies both to adults and children, and is not limited to patients being treated for major depression, but rather, applies to patients being treated with antedepressants for any condition, psychiatric or nonpsychiatric. Clinicians are also advised to observe for the emergence of other symptoms that have been reported in association with antidepressant treatment due to the concern, but not yet proof, for a possible causal link between such symptoms and worsening depression or suicidality. These symptoms include: anxiety, agitation, panic attacks, insomnia, irritability, hostility (aggressiveness), impulsivity, akathisia (psychomotor restlessness), hypomania and mania. The new language also advises families and caregivers of these patients to be alert to the emergence of these symptoms, and to report such symptoms to the health care providers. Finally, the new language alerts clinicians to be particular careful in using these medications in patients with bipolar depression or a family history of bipolar disorder.

The primary focus of our presentations at this meeting will be to provide you with (1) a detailed description of our approach to evaluating and analyzing the pediatric suicidality data, and (2) the results of this work. However, we have also included presentations on related studies, in particular, several pertinent epidemiological studies and TADS (Treatment of Adolescents with Depression Study). Thus, you will hear presentations by both FDA staff and experts in pediatric suicidality from the academic community outside of FDA.

- Dr. Diane Wysowski from the Office of Drug Safety will summarize and comment on findings from several published epidemiological studies that are pertinent to the concerns about suicidality in association with antidepressant drug treatment.

- Dr. John March from Duke University will briefly summarize results from the NIMH-sponsored TADS (Treatment of Adolescents with Depression Study), with an emphasis on findings pertinent to suicidality.

- Dr. Greg Dubitsky from the Division of Neuropharmacological Drug Products will provide an overview of the 23 pediatric antidepressant trials that have been the focus of our review, in order to give you important background information about the structure and conduct of these trials, and about the populations studied.

- Dr. Kelly Posner, from Columbia University, will describe their approach to the blinded classification of suicidality events and their experience in accomplishing this task.

- Dr. Solomon Iyasu from the Office of Counter Terrorism and Pediatrics will provide comments on FDA's independent appraisal of the Columbia approach to classification of suicidality data.

- Dr. Tarek Hammad, from the Safety Group in the Division of Neuropharmacological Drug Products, will present the results of our analysis of the suicidality data, using the events classified by the experts assembled by Columbia University.

- Dr. Andrew Mosholder from the Office of Drug Safety will provide comments based on a comparison of the findings from his initial analysis of pediatric suicidality data that was completed before the results of the Columbia classification of cases was available, with analyses conducted by Dr. Hammad since the classifications were completed.

- You will also hear presentations by several sponsors of antidepressant products who have requested an opportunity to comment on the suicidality data for their products.

There will be an open public session on the afternoon of September 13th, to provide an opportunity for others in the community to make statements pertinent to this concern about a possible causal association between antidepressant drug treatment and emergent suicidality in pediatric patients.

The morning of September 14th has been reserved for your deliberations on this topic.

The background package for this meeting will include the following documents in addition to this cover memo:

- A January 5, 2004 memo written by me in preparation for the February 2, 2004 Advisory Committee meeting. This memo provides a more complete discussion of various events leading up to that earlier meeting and the basis for DNDP's analysis of the suicidality data. It also includes a summary of efficacy findings from the 15 studies in pediatric major depressive disorder (pp. 5-6 and Appendix 1).

- Summary minutes from the February 2, 2004 Advisory Committee Meeting.

- Several published epidemiological studies that are pertinent to the concerns about suicidality in association with antidepressant drug treatment.

- A recent paper (August 18, 2004) from JAMA providing the results of the Treatment for Adolescents with Depression Study (TADS), along with an editorial commenting on the findings from this trial.

- A review by Dr. Greg Dubitsky from DNDP, providing details about the structure and conduct of these trials, and about the populations studied.

- A review by Dr. Solomon Iyasu from OCTAP, describing the methods and results of OCTAP's independent appraisal of the Columbia classification effort. His review includes as appendices several documents from the Columbia University suicidality group describing their approach to the blinded classification of suicidality events.

- A review by Dr. Tarek Hammad from DNDP, providing the detailed results of the analysis of the pediatric suicidality data.

- A review by Dr. Andrew Mosholder from ODS, providing the results of his analysis of the original pediatric suicidality data completed before the results of the classification of cases was available, along with an update on that review to provide a comparison of the findings of that initial analysis, with analyses conducted on the basis of the definitively classified cases.

- Public Health Advisorys on suicidality and antidepressant medications issued by FDA on June 19, 2003, October 27, 2003, and March 22, 2004, and related documents.

- Product labeling for 7 antidepressants that have implemented the labeling changes announced in the March 22, 2004 Public Health Advisory

- Briefing packages from several companies

Additional background information on this general topic of antidepressants and suicidality, including documents generated in relation to the February 2nd advisory committee meeting and those developed in association with FDA's March 22nd Public Health Advisory can be found at the following link: http://www.fda.gov/cder/drug/antidepressants/default.htm. A transcript for the February, 2004 meeting can be found at this link as well.

I would like to draw your attention to some particular issues of interest as you review the package and prepare to answer the questions we will present to you. The data continue to show differences between individual drugs, drug classes, and even across studies within individual drugs, even when the focus is limited to those trials done in patients with major depressive disorder. We have explored a number of possible explanations for such differences, but none has provided a satisfactory answer. Thus, while there remains a "signal" of risk for suicidality for some drugs in some trials, it is important to note that the data are not "black and white" in providing a clear and definitive answer to the question of a link between the drugs and pediatric suicidality. Consequently, we are very interested in hearing comments from committee members on how these data should be interpreted and how these data should be translated into information to guide physicians, patients, and families in the use of these drugs. Now that we have completed our analysis of these data, we would like to move forward to update the labeling of these products to reflect the results from these analyses, and we seek your specific guidance on how best to accomplish this task.

The following are draft questions and topics for discussion at the meeting. These questions and discussion topics may be revised before the meeting.

- Please comment on our approach to classification of the possible cases of suicidality (suicidal thinking and/or behaviors) and our analyses of the resulting data from the 23 pediatric trials involving 9 antidepressant drugs.

- Do the suicidality data from these trials support the conclusion that any or all of these drugs increase the risk of suicidality in pediatric patients?

- If the answer to the previous question is yes, to which of these 9 drugs does this increased risk of suicidality apply? Please discuss, for example, whether the increased risk applies to all antidepressants, only certain classes of antidepressants, or only certain antidepressants.

- If there is a class suicidality risk, or a suicidality risk that is limited to certain drugs in this class, how should this information be reflected in the labeling of each of the products? What, if any, additional regulatory actions should the Agency take?

- Please discuss what additional research is needed to further delineate the risks and benefits of these drugs in pediatric patients with psychiatric illness.

The FDA relies on the knowledge, judgement, experience and wisdom of scientists and practitioners like you to help determine how to move forward and address newly emerging issues related to drug development. We thank you for your time and effort, and we look forward to seeing and hearing from you on September 13th and 14th.

cc:
HFD-120/TLaughren/RKatz/JRacoosin/PDavid
HFD-960/DMurphy/SMurphy/SCummins
HFD-030/PSeligman/ATrontel/MAvignan
HFD-040/RTemple
HFD-020/JJenkins

DOC: PDAC_Sept2004_Memo_Laughren_04.doc

Food and Drug Administration (FDA)
Center for Drug Evaluation and Research (CDER)

Tab 48

Joint Meeting of the
CDER Psychopharmacologic Drugs Advisory Committee
and the FDA Pediatric Advisory Committee

September 13-14, 2004

Questions and Issues

Occurrence of Suicidality in Clinical Trials for Antidepressant Drugs in Pediatric Patients

Questions/Issues for which FDA would like committee discussion and feedback:

1. Please comment on our approach to classification of the possible cases of suicidality (suicidal thinking and/or behaviors) and our analyses of the resulting data from the 23 + 1 pediatric trials involving 9 antidepressant drugs.

2. Do the suicidality data from these trials support the conclusion that any or all of these drugs increase the risk of suicidality in pediatric patients?

3. If the answer to the previous question is yes, to which of these 9 drugs does this increased risk of suicidality apply?
   - Please discuss, for example, whether the increased risk applies to all antidepressants, only certain classes of antidepressants, or only certain antidepressants.

4. If there is a class suicidality risk, or a suicidality risk that is limited to certain drugs in this class, how should this information be reflected in the labeling of each of the products?
   - What, if any, additional regulatory actions should the Agency take?

5. Please discuss what additional research is needed to further delineate the risks and benefits of these drugs in pediatric patients with psychiatric illness.

Press Office
Food and Drug Administration
U.S. Department of Health and Human Services

Tab 49

STATEMENT
September 16, 2004

Media Inquiries: 301-827-6242
Consumer Inquiries: 888-INFO-FDA

FDA STATEMENT ON RECOMMENDATIONS OF THE PSYCHOPHARMACOLOGIC DRUGS AND PEDIATRIC ADVISORY COMMITTEES

The Food and Drug Administration (FDA) generally supports the recommendations that were recently made to the agency by the Psychopharmacologic Drugs and Pediatric Advisory Committees regarding reports of an increased risk of suicidality (suicidal thoughts and actions) associated with the use of certain antidepressants in pediatric patients. FDA has begun working expeditiously to adopt new labeling to enhance the warnings associated with the use of antidepressants and to bolster the information provided to patients when these drugs are dispensed.

In summary, the members of the advisory committees:

- endorsed FDA's approach to classifying and analyzing the suicidal events and behaviors observed in controlled clinical trials and expressed their view that the new analyses increased their confidence in the results;

- concluded that the finding of an increased risk of suicidality in pediatric patients applied to all the drugs studied (Prozac, Zoloft, Remeron, Paxil, Effexor, Celexa Wellbutrin, Luvox and Serzone) in controlled clinical trials;
- recommended that any warning related to an increased risk of suicidality in pediatric patients should be applied to all antidepressant drugs, including those that have not been studied in controlled clinical trials in pediatric patients, since the available data are not adequate to exclude any single medication from an increased risk;
- reached a split decision (15-yes, 8-no) regarding recommending a "black-box" warning related to an increased risk for suicidality in pediatric patients for all antidepressant drugs;
- endorsed a patient information sheet ("Medication Guide") for this class of drugs to be provided to the patient or their caregiver with every prescription;
- recommended that the products not be contraindicated in this country because the Committees thought access

to these therapies was important for those who could benefit; and

- recommended that the results of controlled pediatric trials of depression be included in the labeling for antidepressant drugs.

####

DEPARTMENT OF HEALTH & HUMAN SERVICES

Public Health Service

Food and Drug Administration
Rockville MD 20857

NDA 20-151/S-028/S-030/S-032
NDA 20-699/S-041/S-048/S-052

Tab 50

Wyeth Pharmaceuticals, Inc.
Attention: Kenneth R. Bonk
Director, Worldwide Regulatory Affairs
P.O. Box 8299
Philadelphia, PA 19101-1245

Dear Mr. Bonk:

We acknowledge receipt of your supplemental new drug applications dated April 30, 2004, submitted under section 505(b) of the Federal Food, Drug, and Cosmetic Act for Effexor (venlafaxine hydrochloride) Immediate Release Tablets (NDA 20-151/S-032) and Effexor XR (venlafaxine hydrochloride) Extended Release Capsules (NDA 20-699/S-052).

Your April 30, 2004, submission also constituted a complete response to our action letter dated March 19, 2004 for supplemental applications 20-151/S-028/S-030 and 20-699/S-041/S-048.

Reference is also made to a conference call dated April 28, 2004 between representatives of the Agency and yourself to discuss the Agency's class labeling initiatives.

The above supplemental applications provide for the following changes to product labeling:

NDAs 20-151/S-028 & 20-699/S-041

1. Revisions to the **PRECAUTIONS-Usage in Children** section to denote hostility and suicide related adverse events in pediatric clinical trials.
2. The addition of the term "tinnitus" to the **DOSAGE AND ADMINISTRATION-Discontinuing Effexor** or **Effexor XR** sections.
3. Revisions to the Patient Brief Summary.

We note your agreement to our request to remove your proposed addition of hostility and suicide related adverse events from the **PRECAUTIONS-Usage in Children** section. As discussed during that April 28, 2004 meeting, we continue to feel that it would not be helpful to include the language regarding reports of hostility and suicidality that you have proposed for the **Pediatric Use** section. As currently written, the language is uninterpretable, since it notes that there were increased reports, but without noting with reference to what data. If a reference to placebo data were added, this would suggest a causal association, however, this suggestion would be contradicted by the new language that follows. The difficulty, of course, is that it remains unclear at this point exactly what has been captured under the crude terms used to capture events. The currently proposed language for **WARNINGS** is intended to comprehensively address this complex issue and our current understanding of the available data, and we feel it would be confusing and potentially misleading to maintain your proposed language for the **Pediatric Use** section.

NDAs 20-151/S-030 & 20-699/S-048

These applications provide for revisions to the **DOSAGE and ADMINISTRATION/Discontinuing Effexor** or **Effexor XR** sections of product labeling.

Again, we note your agreement to revise product labeling to incorporate the class labeling initiative for all of the selective serotonin reuptake inhibitors (SSRIs) and serotonin and norepinephrine reuptake inhibitors (SNRIs), to change labeling in regards to discontinuation symptoms and to adverse events occurring in neonates exposed to any of the SSRIs or SNRIs late in the third trimester.

NDAs 20-151/S-032 & 20-699/S-052

These applications provide for antidepressant class labeling revisions to incorporate the following changes to product labeling:

1. The addition of a new subsection under **WARNINGS** entitled **Clinical Worsening and Suicide Risk.**
2. Revisions to the **PRECAUTIONS-Information for Patients** section.
3. Delete the section in **PRECAUTIONS-General** entitled "Suicide".
4. Add a reference to the **WARNINGS** section at the end of the **PRECAUTIONS- Pediatric Use** section, i.e., (see **WARNINGS-Clinical Worsening and Suicide Risk**).

We have completed the review of these supplemental applications and have concluded that adequate information has been presented to demonstrate that the drug product is safe and effective for use as recommended in your labeling submitted on April 30, 2004 and as attached to this letter. Accordingly, these supplemental applications are approved effective on the date of this letter.

If a letter communicating important information about this drug product (i.e., a "Dear Health Care Practitioner" letter) is issued to physicians and others responsible for patient care, we request that you submit a copy of the letter to this NDA and a copy to the following address:

MEDWATCH, HF-2
FDA
5600 Fishers Lane
Rockville, MD 20857

We remind you that you must comply with the requirements for an approved NDA set forth under 21 CFR 314.80 and 314.81.

If you have any questions, call Mr. Paul David, R.Ph., Senior Regulatory Project Manager, at (301) 594-5530.

Sincerely,

{See appended electronic signature page}

Russell Katz, M.D.
Director
Division of Neuropharmacological Drug Products
Office of Drug Evaluation I
Center for Drug Evaluation and Research

Attachment

DEPARTMENT OF HEALTH & HUMAN SERVICES Public Health Service

Food and Drug Administration
Rockville, MD 20857

NDA 20-151/S-024
NDA 20-699/S-030

Tab 51

Wyeth-Ayerst
Attention: Kenneth R. Bonk
Associate Director II, Worldwide Regulatory Affairs
P.O. Box 8299
Philadelphia, PA 19101-1245

Dear Mr. Bonk:

Please refer to your supplemental new drug applications dated September 25, received September 26, 2002, submitted under section 505(b) pursuant to section 505(b)(2) of the Federal Food, Drug, and Cosmetic Act for Effexor (venlafaxine hydrochloride) Immediate Release Tablets (NDA 20-151) and Effexor XR (venlafaxine hydrochloride) Extended Release Capsules (NDA 20-699).

We acknowledge receipt of your submissions dated November 21, and December 4, 9, and 10, 2003.

These "Prior Approval" supplemental new drug applications propose the use of venlafaxine to treat pediatric major depressive disorder (MDD) and pediatric generalized anxiety disorder (GAD).

We have completed our review and find the information presented is inadequate, and the supplemental applications are not approvable under section 505(d) of the Act and 21 CFR 314.125(b)(5). The deficiencies may be summarized as follows:

Specifically, the results from your two studies, Protocols 0600B1-382-US and 0600B1-394-US, failed to demonstrate the efficacy of venlafaxine in pediatric patients with MDD. Given the fact that negative trials are frequently seen, even for antidepressant drugs that we know are effective, we do not feel that it would be useful to describe these negative trials in labeling, since this may be misinterpreted as evidence that venlafaxine does not work in this population. Rather, we feel that the existing language, suggesting simply that efficacy has not been established in this population, is still most appropriate.

In regard to your studies in pediatric GAD, the results from one of your two studies, Study 0600B2-396-US, failed to demonstrate the efficacy of venlafaxine in pediatric patients with GAD. While we consider the second study, Study 0600B2-397-US, to be positive, a single positive study is not sufficient, in our view, to support this new claim in pediatric GAD. We made this point in our April 28, 1999 written request, i.e., that that there is no experience from adequate and well-controlled trials that GAD is essentially the same disorder in adults and children and, as such, two positive studies would be required for approval in this patient population.

Given the fact that negative trials are frequently seen, even for GAD drugs that we know are effective, we also do not feel that it would be useful to describe the one positive and the one negative trial in labeling, since this may be misinterpreted as evidence that venlafaxine either does work in this population, or does not. Rather, we feel that these two studies, by themselves, are essentially uninterpretable. Thus, in the absence of sufficient evidence to support this new claim, we feel that the existing language, suggesting simply that efficacy has not been established in this population, is still most appropriate.

Regarding the PK data, we feel that it is not useful to add these data, given the fact that efficacy has not been established.

However, based upon the safety information reviewed in the pediatric population, a smaller increase in height in children in the pooled GAD studies versus placebo was noted. This was not noted in the MDD group; however, it is surprising that this was noted at all in an 8-week study period. Though height was significantly increased from baseline after 8 weeks of treatment for both venlafaxine ER- treated and placebo- treated patients, the adjusted mean increase at month 2 in the placebo group (1.3 cm) was significantly greater than the venlafaxine ER group (0.4 cm). Mean height in the long term open label treated patients only increased 1.2-cm over 6-months.

Both MDD and GAD patients treated with venlafaxine had mean decreases in weight. The mean weight losses were 0.5 kg (MDD) and 0.6 kg (GAD) over an 8-week period while there was a mean weight gain in the placebo treated MDD and GAD patients. Weight changes in both MDD and GAD patients were statistically significant.

Such information would typically be inserted into the **PRECAUTIONS-Changes in Appetite and Weight** and **PRECAUTIONS-Pediatric Use** sections of labeling.

However, prior to requesting labeling revisions at this point, we are requesting that you submit the following additional information, and a labeling proposal for these sections of labeling.

1. Please provide an analysis of mean height and weight changes from baseline for venlafaxine ER compared to placebo using the data from the pool of four 8-week placebo controlled pediatric studies (396, 397, 382 and 394).

2. Please provide an analysis of mean height and weight changes from baseline for venlafaxine ER compared to placebo using only data from the pediatric GAD studies (396, 397).

3. Please provide an analysis of mean height and weight changes from baseline for venlafaxine ER compared to placebo using only data from the pediatric MDD studies (382, 394).

4. Please repeat the above analyses (#1-3), stratifying on age (<12 years and ≥12 years).

5. Please provide outlier analyses that identify the percentage of pediatric subjects that lost at least 3.5% of their body weight for venlafaxine ER compared to placebo for the following: the pool of four studies; the GAD studies; and the MDD studies.

6. Please provide an analysis of mean height and weight changes from baseline for venlafaxine ER compared to placebo for the following: the pool of four studies; the GAD studies; and the MDD studies.

7. Mean height in the long term open label treated patients only increased 1.2-cm over 6-months. Though this seems like a slow rate of growth, in the absence of comparator data the mean change in height for a group is difficult to interpret since it includes a collection of children of different ages and who started at different height percentiles. Since children grow at different rates depending on their age and gender, growth over a period of time is predicted by gender and the height and weight at the beginning of an observation period. Pediatricians determine whether children are following their growth percentile curve, which is based on normal population data.

   Investigators have used growth curve data to assess growth in open label studies, in some cases by using z-scores. A z-score is the number of standard deviations that one is from their gender/age standardized mean. Investigators determine each subject's z-score at the beginning and then at the end of the observation period. If the mean change in the z-score is negative, then the group did not grow as expected based on normal population data.

   Please provide an electronic data set for the long-term open-label studies that includes one row for each patient and includes the study number, indication, age, gender, baseline height and weight, end study height and weight, baseline height and weight z-scores, end study height and weight z-scores, treatment and assigned dose.

Within 10 days after the date of this letter, you are required to amend the supplemental applications, notify us of your intent to file an amendment, or follow one of your other options under 21 CFR 314.120. In the absence of any such action, FDA may proceed to withdraw the supplemental applications. Any amendment should respond to all the deficiencies listed. We will not process a partial reply as a major amendment nor will the review clock be reactivated until all deficiencies have been addressed.

These products may be considered to be misbranded under the Federal Food, Drug, and Cosmetic Act if they are marketed with these changes prior to approval of these supplemental applications.

If you have any questions, call Paul David, Senior Regulatory Health Project Manager, at (301) 594-5530.

Sincerely,

{See appended electronic signature page}

Russell Katz, M.D.
Director
Division of Neuropharmacological Drug Products
Office of Drug Evaluation I
Center for Drug Evaluation and Research

Results of the Analysis of Suicidality in Pediatric Trials of Newer Antidepressants

Psychopharmacologic Drugs Advisory Committee and the Pediatric Advisory Committee
September 13-14, 2004

Tarek A. Hammad, MD, PhD, MSc, MS

Senior Medical Reviewer

Division of Neuropharmacological Drug Products
Center for Drug Evaluation and Research, FDA

Outline

- Objective
- Data Domain
- Findings
- Limitations
- Summary

Tab 52

Objective

- To investigate the relationship between antidepressants and pediatric suicidality based on:
  - Adverse events reported
  - Suicidality item(s) scores in pertinent depression questionnaires

3

Data Domain

- 25 trials conducted in pediatric patients in nine drug development programs + TADS trial
- Drugs - number of trials:
  - SSRIs
    - Citalopram (Celexa) - 2
    - Fluoxetine (Prozac) - 4 + TADS
    - Fluvoxamine (Luvox) - 1
    - Paroxetine (Paxil) - 6
    - Sertraline (Zoloft) - 3
  - Atypical antidepressants
    - Bupropion (Wellbutrin) - 2
    - Mirtazapine (Remeron) - 1
    - Nefazodone (Serzone) - 2
    - Venlafaxine (Effexor XR) - 4

4

Data Domain, continued ...

- Indications - number of trials
  - Major Depressive Disorder (MDD) - 15 (+ TADS)
  - Anxiety Disorders
    - Obsessive Compulsive Disorder - 5
    - Generalized Anxiety Disorder - 2
    - Social anxiety Disorder/Social Phobia - 1
  - Attention Deficit Hyperactivity Disorder - 2
- Two trials excluded (Paxil 453-relapse prevention, Wellbutrin 41-uncontrolled)
- Trial year: 1983 to 2004
- Duration: 4 to 16 weeks

5

Outline

- Objective
- Data Domain
- Findings
  - Outcomes based on adverse events
  - Outcomes based on suicidality scores
- Limitations
- Summary

Outcomes Based on Adverse Events

Main Outcomes Used in the Analysis

Outcomes	Description	Number
Outcome 1	Suicidal behavior, codes 1 & 2	n=33
Outcome 2	Suicidal ideation, code 6	n=45
Outcome 3 (primary outcome)	Suicidal behavior or ideation (codes 1, 2, & 6)	n=78
Outcome 4	Possible suicidal behavior or ideation (codes 1, 2, 6 + 3, 10)	n=109

8

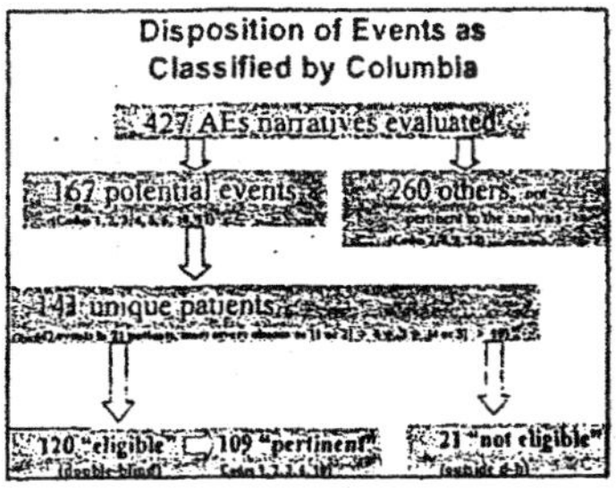

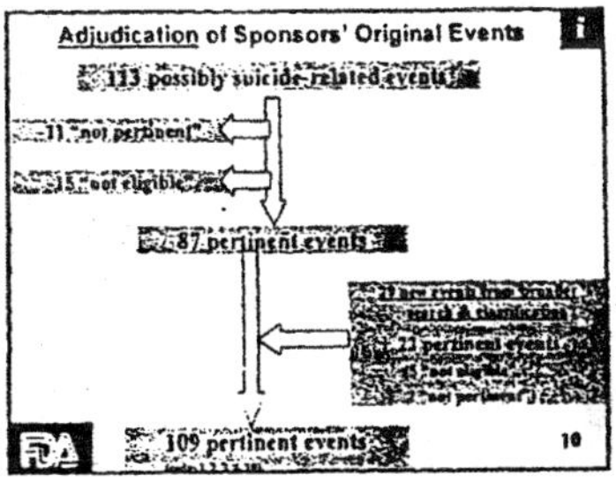

Caveats!

- Possibility for chance finding
  - Post- hoc analyses
  - Multiple outcomes
  - Many sub-analyses
- Difficult to compare across drugs
  - Low power for individual trials
  - Differences in size of drugs' databases
  - Potential role of differences in level of ascertainment of events and completeness of narratives between trials/development programs

11

Examining Effect Modification and Confounding

Examining Effect Modification

> Analysis was done by trial

> Examining effect modification (interaction) was difficult due to small number of events

> Variables examined were:
- Age group (6-11, 12-18)
- Gender
- History of suicide attempt at baseline

> None was found to meaningfully impact the risk estimates

13

Examining Confounding

> Analysis was done by trial

> Examining confounding effect of many variables
- Demographics variables
- Trial-related variables
- Disease-related variables
- Drug-related variables
- Psychiatric history

> None was found to meaningfully impact the risk estimates

14

Suicidal behavior or ideation (codes 1, 2, & 6) by Drug

Celexa

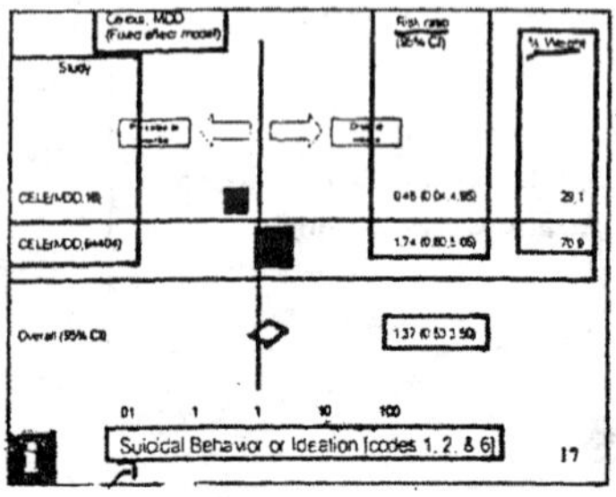

Paxil

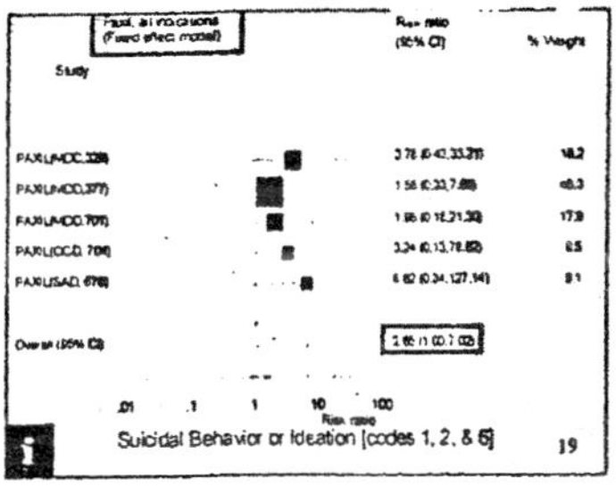

Prozac

FDA

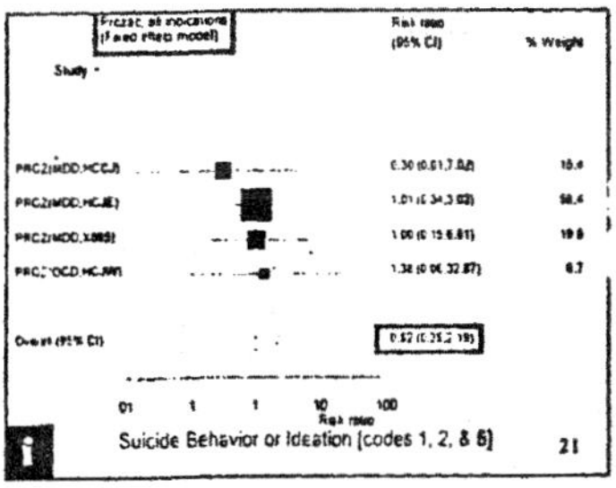

TADS trial

Group	Event code *	Number of events
PROZ (109)	1 (suicidal behavior) 6 (suicidal ideation)	2 7
PBO (112)	6 (suicidal ideation)	2

* Events were classified by the Columbia expert group

FDA 22

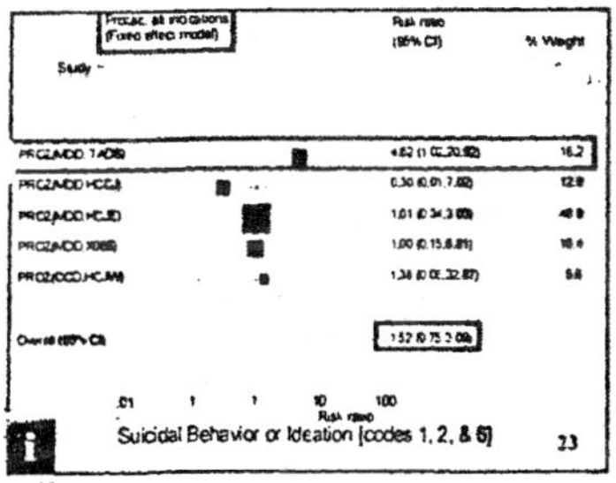

Zoloft

FDA

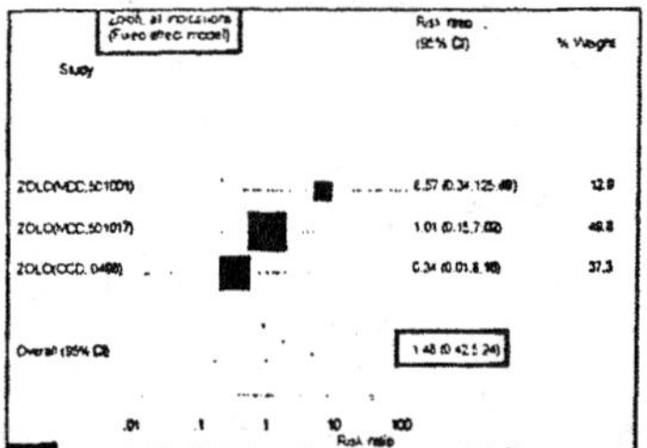

Suicidal Behavior or Ideation [codes 1, 2, & 6] 25

Effexor XR

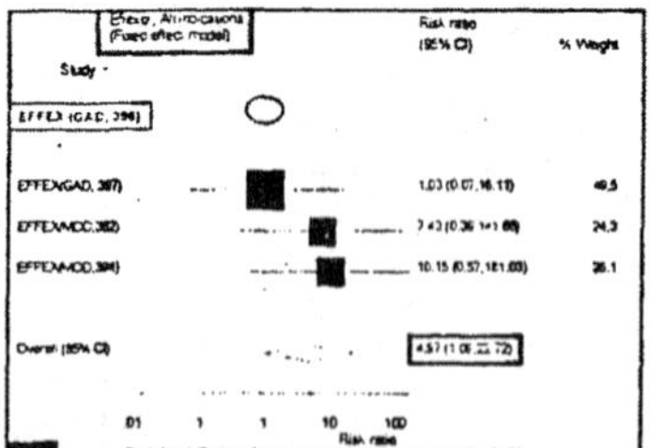

Suicidal Behavior or Ideation [codes 1, 2, & 6] 27

Overall relative risks (RR) of suicidal behavior or ideation (codes 1, 2, & 6) by drug

Drug	Relative Risk (95% CI), MDD trials	Relative Risk (95% CI), all trials, all indications
Celexa	1.37 (0.53, 3.50)	1.37 (0.53, 3.50)
Luvox	No MDD trials	5.52 (0.27, 112.55)
Paxil	2.15 (0.71, 6.52)	2.65 (1.00, 7.02)
Prozac *	1.53 (0.74, 3.16)	1.52 (0.75, 3.09)
Zoloft	2.16 (0.48, 9.62)	1.48 (0.42, 5.24)
Effexor XR	8.84 (1.12, 69.51)	4.97 (1.09, 22.72)
Remeron	1.58 (0.06, 38.37)	1.58 (0.06, 38.37)
Serzone	No events	No events
Wellbutrin	No MDD trials	No events

* Note that TADS data are added to Prozac 28

Trial Design Attributes

- The following trial design attributes were examined:
  - Location (North Am/non-NA)
  - Setting (inpatient/outpatient)
  - Presence of an active control arm
  - Sample size
  - Rate of discontinuation
  - Number of centers
  - Extensive screening
  - Exclusion of placebo respondents
  - Exclusion of treatment-resistant patients
  - Exclusion of baseline suicide risk
  - Exclusion of history of suicide attempt
  - Exclusion of homicide risk
- None was found to consistently explain the observed differences in the risk estimates between trials within/between development programs

29

Components of suicidal behavior or ideation (codes 1, 2, & 6)

- Suicidal Behavior (codes 1 & 2)
- Suicidal Ideation (code 6)

Overall relative risks of suicidal behavior or ideation (codes 1, 2, & 6) by drug in MDD trials

Drug	Relative Risk (95% CI), suicidal behavior (codes 1 & 2)	Relative Risk (95% CI), suicidal ideation (code 6)	Relative Risk (95% CI), suicidal behavior or ideation (codes 1, 2, & 6)
Celexa	2.23 (0.59, 8.46)	0.75 (0.19, 2.95)	1.37 (0.53, 3.50)
Paxil	2.30 (0.67, 7.93)	1.09 (0.24, 5.01)	2.15 (0.71, 6.52)
Prozac *	2.15 (0.50, 9.26)	1.30 (0.59, 2.87)	1.53 (0.74, 3.16)
Zoloft	0.98 (0.17, 5.68)	3.88 (0.44, 34.54)	2.16 (0.48, 9.62)
Effexor XR	2.77 (0.11, 67.10)	7.89 (0.99, 62.59)	8.84 (1.12, 69.51)
Remeron	No events	1.58 (0.07, 38.37)	1.58 (0.06, 38.37)

* Note that TADS data are added to Prozac

FDA 31

Sensitivity Analysis

FDA

Robustness of the risk estimates of suicidal behavior or ideation (codes 1,2, & 6) to event ascertainment: results of outcome 4 "possible suicidal behavior or ideation"

Outcomes	Overall RR (95% CI), all trials, all indications	Overall RR (95% CI), SSRI MDD trials
Suicidal behavior or ideation (codes 1,2, & 6)	1.95 (1.28, 2.98)	1.66 (1.02, 2.68)
Possible suicidal behavior or ideation (codes 1, 2, 6 - 3, 10)	2.19 (1.50, 3.19)	1.91 (1.27, 2.89)

- The signal was slightly altered
- Note that TADS data are added to all analyses

FDA 33

Analysis of Risk Difference (RD)

FDA

Analysis of Risk Difference (RD)

- This analysis estimates the absolute increase in the risk of the event of interest due to treatment
- Risk in the drug grp - risk in the placebo grp
- Overall RD for SSRIs in MDD trials = 2 to 3%
- Out of 100 patients treated, we might expect 2 to 3 patients to have some increase in suicidality due to short-term treatment, i.e., beyond the risk that occurs with the disease being treated

FDA 35

Outcomes Based on Suicidality Scores

FDA

Worsening of Suicidality Score
(Outcome 6, n=434)

- Increase in the suicidality item(s) score of pertinent depression questionnaires relative to baseline, regardless of subsequent change
- Questionnaires used: HAM-D, CDRS-R, MADRS, and K-SADS

Emergence of Suicidality
(Outcome 7, n=349)

- Same concept as above, but with normal baseline score

FDA 37

Worsening of Suicidality
(Outcome6)

- Effect modification and confounding were examined → none was found

FDA

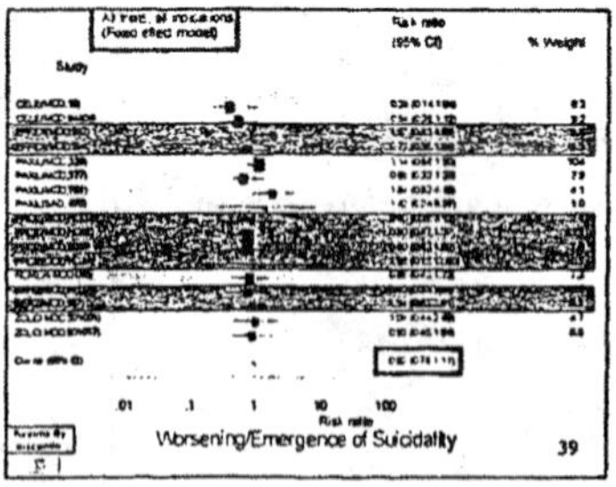

Emergence of Suicidality
(Outcome 7)

- Effect modification and confounding were examined → none was found

FDA

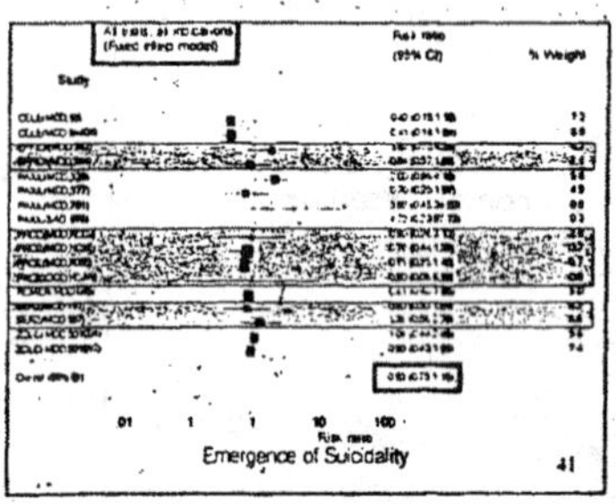

Other Analyses

- Additional sensitivity analysis
  - Fixed-effect vs. random-effects
- Completers analysis
- Time-to-event analysis
  - Kaplan-Meier survival estimates
  - Hazard functions for pooled SSRIs in MDD trials
- Potential "activation" syndrome
- Post-hoc power analysis

42

Limitations

- Post-hoc analyses with multiple outcomes involved, in addition to many sub-analyses. Therefore, caution is warranted in the interpretation of the findings
- Observed differences between drugs
  - Chance finding
  - True differences between drugs (i.e. no class effect)
  - Differences in size of drugs' databases
  - Differences in level of ascertainment of events and completeness of narratives
  - Differences in trial design attributes
- Short-term exposure (4-16 weeks)

FDA 43

Limitations, continued...

- Medication noncompliance may have influenced the occurrence of the events of interest. However, the determination of noncompliance was suboptimal
- Observed rates of suicidality associated with the use of antidepressants might not reflect actual rates among patients in the general population
- Most trials were conducted with a flexible dosing scheme eliminating our ability to examine the dose effect

FDA 44

Summary of Findings

- The broader search for adverse events in various drug development programs and the blinded classification process identified many new events and also eliminated several events that were not appropriately classified
- There were NO completed suicides
- Many individual trials had a RR of 2 or more for suicidality and some CIs of overall estimates did not include 1
- The sensitivity analyses did not yield a meaningful difference in the evaluation of the estimated risks

FDA 45

Summary of Findings, continued...

- None of the examined covariates was found to be an effect modifier or to meaningfully impact the risk estimates as a confounder
- Among the examined trial design attributes, none was found to consistently explain the observed differences in the risk estimates between trials
- No signal was observed in outcomes based on the suicidality scores

FDA 46

FDA

FDA

September 13, 2004
Meeting of Psychopharmacological Drugs Advisory Committee and Pediatric Drugs Advisory Committee

Comparison Between Original ODS and Current DNDP Analyses of Pediatric Suicidality Data Sets

Andrew D. Mosholder, M.D., M.P.H.
Office of Drug Safety

ODS Analysis of Suicidal Events in Pediatric Trials with Antidepressant Drugs

- Same trials as DNDP analysis, except for TADS
- Events determined from responses to July 2003 data requests
  - used sponsor-identified suicide related events that were also classified as serious
  - predated Columbia University reclassification

Tab 53

Differences in Analytic Methods

Analysis	ODS	DNDP
Denominator used	Person-time	# of patients
Post-treatment window for including events	+ 30 days	+ 1 day
Events during down-titration	Included	Excluded
Correction for zero cells	No	Yes

ODS Analysis: Overview of Data

- **Drug N = 2227, patient-years = 406.9**
  - no completed suicides
  - 74 sponsor-defined suicide related events, 54 serious
- **Pbo N = 1936, patient-years = 347.6**
  - no completed suicides
  - 34 sponsor-defined suicide related events, 24 serious

ODS Analysis: Overview of Data, continued

- Definition of "serious" adverse drug experiences (21CFR 312.32):
  - fatal
  - life-threatening
  - involve hospitalization
  - disabling
  - congenital defect
- Sponsor determined whether an adverse event in a clinical trial was serious
- **ODS "serious suicide-related events" will be compared to Columbia University "definitive suicidal behavior/ideation"**

Comparison of Case Classifications

- *ODS Serious, suicide-related events* n=78
  - 61 were classified by Columbia Univ. as "definitive suicidal behavior/ideation"
  - 13 of the remaining 17 cases classified as self-injurious behavior with unknown intent
- *Columbia University "definitive suicidal behavior/ideation* n=95
  - 61 also were ODS serious, suicide-related events
  - 18 new cases
  - 16 sponsor-defined suicide-related events, but nonserious (thus not included in ODS analysis)

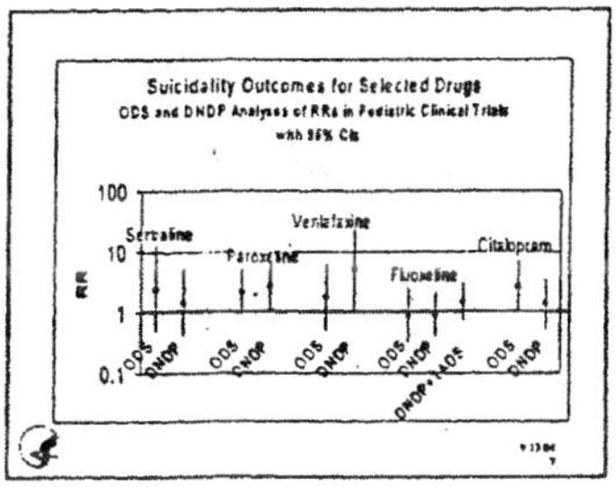

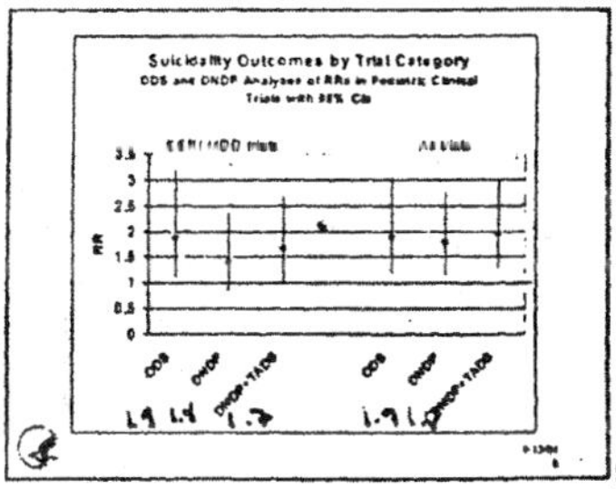

Additional Topics

(reference: March 2004 consult memo)

- Incidence rate difference analysis
- Comparison to adult data for paroxetine
- Discontinuation events

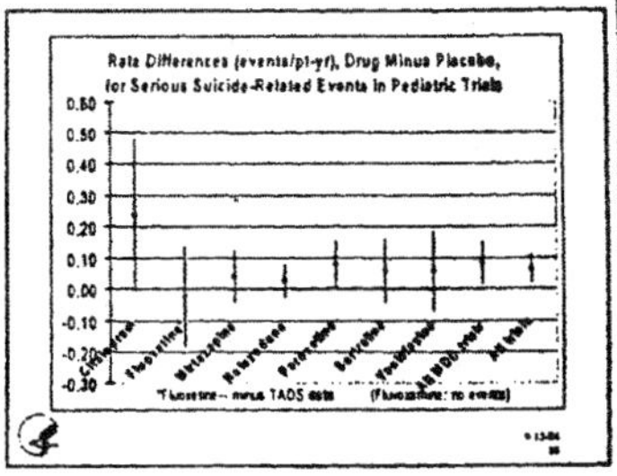

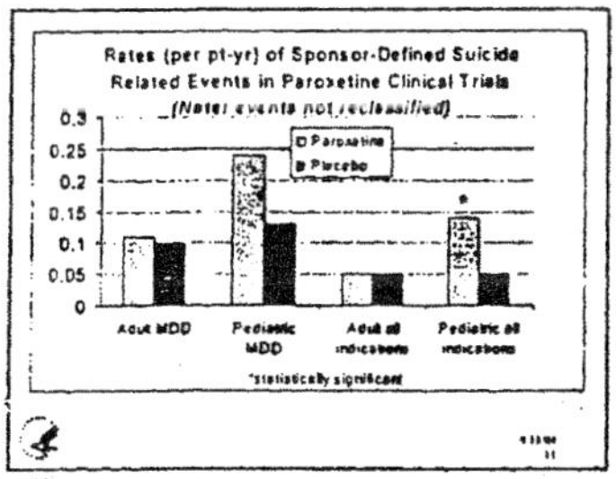

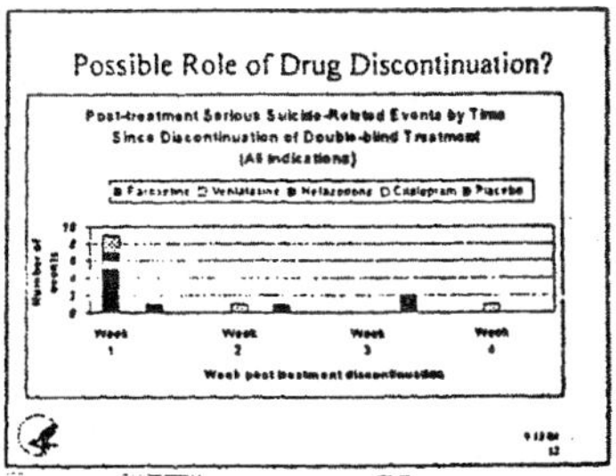

Conclusion

Both the original ODS analysis, and the current DNDP analysis using the Columbia University reclassification of cases, indicate an association of suicidality with antidepressant drug treatment in short-term, placebo-controlled pediatric trials

McCary, Barbara M

From:	Mosholder, Andrew D
nt:	Wednesday, January 28, 2004 12:55 PM
o:	Trontell, Anne E; Willy, Mary E
Subject:	Follow-up to this morning, about the administrative history of the Neuropharm consult

Tab 54

yesterday's reg briefing | RE: Citalopram pediatric suici... | Pediatric Suicide Project

Hi Anne,
Since you raised the question of whether I was supposed to have been looking at these data after the regulatory briefing, I looked back through my email and attached a few that I think will show why I forged ahead with the project. The one from Rusty is a bit vague, I know, but the ones from Paul David, the RPM, are more specific. In one email he is inviting me to a telecon (two months after the regulatory briefing), and in the other he discusses sending me the data from the July requests that I analyzed in the present consult.
I hope this helps provide some perspective on the administrative history of this consult.
-Andy

McCary, Barbara M

From:	Katz, Russell G
ent:	Wednesday, September 17, 2003 8:34 AM
.o:	Mosholder, Andrew D
Subject:	yesterday's reg briefing

Andy-

I had to run out of the meeting yesterday to go to my next meeting, but I just wanted to thank you for a superb presentation (not to mention all the work that went into it). I believe everyone was duly impressed, as they should have been. What the next step is, I don't know yet, but we'll probably get together soon to figure it out. I believe the charge from the group was to "get to the bottom of this", so I guess that's what we'll do.

Anyway, we'll be in touch, but thanks again for all the work and the presentation-it was great.

Rusty

McCary, Barbara M

Erom:	David, Paul A
nt:	Friday, November 14, 2003 11:13 AM
. o:	Mosholdor, Androw D
Subject:	RE: Citalopram pediatric suicidal event narratives

Andy,
Tom, Judy, and myself are meeting this afternoon at 2:30 to discuss the narratives. Would it be possible for you to join us via t-con?
-Paul

-----Original Message-----

From:	Mosholder, Andrew D
Sent:	Friday, November 14, 2003 10:32 AM
To:	David, Paul A; Racoosin, Judith A; Laughren, Thomas P; Stasko, Robert; Hammad, Tarek
Cc:	Willy, Mary E
Subject:	Citalopram pediatric suicidal event narratives

Hello all,

As I was reviewing the Forest submission dated 8-21-03, I realized something about the citalopram narratives. Although we did not request it, Forest included narratives for subjects who discontinued the study or were hospitalized for worsening of depression. This was in addition to the narratives for subjects with suicide-related events. It looks like Forest was the only sponsor to do so.

Here is the list of subjects with worsening of depression but no suicide-related event, in case you want to remove those narratives from the ones to be reviewed blindly:

Study CIT-MD-18: Patients 550, 574
ıdy 94404: Patients 419, 447, 697, 714, 719, 732

Also, I want to point out that for completeness Forest included narratives on three patients from an ongoing study of escitalopram in pediatric depression, study SCT-MD-15 (patients 007-1507, 026-1508, and 033-1509). Of course, these cases can't be part of the analysis, since the treatment is still blinded.

-Andy

McCary, Barbara M

From: David, Paul A
nt: Thursday, September 04, 2003 7:20 AM
: Mosholder, Andrew D
Cc: Racoosin, Judith A; Laughren, Thomas P; Andreason, Paul J
Subject: Pediatric Suicide Project

Andy,
We received the data from Lilly (submission date 9-2-03), and Wyeth (submission date 8-28-03). My desk copy of Wyeth's submission contains the CD ROMs; however, the data is also located in the EDR under the following paths: \\CDSESUB1\N20151\S_024\2003-08-28 & \\CDSESUB1\N20699\S_030\2003-08-28.

I should receive the Serzone submission either today or tomorrow. Therefore, the only one remaining will be Pfizer.

I'll send the Prozac and Effexor desk copies this morning.
-Paul

-----Original Message-----
From: David, Paul A
Sent: Tuesday, September 02, 2003 8:56 AM
To: Mosholder, Andrew D
Cc: Racoosin, Judith A; Laughren, Thomas P; Andreason, Paul J
Subject: RE: JAMA article on Zoloft in pediatric depression

Andy,
I'm sending over hard copies of the following submissions providing for our requested pediatric suicide data: Wellbutrin/Zyban, Celexa/Lexapro, and Remeron. Solvay (Luvox) submitted their data to the EDR, and it can be found at the following path: \\CDSESUB1\N21519\N_000\2003-08-22, and a portion of the Remeron submission was also sent to the EDR with the path: \\CDSESUB1\N20415\N_000\2003-08-13.

..n still awaiting Prozac (due 9/3/03), Zoloft (due 9/12), Effexor/Effexor XR, and Serzone. I'll ding Wyeth and BMS this morning to see if I can scare up a date when then intend to respond to our 7-22-03 request.

-Paul

-----Original Message-----
From: Mosholder, Andrew D
Sent: Wednesday, August 27, 2003 3:20 PM
To: David, Paul A
Subject: RE: JAMA article on Zoloft in pediatric depression

Hi Paul,
You can send them over to me,if you have copies to spare. I've asked my management here if it would be feasible for me to work on phase II of this project; they will consider it since it might require taking me off of other consults for a while. It also might require someone with more statistical skills than I. For starters, I might as well see what you're receiving and take it from there.
I just got the notice about the regulatory briefing; I'll paste it below:

-----Original Appointment-----
From: Mercier, Jennifer L
Sent: Wednesday, August 27, 2003 12:39 PM
To: Mercier, Jennifer L; Hammad, Tarek; Mosholder, Andrew D; Katz, Russell G; Andreason, Paul J; Laughren, Thomas P; Racoosin, Judith A; David, Paul A; Woodcock, Janet; Buehler, Gary J; Bull, Jonca; Chiu, Yuan Yuan; Galson, Steven; Goldberger, Mark J; Harvey, Brian; Houn, Florence; Hussain, Ajaz S; Jacobson-Kram, David; Jenkins, John K; Kweder, Sandra L; Lesko, Lawrence J; Meyer, Robert J; Murphy, Dianne; Nasr, Moheb M; ONeill, Robert T; Seligman, Paul; Sobel, Solomon; Temple, Robert; Winkle, Helen N
Wilkin, Jonathan K; Albrecht, Renata; Allen, Susan S; Anello, Charles; Axelrad, Jane A; Behrman, Rachel E; Beitz, Julie G; Birnkrant, Debra B; Chowdhury, Badrul A; Colangelo, Kim M; Cox, Edward M; Ganley, Charles J; Henderson, Deborah J; Hess, Maureen; Hoiberg, Charles P; Huang, Shiew Mei; Johnson, Susan S; Justice, Robert; Leiderman, Deborah; Love, Patricia Y; Murphy, Shirley; Norden, Janet M; Orloff, David G; Pauls, Lana L; Pazdur, Richard; Phillips, Jerry; Purucker, Mary E; Raczkowski, Victor F; Rappaport, Bob A; Shames, Daniel A; Simon, Lee; Smith, Nancy D (CDER); Soreth, Janice M; Talarico, Lilia; Throckmorton, Douglas C; Trontell,

Anne E; West, Robert L
Subject: Regulatory Briefing - Paxil SPECIAL
When: Tuesday, September 16, 2003 2:00 PM-4:00 PM (GMT-05:00) Eastern Time (US & Canada).
Where: CDER OCD LAPTOP; CDER EOS PROXIMA; CDER WOC2 6FL-G Conf Room

'A 20-031/S-073
_xil (paroxetineHCl) Tablets
This supplement provides for controlled clinical studies in children and adolescents with major depressive disorder (MDD) and obsessive compulsive disorder (OCD). The controlled studies in the pediatric population with MDD demonstrated that pediatric patients who received Paxil had a higher incidence of suicidal ideation/attempts. This supplement received an approvable action on October 10, 2002. GlaxoSmithKline has not submitted a complete response to this action letter.

Andy

> -----Original Message-----
> **From:** David, Paul A
> **Sent:** Wednesday, August 27, 2003 10:00 AM
> **To:** Mosholder, Andrew D
> **Subject:** RE: JAMA article on Zoloft in pediatric depression
>
> Thanks for the reprints Andy. It made for some interesting
> reading. I forwarded them to the peds suicide team as well
> as the psych reviewers.
>
> I've been working with Jennifer Mercier on the Regulatory
> Briefing, and she is going to get back to me in a few days
> with the date. I believe that you are Tarek will be presenting.
>
> We're also starting to get responses from our pediatric
> suicide data request letters, and I believe that Judy is
> going to talk to you about looking at the data. I'm
> receiving lots of desk copies so it should not be a problem
o forward the submissions to you.
>
> -Paul
>
> -----Original Message-----
> **From:** Mosholder, Andrew D
> **Sent:** Wednesday, August 27, 2003 9:30 AM
> **To:** David, Paul A
> **Subject:** JAMA article on Zoloft in pediatric depression
>
> Hi Paul,
> I downloaded the JAMA articles referred to in today's Daily
> Clips. Please share with anyone else over their who's interested.
> As you recall, we turned down this supplement because each
> trial by itself failed. This article combines the two trials
> to show a statistically significant effect. I don't see
> where they've said that the individual trials failed and they
> had to pool them to have a result. Instead, the authors tout
> the combined analysis for having a large sample size...talk
> about spin!
> Andy
>
> << File: Varley editorial JAMA.pdf >> << File: Wagner et al
> JAMA.pdf >>

Katz, Donna

From: Mosholder, Andrew D
Sent: Monday, May 03, 2004 4:26 PM
To: Katz, Donna; McGarey, Patrick; Meister, Karen G
Subject: RE: As we discussed--OIA written statement (attachment only)

Tab 55

Abridged Written Statement 4-1...

Hello all,
In case this is of some help, I am attaching here the abridged version of my Internal Affairs statement, the one I shared with CDER management when I was asked to provide background information on this matter.
You can see that I left out the portions regarding the contacts with Rob Waters, similar to what we discussed today.
Hope this helps.
Andy

-----Original Message-----
From: Mosholder, Andrew D
Sent: Monday, May 03, 2004 2:15 PM
To: Katz, Donna; McGarey, Patrick; Meister, Karen G
Subject: As we discussed--OIA written statement (attachment only)

April 1, 2004

Note: This is a portion of the March 15, 2004 statement I provided to Special Agent Mike Kurisky of the Office of Internal Affairs (OIA). I have only included the sections relevant to the administrative history of this matter.

For context, I reproduce below the request I received from OIA.

> "You can start the statement discussing the previous positions you have had within the FDA and how you came to be the one selected to review this data. Please include how the FDA expanded that review of the data in Aug. '03, how you came to your final conclusion in Nov. '03 and then the fact that the FDA decided in Dec. '03 that this finding was incomplete. You can then discuss the decision by Dr. Katz and others within the Division of Neuropharmacological to pull you from making your presentation at the Advisory Hearing. Finally, please discuss any and all contacts you had with Rob Waters, to include the names of anyone else who was contacted by Waters. Please also include a statement that you did not release any info to Waters."

****

WRITTEN STATEMENT

I, Andrew D. Mosholder, provide the following statement at the request of Special Agent, Michael J. Kurisky of the FDA Office of Internal Affairs:

I am a licensed physician and board certified in child and adolescent psychiatry. I obtained my medical degree from the University of Virginia. I also have a Master of Public Health degree from Johns Hopkins University.

I am currently employed by the U.S. Food and Drug Administration and have been so employed since 1992. During my employment, I have been a medical officer with the Center for Drug Evaluation and Research (CDER) for almost twelve years. For about the past 14 months I have worked as an epidemiologist in the Division of Drug Risk Evaluation, Office of Drug Safety (ODS). Prior to that, I was a medical officer in CDER's Division of Neuropharmacological Drug Products (DNDP) for over 10 years.

My selection for the review of the pediatric suicidality data for antidepressant drugs occurred as follows: As a medical officer in DNDP, I reviewed a number of submissions of pediatric data for antidepressant drugs, including pediatric data submitted for Paxil (paroxetine), manufactured by GlaxoSmithKline (GSK). In May of 2003, after I had transferred to ODS, DNDP received new data analyses from GSK, indicating an increase in suicidal thoughts and behaviors with paroxetine compared to placebo in pediatric clinical trials. On June 2, 2003, Dr. Russell Katz, the Director of DNDP, sent me an email, in which he said, "Given your history with this application and this general issue, we think you would be the right person to help us think about the best way to approach the data in the other NDAs (and their sponsors), as well as to provide ideas for further sources of potentially relevant data...." A consultation request from DNDP to ODS signed June 6, 2003 byg Dr. Katz stated: "Since the original review of the Paxil supplement, as well as the reviews of most other pediatric supplements for SSRIs, was done by Andrew Mosholder, M.D,...we ask that this consult be assigned to him. We seek his advice on further analysis and interpretation of the Paxil results, as well as more general advice on what might be done to re-evaluate the risk of suicidality in the pediatric databases for other SSRIs...."

My managers in ODS agreed to Dr. Katz' request and assigned me to this consultation on June 9, 2003. To determine whether the apparent increase in suicidal events applies to pediatric use of other antidepressant drugs as well, I started to review the pediatric data for other antidepressant drugs. DNDP ultimately decided that the best way to proceed would be to ask the sponsors of other antidepressant drugs to reproduce GSK's analysis of suicidal events for Paxil, with each sponsor applying the same method to their own pediatric trial databases. In July of 2003, DNDP sent requests for such analyses to other antidepressant drug sponsors.

By September of 2003, I had completed an analysis of the paroxetine data and a preliminary analysis of pediatric data on seven other antidepressant drugs. At the request of management, I presented these analyses at a CDER Regulatory Briefing for upper level management on September 16, 2003. During the briefing, I presented the paroxetine pediatric data, along with preliminary findings for other antidepressant drugs. As noted in the briefing minutes, there was discussion about the clinical significance of some of the events in the analysis: "We need to get a better sense of what the events from these studies really are, i.e., are they legitimate, suicide-associated thoughts/actions or self-mutilation acts that are becoming increasingly common in the adolescent population today and are not generally associated with a sincere intent to die." The day following the regulatory briefing, Dr. Katz thanked me by email: "I just wanted to thank you for a superb presentation (not to mention all the work that went into it). I believe everyone was duly impressed, as they should have been. What the next step is, I don't know yet, but we'll probably get together soon to figure it out."

The Federal Register on October 31, 2003 contained this announcement to the public: "The Psychopharmacologic Drugs Advisory Committee and the Pediatric Subcommittee of the Anti-Infective Drugs Advisory Committee will discuss reports of the occurrence of suicidality (both suicidal ideation and suicide attempts) in clinical trials for various antidepressant drugs in pediatric patients with major depressive disorder (MDD). The committee will consider optimal approaches to the analysis of data from these trials, and the results of analyses conducted to date, with regard to the question of what regulatory action may be needed pertinent to the clinical use of these products in pediatric patients.

The committee will also consider further research needs to address questions on this topic."

As DNDP received responses from the other manufacturers to the July information requests, those responses were forwarded to me for review. I then worked on my analysis of these responses over the next couple of months and completed the first written draft of my results in December of 2003. (This document has since been revised, and has not yet received supervisory sign-off in ODS.)[1]

DNDP apparently was reaching a conclusion that the responses from the sponsors to the July requests were not going to be adequate for a definitive analysis. In October of 2003, DNDP sent requests to the manufacturers asking for patient level data sets, to permit a more sophisticated statistical analysis than what I could accomplish using only the responses to the July requests. DNDP also decided that all of the possible suicidal events in these trials should be reclassified by outside experts in suicidology.

On December 10, 2003, the U.K.'s Medicines and Healthcare products Regulatory Agency issued their statement, "Use of Selective Serotonin Reuptake Inhibitors (SSRIs) in children and adolescents with major depressive disorder (MDD) - only fluoxetine (Prozac) shown to have a favourable balance of risks and benefits for the treatment of MDD in the under 18s."

On December 18, 2003, we had one of our planning meetings for the February 2 advisory committee meeting. A draft agenda distributed for the December 18 planning meeting included a 45-minute presentation by me entitled, "Limited Overview of Paxil Controlled Trials and Controlled Trials of Other Antidepressants." At that meeting, I shared a proposed outline of my presentation, which included my finding that suicidal events designated as "serious" in pediatric clinical trials for major depressive disorder were 1.9 times more frequent with antidepressant drug treatment than with placebo, and that this was statistically significant. I recall some discussion of the pros and cons of my analysis.

At a subsequent planning session for the February 2 meeting, an agenda entitled "Proposed Agenda for February 2 As Revised by T. Laughren, 12/30/03," was distributed. It did not include my clinical trial data presentation.

On January 6, 2004, Dr. Katz sent me an email asking to speak with me by phone regarding my presentation at the February 2 Advisory Committee meeting. In our subsequent telephone conversation on that date, he told me that someone else would present the clinical trial data at the February 2 Advisory Committee meeting since I had reached a different view of the clinical trial data from that of DNDP. On January 7, 2004, I sent an email to the team members planning the February 2 meeting, confirming that I would not be giving the presentation as originally planned and attaching a draft of my slides for their use and interest.

---

[1] This consult subsequently received supervisory sign-off on 3-19-04.

On January 12, 2004, the Agency issued a Federal Register notice with a revised agenda for the February 2 meeting. The notice stated, "The committee will not be considering options for definitive regulatory action at this meeting because definitive analyses of the data have not been completed. This topic will be covered in a second meeting to be scheduled by summer 2004."

I cannot pinpoint when I first learned that a reporter was interested in the project, but I believe I first heard of a reporter making inquiries about this project around mid-January...[details regarding contacts with Mr. Waters omitted]...In summary, I kept the agency informed of my contacts from Mr. Waters. In responding to contacts from Mr. Waters, I did not provide Mr. Waters with any information that was not public. I did not share my conclusions from my analysis with him.

I understand that this statement is part of the Office of Internal Affairs investigation and I have been informed that I may be subject to disciplinary proceedings as a result of my statement.

I have read the above statement consisting of 4 pages and represent that the statement made by me is true and accurate to the best of my knowledge and belief.

____
Signature

Signed and affirmed to before me this ______ day of _____________, ______.

____
Special Agent/Date
FDA, Office of Internal Affairs

Authority to administer oaths:
Title 5, U.S. Code, Section 303

____
Witness/Date

Katz, Donna

From:	Mosholder, Andrew D
Sent:	Tuesday, May 04, 2004 8:53 AM
To:	Katz, Donna
Cc:	Meister, Karen G; McGarey, Patrick
Subject:	Abridged Written Statement for tomorrow's meeting with Senate Finance Committee
Importance:	High
Follow Up Flag:	Follow up
Flag Status:	Flagged

Tab 56

Abridged Written Statement 5-4...

Hello Donna,
To expedite things, I took a crack at redacting my Internal Affairs statement in the way we discussed yesterday afternoon. I believe you will find this version acceptable for tomorrow's session with the Finance Committee, based on yesterday's discussion.
Please advise.
Thanks!
Andy

Narrative Portions of Written Statement of Andrew D. Mosholder, M.D., M.P.H.
(For 5-5-04 meeting with Senate Finance Committee)

I am a licensed physician and board certified in child and adolescent psychiatry. I obtained my medical degree from the University of Virginia. I also have a Master of Public Health degree from Johns Hopkins University.

I am currently employed by the U.S. Food and Drug Administration and have been so employed since 1992. During my employment, I have been a medical officer with the Center for Drug Evaluation and Research (CDER) for almost twelve years. For about the past 14 months I have worked as an epidemiologist in the Division of Drug Risk Evaluation, Office of Drug Safety (ODS). Prior to that, I was a medical officer in CDER's Division of Neuropharmacological Drug Products (DNDP) for over 10 years.

My selection for the review of the pediatric suicidality data for antidepressant drugs occurred as follows: As a medical officer in DNDP, I reviewed a number of submissions of pediatric data for antidepressant drugs, including pediatric data submitted for Paxil (paroxetine), manufactured by GlaxoSmithKline (GSK). In May of 2003, after I had transferred to ODS, DNDP received new data analyses from GSK, indicating an increase in suicidal thoughts and behaviors with paroxetine compared to placebo in pediatric clinical trials. On June 2, 2003, Dr. Russell Katz, the Director of DNDP, sent me an email, in which he said, "Given your history with this application and this general issue, we think you would be the right person to help us think about the best way to approach the data in the other NDAs (and their sponsors), as well as to provide ideas for further sources of potentially relevant data...." A consultation request from DNDP to ODS signed June 6, 2003 byg Dr. Katz stated: "Since the original review of the Paxil supplement, as well as the reviews of most other pediatric supplements for SSRIs, was done by Andrew Mosholder, M.D,...we ask that this consult be assigned to him. We seek his advice on further analysis and interpretation of the Paxil results, as well as more general advice on what might be done to re-evaluate the risk of suicidality in the pediatric databases for other SSRIs...."

My managers in ODS agreed to Dr. Katz' request and assigned me to this consultation on June 9, 2003. To determine whether the apparent increase in suicidal events applies to pediatric use of other antidepressant drugs as well, I started to review the pediatric data for other antidepressant drugs. DNDP ultimately decided that the best way to proceed would be to ask the sponsors of other antidepressant drugs to reproduce GSK's analysis of suicidal events for Paxil, with each sponsor applying the same method to their own pediatric trial databases. In July of 2003, DNDP sent requests for such analyses to other antidepressant drug sponsors.

By September of 2003, I had completed an analysis of the paroxetine data and a preliminary analysis of pediatric data on seven other antidepressant drugs. At the request of management, I presented these analyses at a CDER Regulatory Briefing for upper level management on September 16, 2003. During the briefing, I presented the paroxetine pediatric data, along with preliminary findings for other antidepressant drugs. As noted in the briefing minutes, there was discussion about the clinical significance of some of the events in the analysis: "We need to get a better sense of what the events from these studies really are, i.e., are they legitimate, suicide-associated thoughts/actions or self-mutilation acts that are becoming increasingly common in the adolescent population today and are not generally associated with a sincere intent to die." The day following the regulatory briefing, Dr. Katz thanked me by email: "I just wanted to thank you for a superb presentation (not to mention all the work that went into it). I believe everyone was duly impressed, as they should have been. What the next step is, I don't know yet, but we'll probably get together soon to figure it out."

The Federal Register on October 31, 2003 contained this announcement to the public: "The Psychopharmacologic Drugs Advisory Committee and the Pediatric Subcommittee of the Anti-Infective Drugs Advisory Committee will discuss reports of the occurrence of suicidality (both suicidal ideation and suicide attempts) in clinical trials for various antidepressant drugs in pediatric patients with major depressive disorder (MDD). The committee will consider optimal approaches to the analysis of data from these trials, and the results of analyses conducted to date, with regard to the question of what regulatory action may be needed pertinent to the clinical use of these products in pediatric patients. The committee will also consider further research needs to address questions on this topic."

As DNDP received responses from the other manufacturers to the July information requests, those responses were forwarded to me for review. I then worked on my analysis of these responses over the next couple of months and completed the first written draft of my results in December of 2003. (This document has since been revised, and has not yet received supervisory sign-off in ODS.)[1]

DNDP apparently was reaching a conclusion that the responses from the sponsors to the July requests were not going to be adequate for a definitive analysis. In October of 2003, DNDP sent requests to the manufacturers asking for patient level data sets, to permit a more sophisticated statistical analysis than what I could accomplish using only the responses to the July requests. DNDP also decided that all of the possible suicidal events in these trials should be reclassified by outside experts in suicidology.

On December 10, 2003, the U.K.'s Medicines and Healthcare products Regulatory Agency issued their statement, "Use of Selective Serotonin Reuptake Inhibitors (SSRIs) in children and adolescents with major depressive disorder (MDD) - only fluoxetine (Prozac) shown to have a favourable balance of risks and benefits for the treatment of MDD in the under 18s."

On December 18, 2003, we had one of our planning meetings for the February 2 advisory committee meeting. A draft agenda distributed for the December 18 planning meeting included a 45-minute presentation by me entitled, "Limited Overview of Paxil Controlled

[1] This consult subsequently received supervisory sign-off on 3-19-04.

Trials and Controlled Trials of Other Antidepressants." At that meeting, I shared a proposed outline of my presentation, which included my finding that suicidal events designated as "serious" in pediatric clinical trials for major depressive disorder were 1.9 times more frequent with antidepressant drug treatment than with placebo, and that this was statistically significant. I recall some discussion of the pros and cons of my analysis.

At a subsequent planning session for the February 2 meeting, an agenda entitled "Proposed Agenda for February 2 As Revised by T. Laughren, 12/30/03," was distributed. It did not include my clinical trial data presentation.

On January 6, 2004, Dr. Katz sent me an email asking to speak with me by phone regarding my presentation at the February 2 Advisory Committee meeting. In our subsequent telephone conversation on that date, he told me that someone else would present the clinical trial data at the February 2 Advisory Committee meeting since I had reached a different view of the clinical trial data from that of DNDP. On January 7, 2004, I sent an email to the team members planning the February 2 meeting, confirming that I would not be giving the presentation as originally planned and attaching a draft of my slides for their use and interest.

On January 12, 2004, the Agency issued a Federal Register notice with a revised agenda for the February 2 meeting. The notice stated, "The committee will not be considering options for definitive regulatory action at this meeting because definitive analyses of the data have not been completed. This topic will be covered in a second meeting to be scheduled by summer 2004."

I cannot pinpoint when I first learned that a reporter was interested in the project, but I believe I first heard of a reporter making inquiries about this project around mid-January...[details regarding contacts with Mr. Waters omitted]...In summary, I kept the agency informed of my contacts from Mr. Waters. In responding to contacts from Mr. Waters, I did not provide Mr. Waters with any information that was not public. I did not share my conclusions from my analysis with him.

Katz, Donna

From: Katz, Donna
Sent: Tuesday, May 04, 2004 2:37 PM
To: Mosholder, Andrew D
Cc: Dettelbach, Kim; McGarey, Patrick; Meister, Karen G
Subject: statement

Tab 57

Written Statement DKMay4L.doc

Andy: I've taken a look at your written statement and made some suggested edits. Given that this will be a new document created to give to the Senate Finance Committee (albeit, based on an earlier document), I think it's cleaner to make this a stand alone document--ie, to include everything in it that is current and you would like to include, and just to leave out anything you would like to leave out. I don't think it's necessary to indicate that this document represents a version of the earlier one by noting that things have been omitted; that simply invites the committee to ask further questions about what was omitted and the earlier document.

Please let me know if you have any questions (301-827-7136). I can give you a clean version incorporating my edits if you would like.

Thanks,
Donna

Andrew D. Mosholder, M.D., M.P.H.
(For 5-5-04 meeting with Senate Finance Committee)~~WRITTEN STATEMENT~~

~~I, Andrew D. Mosholder, provide the following statement at the request of Special Agent, Michael J. Kurisky of the FDA Office of Internal Affairs.~~

I am a licensed physician and board certified in child and adolescent psychiatry. I obtained my medical degree from the University of Virginia. I also have a Master of Public Health degree from Johns Hopkins University.

I am currently employed by the U.S. Food and Drug Administration and have been so employed since 1992. During my employment, I have been a medical officer with the Center for Drug Evaluation and Research (CDER) for almost twelve years. For about the past 14 months I have worked as an epidemiologist in the Division of Drug Risk Evaluation, Office of Drug Safety (ODS). Prior to that, I was a medical officer in CDER's Division of Neuropharmacological Drug Products (DNDP) for over 10 years.

My selection for the review of the pediatric suicidality data for antidepressant drugs occurred as follows: As a medical officer in DNDP, I reviewed a number of submissions of pediatric data for antidepressant drugs, including pediatric data submitted for Paxil (paroxetine), manufactured by GlaxoSmithKline (GSK). In May of 2003, after I had transferred to ODS, DNDP received new data analyses from GSK, indicating an increase in suicidal thoughts and behaviors with paroxetine compared to placebo in pediatric clinical trials. On June 2, 2003, Dr. Russell Katz, the Director of DNDP, sent me an email, in which he said, "Given your history with this application and this general issue, we think you would be the right person to help us think about the best way to approach the data in the other NDAs (and their sponsors), as well as to provide ideas for further sources of potentially relevant data...." A consultation request from DNDP to ODS signed June 6, 2003 byg Dr. Katz stated: "Since the original review of the Paxil supplement, as well as the reviews of most other pediatric supplements for SSRIs, was done by Andrew Mosholder, M.D,...we ask that this consult be assigned to him. We seek his advice on further analysis and interpretation of the Paxil results, as well as more general advice on what might be done to re-evaluate the risk of suicidality in the pediatric databases for other SSRIs...."

My managers in ODS agreed to Dr. Katz' request and assigned me to this consultation on June 9, 2003. To determine whether the apparent increase in suicidal events applies to pediatric use of other antidepressant drugs as well, I started to review the pediatric data for other antidepressant drugs. DNDP ultimately decided that the best way to proceed would be to ask the sponsors of other antidepressant drugs to reproduce GSK's analysis of suicidal events for Paxil, with each sponsor applying the same method to their own pediatric trial databases. In July of 2003, DNDP sent requests for such analyses to other antidepressant drug sponsors.

By September of 2003, I had completed an analysis of the paroxetine data and a preliminary analysis of pediatric data on seven other antidepressant drugs. At the request of management, I presented these analyses at a CDER Regulatory Briefing for upper level management on September 16, 2003. During the briefing, I presented the paroxetine pediatric data, along with preliminary findings for other antidepressant drugs. As noted in the briefing minutes, there was discussion about the clinical significance of some of the events in the analysis: "We need to get a better sense of what the events from these studies really are, i.e., are they legitimate, suicide-associated thoughts/actions or self-mutilation acts that are becoming increasingly common in the adolescent population today and are not generally associated with a sincere intent to die." The day following the regulatory briefing, Dr. Katz thanked me by email: "I just wanted to thank you for a superb presentation (not to mention all the work that went into it). I believe everyone was duly impressed, as they should have been. What the next step is, I don't know yet, but we'll probably get together soon to figure it out."

The Federal Register on October 31, 2003 contained this announcement to the public: "The Psychopharmacologic Drugs Advisory Committee and the Pediatric Subcommittee of the Anti-Infective Drugs Advisory Committee will discuss reports of the occurrence of suicidality (both suicidal ideation and suicide attempts) in clinical trials for various antidepressant drugs in pediatric patients with major depressive disorder (MDD). The committee will consider optimal approaches to the analysis of data from these trials, and the results of analyses conducted to date, with regard to the question of what regulatory action may be needed pertinent to the clinical use of these products in pediatric patients. The committee will also consider further research needs to address questions on this topic."

As DNDP received responses from the other manufacturers to the July information requests, those responses were forwarded to me for review. I then worked on my analysis of these responses over the next couple of months and completed the first written draft of my results in December of 2003. This consult subsequently received supervisory sign-off on March 19, 2004. ~~(This document has since been revised, and has not yet received supervisory sign-off in ODS.)~~

DNDP apparently was reaching a conclusion that the responses from the sponsors to the July requests were not going to be adequate for a definitive analysis. In October of 2003, DNDP sent requests to the manufacturers asking for patient level data sets, to permit a more sophisticated statistical analysis than what I could accomplish using only the responses to the July requests. DNDP also decided that all of the possible suicidal events in these trials should be reclassified by outside experts in suicidology.

On December 10, 2003, the U.K.'s Medicines and Healthcare products Regulatory Agency issued their statement, "Use of Selective Serotonin Reuptake Inhibitors (SSRIs) in children and adolescents with major depressive disorder (MDD) - only fluoxetine (Prozac) shown to have a favourable balance of risks and benefits for the treatment of MDD in the under 18s."

On December 18, 2003, we had one of our planning meetings for the February 2 advisory committee meeting. A draft agenda distributed for the December 18 planning meeting included a 45-minute presentation by me entitled, "Limited Overview of Paxil Controlled Trials and Controlled Trials of Other Antidepressants." At that meeting, I shared a proposed outline of my presentation, which included my finding that suicidal events designated as "serious" in pediatric clinical trials for major depressive disorder were 1.9 times more frequent with antidepressant drug treatment than with placebo, and that this was statistically significant. I recall some discussion of the pros and cons of my analysis.

At a subsequent planning session for the February 2 meeting, an agenda entitled "Proposed Agenda for February 2 As Revised by T. Laughren, 12/30/03," was distributed. It did not include my clinical trial data presentation.

On January 6, 2004, Dr. Katz sent me an email asking to speak with me by phone regarding my presentation at the February 2 Advisory Committee meeting. In our subsequent telephone conversation on that date, he told me that someone else would present the clinical trial data at the February 2 Advisory Committee meeting since I had reached a different view of the clinical trial data from that of DNDP. On January 7, 2004, I sent an email to the team members planning the February 2 meeting, confirming that I would not be giving the presentation as originally planned and attaching a draft of my slides for their use and interest.

On January 12, 2004, the Agency issued a Federal Register notice with a revised agenda for the February 2 meeting. The notice stated, "The committee will not be considering options for definitive regulatory action at this meeting because definitive analyses of the data have not been completed. This topic will be covered in a second meeting to be scheduled by summer 2004."

I cannot pinpoint when I first learned that a reporter was interested in the project, but I believe I first heard of a reporter making inquiries about this project around mid-January. I also recall that some of my co-workers mentioned such contacts. ~~To the best of my recollection, those employees were Syed Rizwanuddin Ahmad, Renan Bonnel, Evelyn Farinas, Kate Gelperin, David J. Graham, Rita Ouellet-Hellstrom, Anne Trontell, and Mary Willy, although there may have been others that I do not recall.~~

I believe that my first contact from Mr. Rob Waters was on January 22, 2004. Mr. Waters telephoned me at the office to ask to interview me about my work on the issue of pediatric use of antidepressant drugs. I told him that I was not interested in being interviewed unless it was approved through our Public Affairs office. I did inform him of the upcoming advisory committee meeting, referred him to the agency's Public Affairs office, and then notified my managers and our Public Affairs office by email of his telephone call.

On January 27, 2004, I received (at my home address in West Virginia) a letter from Mr. Waters by FedEx, in which he asked me to reconsider speaking to him about this project, independently of the agency's Public Affairs office. I believe I sent Mr. Waters an e-mail from my home email account, telling him that I had no comment and I again ask him to contact the Public Affairs office. I unfortunately did not keep a copy of the e-mail since I did not view his contact of me as important.

On or around January 29, 2004, I received another telephone call from Mr. Waters, asking me to review his story on this issue to make sure that it was factual. Mr. Waters did not send me his proposed article. I informed my Division Director of the contact and, at the direction of my Division Director, I emailed Mr. Waters to suggest that he contact the Public Affairs office for Agency comments on the story. Mr. Waters replied by email to say he was not thinking of sending the entire story, but that he would consider my suggestion.

After the story ran on February 1, 2004 in the San Francisco Chronicle, I sent Mr. Waters an email thanking him for properly reporting that I declined to provide any information for his article, and I believe he sent a reply asking if I had any comments about the article. I met Mr. Waters in person at the February 2 Advisory Committee meeting, where I was one of the presenters (although not as to my findings from the analysis in question). I again thanked him for respecting my rejection of his requests. I may have sent him another email suggesting he could have emphasized the information posted on the British regulatory agency's web site, which I felt should have been more of a focus for his article, but I cannot recall the exact timing of that email. Following the February 2 Advisory Committee meeting, I went on leave to assist my wife, who was hospitalized for a surgical procedure February 3. [[Andy: if you want to leave out the highlighted portion, it's fine; it's also ok to leave it in if you would like.]

In summary, I kept the agency informed of my contacts from Mr. Rob Waters. In responding to contacts from Mr. Waters, I did not provide Mr. Waters with any information that was not public. I did not share my conclusions from my analysis with him.

~~I understand that this statement is part of the Office of Internal Affairs investigation and I have been informed that I may be subject to disciplinary proceedings as a result of my statement.~~

~~I have read the above statement consisting of 4 pages and represent that the statement made by me is true and accurate to the best of my knowledge and belief.~~

~~Signature~~

~~Signed and affirmed to before me this~~ ______ ~~day of~~ ______________, ________.

~~Authority to administer oaths: Title 5, U.S. Code, Section 303~~

~~Special Agent/Date~~
~~FDA, Office of Internal Affairs~~

Mosholder, Andrew D

From:	Mosholder, Andrew D
Sent:	Tuesday, May 04, 2004 3:17 PM
To:	Katz, Donna
Cc:	Dettelbach, Kim; McGarey, Patrick; Meister, Karen G
Subject:	RE: statement

Tab 58

Abridged
n Statement

Thanks very much, Donna. Your version is actually very similar to the one I came up with on my own this am (see attached).

Although it might be cleaner to do so, as you say, I am uncomfortable with concealing from the Committee the fact that this is not a new document. Accordingly, I prefer to use the version I edited (as in the attached email), which otherwise incorporates all the edits we've discussed.

Thanks,
Andy

-----Original Message-----
From: Katz, Donna
Sent: Tuesday, May 04, 2004 2:37 PM
To: Mosholder, Andrew D
Cc: Dettelbach, Kim; McGarey, Patrick; Meister, Karen G
Subject: statement

Andy: I've taken a look at your written statement and made some suggested edits. Given that this will be a new document created to give to the Senate Finance Committee (albeit, based on an earlier document), I think it's cleaner to make this a stand alone document--ie, to include everything in it that is current and you would like to include, and just to leave out anything you would like to leave out. I don't think it's necessary to indicate that this document represents a version of the earlier one by noting that things have been omitted; that simply invites the committee to ask further questions about what was omitted and the earlier document.

Please let me know if you have any questions (301-827-7136). I can give you a clean version incorporating my edits if you would like.

Thanks,
Donna

Mosholder, Andrew D

From:	Meister, Karen G
ent:	Tuesday, May 11, 2004 11:18 AM
o:	Henig, Anne M
Cc:	Mosholder, Andrew D; McGarey, Patrick; Katz, Donna; Dettelbach, Kim; Torres, Abelardo (OS)
Subject:	Times for interview

The OIA investigation has been closed. We have told the committee that we are ready to schedule the interview with Dr. Mosholder and are waiting to hear back. Please let us know what times in the next week Dr. Mosholder is available. Also, Dr. Mosholder may bring and use the affidavit he used for OIA with the names of the other FDA employees redacted. Thanks.

Tab 59

Karen G. Meister
Legislative Analyst
FDA Office of Legislation
(301) 827-0101
(301) 827-1955 fax

WRITTEN STATEMENT

Tab 60

I, Andrew D. Mosholder, provide the following statement at the request of Special Agent, of the FDA Office of Internal Affairs:

I am a licensed physician and board certified in child and adolescent psychiatry. I obtained my medical degree from the University of Virginia. I also have a Master of Public Health degree from Johns Hopkins University.

I am currently employed by the U.S. Food and Drug Administration and have been so employed since 1992. During my employment, I have been a medical officer with the Center for Drug Evaluation and Research (CDER) for almost twelve years. For about the past 14 months I have worked as an epidemiologist in the Division of Drug Risk Evaluation, Office of Drug Safety (ODS). Prior to that, I was a medical officer in CDER's Division of Neuropharmacological Drug Products (DNDP) for over 10 years.

My selection for the review of the pediatric suicidality data for antidepressant drugs occurred as follows: As a medical officer in DNDP, I reviewed a number of submissions of pediatric data for antidepressant drugs, including pediatric data submitted for Paxil (paroxetine), manufactured by GlaxoSmithKline (GSK). In May of 2003, after I had transferred to ODS, DNDP received new data analyses from GSK, indicating an increase in suicidal thoughts and behaviors with paroxetine compared to placebo in pediatric clinical trials. On June 2, 2003, Dr. Russell Katz, the Director of DNDP, sent me an email, in which he said, "Given your history with this application and this general issue, we think you would be the right person to help us think about the best way to approach the data in the other NDAs (and their sponsors), as well as to provide ideas for further sources of potentially relevant data...." A consultation request from DNDP to ODS signed June 6, 2003 byg Dr. Katz stated: "Since the original review of the Paxil supplement, as well as the reviews of most other pediatric supplements for SSRIs, was done by Andrew Mosholder, M.D,...we ask that this consult be assigned to him. We seek his advice on further analysis and interpretation of the Paxil results, as well as more general advice on what might be done to re-evaluate the risk of suicidality in the pediatric databases for other SSRIs...."

My managers in ODS agreed to Dr. Katz' request and assigned me to this consultation on June 9, 2003. To determine whether the apparent increase in suicidal events applies to pediatric use of other antidepressant drugs as well, I started to review the pediatric data for other antidepressant drugs. DNDP ultimately decided that the best way to proceed would be to ask the sponsors of other antidepressant drugs to reproduce GSK's analysis of suicidal events for Paxil, with each sponsor applying the same method to their own pediatric trial databases. In July of 2003, DNDP sent requests for such analyses to other antidepressant drug sponsors.

By September of 2003, I had completed an analysis of the paroxetine data and a preliminary analysis of pediatric data on seven other antidepressant drugs. At the request of management, I presented these analyses at a CDER Regulatory Briefing for upper level management on September 16, 2003. During the briefing, I presented the paroxetine pediatric data, along with preliminary findings for other antidepressant drugs. As noted in the briefing minutes, there was discussion about the clinical significance of some of the events in the analysis: "We need to get a better sense of what the events from these studies really are, i.e., are they legitimate, suicide-associated thoughts/actions or self-mutilation acts that are becoming increasingly common in the adolescent population today and are not generally associated with a sincere intent to die." The day following the regulatory briefing, Dr. Katz thanked me by email: "I just wanted to thank you for a superb presentation (not to mention all the work that went into it). I believe everyone was duly impressed, as they should have been. What the next step is, I don't know yet, but we'll probably get together soon to figure it out."

The Federal Register on October 31, 2003 contained this announcement to the public: "The Psychopharmacologic Drugs Advisory Committee and the Pediatric Subcommittee of the Anti-Infective Drugs Advisory Committee will discuss reports of the occurrence of suicidality (both suicidal ideation and suicide attempts) in clinical trials for various antidepressant drugs in pediatric patients with major depressive disorder (MDD). The committee will consider optimal approaches to the analysis of data from these trials, and the results of analyses conducted to date, with regard to the question of what regulatory action may be needed pertinent to the clinical use of these products in pediatric patients. The committee will also consider further research needs to address questions on this topic."

As DNDP received responses from the other manufacturers to the July information requests, those responses were forwarded to me for review. I then worked on my analysis of these responses over the next couple of months and completed the first written draft of my results in December of 2003. (This document has since been revised, and has not yet received supervisory sign-off in ODS.)

DNDP apparently was reaching a conclusion that the responses from the sponsors to the July requests were not going to be adequate for a definitive analysis. In October of 2003, DNDP sent requests to the manufacturers asking for patient level data sets, to permit a more sophisticated statistical analysis than what I could accomplish using only the responses to the July requests. DNDP also decided that all of the possible suicidal events in these trials should be reclassified by outside experts in suicidology.

On December 10, 2003, the U.K.'s Medicines and Healthcare products Regulatory Agency issued their statement, "Use of Selective Serotonin Reuptake Inhibitors (SSRIs) in children and adolescents with major depressive disorder (MDD) - only fluoxetine (Prozac) shown to have a favourable balance of risks and benefits for the treatment of MDD in the under 18s."

On December 18, 2003, we had one of our planning meetings for the February 2 advisory committee meeting. A draft agenda distributed for the December 18 planning meeting included a 45-minute presentation by me entitled, "Limited Overview of Paxil Controlled

Trials and Controlled Trials of Other Antidepressants." At that meeting, I shared a proposed outline of my presentation, which included my finding that suicidal events designated as "serious" in pediatric clinical trials for major depressive disorder were 1.9 times more frequent with antidepressant drug treatment than with placebo, and that this was statistically significant. I recall some discussion of the pros and cons of my analysis.

At a subsequent planning session for the February 2 meeting, an agenda entitled "Proposed Agenda for February 2 As Revised by 12/30/03," was distributed. It did not include my clinical trial data presentation.

On January 6, 2004, Dr. Katz sent me an email asking to speak with me by phone regarding my presentation at the February 2 Advisory Committee meeting. In our subsequent telephone conversation on that date, he told me that someone else would present the clinical trial data at the February 2 Advisory Committee meeting since I had reached a different view of the clinical trial data from that of DNDP. On January 7, 2004, I sent an email to the team members planning the February 2 meeting, confirming that I would not be giving the presentation as originally planned and attaching a draft of my slides for their use and interest.

On January 12, 2004, the Agency issued a Federal Register notice with a revised agenda for the February 2 meeting. The notice stated, "The committee will not be considering options for definitive regulatory action at this meeting because definitive analyses of the data have not been completed. This topic will be covered in a second meeting to be scheduled by summer 2004."

I cannot pinpoint when I first learned that a reporter was interested in the project, but I believe I first heard of a reporter making inquiries about this project around mid-January. I also recall that some of my co-workers mentioned such contacts. To the best of my recollection, those employees were,

although there may have been others that I do not recall.

I believe that my first contact from Mr. Rob Waters was on January 22, 2004. Mr. Waters telephoned me at the office to ask to interview me about my work on the issue of pediatric use of antidepressant drugs. I told him that I was not interested in being interviewed unless it was approved through our Public Affairs office. I did inform him of the upcoming advisory committee meeting, referred him to the agency's Public Affairs office, and then notified my managers and our Public Affairs office by email of his telephone call.

On January 27, 2004, I received (at my home address) a letter from Mr. Waters by FedEx, in which he asked me to reconsider speaking to him about this project, independently of the agency's Public Affairs office. I believe I sent Mr. Waters an e-mail from my home email account, telling him that I had no comment and I again ask him to contact the Public Affairs office. I unfortunately did not keep a copy of the e-mail since I did not view his contact of me as important.

On or around January 29, 2004, I received another telephone call from Mr. Waters, asking me to review his story on this issue to make sure that it was factual. Mr. Waters did not send me his proposed article. I informed my Division Director of the contact and, at the direction of my Division Director, I emailed Mr. Waters to suggest that he contact the Public Affairs office for Agency comments on the story. Mr. Waters replied by email to say he was not thinking of sending the entire story, but that he would consider my suggestion.

After the story ran on February 1, 2004 in the San Francisco Chronicle, I sent Mr. Waters an email thanking him for properly reporting that I declined to provide any information for his article, and I believe he sent a reply asking if I had any comments about the article. I met Mr. Waters in person at the February 2 Advisory Committee meeting, where I was one of the presenters (although not as to my findings from the analysis in question). I again thanked him for respecting my rejection of his requests. I may have sent him another email suggesting he could have emphasized the information posted on the British regulatory agency's web site, which I felt should have been more of a focus for his article, but I cannot recall the exact timing of that email. Following the February 2 Advisory Committee meeting, I went on leave to assist my wife,

In summary, I kept the agency informed of my contacts from Mr. Waters. In responding to contacts from Mr. Waters, I did not provide Mr. Waters with any information that was not public. I did not share my conclusions from my analysis with him.

I understand that this statement is part of the Office of Internal Affairs investigation and I have been informed that I may be subject to disciplinary proceedings as a result of my statement.

I have read the above statement consisting of 4 pages and represent that the statement made by me is true and accurate to the best of my knowledge and belief.

____
Signature

Signed and affirmed to before me this ______ day of ____________, _______.

____
Special Agent/Date
FDA, Office of Internal Affairs

Authority to administer oaths:
Title 5, U.S. Code, Section 303

____
Witness/Date

Home | Previous Page

U.S. Securities and Exchange Commission

Whistleblower Protection Act Information

Tab 61

A federal agency violates the Whistleblower Protection Act if it takes or fails to take (or threatens to take or fail to take) a personnel action with respect to any employee or applicant because of any disclosure of information by the employee or applicant that he or she reasonably believes evidences a violation of a law, rule or regulation; gross mismanagement; gross waste of funds; an abuse of authority; or a substantial and specific danger to public health or safety.

The U.S. Office of Special Counsel (OSC) has jurisdiction over allegations of whistleblower retaliation for made by employees of the SEC.

- Whistleblower Protection Act Complaints should be sent to

  U.S. Office of Special Counsel
  Complaints Examining Unit
  1730 M Street, NW, Suite 201
  Washington, DC 20036-4505

The required Whistleblower complaint form is available online at

OSC (www.osc.gov)

http://www.sec.gov/eeoinfo/whistleblowers.htm

Home | Previous Page

Modified: 01/30/2004

Food and Drug Administration
Office of Internal Affairs

Statement of Rights and Obligations
(ADMINSTRATIVE WARNING)

Tab 62

Before we ask you any questions, it is my obligation to inform you of the following:

You are here to be asked questions pertaining to your employment with FDA and the duties you perform for FDA. You have a duty to reply to these questions, and Agency disciplinary proceedings resulting in discipline up to and including discharge may be initiated as a result of your answers. You are also advised that you may be subject to criminal prosecution for any false answers given in response to my questions. You may be subject to discharge if you refuse to answer or fail to respond truthfully to any relevant questions.

Acknowledgement of Receipt by Employee

I have been given the above statement of rights and obligations at the beginning of the interview held on March 3, 2004.

[signature]	3/3/04
Signature of Employee	Date
Mike J. King	3·3·04
Witness Signature	Date
Mark S. McCormack	3/3/04
Witness Signature	Date

From: Mosholder, Andrew D
Sent: Wednesday, March 03, 2004 10:16 AM
To: Addy, Rosemary; Murphy, Dianne; Cummins, Susan; Iyasu, Solomon; Laughren, Thomas P; Katz, Russell G; Trontell, Anne E; Seligman, Paul; Temple, Robert; Racoosin, Judith A; Willy, Mary E; Avigan, Mark I; CDER-DNDP-PSYCHOPHARM; David, Paul A
Cc: Cruzan, Susan M
Subject: Inquiry regarding Feb. 2 AC meeting

Hello,

Those of you who were involved in planning the February 2 AC meeting may want to know that there is now an FDA Internal Affairs investigation of the "leak" which generated the February 1 San Francisco Chronicle article. As it seems probable that many of you will also be contacted as part of this inquiry, I thought I should let everyone have a "heads up" about this.

Regards,

Andy

Tab 63

Mosholder, Andrew D

From:	Meister, Karen G
Sent:	Thursday, April 29, 2004 4:26 PM
To:	Mosholder, Andrew D
Cc:	Henig, Anne M; Katz, Donna; Dettelbach, Kim
Subject:	Meeting on Mon. at 1 pm

This is to confirm that we will meet again on Monday at 1 pm (May 3) in Patrick's office. Anne, Donna, and Kim, can you join us? Thanks.

Karen G. Meister
Legislative Analyst
FDA Office of Legislation
(301) 827-0101
(301) 827-1955 fax

Tab 64

Doyle, Thomas

Tab 65

rom:	Seligman, Paul
nt:	Tuesday, February 10, 2004 1:44 PM
o:	Coleman, Horace; Doyle, Thomas
Subject:	Inappropriate Disclosure

Per my conversation earlier today with Mr. Doyle, I am emailing you both regarding a circumstance in my office which I believe may merit further follow up from your office.

During the course of the preparation for an FDA advisory committee meeting that was held on February 2, 2004, on the potential relationship between a risk of suicide in children and the use of anti-depressant drugs in a class called selective serotonin reuptake inhibitors (SSRIs), I believe that an inappropriate disclosure of sensitive information may have occurred to a reporter working for the San Francisco Chronicle.

This disclosure resulted in staff members in the Office of Drug Safety being called at home on evenings and weekends by the reporter, and the publication of information in the Chronicle on February 1st that was not publicly available.

The article (attached) cites unnamed FDA sources and includes the following statement, "His preliminary analysis, according to two FDA sources familiar with the report's contents, concluded that there was an increased risk of suicidal behavior among children being treated for depression with Paxil and several other antidepressants."

As the consult upon which this disclosure was based had not been completed, I am concerned that a member or members of the staff of the Office of Drug Safety may have inappropriately disclosed information of a sensitive nature.

I look forward to discussing this matter further with you regarding the best way to proceed.

Thank you for your consideration.

aul Seligman, MD, MPH
cting Director, Office of Drug Safety

San Francisco
Chronicle Articl...

Scientist links antidepressants to suicide in kids
Rob Waters, Special to the Chronicle
Sunday, February 1, 2004

URL: sfgate.com/article.cgi?file=/c/a/2004/02/01/MNFDA.TMP

A scientist at the Food and Drug Administration has been barred from publicly presenting his finding that several leading antidepressants may increase the risk of suicidal behaviors among children, according to sources inside the FDA.

FDA medical officer Andrew Mosholder was to present his report Monday at an FDA advisory hearing in Washington that promises to be a contentious affair involving competing medical experts and parents whose children took their own lives while on the medications.

A senior FDA official said the study wouldn't be presented because it wasn't "finalized." But critics fear that the agency's action indicates it is not prepared to take stronger action against the drugs, despite warnings about their possible effects on children.

Mosholder had been asked by the agency to perform a safety analysis of antidepressants after reports emerged this summer of high rates of suicidal behavior among children enrolled in clinical trials for Paxil, Effexor and other antidepressants.

Mosholder, a child psychiatrist, reviewed data from 20 clinical trials involving more than 4,100 children and eight different antidepressants. His preliminary analysis, according to two FDA sources familiar with the report's contents, concluded that there was an increased risk of suicidal behavior among children being treated for depression with Paxil and several other antidepressants.

An initial agenda for Monday's hearing listed Mosholder and his findings, but his presentation was removed from a revised agenda, and Mosholder was told that he could not present his findings at the hearing, one FDA official, who wished to remain anonymous, told The Chronicle.

According to the official, in early January, Russell Katz, director of the division of neuropharmacological drug products, called Mosholder in for a meeting. "He told him that he was sorry, but he wasn't going to be able to present (his report) because he had reached a conclusion and therefore was biased," the official said.

Mosholder declined several requests to be interviewed and was not made available despite repeated requests to FDA's press office. Katz was unavailable to comment on the charges.

In a telephone interview Friday with The Chronicle, Anne Trontell, deputy director of the agency's Office of Drug Safety, who is Mosholder's direct supervisor, said the analysis would not be presented because it had not yet been approved within her office.

"The consult on that is not finalized. It's not a final document within the Office of Drug Safety," Trontell said.

However, Trontell said that at Monday's hearing, Mosholder would provide a rundown of reports of suicidal behavior received by the agency from doctors and other professionals.

While Mosholder's safety analysis report may eventually be completed and made public, some FDA insiders fear that withholding it from Monday's hearing indicates that the agency may be siding with the pharmaceutical industry in its long-running battle with critics of antidepressants.

"Why is the agency sitting on its hands and acting as if there isn't a risk when their own scientists have looked at the data and concluded that there is?" one FDA official remarked.

The use of antidepressants and other psychiatric medication among children has more than tripled in recent years and now approaches adult usage rates, according to a January 2003 study in the Archives of Pediatric and Adolescent Medicine. Study author Julie Zito, an associate professor of pharmacy and medicine at the University of Maryland, estimates that more than 1 million American children used antidepressants in 2000.

Advocates of the drugs argue that they are imperfect but necessary weapons against a rising tide of mental illness among children.

Last month, a task force of the American College of Neuropsychopharmacology released its own preliminary review of published studies on antidepressants and suicide and stated it found no statistically significant increase in suicide attempts among children taking the drugs.

"The most likely explanation for the episodes of attempted suicide while taking SSRIs (selective serotonin reuptake inhibitors) is the underlying depression, not the SSRIs," said Graham Emslie, a child psychiatrist and researcher at the University of Texas Southwestern Medical Center in Dallas.

But critics, including consumer advocates and mental health professionals contend, based on other studies, that the drugs are often ineffective and sometimes dangerous and that the FDA has failed to vigorously investigate the risks and protect children's safety.

"The FDA is shielding the industry," said Vera Sharav, president of the Alliance for Human Research Protection, a consumer advocacy group.

Mosholder's analysis appears to be similar to the conclusions reached by British regulators, who told doctors in December to stop prescribing Paxil, Zoloft, Effexor and three other antidepressants to children because of an apparent "increased rate of self-harm and suicidal thoughts."

British regulators took action against Paxil in early June after new data presented to U.S. and British authorities showed that children taking the drug were nearly three times as likely to consider or attempt suicide as children taking placebos.

Later that month, the FDA issued a similar warning, urging doctors not to prescribe Paxil to children and announced that it would conduct a detailed review of pediatric trials of Paxil. The review was subsequently broadened to include seven other antidepressants, including top sellers Prozac, Zoloft and Effexor.

In October, the agency wrote to physicians to "call to (their) attention" reports of suicide among children in antidepressant trials. The agency did not, however, urge doctors to stop prescribing the drugs.

Several current and former FDA staff members interviewed by The Chronicle said the dispute over Mosholder's report highlights a lack of assertiveness within the agency over safety issues. They spoke of a split between the Office of Drug Safety - Mosholder's office - and the FDA's drug-reviewing divisions.

As an example, they cite a hearing last March on a rheumatoid arthritis drug, Arava, which had generated numerous reports of adverse effects, including nine deaths, after being approved by the FDA.

Members of the Office of Drug Safety, who had prepared a 37-page safety report, were present at the hearing but were not allowed to speak. A representative of the FDA division that originally approved the drug, along with the pharmaceutical company that makes the drug, did most of the talking.

A documentary crew from the PBS series Frontline filmed the meeting and afterward, in the hallway, caught up with David Graham, a senior epidemiologist with the Office of Drug Safety. The producers had been denied previous requests to interview Graham, but the government scientist gave a brief interview without permission.

"We had a different perspective, and we really weren't given an opportunity to present our side of the story," Graham, on camera, told the producers. "And the people who did present, the reviewing division and the company, you know, they didn't see a problem. This was a very hostile process. And let's just leave it at that."

Paul Stolley, a professor and former chairman of the department of epidemiology at the University of Maryland, spent a sabbatical year as a senior consultant in the Office of Drug Safety in 2000 and 2001. While there, he recalls, he tussled with agency managers over the safety of Lotronex, a drug used to treat irritable bowel syndrome, a chronic but usually not serious disease.

Stolley said his investigation uncovered high rates of negative side effects, including a number of deaths, among patients using the drug and led the company to withdraw the drug from the market.

A few months later, over Stolley's objections, the agency allowed the drug back on the market with a "risk management" program aimed at educating patients and doctors about the drug's risks. Stolley said he was excluded from internal FDA meetings on the issue.

"I'm worried about the agency," he says. "I didn't expect people to think I was right just because I was very senior. What I did expect was a vigorous debate and instead of having a vigorous debate, they made a policy decision and then excluded me."

Rob Waters' article, "A Suicide Side Effect? What parents aren't being told about their kids' antidepressants," appeared in the Jan. 4 edition of The Chronicle Magazine. (Read it here) E-mail Waters at robw001@pacbell.net.

Food and Drug Administration
Office of Internal Affairs (HFH-560)

MEMORANDUM

Date: March 10, 2004

Tab 66

From: Special Agent in Charge
Office of Internal Affairs (HFH-560)

Subject: Report of Investigation on the CDER, Office of Drug Safety E-mail, dated 5/10/04
(OIA Case Control Number)

To: Dr. Paul Seligman, Director, Office of Pharmacoepidemiology & Statistical Science, Center for Drug Evaluation and Research (HFD-030)

Attached is our report of investigation in response to allegations of misconduct reported to the Office of Internal Affairs.

We have provided you a copy of this report for your information. Management review is necessary to determine whether personnel action is warranted based upon the facts of the case. This report remains the property of the Office of Internal Affairs and should not be disseminated without prior approval. It must be returned within 30 days of receipt.

Please advise OIA of your decision regarding the necessity for and details of any administrative actions taken based upon the results of this investigation.

If you have any questions, please contact SA at (301) 827-0243. The cooperation and courtesies extended to my staff during the investigation are appreciated.

Horace L. Coleman

Attachment

Cc:
Chron
Case File

Food and Drug Administration
Office of Internal Affairs (HFH-560)

MEMORANDUM

Date: March 10, 2004

From: Special Agent in Charge
Office of Internal Affairs (HFH-560)

Subject: Report of Investigation on the CDER, Office of Drug Safety E-mail, dated 5/10/04
(OIA Case Control Number)

To: Mr. Michael Shane
Attorney, Office of Chief Counsel (GCF-1)

Attached is our report of investigation in response to allegations of misconduct reported to the Office of Internal Affairs.

We have provided you a copy of this report for your information. This report remains the property of the Office of Internal Affairs and should not be disseminated without prior approval. It must be returned within 30 days of receipt.

If you have any questions, please contact SA at (301) 827-0243. The cooperation and courtesies extended to my staff during the investigation are appreciated.

Horace L. Coleman

Attachment

Cc:
Chron
Case File

Food and Drug Administration
Office of Internal Affairs

REPORT OF INVESTIGATION

****

TITLE: CDER Office of Drug Safety Email **CASE NO:** 04-OIA-971-043

TYPE OF CASE: 971.000 Unauthorized Release of Information

INVESTIGATION MADE AT: Rockville, MD

PERIOD COVERED: 02/12/04 to 05/10/04

INVESTIGATION MADE BY: SA Michael Kurisky and SA Mark McCormack

REPORTING AGENT: SA Michael Kurisky

STATUS OF CASE: ( ) CONTINUING INVESTIGATION
( ) SIGNIFICANT DEVELOPMENT
( ) PENDING ADMINISTRATIVE ACTION
( ) PENDING JUDICIAL ACTION
( ) REFERRAL TO ANOTHER AGENCY
(X) CLOSED

/ 5/10/04 5/10/04

Signature / Date	Approval Signature / Date
Michael J. Kurisky	Horace L. Coleman
Special Agent	Special Agent in Charge

****

RESTRICTED INFORMATION

This report is furnished on an official need-to-know basis and must be protected from dissemination which might compromise the best interests of the Food and Drug Administration, Office of Internal Affairs. This report shall not be released in response to a Freedom of Information Act or Privacy Act request or disseminated to other parties without prior consultation with the FDA Office of Internal Affairs. UNAUTHORIZED RELEASE MAY RESULT IN CRIMINAL PROSECUTION.

DISTRIBUTION:

OIA: Orig & 1cc
Ms. Cindy Lepson, Deputy Director, Employee and Labor Relations Branch: 1cc
Dr. Paul Seligman, Director, Office of Pharmacoepidemiology & Statistical Science, Center for Drug Evaluation and Research: 1cc
Mr. Michael Shane, Attorney, Office of Chief Counsel: 1cc

1. INTRODUCTION:

This case originated on 02/10/04 based on a telephone call from Dr. Paul Seligman, Director – Office of Pharmacoepidemiology & Statistical Science, Center for Drug Evaluation and Research, 5600 Fishers Lane, Room 15B03, Rockville, MD, 301-827-3219. Dr. Seligman alleged that while preparing for a FDA Advisory Committee meeting held on February 2, 2004 that discussed the potential relationship between the risk of suicide in children and the use of anti-depressant drugs in a class called selective serotonin reuptake inhibitors (SSRI's), an FDA employee might have made an inappropriate disclosure of sensitive information to a newspaper reporter from the San Francisco Chronicle; Rob Waters. This incident resulted in FDA employees being contacted at home by the reporter and the publication of information in the Chronicle newspaper that was not publicly available.

2. SYNOPSIS:

Interviews have been conducted with all known FDA employees who were contacted by Waters. Investigation has revealed that there does not appear to have been any release of any proprietary or sensitive data.

Case is closed.

3. DETAILS OF INVESTIGATION:

Background

In May 2003, the Center for Drug Evaluation and Research's Division of Neuropharmacological Drug Products (DNDP) had received some new data analysis from GlaxoSmithKline (GSK) indicating an increase in suicidal thoughts and behaviors with paroxetine (Paxil) compared to the placebo in pediatric clinical trials. In June 2003, Dr. Andrew Mosholder was selected to analyze and interpret this data. DNDP eventually decided to request data from 22 short-term placebo controlled trials involving 9 different antidepressant drugs* to see if there appeared to be an increase in suicidality in those individuals taking the drugs.

In September 2003, Mosholder had completed the analysis of the paroxetine data and a preliminary analysis of the data on the other antidepressant drugs. These finding were presented at a CDER Regulatory Briefing for upper level management on September 16, 2003. During this meeting, the issue was brought up that some of the acts identified during the trials as suicidal behavior/ideations might not actually truly be that type of behavior, but rather self-mutilation behavior which is common in today's adolescents.

In October 2003, the decision was made within DNDP that all of the possible suicidal events in these trials should be re-classified by outside experts in suicidology.

---

* Drugs included paroxetine, sertraline, venlafaxine, fluoxetine, fluvoxamine, citalopram, nefazodone, mirtazapine and bupropion.

On October 31, 2003, The Federal Register contained the announcement that "The Psychopharmacologic Drugs Advisory Committee and the Pediatric Subcommittee of the Anti-Infective Drugs Advisory Committee will discuss reports of the occurrence of suicidality in clinical trials for various antidepressant drugs in pediatric patients with major depressive disorder (MDD). This meeting was the one that took place on February 2, 2004.

In December 2003, the United Kingdom's Medicines and Healthcare products Regulatory Agency issued a statement that only fluoxetine (Prozac) was the only antidepressant shown to have a favorable balance of risks and benefits for the treatment of MDD in individuals less than 18 years of age.

On December 18, 2003, a planning meeting was held to prepare for the Advisory Committee meeting scheduled on February 2, 2004. A draft agenda for the February 2, 2004 meeting included a 45 minute presentation by Dr. Mosholder entitled "Limited Overview of Paxil Controlled Trials and Controlled Trials of Other Antidepressants." This presentation included Mosholder's finding that "suicidal events designated as "serious" in pediatric clinical trials for major depressive disorder were 1.9 times more frequent with antidepressant drug treatment then with placebo." According to Mosholder, at a subsequent planning session, an agenda entitled "Proposed Agenda for February 2 as Revised by T. Laughren, 12/30/03" was distributed that did not include Mosholder's presentation.

On January 6, 2004, Mosholder was contacted by Dr. Russell Katz, Director of DNDP, and was told that he would not be making his presentation at the February 2, 2004 Advisory Committee meeting since he had reached a different view of the clinical trial data from that of the DNDP.

In the early part of January 2004, San Francisco Chronicle reporter Rob Waters contacted five FDA employees within the Office of Drug Safety at their residences in regards to the study into the possible relationship between adolescents on antidepressants and an increased risk of suicide.

On February 1, 2004, an article entitled *"Drug Report barred by the FDA – Scientist links antidepressants to suicide in kids"*, written by Rob Waters, was published in the San Francisco Chronicle.

On February 2, 2004, the Psychopharmacologic Drugs Advisory Committee with the Pediatric Subcommittee of the Anti-Infective Drugs Advisory Committee met at the Holiday Inn, Bethesda, Maryland. A review of the transcripts (www.fda.gov/ohrms/dockets/ac/04/transcripts/4006T1.htm) from this meeting show that Dr. Mosholder made a presentation in regards to the Office of Drug Safety's Data Resources for the Study of Suicidal Events, but did not present any findings in regards to his review of the data examined in 2003. At the beginning of the Advisory Committee meeting Dr. Russell Katz, Director of the DNDP stated the following:

> *"It should be noted that this view of the data has not been a unanimous one among Agency staff. Some within the Agency have examined the data and concluded that the data, as currently submitted, do permit definitive analysis and that these analysis support the conclusion that this class of drugs is associated with a risk of suicidal behavior in pediatric patients.*
>
> *However, the staff of the Neuropharmacological Drugs Division has examined the individual cases reported by the sponsors that allegedly represent suicidal behavior, and we are convinced*

that the categorization of these events, as performed idiosyncratically by the individual sponsors, is not entirely reliable."

Investigation

On February 10, 2004, Dr. Paul Seligman contacted the Office of Internal Affairs Special Agent in Charge; Thomas P. Doyle, via telephone, to discuss his concern over the possibility that an FDA employee had disclosed sensitive information to Waters.

On February 19, 2004, SA Kurisky interviewed Dr. Seligman at his office, Rm. 15B03, Parklawn building. The purpose of this meeting was to obtain more details in regards to the allegations. Seligman advised that after January 6, 2004, five employees within the Office of Drug Safety had been called at home by Waters. The five employees were identified as Andrew Mosholder, Mary Willy, Anne Trontell, Evelyn Farinas, and Renan Bonnel. Seligman indicated that Mosholder had been pulled from presenting because his findings were different from that of the Advisory Committee. He further indicated that there had been at least one prior incident of information being released to the press prior to an Advisory Committee meeting. When questioned as to whom he thought might have made this disclosure, Seligman indicated that FDA employee David Graham had been very vocal in the past in regards to scientist findings being suppressed. Seligman also stated that Russell Katz was the individual who made the decision that Mosholder's views were not concurrent with the committees.

On March 2, 2004, Andrew Mosholder was contacted and requested to come to the Office of Internal Affairs for an interview the following day. On March 3, 2004, Mosholder appeared at the office for an interview. Also present was National Treasury Employees Union representative Stefan Monica. Mosholder was provided and signed a Statement of Rights and Obligations (**Attachment 1**). During the interview, Mosholder was advised of the protections afforded by the Whistleblower Protection Act in regards to disclosures of information made by employees that they reasonably believe evidences a substantial or specific danger to public health or safety. Mosholder was further advised that if he had made disclosures the interview would be terminated in order to protect his rights under the law. In response to questions presented by SA Kurisky, Mosholder provided an overview of his involvement in this study to include when and why he was selected to review this data, when he had come to his preliminary and final conclusions, when and why he was pulled from making the presentation at the advisory committee meeting as well as a discussion of his contacts with Waters. During this interview, Mosholder was told that he was not a suspect, based on his full disclosure of his contacts with Waters to include a January 27, 2004 e-mail addressed to Anne Trontell, Mark Avigan and Mary Willy that disclosed a letter from Waters to Mosholder (**Attachment 2**). It was also learned during this interview that Mosholder was contacted on his unlisted home telephone number. Mosholder was given the opportunity to prepare a written statement over the course of several days in order to be both thorough and accurate. Mosholder signed this statement on March 15th, 2004 (**Attachment 3**).

On March 15, 2004, Evelyn Farinas was interviewed at her office located in Room 15B18 of the Parklawn building. Present for this interview was National Treasury Employees Union Representative Michael Theodorakis. Farinas was provided and signed a Statement of Rights and Obligations (**Attachment 4**). In response to questions presented by SA Kurisky, Farinas discussed her position and duties with the FDA, her contacts with Waters and her involvement with Mosholder's study. Farinas indicated that she was not involved in Mosholder's study and that she thought Waters was calling in regards to a previous consult she was assigned that involved the drug mifepristone (RU-486). Farinas instructed Waters to contact her only at work and notified her supervisor the following day. Farinas was given the opportunity to prepare a written statement over the course of several days in order to be both thorough and accurate. She signed this statement on March 23rd, 2004 (**Attachment 5**).

On March 23, 2004, Mary Willy was interviewed at her office located in Room 15B18 of the Parklawn building. Willy was provided and signed a Statement of Rights and Obligations (**Attachment 6**). Willy was Mosholder's Team Leader in the Division of Drug Risk Evaluation (DDRE) and was responsible for assigning the various consults to epidemiologists within DDRE and monitoring the progress of these assignments. Willy viewed Mosholder as a very competent worker requiring very little supervision. Willy was in agreement with Mosholder's findings in regards to the risk associated with the use of antidepressants in adolescents with MDD. Willy also discussed her brief telephone conversation with a reporter at her house in early January. Willy was given the opportunity to prepare a written statement over the course of several days in order to be both thorough and accurate. She signed this written statement (**Attachment 7**) on April 6, 2004.

On April 16, 2004, Dr. Russell Katz was interviewed at the Office of Internal Affairs. Katz was provided and signed a Statement of Rights and Obligations (**Attachment 8**). The purpose of this interview was to establish why Mosholder had been prevent from presenting his findings at the February 2, 2004 Advisory Committee meeting. Katz discussed why Mosholder had been chosen to review that Paxil data and then the reasons for expanding the review to include other SSRI's. As the study progressed, it was found that there was no uniformity among the drug companies as to the behaviors they classified as suicidal. Katz indicated that he and others on the Advisory Committee felt that many things labeled as suicidal behavior were not truly suicidal acts. Katz advised that in September 2003 there was a regulatory briefing in which this issue was discussed. At this meeting, Katz advised that it was decided to bring in outside experts (from Columbia University) to review the data and determine if the behaviors could truly be classified as a suicidal event. Katz also discussed his conversation with Mosholder in January 2004, when he was informed that he would not be presenting his findings at the Advisory Committee meeting. Katz was given the opportunity to prepare a written statement over the course of several days in order to be both thorough and accurate. He signed this written statement (**Attachment 9**) on May 6, 2004.

On April 19, 2004, SA Kurisky left a message with Dr. David Graham in regards to providing a statement about his knowledge of any unauthorized disclosures regarding Mosholder being pulled from presenting his data at the Advisory Committee meeting. On the same day, SA Kurisky received a call from Tom Devine, Legal Director of the Government Accountability Project (202-408-0034 x124). According to the organizations website (www.whistleblower.org), the Government Accountability Project's mission is to protect the public interest by promoting government and corporate accountability through advancing occupational free speech and ethical conduct, defending whistleblowers, and empowering citizen activists. Devine indicated that he was calling on behalf of Graham. After verifying with Graham that Devine was calling on his behalf, SA Kurisky informed him as to the nature of this investigation. Devine was informed that Internal Affairs was trying to determine several things. First; if classified or proprietary data had been disclosed, second; if someone had released personal information about FDA employees (i.e. Mosholder's unlisted telephone number) and third; why Mosholder had been pulled from presenting his finding at the Advisory Committee meeting. Devine recited numerous US Codes and statutes to include 5 USC §2302(b)(8) and Section 620 of the

Consolidated Appropriations Act, 2004, (Public Law 108-199, signed 01/23/04), that would protect any individual who might have disclosed to the media that Mosholder had been prevented from presenting his findings at the Advisory Committee meeting. Furthermore, Devine indicated that 5 USC §2302 has no restriction on the avenue in which the disclosure is made, thereby allowing disclosure to the media. Devine was requested to send over all relevant statutes for further review by the FDA's Office of Chief Counsel.

On April 22, 2004, Devine faxed over the requested documents which were forwarded to Michael Shane in the Office of Chief Counsel for review.

On April 26, 2004, SA Kurisky spoke to Michael Shane. Shane indicated that if the material released to the reporter was not classified or proprietary, then the individual who released the information would have protections under the Whistleblower Protection Act. Shane was informed that to date; no evidence had been uncovered to show that the information released was classified or proprietary in nature.

On April 26, 2004, Dr. Anne Trontell was interviewed at her office in Room 15B-33 of the Parklawn building. Trontell is the Deputy Director of the Office of Drug Safety. Trontell discussed her phone conversation with Waters that occurred at her residence on the morning of Saturday, January 10, 2004. Trontell was given the opportunity to prepare a written statement over the course of several days in order to be both thorough and accurate. She signed this written statement (**Attachment 10**) on May 10, 2004.

On April 28, 2004, Renan Bonnel appeared at the Office of Internal Affairs to sign her written statement (**Attachment 11**) that discussed her telephone conversation with Waters that occurred in January 2004.

On May 3, 2004, SA Kurisky and Internal Affairs Special Agent in Charge Horace Coleman met with Dr. Paul Seligman to discuss our findings in this investigation.

Conclusions

After speaking to all individuals who were contacted at home by Waters and a review of the articles written by Waters, no evidence was found indicating that classified or proprietary information from the FDA was released. Furthermore, according to Bonnel's statement, Waters had said that he had received an anonymous phone message stating that the FDA was not handling the safety information of antidepressants in children properly for the preparation of the Advisory Committee meeting in the coming weeks.

In regards to the release of a FDA employee's unlisted telephone number, investigation showed that this number could easily be obtained through any number of fee based information services. An intelligence research specialist from the Investigative Analysis Branch was asked to try and find as much information about Andrew Mosholder as possible using only his name. A query with the Autotrack database provided Mosholder's unlisted home number and address. These information services are not restricted to law enforcement and often subscribe to by media organizations.

Finally, the decision to have the data further reviewed by specialists at Columbia University was something that had been discussed as early as September 2003. The fact that some scientists at the FDA did believe there was an increased risk of suicide among adolescents taking these SSRI's was mentioned at the February 2 Advisory Committee meeting. As the Director of the Division of Neuropharmacological Drug Products, Katz did have the final say so in whether or not Mosholder's findings would be presented. However, he felt that Mosholder had based his findings on data that was not accurately coded during the clinical trials.

Case is closed.

4. OTHER INVESTIGATIONS:

None

5. JUDICIAL/ADMINISTRATIVE ACTION:

None

6. DISPOSITION OF EVIDENCE, CONTRABAND, AND PERSONAL PROPERTY:

None

7. DISPOSITION STATUS:

Case is closed

8. INFORMATION TO BE INDEXED:

None

9. ATTACHMENTS:

No.	Description
1.)	Statement of Rights and Obligations, dated 3/3/04, signed by Andrew Mosholder
2.)	E-mail from Mosholder to Trontell, dated 1/27/04, with attached letter from Waters
3.)	Statement of Andrew Mosholder, dated 03/15/04
4.)	Statement of Rights and Obligations, dated 03/15/04, signed by Evelyn Farinas
5.)	Statement of Evelyn Farinas, dated 03/23/04
6.)	Statement of Rights and Obligations, dated 03/23/04, signed by Mary Willy
7.)	Statement of Mary Willy, dated 04/06/04
8.)	Statement of Rights and Obligations, dated 4/16/04, signed by Russell Katz
9.)	Statement of Russell Katz, dated 5/6/04
10.)	Statement of Anne Trontell, dated 5/10/04
11.)	Statement of Renan Bonnel, dated 04/28/04

The originals of the attachments are being maintained by the FDA Office of Internal Affairs, Rockville, MD.

WRITTEN STATEMENT **Tab 67**

I, Andrew D. Mosholder, provide the following statement at the request of Special Agent, Michael J. Kurisky of the FDA Office of Internal Affairs:

I am a licensed physician and board certified in child and adolescent psychiatry. I obtained my medical degree from the University of Virginia. I also have a Master of Public Health degree from Johns Hopkins University.

I am currently employed by the U.S. Food and Drug Administration and have been so employed since 1992. During my employment, I have been a medical officer with the Center for Drug Evaluation and Research (CDER) for almost twelve years. For about the past 14 months I have worked as an epidemiologist in the Division of Drug Risk Evaluation, Office of Drug Safety (ODS). Prior to that, I was a medical officer in CDER's Division of Neuropharmacological Drug Products (DNDP) for over 10 years.

My selection for the review of the pediatric suicidality data for antidepressant drugs occurred as follows: As a medical officer in DNDP, I reviewed a number of submissions of pediatric data for antidepressant drugs, including pediatric data submitted for Paxil (paroxetine), manufactured by GlaxoSmithKline (GSK). In May of 2003, after I had transferred to ODS, DNDP received new data analyses from GSK, indicating an increase in suicidal thoughts and behaviors with paroxetine compared to placebo in pediatric clinical trials. On June 2, 2003, Dr. Russell Katz, the Director of DNDP, sent me an email, in which he said, "Given your history with this application and this general issue, we think you would be the right person to help us think about the best way to approach the data in the other NDAs (and their sponsors), as well as to provide ideas for further sources of potentially relevant data...." A consultation request from DNDP to ODS signed June 6, 2003 byg Dr. Katz stated: "Since the original review of the Paxil supplement, as well as the reviews of most other pediatric supplements for SSRIs, was done by Andrew Mosholder, M.D,...we ask that this consult be assigned to him. We seek his advice on further analysis and interpretation of the Paxil results, as well as more general advice on what might be done to re-evaluate the risk of suicidality in the pediatric databases for other SSRIs...."

My managers in ODS agreed to Dr. Katz' request and assigned me to this consultation on June 9, 2003. To determine whether the apparent increase in suicidal events applies to pediatric use of other antidepressant drugs as well, I started to review the pediatric data for other antidepressant drugs. DNDP ultimately decided that the best way to proceed would be to ask the sponsors of other antidepressant drugs to reproduce GSK's analysis of suicidal events for Paxil, with each sponsor applying the same method to their own pediatric trial databases. In July of 2003, DNDP sent requests for such analyses to other antidepressant drug sponsors.

By September of 2003, I had completed an analysis of the paroxetine data and a preliminary analysis of pediatric data on seven other antidepressant drugs. At the request of management, I presented these analyses at a CDER Regulatory Briefing for upper level management on September 16, 2003. During the briefing, I presented the paroxetine pediatric data, along with preliminary findings for other antidepressant drugs. As noted in the briefing minutes, there was discussion about the clinical significance of some of the events in the analysis: "We need to get a better sense of what the events from these studies really are, i.e., are they legitimate, suicide-associated thoughts/actions or self-mutilation acts that are becoming increasingly common in the adolescent population today and are not generally associated with a sincere intent to die." The day following the regulatory briefing, Dr. Katz thanked me by email: "I just wanted to thank you for a superb presentation (not to mention all the work that went into it). I believe everyone was duly impressed, as they should have been. What the next step is, I don't know yet, but we'll probably get together soon to figure it out."

The Federal Register on October 31, 2003 contained this announcement to the public: "The Psychopharmacologic Drugs Advisory Committee and the Pediatric Subcommittee of the Anti-Infective Drugs Advisory Committee will discuss reports of the occurrence of suicidality (both suicidal ideation and suicide attempts) in clinical trials for various antidepressant drugs in pediatric patients with major depressive disorder (MDD). The committee will consider optimal approaches to the analysis of data from these trials, and the results of analyses conducted to date, with regard to the question of what regulatory action may be needed pertinent to the clinical use of these products in pediatric patients. The committee will also consider further research needs to address questions on this topic."

As DNDP received responses from the other manufacturers to the July information requests, those responses were forwarded to me for review. I then worked on my analysis of these responses over the next couple of months and completed the first written draft of my results in December of 2003. (This document has since been revised, and has not yet received supervisory sign-off in ODS.)

DNDP apparently was reaching a conclusion that the responses from the sponsors to the July requests were not going to be adequate for a definitive analysis. In October of 2003, DNDP sent requests to the manufacturers asking for patient level data sets, to permit a more sophisticated statistical analysis than what I could accomplish using only the responses to the July requests. DNDP also decided that all of the possible suicidal events in these trials should be reclassified by outside experts in suicidology.

On December 10, 2003, the U.K.'s Medicines and Healthcare products Regulatory Agency issued their statement, "Use of Selective Serotonin Reuptake Inhibitors (SSRIs) in children and adolescents with major depressive disorder (MDD) - only fluoxetine (Prozac) shown to have a favourable balance of risks and benefits for the treatment of MDD in the under 18s."

On December 18, 2003, we had one of our planning meetings for the February 2 advisory committee meeting. A draft agenda distributed for the December 18 planning meeting included a 45-minute presentation by me entitled, "Limited Overview of Paxil Controlled

Trials and Controlled Trials of Other Antidepressants." At that meeting, I shared a proposed outline of my presentation, which included my finding that suicidal events designated as "serious" in pediatric clinical trials for major depressive disorder were 1.9 times more frequent with antidepressant drug treatment than with placebo, and that this was statistically significant. I recall some discussion of the pros and cons of my analysis.

At a subsequent planning session for the February 2 meeting, an agenda entitled "Proposed Agenda for February 2 As Revised by T. Laughren, 12/30/03," was distributed. It did not include my clinical trial data presentation.

On January 6, 2004, Dr. Katz sent me an email asking to speak with me by phone regarding my presentation at the February 2 Advisory Committee meeting. In our subsequent telephone conversation on that date, he told me that someone else would present the clinical trial data at the February 2 Advisory Committee meeting since I had reached a different view of the clinical trial data from that of DNDP. On January 7, 2004, I sent an email to the team members planning the February 2 meeting, confirming that I would not be giving the presentation as originally planned and attaching a draft of my slides for their use and interest.

On January 12, 2004, the Agency issued a Federal Register notice with a revised agenda for the February 2 meeting. The notice stated, "The committee will not be considering options for definitive regulatory action at this meeting because definitive analyses of the data have not been completed. This topic will be covered in a second meeting to be scheduled by summer 2004."

I cannot pinpoint when I first learned that a reporter was interested in the project, but I believe I first heard of a reporter making inquiries about this project around mid-January. I also recall that some of my co-workers mentioned such contacts. To the best of my recollection, those employees were Syed Rizwanuddin Ahmad, Renan Bonnel, Evelyn Farinas, Kate Gelperin, David J. Graham, Rita Ouellet-Hellstrom, Anne Trontell, and Mary Willy, although there may have been others that I do not recall.

I believe that my first contact from Mr. Rob Waters was on January 22, 2004. Mr. Waters telephoned me at the office to ask to interview me about my work on the issue of pediatric use of antidepressant drugs. I told him that I was not interested in being interviewed unless it was approved through our Public Affairs office. I did inform him of the upcoming advisory committee meeting, referred him to the agency's Public Affairs office, and then notified my managers and our Public Affairs office by email of his telephone call.

On January 27, 2004, I received (at my home address in West Virginia) a letter from Mr. Waters by FedEx, in which he asked me to reconsider speaking to him about this project, independently of the agency's Public Affairs office. I believe I sent Mr. Waters an e-mail from my home email account, telling him that I had no comment and I again ask him to contact the Public Affairs office. I unfortunately did not keep a copy of the e-mail since I did not view his contact of me as important.

On or around January 29, 2004, I received another telephone call from Mr. Waters, asking me to review his story on this issue to make sure that it was factual. Mr. Waters did not send me his proposed article. I informed my Division Director of the contact and, at the direction of my Division Director, I emailed Mr. Waters to suggest that he contact the Public Affairs office for Agency comments on the story. Mr. Waters replied by email to say he was not thinking of sending the entire story, but that he would consider my suggestion.

After the story ran on February 1, 2004 in the San Francisco Chronicle, I sent Mr. Waters an email thanking him for properly reporting that I declined to provide any information for his article, and I believe he sent a reply asking if I had any comments about the article. I met Mr. Waters in person at the February 2 Advisory Committee meeting, where I was one of the presenters (although not as to my findings from the analysis in question). I again thanked him for respecting my rejection of his requests. I may have sent him another email suggesting he could have emphasized the information posted on the British regulatory agency's web site, which I felt should have been more of a focus for his article, but I cannot recall the exact timing of that email. Following the February 2 Advisory Committee meeting, I went on leave to assist my wife, who was hospitalized for a surgical procedure February 3.

In summary, I kept the agency informed of my contacts from Mr. Waters. In responding to contacts from Mr. Waters, I did not provide Mr. Waters with any information that was not public. I did not share my conclusions from my analysis with him.

I understand that this statement is part of the Office of Internal Affairs investigation and I have been informed that I may be subject to disciplinary proceedings as a result of my statement.

I have read the above statement consisting of 4 pages and represent that the statement made by me is true and accurate to the best of my knowledge and belief.

[signature]
Signature

Signed and affirmed to before me this 15th day of March, 2004.

[signature] 3/15/04
Special Agent/Date
FDA, Office of Internal Affairs

Authority to administer oaths:
Title 5, U.S. Code, Section 303

____
Witness/Date

WRITTEN STATEMENT **Tab 68**

I, Russell Katz, employed at the Food and Drug Administration, make the following statement freely and voluntarily:

This statement describes my understanding of the Agency's review of possibly suicide related events in children and adolescents treated with antidepressant drugs, and in particular to events related to a review of these data by Dr. Andrew Mosholder of the Office of Drug Safety (ODS) and reports in the media that the Agency suppressed Dr. Mosholder's presentation at a meeting of the Psychiatric Drugs Advisory Committee on February 2, 2004.

The relevant events date back to 2002, when Dr. Mosholder, then a medical reviewer in the Division of Neuropharmacological Drug Products (DNDP; I was then, and am now, the director of that division), was the primary reviewer of the new drug application for Paxil (paroxetine) for use in children and adolescents with depression. Dr. Mosholder noticed that a number of adverse events that appeared to be possibly suicide related were categorized by the sponsor, SmithKline, as "emotional lability", a classification that seemed unusual. In a letter to the sponsor, the division asked the sponsor to further clarify these events, and to explain why they had made this particular classification.

The next relevant event occurred at the end of May, 2003, when we received a phone call from the UK regulatory agency, asking us our opinion of the increased signal for possibly suicide related events with Paxil. As it turned out, the sponsor had submitted a report to the UK (unbeknownst to us) in which they had determined (based on analyses they did in response to our request) that there was an increase in the incidence of these events on drug compared to placebo. The sponsor soon thereafter submitted a response to our letter, in which they reported this increased incidence of possibly suicide-related events. After an initial review of their analyses, we asked other sponsors of antidepressant drug trials in pediatric patients to submit similar analyses.

When the data from the other sponsors came into the Agency, we decided that Dr. Mosholder should review these data, although by this time, he was a reviewer in ODS. Dr. Mosholder had been the primary reviewer for many of these applications when he was employed in DNDP, and we agreed that he would be the appropriate reviewer for these data.

While Dr.. Mosholder was the primary reviewer of the suicide data, others in our division continued to examine the data as well. As we examined the data closely over time, it became clear to us, and to others in the Agency, that the idiosyncratic classification of behaviors performed by the sponsors called into question the reliability of the analyses as presented by the various sponsors. For example, one sponsor classified as a possibly suicide related event an event in which a young girl slapped herself in the head. On multiple occasions, sponsors classified behaviors characterized by superficial cutting of the skin as possibly suicide related. It was clear to us, as well as to others in the Agency, that these behaviors, as well as some others, were clearly not suicide related, despite the sponsors' reporting them as such. Meanwhile, although these questions about the validity of the sponsors' characterizations of these behaviors were becoming obvious and were being discussed widely at several meetings, Dr. Mosholder continued to perform his analyses based on the events as categorized by the sponsors. His preliminary analyses demonstrated an increase in the incidence of possibly suicide-related events on the drugs compared to placebo (he analyzed the individual drugs and also performed analyses in which he combined the data from all of the drugs). His preliminary analyses were discussed at a meeting with the Director of the Office of New Drugs as well as other high ranking members of OND in September, 2003; at that meeting, the unreliable classifications of events as performed by the sponsors was also discussed, and the suggestion was made that the Agency should ask a group of outside experts to re-classify the events based on a blinded examination of the descriptions of the actual behaviors in the patients as reported by the investigators (a suggestion that we ultimately took; that effort is currently on-going). Despite these serious reservations about the reliability of the events as reported by the sponsors, Dr. Mosholder continued to perform his analyses relying on the sponsor classifications.

The Agency decided to discuss our continuing analyses and our plans for future analyses in a combined public meeting of the Psychopharmacologic Drugs Advisory Committee and the Pediatric Sub-committee of the Anti-Infective Drugs Advisory Committee. There was wide agreement within the Agency that we were not in a position to present definitive analyses of the data primarily for the reasons stated; that is, we did not believe that (some, perhaps large, proportion of) the events the sponsors called possibly suicide related were actually suicide related, and that definitive analyses must await an objective re-classification of these events (as noted, this is currently being done by a group of international experts, coordinated by Columbia University). Indeed, the Federal Register notice announcing the meeting explicitly stated that we would not present definitive results, because definitive analyses had not been performed.

Dr. Mosholder had originally been on a preliminary agenda for the meeting; he was to present his analyses. However, as it became increasingly clear that his analyses relied on the events as classified by the sponsors, it became increasingly clear that his conclusion, which he considered at that point essentially definitive, was not supported by the data. At a meeting in late December, 2003, attended by Dr. John Jenkins, Director of the Office of New Drugs, Dr. Robert Temple, Director of the Office of Medical Policy, Jane Axelrad of the Office of Regulatory Policy, Dr. Thomas Laughren, Psychiatric Drugs Team Leader of DNDP, and myself, there was unanimous agreement that Dr. Mosholder should not present these analyses at the meeting, because we agreed that it would be misleading to have an Agency representative present definitive analyses, given that the division responsible for this drug (DNDP) as well as essentially all other Agency officials (listed above, as well as others) concluded that definitive analyses could not be performed at that time.

Shortly thereafter, in early January, 2004, I called Dr. Mosholder and informed him that he could not present the results of his analyses at the meeting, because he had reached a definitive decision (he agreed that he had reached a conclusion) and we in the division, as well as the Center hierarchy, concluded that definitive analyses were not possible at that time. I informed Dr. Mosholder that when definitive analyses had been performed, they would be presented at another public Advisory Committee meeting, and if, at that time, Dr. Mosholder still felt his analyses were supportable (and they differed from those to be yet done by the Agency with the re-classified data), he would be given the opportunity to present his results at such a meeting. When I told Dr. Mosholder about our reservations about the data as presented by the sponsor and the fact that we were going to wait until we got the re-classified data from Columbia before we performed definitive analyses, he stated that he was confident that these analyses would confirm his analyses. I did not ask him how he knew that this would be the case.

I became aware that the press had found out about the decision to not permit Dr. Mosholder to present his analyses at the meeting the morning of the meeting, February 2, 2004. That morning, I was told by numerous people that the San Francisco Chronicle had reported the story the day before (in fact, Dr. Mosholder had sent an e-mail the previous day [which I had not read before 2/2/04] alerting me to the fact that a story had appeared, so that I would not be taken by surprise). Subsequent to this story, there have been numerous stories related to this issue (I have been interviewed by numerous reporters about this aspect of the story, as well as about the larger issue of antidepressants and possible suicide related behaviors in pediatric patients). In addition, I am aware that Dr. Mosholder's final review (which was finalized in March, 2004, I believe, and which comes to the same conclusion as his preliminary review) has also found its way into the hands of reporters.

The Advisory Committees agreed with our view that the data, as currently submitted by the sponsors, is unreliable, and they agreed with our plan to have outside experts re-classify the cases. At the meeting, Dr. Laughren presented the data as submitted by the sponsors (essentially the same numbers on which Dr. Mosholder based his review), and pointed out that, when these data are analyzed as submitted by the sponsors, an increased incidence of possibly suicide related behaviors on the drugs as compared to placebo, was seen (essentially the same results as obtained by Dr. Mosholder). Dr. Laughren pointed out, however, that we believed these classifications were unreliable, for the reasons stated above. I also stated, in my opening remarks, that there were reviewers in the Agency who felt that the data supported definitive analyses and conclusions at that time, but that the Agency view was that this was not so, again, for the reasons stated.

I have no personal knowledge of how the press became aware of our decision to not permit Dr. Mosholder to present his conclusions, nor do I have any knowledge of how Dr. Mosholder's review was released to the press. I have not been in contact with Dr. Mosholder recently, and have not discussed the issue of the "leaking" of our decision or his review to the press with him. Subsequent reports in the press allege that one or several of Dr. Mosholder's supervisors asked and/or required him to "soften" his conclusions. It is Agency policy and practice that medical reviewers are to arrive at independent conclusions based on their review and interpretation of the relevant data. Supervisors are not to instruct reviewers to arrive at particular conclusions. I have no knowledge about any of Dr. Mosholder's supervisors directing him to reach any particular conclusions.

I have read/have had read to me the above statement consisting of 4 pages, and the statement made by me is true and accurate to the best of my knowledge and belief.

No threats or promises have been made to me and no pressure or coercion of any kind has been used against me.

Signature

Signed and sworn to before me this 6 day of May, 2004.

5-6-04
Special Agent/Date
FDA, Office of Internal Affairs

Authority to administer oaths:
Title 5, U.S. Code, Section 303

Mark S. McLamach 5/6/04
Witness/Date

To FILE 04-OIA-971-043

Tab 69

Food and Drug Administration
Office of Internal Affairs (HFH-560)

MEMORANDUM

Date: June 1, 2004

From: Special Agent in Charge
Office of Internal Affairs (HFH-560)

Subject: OIA Investigative Reports in Response to Request of Senate Chairman Grassley

To: Karen Meister
FDA Office of Legislative Affairs (HFW-14)

Per your 05/25/04 request I have enclosed three copies (one un-redacted and two redacted) of the above described reports. Please let me know if you will need any additional items.

Regards,

Horace L. Coleman

Enclosures: (3)

Date: May 28, 2004

From: Director
Office of Pharmacoepidemiology and Statistical Science (HFD-030)

Subject: Report on Investigation on the CDER, Office of Drug Safety, dated 5/10/04 (OIA Case Control Number 04-OIA-971-043)

To: Horace L. Coleman
Special Agent in Charge
Office of Internal Affairs (HFH-560)

Per your cover memo, I am returning the copy of this report that you shared with me.

After carefully and thoroughly reviewing its content and conclusions, I have no plans at present to take any administrative actions based upon the results of this investigation.

Thank you for your prompt and careful attention to this matter. In particular, I want to commend Special Agent Kurisky for his thorough and sensitive handling of the investigation.

Paul J. Seligman, MD, MPH

Attachment

Food and Drug Administration
Office of Internal Affairs (HFH-560)

MEMORANDUM

5-14-04

Date: May 14, 2004

From: Special Agent Michael Kurisky MJK
Office of Internal Affairs (HFH-560)

Subject: Memo to Report of Investigation on the CDER, Office of Drug Safety E-mail, dated 5/10/04

To: Official Office File - OIA Case Control Number 04-OIA-971-043

On today's date I received a telephone call from Dr. Paul Seligman indicating that he had reviewed the Report of Investigation in this case. Dr. Seligman indicated that on page 4 of the ROI, the following sentence appeared:

"Seligman indicated that Mosholder had been pulled from presenting because his findings were different from that of the Advisory Committee."

Seligman stated that instead of "Advisory Committee", the proper term should have been "Reviewing Division". I acknowledged that I was in fact referring to the "reviewing division" when writing the ROI, but unfortunately used the term "Advisory Committee". For clarification purposes, the Psychopharmacologic Drugs Advisory Committee that met on February 2, 2004 was not the group referenced in this sentence, it was the review division within the Office of Drug Safety that had come to a different set of findings from Dr. Mosholder.

cc:
Chron
Case File

05/07/04

Case Notes: 04-OIA-971-043

Mike,

Per the Director, I spoke with Dr. Seligman to inquire if he had talked with Dr. Mosholder concerning our 05/03/04 debriefing/meeting regarding the status of this case. Dr. Seligman responded in the negative, but advised that he did talk to Dr. Mosholder who had expressed some concerns regarding changes that OGC and OLA wanted him to make on the statement he wanted to present to the Senate Committee (privacy issues and portions of his conversation with Rob Waters). Dr. Mosholder was not comfortable with the changes and felt that it changed the flavor of his initial statement he previously provided to OIA.

I then advised Dr. Seligman of the receipt of information (Pat McGarey - OLA, Donna Katz - OGC, and more recently Director Vermillion [via the ACRA]) that Dr. Mosholder believes that he is the subject of this investigation (note: I previously advised all concerned parties that you and SA McCormack had personally advised the good doctor that he was not the target of this case and documented such in the ROI).

I reiterated the focus of our investigation to Dr. Seligman and requested that he personally contact Dr. Mosholder to assure him of the following facts:

- Dr. Mosholder was not/is not a target of this investigation
- OIA's focus was to determine if there had been any release of proprietary or sensitive information
- To determine through witness interviews (all persons contacted by Waters) if through their conversations with Waters if it appeared that he might have had or discussed any sensitive FDA data.
- OIA was satisfied that no evidence was found to indicate that classified or proprietary information had been released.
- OIA is in the process of closing its investigation.

I advised Dr. Seligman that I would also contact CDER Center Director Steve Galson to advise of the above information (note: that Mr. Galson left the office to attend the FDA Awards Ceremony.

I contacted Director Vermillion, debriefed him on the above facts and requested that he reach out to Mr. Galson if possible

Horace Coleman

*************** -COMM. : VAL- ****************** DATE FEB-12-200 *** TIME 17:01 *** P.01

MODE = MEMORY TRANSMISSION START=FEB-12 16:59 END=FEB-12 17:01

FILE NO.= 079

STN NO.	COM	ABBR NO.	STATION NAME/TEL.NO.	PAGES	DURATION
001	OK	<03>	WILSON/OIG	003/003	00:00'24"
002	OK	<17>	PAT DOYLE/OIG	003/003	00:00'47"

************************************* - - ***** - 111111111- *********

Food and Drug Administration
Office of Regulatory Affairs
OCI/Office of Internal Affairs
One Church Street, Suite 700
Rockville, MD 20850
Phone: 301/827-0243 Fax: 301/827-0273

Facsimile Transmittal

To: Pat Doyle
Tawnia Wilson

Fax:

From: Jen Kowaleski

Date: 2/12/04

Subject: new case

Pages: 3

CC:

☐ Urgent ☐ For Review ☐ Please Sign ☐ Please Reply ☐ Please Handle

Notes:

04-OIA-971-041
CDER OFFICE OF DRUG SAFETY EMAIL
SA Mike Kurisky

Cruzan, Susan M

From:	Mosholder, Andrew D
Sent:	Tuesday, January 27, 2004 6:13 PM
To:	Trontell, Anne E; Avigan, Mark I; Willy, Mary E
Cc:	Cruzan, Susan M
Subject:	Feb 2 AC meeting/letter from Rob Waters, freelance reporter

Hello all,
FYI, I received the attached letter today from Rob Waters, the reporter who writes for the San Francisco Chronicle. (It was FedEx-ed to my house.)
-Andy

Rob Waters letter.pdf

Tab 70

Rob Waters

1250 Addison Street, suite 211A
Berkeley, CA 94702
(510) 849-1199
fax: (510) 540-7197
email: robw001@pacbell.net

Dear Dr. Mosholder,

I understand why you declined to speak with me last week when I phoned you and referred me to the press office. Nonetheless, I wanted to appeal to you privately one more time and to give you a little more background on who I am and what I do. I've also included copies of some of my articles so you can see my work.

I write a lot about children's health and mental health issues, and have been doing so for years. I've written several stories on antidepressant safety for children and have a fair amount of background on this topic.

As a journalist (and a parent), I want to find out as much as possible about the safety of these medications which are being taken by so many children. I want to know–and I want the public to know–what the experts who have looked closely at these issues and have reviewed the data, have learned. You at the FDA are the guardians of the public health and the public needs the benefit of your knowledge and experience.

I will be coming to Washington to cover the advisory committee hearing, but I also want to report on what is now going on at the agency with regards to your safety review. I have been told by various sources that you have been working on this review for several months, and that (like the British regulators) you had reached a conclusion that these drugs have an unfavorable safety profile with children and do seem to be associated with an elevated suicide risk. I was also told that you were informed a couple of weeks ago that you would not be allowed to present your findings because you had reached a conclusion and were therefore biased, and that you were being pressed to tone down your findings. I understand also that your safety review will not be presented to the committee and that your expertise and hard work on this issue is essentially being discarded and ignored so that a new group of experts at Columbia can now start from scratch and review the same data.

If this is true, I would like to appeal to you to help me get the word out. I very much respect the delicate position you are in and I don't want to get you in trouble. I respect the fact that you did what you've been instructed to do by referring me to the press office and I have put in a request to be allowed to interview you. However, I know from past practice that, in the unlikely event they allow you to talk to me, a press officer will probably be on the phone with us, monitoring the conversation and steering it when necessary.

So, I am hoping that you will agree to speak with me on background. That means that I would quote your words but not identify you by name or in any way that would make it clear that you have spoken with me. The truth is I feel obligated to do a story on the safety review even if my appeal to speak with you is not successful. It would be so much better and more informed if I did have that opportunity. We could set up specific ground rules about the things I could report and not report so that I wouldn't report anything that was known only to you. As you may know, I have called a number of other people from the agency at their offices or homes and they have reported my calls to their superiors or to the press office. You can obviously do the same. No one can prove who spoke to me and who did not.

Of course, if the information I have been given is not true, I very much want to know that. I certainly do not want to report anything that is not accurate. If FDA management officials tell me my information is inaccurate, I would be highly skeptical as to whether it is the truth; if you tell me that, it would be quite another thing.

So, I am hoping you will decide to speak with me and will contact me. You can call me at my office (510-849-1199), on my cell phone (510-703-1199) or at home (510-549-1188). You can email me at robw001@pacbell.net. You can fax me at 510-540-7197. Call me any time, but I would need to speak with you by Wednesday or Thursday. If necessary, I could probably come to Washington early to meet you. (I am now planning to come on Sunday.)

Whatever your decision, I respect it and wish you the best.

Sincerely,

Rob Waters

03/19/96 10:18 ☎301 594 2859 FDA-NEUROPHARM 001

Tab 71

MR

FOOD AND DRUG ADMINISTRATION
DIVISION OF NEUROPHARMACOLOGICAL DRUG PRODUCTS (HFD-120)
5800 FISHERS LANE
ROCKVILLE, MARYLAND 20857
FAX #'s (301) 594-2858/594-2859
TELECOPIER COVER SHEET

NOTE: THIS DOCUMENT IS INTENDED ONLY FOR THE USE OF PARTY TO WHOM IT IS ADDRESSED AND MAY CONTAIN INFORMATION THAT IS PRIVILEGED, CONFIDENTIAL, AND PROTECTED FROM DISCLOSURE UNDER APPLICABLE LAW. If you are not the addressee, or a person authorized to deliver the document to the addressee, you are hereby notified that any review, disclosure, dissemination, copying, or other action based on the content of this communication is not authorized. If you have received this document in error, please immediately notify us by telephone at (301) 594-2775 and return it to us at the above address by mail, Attn: (HFD-120). Thank you.

DATE: March 19, 1996

TIME: 10 AC

FOR INCLUSION IN YOUR FILE(S)
✓ NDA 19-839
☐ IND
☐ CERT.
☐ MF

PLEASE DELIVER THE FOLLOWING PAGE(S) TO:

Martha A. Brumfield, Ph.D
Senior Associate Director
Pfizer Inc.

COPY 1 - 786

FAX # 212-573-1563 (Telephone #. 212-573-5406)

FROM;

James F. Knudsen
F.D.A

Total number of pages, including cover page: 2

If you do not receive all pages or have any problems with receiving, call (301) 594-2850.

MESSAGE:

03/19/96 10:18 ☎301 594 2659 FDA-NEUROPHARM 002

DEPARTMENT OF HEALTH & HUMAN SERVICES Public Health Service

Food and Drug Administration
Rockville MD 20857

19 March 1996
(301)594-2648

Martha A. Brumfield, Ph.D.
Senior Associate Director
Regulatory Affairs
Pfizer, Inc.
235 East 42nd Street
New York, NY 10017-5755

Dear Dr. Brumfield:

Reference is made to NDA 19-839, supplement S-002, fur Zoloft® (sertraline) Tablets in the treatment of OCD mid to the Safety Update submitted on December 7, 1995.

To address the issue of suicidality, we believe two *summary* tables would be helpful. One table would consist of data from the adult OCD safety update and include all completed and ongoing studies for all treatment groups. The second table would be a similar one for the pediatric/adolescent database. The columns in these tables should consist of the following: protocol number, study and patient numbers, age, gender, dose at time of event if sertraline or a active control, duration of exposure to therapy prior to event, and a comment section The comment section should note. past medical history with respect to depression, drug use. family history if known, type of suicidality (ideation, gesture, attempt, etc.), and outcome with respect to patient's disposition.

The development of intense self-injuriousideation and/or behavior in children and adolescents diagnosed with OCD who received treatment with fluoxetine has been described (King etal. J AM. Acad Child Adolesc. Psychiatry 30:2. 179, 1991).

We note that there appears to be an increase frequency of reports of suicidally in the pediatric/adolescent patients exposed to sertraline compared to either placebo or sertraline-treated adult OCD patients. If this is in fact the case what would be a plausible explanation?

Sincerely Yours,
James F. Knudsen, M.D., Ph.D

: 3-19-96 : 12:10 : .... DRAD- SAFETY ASSURANCE

DEPARTMENT OF HEALTH & HUMAN SERVICES

Public Health Service

Food and Drug Administration
Rockville MD 20857

Tab 72

19 March 1996
(301)594-2648

Martha A. Brumfield, Ph.D.
Senior Associate Director
Regulatory Affairs
Pfizer, Inc.
235 East 42nd Street
New York, NY 10017-5755

Dear Dr. Brumfield:

Reference is made to NDA 19-839, supplement S-002, for Zoloft® (sertraline) Tablets in the treatment of OCD and to the Safety Update submitted on December 7, 1995.

To address the issue of suicidality, we believe two summary tables would be helpful. One table would consist of data from the adult OCD safety update and include all completed and ongoing studies for all treatment groups. The second table would be a similar one for the pediatric/adolescent database. The columns in these tables should consist of the following: protocol number, study and patient numbers, age, gender, dose at time of event if sertraline or a active control, duration of exposure to therapy prior to event, and a comment section. The comment section should note: past medical history with respect to depression, drug use, family history if known, type of suicidality (ideation, gesture, attempt, etc.), and outcome with respect to patient's disposition.

The development of intense self-injurious ideation and/or behavior in children and adolescents diagnosed with OCD who received treatment with fluoxetine has been described (King et al., J. AM. Acad Child Adolesc. Psychiatry 30:2, 179, 1991).

We note that there appears to be an increase frequency of reports of suicidally in the pediatric/adolescent patients exposed to sertraline compared to either placebo or sertraline-treated adult OCD patients. If this is in fact the case what would be a plausible explanation?

Sincerely Yours,

James F. Knudsen, M.D., Ph.D

Regulatory Affairs Division
Pfizer Inc
235 East 42nd Street
New York, NY 10017-5755
Tel 212 573 5406 Fax 212 573 1563

FOR INCLUSION IN YOUR FILE(
NDA 19-839
IND
CERT

COPY 1 - 816

Martha A. Brumfield, PhD
Senior Associate Director—Regulatory Affairs

May 28,1996

Tab 73

Paul Leber, M.D. Director
Division of Neuropharmacological
Drug Products (HFD-120)
Center for Drug Evaluation & Research
Office of Drug Evaluation I
Attn: DOCUMENT ROOM #10B-34
Food and Drug Administration
5600 Fishers Lane
Rockville, Maryland 20857

RE: NDA # 19-839 - Zoloft Tablets
S-002 - Obsessive Compulsive Disorder

Dear Dr. Leber:

Please refer to our supplemental application (S-002) for Obsessive Compulsive Disorder filed to NDA 19-839 Zoloft Tablets on May 14, 1992 and the Final Safety Update submitted December 7, 1995. Reference is also made to Dr. Knudsen's correspondence of March 19, 1996.

Attached is our response to the March 19, 1996 letter. The response is organized as follows:

SUMMARY (1 page)

Enclosure I - Document addressing suicidal behavior in children and adolescents

Enclosure II - Document addressing suicidal behavior in adults

The two summary tables you requested (one containing data from the adult OCD safety update database and one containing data from the pediatric/adolescent OCD safety update database) are included. The adult table can be found in Enclosure II and the pediatric/adolescent table can be found in Enclosure I.

C:\wpwin\mb052896

In reviewing available data with respect to suicidality in pediatric/adolescent patients being treated with sertraline for OCD we expanded our search beyond the data previously submitted in the Safety Update to include (1) any nonserious suicide related events including those not meeting the criteria for "serious events", (2) an analysis of Pfizer's early alert safety database and (3) a review of the epidemiologic literature regarding suicidal behavior in children and adolescents.

It should be noted that in the OCD FSU Volume I, Page 2-26 indicated that there were eight cases of suicidal ideation or self-destructive thoughts, 6 on sertraline therapy and 2 on blinded therapy; in fact, there were **5** on sertraline therapy and **3** on blinded therapy. The total number of SAEs and the total number of cases of suicidality are unaffected by this change.

Please include this information in our file for Zoloft Tablets NDA # 19-839.

Sincerely,

Paula R DiCola for
Martha A. Brumfield, Ph.D.
MAB:kc
OCD/sum 1-2

Desk copy: Dr. James Knudsen

CONFIDENTIAL/TRADE SECRET INFORMATION SUBJECT TO 18-USC-1905 AND TO WHICH ALL CLAIMS OF PRIVILEGE AND CONFIDENTIALITY ARE ASSERTED IN BOTH STATUTORY AND COMMON LAW.

C:\wpwin\mb05289€

DEPARTMENT OF HEALTH AND HUMAN SERVICES
PUBLIC HEALTH SERVICE
FOOD AND DRUG ADMINISTRATION

APPLICATION TO MARKET A NEW DRUG FOR HUMAN USE OR AN ANTIBIOTIC DRUG FOR HUMAN USE

(TITLE 21, Code of Federal Regulations, 374)

Form approved OMB No 0910-0001.
Expiration Date December 31, 1995
See OMB Statement on Page 3

FOR FDA USE ONLY	
DATE RECEIVED	DATE FILED
DIVISION ASSIGNED	NDA/ANDA NO. ASS.

NOTE: No application may be filed unless a completed application form has been received (21 CFR Part 314).

NAME OF APPLICANT
Pfizer, Inc.

ADDRESS (*Number, Street, City, State, and Zip Code*)
235 East 42nd Street
New York, NY 10017

DATE OF SUBMISSION
05/28/96

TELEPHONE NO. (Include Area Code)
(212) 573-2323

NEW DRUG OR ANTIBIOTIC APPLICATION NUMBER (*If previously issued*)
NDA #19-839

ESTABLISHED NAME (e.g., USP/USAN)	PROPRIETARY NAME (If any)
Sertraline HCl	Zoloft

CODE NAME (If any)	CHEMICAL NAME
CP-51, 974-1	(1S-cis)-4-(3,4-dichlorophenyl)-1,2,3,4-tetrahydro-N-methyl-1-naphthalenamine hydrochloride)

DOSAGE FORM	ROUTE OF ADMINISTRATION	STRENGTH(S)
Tablets	Oral	50 mg, 100 mg, 200 mg

PROPOSED INDICATIONS FOR USE

NAME OF DRUG	HOLDER OF APPROVED APPLICATION

TYPE SUBMISSION (*Check one*)

- ☐ PRESUBMISSION
- ☐ ORIGINAL APPLICATION
- ☐ AN AMENDMENT TO A PENDING APPLICATION
- ☐ RESUBMISSION
- ☐ SUPPLEMENTAL APPLICATION

SPECIFIC REGULATION(S) TO SUPPORT CHANGE OF APPLICATION (e.g., Part 314.70(b)(2)(iv))

PROPOSED MARKETING STATUS (*Check one*)

- ☒ APPLICATION FOR A PRESCRIPTION DRUG PRODUCT (Rx)
- ☐ APPLICATION FOR AN OVER-THE-COUNTER PRODUCT (OTC)

CONTENTS OF APPLICATION

This application contains the following items: (Check *all that apply*)

	1. Index
	2. Summary (21 CFR 314.50(c))
	3. Chemistry, manufacturing, and control section (21 CFR 314.50 (d) (1))
	4. a. Samples (21 CFR 314.50 (e) (1)) (Submit only upon FDA's request)
	b. Methods Validation Package (21 CFR 314 50 (e) (2) (i))
	c. Labeling (21 CFR 314.50 (e) (2) (ii))
	i. draft labeling *(4 copies)*
	ii. final printed labeling (12 copies)
	5. Nonclinical pharmacology and toxicology section (21 CFR 314.50 (d) (2))
	6. Human pharmacokinetics and bioavailability section (21 CFR 314.50 (d) (3))
	7. Microbiology section (21 CFR 314.50 (d) (4))
	8. Clinical data section (21 CFR 314.50 (d) (5))
	9. Safety update report (21 CFR 314.50 (d) (5) (vi) (b))
	10. Statistical section (21 CFR 314.50 (d) (6))
	11. Case report tabulations (21 CFR 314.50 (f) (1))
	12. Case reports forms (21 CFR 314.50 (9 (1))
	13. Patent information on any patent which claims the drug (21 U.S.C. 355 (b) or (c))
	14. A patent certification with respect to any patent which claims the drug (21 U.S.C. 355 (b) (2) or (j) (2) (A))
	15. OTHER *(Specify)*

I agree to update this application with new safety information about the drug that may reasonably affect the statement of contraindications, warnings, precautions, or adverse reactions in the draft labeling. I agree to submit these safety update reports as follows: (1) 4 months after the initial submission, (2) following receipt of an approvable letter and (3) at other times as requested by FDA. If this application is approved, I agree lo comply with all laws and regulations that apply to approved applications, including the following:

1. Good manufacturing practice regulations in 21 CFR 210 and 211.
2. Labeling regulations 21 CFR 201.
3. In the case of a prescription drug product, prescription drug advertising regulations in 21 CFR 202.
4. Regulations on making changes in application in 21 CFR 314.70. 314.71, and 314.72.
5. Regulations on reports in 21 CFR 314.80 and 314.81.
6. Local, state, and Federal environmental impact laws.

If this application applies to a drug product that FDA has proposed for scheduling under the controlled substances Act I agree not to market the product until the Drug Enforcement Administration makes a final scheduling decision.

NAME OF RESPONSIBLE OFFICIAL OR AGENT	SIGNATURE OF RESPONSIBLE OFFICIAL OR AGENT	DATE
Margaret A. Longshore, Ph.D., Director	[signature]	5/28/96
ADDRESS *(Street, City, State, Zip Code)* 235 East 42nd Street, New York, NY 10017		TELEPHONE NO. *(Include Area Code)* (212) 573-2556

(WARNING: A willfully false statement is a criminal offense. U.S.C. Title 18, Sec. 1001.)

Summary: *During the sertraline clinical development program for obsessive-compulsive disorder (OCD) there were eight serious suicide-related events (gestures, attempts or ideation) among 1,581 adult patients treated with sertraline (0.51%) and six serious suicide-related events among 220 children or adolescents treated with sertraline (2.7%) as of June 30, 1995 and discussed in the Final Safety Update (FSU).*

The issue of suicide-related behavior among children and adolescents has been considered in detail in one of the enclosed documents and placed in perspective using other data specific to young people. The adult group does not provide an adequate comparison group for several reasons. There were substantial differences between the adult and pediatric databases in (1) psychiatric/neurologic comorbidity, (2) duration of exposure to sertraline, and (3) dose of sertraline given.

The most important difference between the two databases was the frequency of concomitant psychiatric diseases. The entrance criteria were significantly less restrictive with regard to concomitant diagnoses in the pediatric studies as compared to the adult studies. Many of the pediatric patients carried concomitant psychiatric diagnoses. As noted in the attached pediatric document, at least 45 of the young patients had major depressive disorder, which is an extremely strong risk factor for suicidal behavior. Many of the others also had concomitant diagnoses such as attention deficit hyperactivity disorder, oppositional defiant disorder, post-traumatic stress disorder, and dysthymia.

With respect to duration of exposure, most of the adult protocols were 10-18 weeks in duration while most of the pediatric/adolescent patients entered protocols providing a total of 31-64 weeks of sertraline treatment.

Titration schedules differed between the two databases. Most adult patients were flexibly titrated over the 50-200 mg dose range. Pediatric sertraline patients were initially either force-titrated to 200 mg or titrated to their maximum tolerated dose up to 200 mg. The average maximum dose among children/adolescents in completed studies was 184.8 mg/day while it was 148 mg/day in adults.

For these reasons, suicide-related behavior in children and adolescents has been extensively reviewed separately in one of the enclosed documents. The other enclosed document provides details on the eight serious suicide-related events in adults treated with sertraline.

SUICIDE-RELATED BEHAVIOR IN CHILDREN AND ADOLESCENTS SERTRALINE OCD CLINICAL DEVELOPMENT PROGRAM

Abstract: *The purpose of this report is to review the frequency of suicidal behavior in children and adolescents in the sertraline obsessive-compulsive disorder (OCD) clinical development program. The frequency of suicide attempts or suicidal ideation leading to hospitalization among children and adolescents in this program is 2.7% (6/220) among individuals treated with sertraline. This is identical to the rate of 2.7% reported for suicide attempts requiring medical care in a nationwide sample of adolescents unselected for any psychiatric or behavioral problem." All of the six patients exhibiting serious suicidal ideation or attempts during the clinical development program had multiple risk factors for suicidal behavior.*

In the placebo-controlled portion of the development program there were no serious suicide-related events among 92 patients treated with sertraline, and one serious suicide-related event among the 95 patients receiving placebo. When considering the entire clinical development program, the larger number of reports of suicidal behavior in children and adolescents treated with sertraline compared to those receiving placebo may be explained by: (1) larger sample size in the sertraline group, (2) longer exposure time (and consequently longer period at risk during follow-up) in the sertraline group and (3) the greater inherent risk of the patients receiving sertraline, due to the large number with major depression, without a comparable control group. All rates observed are within the range described in normal population samples of adolescents and are below the range described in the epidemiologic literature for adolescents with major psychiatric illness.

Introduction

This document was prepared in response to questions regarding suicidality raised by the United States Food and Drug Administration (FDA) as stated in correspondence dated March 19, 1996. The purpose of the report is to review the frequency of suicidal behavior (suicidal ideation and/or suicide attempts) in children and adolescents receiving sertraline for the treatment of obsessive-compulsive disorder (OCD). This report includes a discussion of suicide-related events in children and adolescents reported during the OCD clinical development program, an analysis of Pfizer's early alert safety database, and a review of the epidemiologic literature regarding suicidal behavior in children and adolescents.

Description of the Pediatric/Adolescent OCD Clinical Program

The pediatric section of the sertraline OCD Final Safety Update (FSU) reviewed all safety data collected from children (6-12 years old) and adolescents (13-17 years old) who were treated in any completed OCD study as of June 30, 1995 (Protocols 90CE21-0498 and 90CK21-0525). The review of serious adverse events in the FSU included events from all ongoing studies (Protocols 550 and 536) as well as the completed studies.

Protocol 498 was a 12-week, multicenter, double-blind. parallel. placebo-controlled study designed to examine the efficacy and safety of sertraline in the treatment of non-depressed pediatric (6-12 years old) and adolescent (13-17 years old) outpatients with OCD. Ninety-two patients were treated with sertraline and 95 with placebo. All participants had OCD.

Protocol 525 was a 51-day open-label parallel study designed to determine the pharmacokinetics of and tolerance to sertraline after single and multiple dose administration to children and adolescents with OCD or depression. Sixty-one patients were included; forty-four patients had depression, 15 had OCD without a known diagnosis of depression. one had both OCD and depression and one had both OCD and dysthymia. All subjects received sertraline. There was no comparative group of young people with depression treated with placebo or comparative agent.

The additional safety data examined in the FSU were provided from two open-label extension studies that were ongoing as of June 30, 1995. An estimated 67 placebo patients from Protocol 498 were subsequently treated with sertraline in an extension study (Protocol 536), bringing the total safety denominator for sertraline-treated pediatric patients in the OCD FSU to 220. The number of new sertraline exposures in Protocol 536 is an estimate based on the assumption that patients entering the open extension included an equal number of sertraline and placebo patients from Protocol 498, Protocol 550 is a flexible dose, open label extension to Protocol 525. This study adds no newly-exposed patients to the sertraline safety database. as all subjects initially received sertraline in the pharmacokinetics study.

Suicide-related behavior among children and adolescents in the OCD program

There were six cases of suicidal ideation and/or attempt among sertraline treated patients that met the criteria for being a "serious" event in the FSU (Table 1). The overall incidence of serious suicidal behavior among sertraline-treated patients in the clinical trials is *2.7%* (6/220). The disease-specific incidence rates of suicide-related events in children and adolescents treated with sertraline are 8.9% (4/45) in subjects with depression and 1.1% (2/175) in non-depressed subjects with OCD.

The six events were distributed among the individual protocols as follows. In Protocol 498, there were no serious suicide-related events among 92 subjects with OCD treated with sertraline. In contrast. there was one suicide-related event among 95 placebo patients with OCD. During the long-term open-label extension to this study (Protocol *536)* there were two suicide-related events among the total of 133 patients with OCD treated with sertraline (an estimated 66 of the 133 were previously treated with sertraline in Protocol 498 and contribute to the denominator of 92 previously mentioned). In Protocols *525* and *550* there were four events: three among the 45 subjects with depression in Protocol *525*, and one among the *33* with major depression who continued on to the long-term extension study (Protocol *550)*.

All of the six young people experiencing serious suicide-related events had several risk factors for suicidal behavior including multiple psychiatric diagnoses. familial dysfunction, family history of psychiatric disorders, histories of sexual or child abuse, and early onset and long duration of their primary psychiatric disorder. Four had primary diagnoses of major depression. Of the two without major depression, both also had other risk factors. Patient #217 carried diagnoses of OCD and attention deficit hyperactivity disorder (ADHD) and had been treated with multiple medications in the past. The investigator attributed the event to life stress and underlying disease. Patient # 221 had post-traumatic stress disorder as well as OCD. She has a family history of both depression and ADHD and her suicidal ideation emerged when she regained memories of having been raped. Risk factors for suicide-related behavior in all six individuals are included in Table 1 and summarized in Table 2.

In addition to reviewing serious cases discussed in the FSU, the sertraline OCD pediatric/adolescent databases were searched for cases of suicidal behavior not meeting the criteria for "serious" events. As of March 21, 1996, there were *two* additional cases of non-serious "suicidal ideation" reported during the clinical development program; one in a patient with OCD and one in a patient with depression. Both were during the pharmacokinetic trial (Protocol 525). Patient 92-N-0058 # 228 was a 16 year old male with OCD treated with Anafranil, Loxitane, and Ritalin over the past 3 years (until 10 days prior to the study). Family history was significant for affective disorders in his mother and maternal grandmother, OCD in a maternal aunt and maternal grandfather and substance abuse in a paternal uncle and brother. The patient lived in a boarding home. He developed non-serious suicidal ideation (lasting two days) after approximately 2 weeks on the study. The investigator felt the event was due to study drug, but the patient continued on the study and recovered from the suicidal ideation. The second case (92-N-0058 #24) was a 12 year old male with major depression and attention deficit hyperactivity disorder who had been treated with Ritalin for 7 years (until one week prior to study). Family history was significant for affective disorders in his mother and maternal grandmother. He developed non-serious suicidal thoughts (for a period of one week) after approximately one month on study. The investigator listed the causality as "uncertain" and continued the patient on the study without any re-emergence of suicidal ideation.

Spontaneous reports of suicide-related behavior in children and adolescents

Pfizer's early alert safety database was also reviewed in order to identify non-clinical study cases that may have been spontaneously reported to Pfizer. This database contains case reports of all adverse events spontaneously reported directly to Pfizer, cases of serious adverse events reported from clinical trials regardless of causality, cases of serious adverse events reported to adverse event registries, and reports of serious adverse events published in the medical literature. The database was reviewed for all non-clinical trial sertraline cases in individuals under the age of 18 coded to the WHO-ART adverse event terms "suicide attempt," "suicidal ideation." "suicide gesture," "drug overdose,, intentional," or "death by suicide."

As of March 28, 1996, 25 cases were identified. In four cases, individuals who were not previously taking sertraline were reported to have stolen the drug from someone else for purposes of suicide attempt or abuse (these cases are not included in this report, leaving 21 cases). One domestic spontaneous report (R-42B792) is the same individual as study case 91-N-0242 #217 (included in Table 1). After finishing the study she continued on sertraline and made a subsequent attempt. Another case was that of an 11-year-old boy whose mother reported the event (9511941). Follow-up from the physician revealed that the mother (reporter) was a paranoid schizophrenic who had little contact with the son. The physician claims that none of the events reported by the mother actually happened. The two preceding cases (R-42B792 and 9511941) will not be further discussed in this section, but the CIOMS forms are included in Appendix A. Of the remaining 19 cases, twelve were females, seven were males, ranging in age from 9 to 17 with a mean age of 14. The indication for drug was reported to be depression in nine cases, OCD/dysthymia/explosive disorder in one case, anxiety and oppositional defiant disorder in one case each, and was not stated in the remaining cases. In several of these cases it was not clear that the individual was actually receiving sertraline prior to the event; however, these are included, since there is no explicit information stating that the individual took or ingested someone else's medication. None of the spontaneous reports resulted in successful suicide. There is minimal information in most reports about the individual's history or course of treatment that would allow one to characterize these cases. In one case of an 11-year-old boy with oppositional defiant disorder (9402535). the reporter felt that activation due to sertraline was the cause of the event. In one other case of a 9-year-old boy with depression (9403519), the event occurred after an increase in dose, and abated with a return to his previous dose of sertraline.

All other non-clinical trial cases with WHO-ART adverse event terms coding to the "psychiatric" body system were reviewed as well, to ensure that no cases (possibly coded to other terms) were missed. No additional cases were found by this method. Individual spontaneous reports are attached in Appendix **A.**

Epidemiology of suicidal behavior in children and adolescents

The frequency of suicidal behavior among adolescents: A review of the epidemiology of suicidal behavior in general population samples is useful to place the observed events in perspective. Most studies have been conducted in non-clinical general samples designed to be representative of all individuals in the population without regard to history of psychiatric diagnosis or mental disorder. Samples drawn from clinical populations (or those referred for mental health care) have higher rates of such events by virtue of the strong association between psychiatric disorders and suicidal behavior. One would expect a clinical trial sample (such as discussed in the FSU) to have higher rates of suicidal behavior than the general population. At best, a clinical trial sample would have similar rates to the range observed in psychiatrically-referred clinical samples in the literature (depending upon how similar the clinical trial population is to the literature sample).

Suicidal behavior (suicidal ideation. suicide gestures, and attempts) is extremely common during adolescence. The Centers for Disease Control (CDC) Youth Risk Behavior Surveillance Survey (YRBSS) is a population-based survey that is designed to be nationally representative of all students in grades 9 through 12 in the United States. Participants were selected without regard to any psychiatric, mental health or physical health history. During the 1993 survey, 24% of all students nationwide reported that they had considered attempting suicide during the year preceding the survey. Nineteen percent of all students reported more serious suicidal ideation (SI) in that they had formulated a specific plan to attempt suicide. Nationwide, 8.6% of all students had actually made a suicide attempt, and 2.7% of all students reported a suicide attempt that required medical attention during the past year.[20] The magnitude of these estimates are stable across several years of the YRBSS.[2,3]

The National Adolescent Student Health Survey (NASHS) is another population-based survey designed to be nationally representative of eighth and tenth grade students in the entire U.S. (American School Health Association).' More than one-third of the students (34%) report that they had "seriously thought" about committing suicide, and 14% report that they had "actually tried" to commit suicide.

While the YRBSS and NASHS are designed to be representative of the entire U.S. population of students in eighth grade and high school, there are a number of other smaller population-based epidemiologic studies of non-psychiatric samples drawn from a variety of geographic. socioeconomic, and ethnic groups. Estimates vary depending upon the specific population sampled, the age of participants, the methods used for measurement, and the definitions used; however. rates are similar to the YRBSS and NASHS. The prevalence of suicidal thoughts or ideation during the past six months to one year among adolescents ranges from about 3% to 27%.[15,16,18,19,24,25,29,30] The same studies found that from 1.7% to 15% of adolescents report that they have actually made a suicide attempt (SA). Garrison and associates report that 18% of suicide attempts were "impulsive." that is, no specific thought or plan had been formulated in the year prior to the attempt.[15]

Cappelli and associates report on a sample of individuals referred to an adolescent health clinic.'' One quarter were referred for a physical complaint. one half for a mental health complaint and one quarter for both a physical and mental complaint. Twenty-three percent of the entire sample were assessed as having a "suicidal probability" and half of those presenting with a psychological problem were suicidal.

Risk factors for adolescent suicidal behavior: Beyond describing the frequency of suicide-related behavior in adolescents. one can describe risk factors for adolescents who exhibit such behavior. The most frequent epidemiologic study design used for these purposes is a case-control study, in which cases (adolescents with suicidal behavior) are compared to controls (adolescents who have not displayed suicidal behavior). The resulting measure of association is the odds ratio (OR) which estimates the frequency of the specific risk factor in suicidal adolescents compared to the frequency in non-suicidal adolescents. An odds ratio of one (1) indicates no association (identical frequencies in both cases and controls); the higher the odds ratio. the more frequent the risk factor among cases compared to controls.

Depression is the risk factor for suicidal ideation found most consistently across studies and is associated with the highest odds ratio. Odds ratios for depression and suicidal ideation (SI) in adolescents range from 5.9 to 22.[16,25,29,30] Other risk factors for SI include family dysfunction,[19,29] early onset (prior to age 14) of one or more psychiatric disorders,[26,29] panic attacks/disorder,[38] and hyperactivity.''

Risk factors for suicide attempt (SA) and odds ratios relating depression to SA are similar to those for suicidal ideation; the odds ratios for depression range from 9.8 to 15.6.[25,29] The odds ratio for post-traumatic stress disorder and SA in one study is reported as 21.[29] Other risk factors include: early onset of one or more psychiatric disorders,'' comorbidity consisting of more than one DSM (Diagnostic and Statistical Manual of Mental Disorders) diagnosis?' family history of SA,[18] sexual abuse,[18,21,35] behavioral problems,[35] family history of depression or other emotional problem.[35,37] panic attacks/disorders.[38] and family problems or stressful life events.[14,21,34]

With respect to family history, Weissman and associates[37] conducted a longitudinal cohort study of offspring of depressed parents and found that 7.8% attempted suicide over a two-year period. This was 5.6 times the rate observed in offspring of non-depressed parents.

Risk factors for completed suicide are similar to those for suicide attempt and suicidal ideation; major depression, family history of affective illness, previous suicidal behavior, stressful life events, and psychiatric comorbidity.[6-9] The odds ratio for major depression in those completing suicide was reported as 27 by Brent and associates.[7]

The risk of suicidal behavior among adolescents with depression or OCD: Few studies allow one to estimate the absolute risk over time of suicidal behavior in adolescents with psychiatric illness. Rao reported on a longitudinal study of individuals identified as having depression during childhood and found that **4.4%** killed themselves over the subsequent 10 years.[28]

Individuals who are suicidal tend to repeat their suicide attempts over time. Larsson et al. found that half of adolescents who had made a suicide attempt reported that they had made more than one attempt.[24] Brent followed a group of adolescent psychiatric inpatients for six months following discharge.[6] The original reason for admission was suicide attempt in **48** patients. SI in 33. other psychiatric reason in 53. At **six** months, 9.7% had made a subsequent SA and 26.8% had made a plan to attempt suicide. Almost all (92%) of those who made a subsequent SA were suicidal while in the hospital.

Ryan found that adolescents whose depression had existed for longer than *2* years were at higher risk of suicidal behavior than adolescents with a shorter duration.'' Sixty-percent of their sample of childredadolescents with major depression had SI; *25%* of children and **34%** of adolescents with major depression had attempted suicide during the current episode of depression.

Few epidemiologic studies specific to OCD and suicidal behavior have been conducted. It is known that those with OCD very frequently have one or more comorbid psychiatric conditions that are themselves independent risk factors for suicidal behavior, such as depression, dysthymia, substance abuse and anxiety disorders.[23] Forty-five percent of the community sample of adolescents with OCD studied by Valleni-Basile and associates had major depression.[36] Twenty-three percent of those with OCD had suicidal ideation and *5%* reported suicidal acts. Of those with subclinical OCD, 10% reported suicidal ideation. Suicidal ideation in those with DSM defined OCD **was 3.8** times more frequent than in the group without either OCD or subclinical OCD and suicidal acts were 2.5 times more frequent (Personal communication. JL Waller, University of South Carolina).

Discussion

The fact that numerically more suicidal events occurred in patients receiving sertraline than in those receiving placebo in the FSU may be explained by several factors. In Protocol **498,** which was the only placebo-controlled study, there were no suicide-related events in the sertraline group, but there was one such event in the placebo group. In this study, individuals with depression were excluded. Two events were observed during the open-label sertraline follow up phase of the study. The majority of suicidal events occurred during Protocols 525 and *550.* Not only were individuals with depression allowed, but in fact, almost three quarters of the participants did have depression, conferring an inherently higher risk of suicidal behavior in these studies compared with Protocols 498 and 536. There is no placebo comparison group available for children and adolescents with depression: therefore. the expected rate in a comparable group receiving placebo cannot be estimated. **As** previously mentioned, the observed rates of suicidal behavior are well below what one would expect in a depressed population based on the literature.

The pediatric/adolescent clinical program described in the FSU is weighted towards longer time at-risk in the sertraline exposed group (although the exact person-time of exposure is not yet available since studies are ongoing) and weighted towards more severe psychiatric comorbidity in the sertraline group compared to the placebo group. An estimated 176 individuals (at least 45 of whom have major depression) of the 220 receiving sertraline were treated on long-term open label extension studies of 24 weeks (Protocol 550) or 52 weeks (protocol 536) compared to approximately 44 individuals, none of whom had depression, treated only with placebo for shorter periods of time (up to 12 weeks in Protocol 498).

At least 45 of the 220 individuals treated with sertraline were known to have a diagnosis of depressive disorder, and four of the six reports of serious suicidal behavior are from this group. Of the two individuals without major depression reporting suicidal behavior, both had other risk factors.

All of the six young people with serious suicide-related events had at least one other risk factor for suicidal behavior including multiple psychiatric diagnoses, familial dysfunction, family history of psychiatric disorders, histories of sexual or child abuse, and early onset and long duration of psychiatric disorders. Patient #4 was the only one of the six cases in which the investigator attributed the event to sertraline. Both of the individuals with non-serious suicidal ideation also had multiple risk factors for suicidal behavior.

Pfizer has received 19 spontaneous reports of suicidal behavior in individuals under the age of 18 treated with sertraline. Most reports do not contain sufficient information to allow one to draw conclusions or characterize the events, but few of the reports are particularly striking. It is well known that spontaneous reports are not a good indication of the true frequency of events. There has been substantial publicity over the past five years regarding the possibility of suicidal behavior in relation to SSRI's. In light of this, as well as the high emotional content of suicidal events in children and adolescents, one might postulate that health care providers would be relatively more likely to report these events compared to other types of events. This does not appear to be an unusual number of spontaneous reports given that approximately 4% of the estimated 11.5 million individuals in the U.S. that have received sertraline since marketing are under the age of 18 (source: Scott-Levin Associates, Physician Drug and Diagnosis Audit), and that individuals taking antidepressants are at inherently high risk of suicidal behavior.

Beasley et al. report on placebo-controlled data of fluoxetine in OCD.[5] They include 266 patients with OCD treated with fluoxetine and 89 receiving placebo. Patients were age 14-70, with a mean age of mid to late 30's. The emergence of substantial suicidal ideation was numerically greater with placebo (3.6%) than with fluoxetine (1.7%), but was not statistically significant. The rate observed in the Pfizer OCD clinical development program among children and adolescents with OCD is consistent with this rate (1.1%, 2/175).

King and associates" present three hypotheses for the apparent association between fluoxetine and suicidal behavior in their uncontrolled study: (1) coincidence (under which they include the high degree of psychiatric comorbidity in the OCD population and the large numbers of risk factors in these patients), (2) disorganization of vulnerable individuals secondary to drug-induced activation. and (3) a specific serotonergic-mediated effect on the regulation of aggression.

Drug-induced activation is a plausible explanation for the emergence of suicidal behavior in our patient #4, who had few risk factors for this behavior other than early onset of disease and family history of depression and suicide. In all other cases, these events occurred in individuals with severe psychiatric illness who also had a number of social and familial risk factors for self-destructive behavior. Given the size, duration of treatment, and the severity of illness and comorbidity in the sertraline group compared to the placebo group, a plausible explanation for the remaining cases lies with what King calls "coincidence." but we would explain as "severity and type of underlying disease."

Summary and conclusions

The frequency of suicide attempts or suicidal ideation leading to hospitalization among children and adolescents treated with sertraline in the **FSU** is **2.7%** (6/220). This is identical to the rate of 2.7% reported for suicide attempts requiring medical care in a nationwide sample of adolescents unselected for any psychiatric or behavioral problem (YRBSS).[20] Since suicidal behavior is highly correlated with psychiatric illness, a higher rate in a psychiatric clinical trial population than that seen in the non-psychiatric, non-referred population would be expected, but that was not found in this case. The observed frequency is well below that reported for adolescents with serious psychiatric illness in the epidemiologic literature.

The six young people with serious suicide-related events all had at least one other risk factor for suicidal behavior including multiple psychiatric diagnoses, familial dysfunction, family history of psychiatric disorders, histories of sexual or child abuse, and early onset and long duration of psychiatric disorder. In only one of the six was the event attributed to sertraline by the investigator.

In conclusion, the differences in the crude numbers of suicidal behavior between children and adolescents treated with sertraline and those receiving placebo may be related to the longer exposure time (and consequently longer period at risk during follow-up) in the sertraline group and the greater inherent risk of these patients (due to the large number with major depression. without a comparable control group). All rates observed are within the range described in normal population samples of adolescents and are below the range described in the epidemiologic literature for adolescents with major psychiatric illness.

M E M O R A N D U M

DEPARTMENT OF HEALTH AND HUMAN SERVICES
PUBLIC HEALTH SERVICE
FOOD AND DRUG ADMINISTRATION
CENTER FOR DRUG EVALUATION AND RESEARCH

Tab 74

DATE: September 30, 1996

FROM: Thomas P. Laughren, M.D. TPL
Team Leader, Psychiatric Drug Products
Division of Neuropharmacological Drug Products
HFD-120

SUBJECT: Recommendation for Approval Action for Zoloft (sertraline) for Obsessive Compulsive Disorder (OCD)

TO: File NDA 19-839/S-002
[**Note:** This overview should be filed with the 12-7-95 response to the approvable letter.]

1.0 BACKGROUND

An approvable letter for this supplement was issued 8-1-95, and a response was submitted 12-7-95. Subsequent submissions critical to this approval recommendation were study reports for in vivo interaction studies of sertraline with carbamazepine (3-22-96) and terfenadine (8-13-96). All of the issues in our approvable letter have now been addressed, including our concern about the potential for sertraline to interact with certain substrates of the P450 enzyme 3A4 (see Biopharmaceutics below).

Through an exchange of faxes, we achieved agreement on most remaining labeling issues, however, we were unable to reach agreement on several clinical issues that are discussed later in more detail under 6.0 Labeling. Faxes from the Agency to Pfizer were sent 9-6-96 and 9-20-96, and faxes from Pfizer to the Agency were sent 9-13-96 and 9-27-96. The labeling attached to the approval letter represents labeling agreements achieved at a Team Leader level, along with proposed language in those clinical sections where agreement could not be reached.

2.0 CHEMISTRY

The environmental assessment issue raised in our 8-1-96 approvable letter has now been satisfactorily resolved.

3.0 PHARMACOLOGY

The sponsor has accepted our recommendation for a pregnancy category C.

4.0 BIOPHARMACEUTICS

The data supporting the "changes being effected" submitted in SLR-003 have been reviewed by the Division of Biopharmaceutics and this supplement was approved in an agency letter dated 9-14-95.

In vivo interaction studies of sertraline with carbamazepine and terfenadine, both 3A substrates, have demonstrated no effect of sertraline on the pharmacokinetics of these substances. In fact, the data were suggestive of slight induction by sertraline, resulting in a slight increase in the clearance of these substrates. Consequently, I don't see any need to ask for additional in vitro assays for other potentially important 3A substrates, e.g., astemizole, cisapride, etc. I believe the labeling proposed by Pfizer to address this issue in the 8-13-96 submission is adequate, and I have incorporated this language into the Precautions section of the final labeling proposal.

5.0 CLINICAL DATA

5.1 Efficacy Update

5.1 1 Age and Gender Analyses

In their 12-7-95 response to our approvable letter, the sponsor provided the results of age and gender analyses. These included individual analyses of studies 248, 272, and 546, as well as analyses of a pool of all three studies. Overall, the pattern of results was not suggestive of age or gender effects, and a statement to this effect will be included in labeling.

5.1.2 Relapse Prevention Trial

In their 12-7-95 response to our approvable letter, the sponsor acknowledged the request in our approvable letter to commit to an adequate and well controlled relapse prevention trial for Zoloft in the treatment of OCD. In fact, enrollment is complete for study 93CE21-0615 and they expect the study to be completed in about 18 months.

5.1.3 Pediatric OCD Studies

In their 12-7-95 response to our approvable letter, the sponsor acknowledged the request in our approvable letter to commit to studies of the efficacy and safety of Zoloft in the treatment of OCD in children and adolescents. In fact, the sponsor has completed 2 pertinent studies, i.e., study 90CE21-0498 (A double-blind comparison of sertraline and placebo in children and adolescents with OCD) and study 90CK21-0525 (Tolerance and PK of sertraline in an children and adolescents with OCD or depression). Analyses are underway for these studies, as are extension phases for both.

5.2 Safety Update

The sponsor's obsessive compulsive disorder final safety update (OCD-FSU) had a cutoff date of 6-30-95 and included as a subset all the data from the original OCD-NDA, for which the cutoff date was 4-17-91. For the FSU, the integrated database included only patients from completed studies, however, the serious adverse events (SAE) events listing included any SAEs from ongoing studies as well (same 6-30-95 cutoff date). A summary enumeration of the adult sertraline exposed OCD patients in the OCD development program follows:

	OCD-FSU	OCD-NDA
Completed Studies	627	290[1]
Ongoing Studies[2]	954	
Total	1581	

1 The 290 patients are included in the FSU total of 627
2 This is an estimate, since many patients are still unblinded

In addition to the adult patients, the FSU included pediatric OCD patients exposed to sertraline. A summary enumeration of the pediatric sertraline exposed OCD patients in the OCD development program follows:

	Ped-OCD
Completed Studies	153
Ongoing Studies[1]	67
Total	220

1 This is an estimate, since many patients are still unblinded

The sponsor's strategy in conducting the safety update was to compare the findings from the OCD-FSU total adult database with the original OCD-NDA database, and also to compare the OCD-FSU adult database with the pediatric OCD database.

For the adult databases, the sertraline exposure and demographics were comparable, as were the overall rates of discontinuation for adverse events. Overall, there were 57 patients with serious adverse events among the adult patients in the OCD-FSU, including 30 for sertraline, 11 for placebo, 8 for active control, and 8 unblinded. There were no deaths among these patients, several suicide attempts, and 1 seizure. The overall adverse event profiles for the FSU and NDA databases were the same, and were similar to the recognized profile for sertraline in depression. There were no obvious age or gender differences in adverse events. There were also no patterns of laboratory, VS, or ECG findings suggestive of any clinically important sertraline related effects.

For the pediatric patients, the average maximum sertraline dose was somewhat higher than in the adult FSU population (185 vs 148 mg/day). Sixteen of the pediatric patients experienced serious adverse events, all among sertraline patients. The adverse event profile in the pediatric OCD patients was similar to that seen in adults. The one difference worth noting was the finding of 3 seizures among the pediatric patients (3/220; 1.4%). That seizure rate compares with an estimated rate of 0.06% (1/1581) in the adult OCD population. However, the 3 pediatric patients with seizures were aged 14, 15, and 15, i.e., they might reasonably be grouped with the adults, yielding a seizure risk of 4/1800 (0.2%). It is also important to note that 2 of the three children with seizures likely had coexisting seizures disorders, and the third had a strong family history of seizure disorder. Nevertheless, this finding needs to be noted in labeling.

The safety update also included an update on spontaneous reports. There were 114 such reports in patients identified as being treated with sertraline for OCD. Of these, 11 were considered serious. These serious reports included a suicide, a seizure, and a patient having a hypomanic episode. Overall, there was no pattern of findings among these reports suggestive of a different profile of adverse events for sertraline in OCD patients compared to other patients treated with this drug.

Dr. James Knudsen concluded in his 3-28-96 review of this safety update that there were no findings that would preclude the approval of this supplement, and I agree.

6.0 LABELING

I examined the foreign labeling provided with the 12-7-95 response to our approvable letter, and my impression was that our labeling is generally more complete and stronger than foreign labeling.

As noted above, through an exchange of faxes, we were able to reach agreement on most remaining labeling concerns, but we were unable to reach agreement on the precise wording in two sections of the labeling:

Clinical Trials Subsection of Clinical Pharmacology

Inclusion of Information about Mean Dose Achieved in Flexible Dose Trials

Pfizer objected to the inclusion of data regarding the mean dose utilized in the flexible dosing design depression and OCD trials. They argued that patients in these trials may have been titrated more rapidly than necessary, thereby achieving higher doses than was necessary or would likely be utilized in usual clinical practice. They expressed concern that the inclusion of such information may mislead clinicians into believing that these doses are the optimally effective doses.

Ordinarily, information about optimal dosing would be expected to come from adequate and well controlled fixed dose studies. Unfortunately, neither of the fixed dose studies conducted, i.e., 1 for depression and 1 for OCD, is readily interpretable. Consequently, there is no information directly pertinent to the issue of optimal dose, for either indication. Nevertheless, truth in labeling requires that the studies supporting a claim be accurately described. There is no suggestion in our proposed descriptions that the mean doses were the optimal doses. Rather, the proposed trial summaries simply state the facts, both regarding mean dose in the flexible dose trials and the fact that the fixed dose studies did not provide clear advice about optimal dose. Moreover, the Dosage and Administration section, ordinarily relied on by clinicians as a source of advice about dosing, recommends 50 mg as the starting dose for both indications, with further titration within a dose range of 50-200 mg/day being left up to the judgement of clinicians.

On the basis of the above arguments, I have not deleted information about mean doses for the flexible dose depression and OCD trials.

Lack of Interpretability of Fixed Dose Depression Study

Pfizer objected to our proposed statement regarding the fixed dose depression study as not being readily interpretability due to high dropouts at the higher doses. They argued that this statement does not provide clear guidance to clinicians and is "potentially confusing, inaccurate, and misleading." Alternatively, they proposed a statement suggesting that "there was no clear indication of a dose response relationship for effectiveness." I disagree, again from the standpoints of truth in labeling and what useful information can be gleaned from a clinical trial. To state that there was no indication of a dose response relationship suggests that the data from the fixed dose study were interpretable, when they were not. Alternatively, I have proposed a revised statement to simply indicate that the study was not readily interpretable regarding dose response for efficacy, rather than getting into speculation about the reasons.

Dosage and Administration Section

Pfizer indicated that they feel it is important for them to be able to refer to the results of continuation trials for OCD suggesting no loss of benefit in responding patients for periods of up to 1 year. They argued that this is important information to provide to clinicians. I disagree with including these data, since, as noted previously, it is my view that studies of this design are basically flawed, i.e., the randomization is violated, since only responding patients are continued in the extension phase. Consequently, these studies cannot provide definitive data pertinent to the question of long-term efficacy, and to include these data undermines our current approach to labeling on this matter. While it is true that examples can be found for previously approved labeling where this principle is violated, labeling policy is constantly evolving, and our current approach is to not include such data. In any case, the labeling acknowledges the usual practice of continuing responding patients, so that including this information does not strengthen labeling in any way from the clinician's standpoint.

On the basis of the above arguments, I have not further modfied this section as proposed in Pfizer's September 27, 1996 fax.

7.0 WORLD LITERATURE

In their 12-7-95 response to our approvable letter, the sponsor provided details of their world wide literature update, including copies of all pertinent papers, and they warranted that no findings adversely affected their conclusions about the safety of sertraline in the treatment of OCD. Dr. Knudsen reviewed this material as well and he did not discover any previously unrecognized important safety concerns for this drug.

8.0 FOREIGN REGULATORY ACTIONS

According the the 12-7-95 response to our approvable letter, Zoloft has been approved for the treatment of OCD in 12 countries and applications are under review in 34 additional countries. The response included a listing of what other regulatory agencies considered interim deficiencies, none of which we were not also aware of.

9.0 APPROVAL LETTER

The approval letter acknowledges the areas of disagreement in the clinical sections of labeling and provides discussion of why we have not agreed to Pfizer's proposed changes in these sections.

10.0 CONCLUSIONS AND RECOMMENDATIONS

I believe that Pfizer has submitted sufficient data to support the conclusion that Zoloft is effective and acceptably safe in the treatment of OCD. I recommend that we issue the attached approval letter with our proposal for final labeling.

cc:
Orig NDA 19-839/S-002
HFD-120/Div File
HFD-120/TLaughren/PLeber/AMosholder/HLee/JKnudsen/PDavid

DOC: MEMZLOCD.AP1

M E M O R A N D U M

DEPARTMENT OF HEALTH AND HUMAN SERVICES
PUBLIC HEALTH SERVICE
FOOD AND DRUG ADMINISTRATION
CENTER FOR DRUG EVALUATION AND RESEARCH

Tab 75

DATE: October 25, 1996

FROM: Thomas P. Laughren, M.D.
Team Leader, Psychiatric Drug Products
Division of Neuropharmacological Drug Products
HFD-120

SUBJECT: Comment on data in the OCD database pertinent to the emergence of suicidal ideation, gestures, and attempts in association with sertraline use

TO: File NDA 19-839/S-002
[**Note:** This overview should be filed with the 12-7-95 response to the approvable letter.]

A concern about the possibility of a signal of emergent suicidality (suicide attempts, gestures, or ideation) associated with sertraline use in pediatric patients was raised in the 3-28-96 review by Dr. James Knudsen. In his review, Dr. Knudsen reported a crude incidence of suicidality for adults taking sertraline of 9/1581 (0.6%) compared to 1/426 (0.2%) for placebo patients. The comparable crude incidence data for pediatric patients were 6/220 (3.0%) for sertraline and 0/95 for placebo. There were no suicides, and only 2 attempts among adults and 1 among pediatric patients. Dr. Knudsen provided person-time data only for the sertraline exposed patients, yielding adjusted estimates of 0.035/PEY for adults and 0.25/PEY for pediatric patients. He commented on the 7-fold greater incidence of suicidality in children taking sertraline compared to adults taking sertraline, but concluded that this finding may have been a result of a higher incidence of comorbid depression in the pediatric patients.

I agree that the adult and pediatric populations may have differed regarding comorbid depression, and that is one reason why the comparison of incidence data for sertraline exposed patients in these 2 databases may not have been appropriate. Four pediatric studies contributed patients to the pediatric database, two of which permitted the entry of patients with either OCD or major depression. **In fact,** 4 of the 6 pediatric subjects having suicidality had diagnoses of major depression. OCD was required for all the adult studies, and my impression is that there was minimal comorbid major depression. Thus, it is not reasonable, in my view, to compare adults to children on the incidence of suicidality in sertraline exposed patients. It would have been more informative to compare the risk ratios, i.e., drug to placebo, after adjusting for persone-time, within each of the adult and pediatric strata. Unfortunately, person-time data were provided only for sertraline exposed subjects, and not placebo. In fact, 3 of the 4 pediatric studies were open label, and 2 of these were long-term, thus drug exposed patients had a much greater opportunity for having events than placebo exposed patients.

In summary, I don't consider these data to represent a signal of risk for suicidality for either adults or children. Supplements are planned for both depression and OCD in pediatric patients, and when we have more complete data, including HAMD data, we can look more critically at this issue, using the now standard approach of comparing the proportions of drug and placebo exposed patients who show worsening on Item 3 (suicidality item) of the HAMD during treatment. At the present time, current labeling simply notes that Zoloft has not been adequately evaluated for safety and effectiveness in pediatric patients.

cc:
Orig NDA 19-839/S-002
HFD-120/Div File
HFD-120/TLaughren/PLeber/AMosholder/PDavid

DOC: MEMZLOCD.AP2

Memorandum

Tab 76

Department of Health and Human Services
Public Health Service
Food and Drug Administration
Center for Drug Evaluation and Research

DATE: October 25, 1996

FROM: Paul Leber, M.D.
Director,
Division of Neuropharmacological Drug Products
HFD-120

SUBJECT: Zoloft™ [sertraline hydrochloride] for OCD
NDA 19-839/S-002 Approval Action Memorandum

TO: File NDA 19-839

This memorandum documents for the administrative file the basis for my decision to approve NDA 19-839/ S-002 for Zoloft's use in OCD. The basis for my affirmative conclusions about sertraline's safety for use and effectiveness in use as a treatment for OCD are explicated in my 8/1/95 approvable action memorandum.

Post-approvable Action Issues and their Resolution:

The approvable action letter (issued 8/1/95) informed Pfizer Pharmaceuticals that final approval of the Zoloft OCD effectiveness supplement was conditioned upon the acceptability of their response to a number of requests enumerated in our letter.

In his comprehensive supervisory memorandum (9/30/96) recommending approval of the Zoloft OCD effectiveness supplement, Dr. Laughren reviews the regulatory issues pending at the time the approvable action was taken in regard to whether or not they have been satisfactorily resolved from the agency's perspective.

There are 3 issues concerning product labeling about which the sponsor and the Division review team have, despite extensive negotiations, failed to agree. In his memorandum, Dr. Laughren explicates the basis for these disagreements, and explains why he believes the Division Review Team's position on them should prevail.

I have discussed each of these issues in detail with Dr. Laughren, and I am persuaded that the Review Team's proposals for labeling are preferable (more accurate, less misleading, and/or better substantiated by the evidence) to the firm's.

For the record, I should also note that I am in full agreement with the manner in which the Review team and Pfizer have resolved all other issues[1] affecting the final approval of the supplement.

I note, in particular, that the evidence relied upon to support the text and placement of the sections of Zoloft product labeling about sertraline's lack of effect on the clearance of two drug products metabolized by CYP450 3A4 derives from reports made in other supplements and/or submissions[2] to the NDA.

I take note also of the fact that the firm has agreed, as requested, to make commitments to 1) conduct a "relapse prevention trial, " and to 2) conduct, and/or report the results of already completed, clinical trials evaluating sertraline's safety and efficacy as a treatment for OCD in children and adolescents.

Finally, I note that the set of reports ordinarily made by a sponsor following the receipt of an approvable action (i.e., Safety Update, archival literature review and summary of adverse foreign regulatory actions) have, upon review, been found to provide no new evidence that would cause the Division to revise and/or substantively modify its conclusion that Zoloft will be safe for use and effective in use as a treatment for OCD

---

[1] A minor concern that I had about the possible misinterpretation of a comparison of suicide rates in adults and children offered in the medical officer's review has been satisfactorily clarified by Dr. Laughren in his memorandum to the file of October 25, 1996.

[2] The matter of 3A4 enzyme inhibition was not immediately critical to the OCD approvable action decision. For technical regulatory reasons, however, it had to be considered in the approvable action letter because a "changes being effected" labeling supplement bearing on this PK/safety issue was pending at the time that action was taken.

provided that Zoloft is marketed under the conditions of use described in the version of labeling developed by the Division. Mention of this linkage is made in the approval action letter which advises the sponsor that marketing of Zoloft under labeling other than that incorporated in the approval action letter would make the product misbranded and subject it to a new drug charge.

Approval in the face of unresolved disputes concerning drug product labeling:

Although the labeling under which a new drug is marketed is viewed as "belonging to" the drug's sponsor, the content of that labeling is ordinarily developed jointly by the agency's review team and the sponsor's representatives. Joint labeling development is the rule rather than the exception, not because FDA regulation requires it, but because experience has shown that joint development speeds the process of negotiation through which accurate and informative product labeling is ordinarily developed at the end of a review cycle.

There are occasions, however, when, despite extended negotiations, agreement on the precise wording of one or more sections of labeling cannot be reached. In such circumstances, the agency has two choices: 1) to disapprove the application on the grounds that product labeling is false or misleading, or 2) to approve the application, but under a version of labeling that the agency determines will allow the product to be marketed under conditions that satisfy the requirements of law. The latter choice, in my view, is invariably superior to the former.

I make note of this because the Division's Review Team and Pfizer's representatives, despite extensive efforts to resolve their differences, have failed to reach agreement on what I believe to be three relatively minor labeling issues. Two concern details about the text[3] best used to describe the clinical trials from which substantial evidence of sertraline's effectiveness have been adduced. The third concerns whether or not the firm, in the absence of evidence from valid clinical trials, may

---

[3] presented in the Clinical Trials subsection of the Clinical Pharmacology Section

assert that sertraline, in extended use, has a sustained effect on OCD phenomena.

In my judgment, the Division Review Teams's proposed labeling is unquestionably more accurate and less subject to misleading interpretation than the firm's. Moreover, I find nothing in the labeling text advanced by the Division Review Team that promotes anything that is at odds with the facts or undermining of the product.

Accordingly, I have concluded that Pfizer's OCD supplement should be approved, but under the labeling that has been developed by the Division. If Pfizer finds this version of labeling unacceptable, they are not compelled to market Zoloft for OCD.

It is my understanding, in approving the supplement under these conditions, that the marketing of Zoloft under any labeling other than that attached to the approval action letter (with the obvious exception of currently approved product labeling) would be in violation of the requirements of the FD&C Act and would, therefore, be a basis for adverse regulatory action.

Conclusion and Action:

For the reasons explicated, I have determined that NDA 19-839/S002 may be approved under the conditions of use recommended in the version of labeling attached to the approval action letter that is issuing under my signature.

Paul Leber, M.D.
October 25, 1996

cc
NDA 19-839, HFD-120/DIV FILE
HFD-100 Temple
HFD-120 TLaughren/AMosholder
HFD-120/BRosloff/GFitzgerald
HFD-120/MZarifa/SBlum/PDavid
HFD-713/TSahlroot
HFD-860/RBaweja/SIbrahim

NOV 13 1996

REVIEW AND EVALUATION OF CLINICAL DATA

NDA	20-243
SPONSOR:	Solvay Pharmaceuticals
DRUG:	Fluvoxamine maleate (Luvox)
MATERIAL SUBMITTED:	Supplement 6 for Pediatric Labeling
DATE SUBMITTED:	12/21/95
DATE RECEIVED:	12/26/95
MEDICAL OFFICER:	Andrew Mosholder, M.D.
REVIEW COMPLETED:	8/27/96

Tab 77

Contents of Review

1.0 Material Utilized in Review

1.1 Material from NDA/IND

This review encompassed the 10 volumes of the 12/21/95 submission to NDA 20-243, supplement 6. In addition, at my request conveyed by telephone on 8/26/96, Solvay FAXed EKG data regarding patient 65856.

1.2 Related Reviews

Clinical review for NDA 20-243 by Dr. Gregory Dubitsky (10/22/93).

2.0 Background

2.1 Indication

Obsessive-compulsive disorder (OCD), as defined in DSM-IV, involves either obsessions or compulsions that are severe enough to be time consuming or that cause significant impairment or distress.

With respect to pediatric patients, recognition of the abnormality of these symptoms is not required for the diagnosis (unlike adults).

Fluvoxamine is a selective serotonin reuptake inhibitor currently marketed in the U.S. for the treatment of OCD. However, the current labeling for fluvoxamine does not incorporate any pediatric clinical data. At the time of approval in December 1994, Solvay pledged to provide clinical data on the use of fluvoxamine in pediatric patients with OCD.

Currently, two other drugs are approved for the treatment of OCD: fluoxetine (Prozac) and clomipramine (Anafranil). Of these two, only Anafranil labeling includes information on use in children and adolescents: In an 8 week controlled trial in patients aged 10-17 years, clomipramine treated patients achieved a mean decrease of 10 points on the Yale Brown Obsessive Compulsive Scale (YBOCS), compared to negligible improvement on average for placebo treated patients.

2.2 Important Information from Related INDs and NDAs and from Pharmacologically Related Agents

I am not aware of any critical data from these which would not be found in the present submission.

2.3 Administrative History

Solvay sponsors commercial IND 11,925 for fluvoxamine, under which studies of OCD and depression were conducted. NDA 19-189, which was not approved, provided for the use of fluvoxamine in depression, while NDA 20-243, approved on 12/5/94, provides for use of fluvoxamine to treat OCD.

2.4 Directions for Use

Current labeling for use in adults with OCD recommends a starting dose of 50 mg QHS, increased by 50 mg increments every 4-7 days to a suggested range of 100-300 mg/day. Doses above 100 mg daily should be divided.

The proposed labeling for this supplement recommends a starting dose of 25 mg in pediatric patients (i.e., aged 8-17). The dose should be increased in 25 mg increments every 4-7 days, up to a maximum of 200 mg/day. Daily doses more than 50 mg should be divided, with the larger dose given at bedtime if the doses are unequal.

2.5 Foreign Marketing

Luvox is marketed in over 40 countries worldwide, with an estimated worldwide exposure of over 9 million as of August 1995 according to Solvay. No information on approval for pediatric use in other countries was provided in this supplement.

3.0 Chemistry

There are no applicable chemistry manufacturing and controls issues. To achieve dosing in 25 mg increments, the tablets, which are scored, will have to be broken.

4.0 Animal Pharmacology

Solvay conducted no new animal studies for this supplement.

5.0 Description of Clinical Data Sources

The clinical data source for this supplement consists of a single study, Protocol RH 114.02.01, which was a randomized, double blind, multicenter, ten week placebo controlled trial. 120 subjects with OCD, aged 8-17 years, participated (57 received fluvoxamine and 63 placebo). The study is completed; however, an

There were no adverse drug effects noted for this system.

8.2.4 Metabolic and Endocrine

Weight loss was more frequently noted in the fluvoxamine treated group, and weight gain was more frequent in the placebo group. With a sample size this small, it is difficult to draw conclusions, but if this is a true drug effect it may be related to the gastrointestinal symptoms mentioned above such as anorexia.

8.2.5 Musculoskelatal

In the extension/humanitarian phase, one child had surgery for scoliosis and two children sustained fractures. These events do not appear drug related.

8.2.6 Nervous

Agitation, depression and insomnia were common and drug related adverse events. There was one premature discontinuation for a manic reaction and one for agitation; also, one subject in the extension/humanitarian phase was hospitalized at a psychiatric facility for suicidality. Agitation was not a common, drug related event in adult fluvoxamine clinical trials. Pediatric behavioral disturbances with SSRI compounds have been reported in the literature (for review, see DeVane CL and Sallee FR, J Clin Psychiatry 1996;57:55-66).

8.2.7 Respiratory

There were no adverse drug effects noted for this system.

8.2.8 Dermatologic

One subject dropped out for exacerbation of eczema.

8.2.9 Special Senses

There were no adverse drug effects noted for this system.

8.2.10 Genitourinary

Abnormal urinalyses were reported more frequently in the fluvoxamine group, as shown in the table of laboratory findings above. The specific abnormalities involved hematuria (attributed to menstruation), bactiuria and presence of white blood cells. These findings are, in my opinion, not likely to be drug related. Dysmennorhea was observed in 7% of females, but due to the small number of female subjects this figure represented only two patients.

8.3 Summary of Key Adverse Findings

In my judgement, the key adverse events associated with fluvoxamine in this study involve gastrointestinal disturbances, weight loss, and behavioral symptoms centering on activation, mania or agitation. However, it is difficult to draw firm conclusions about the adverse reaction profile in the pediatric age group when dealing with a sample this small.

9.0 Labeling Review

The proposed labeling includes an addition to the Clinical Trials subsection describing this study, including a table of results on the CGI similar to that appearing in the current labeling for adults. Also, the Pediatric Use subsection has been revised. Under Adverse Reactions, a "one percent" table of adverse event incidence rates for this study has been added, and the Dosage and Administration section has been revised to include dosing recommendations that parallel the dosing in this clinical trial.

I propose adding a statement to the current Precautions/Activation of Mania/Hypomania subsection, as follows: "In a pediatric OCD clinical trial, 2 out of 57 (3.5%) of fluvoxamine treated patients experienced a manic reaction, compared to none out of 63 placebo patients."

Under Pediatric Use, I am not entirely comfortable with the statement that there were no observed differences in safety between children and adults. Generally, there seem to be more behavioral adverse events among the pediatric patients; also, weight loss was more prominent in the pediatric group. I propose adding a recommendation under Pediatric Use for monitoring growth in young patients: "Weight loss was observed in a few patients in the pediatric OCD study, therefore, regular monitoring of weight and growth is recommended if treatment of a child is continued long term."

10.0 Conclusions

This study provides evidence that fluvoxamine is effective in the treatment of children and adolescents with OCD. No critical safety findings emerged during this study that would preclude approval for this age group; however, the size of the study limits the degree of confidence regarding safety in this population.

11.0 Recommendations

With the slight modifications to the proposed labeling outlined above, I believe that this supplement can be approved. This supplement appears to fulfill the sponsor's obligation under the recently revised Pediatric Labeling regulations (21 CFR 201.57, amended 12/13/94).

Consideration should be given to asking Solvay for some additional information, such as a literature search regarding pediatric use of fluvoxamine, and a survey of their postmarketing spontaneous reports involving pediatric patients; the submission did not include such material.

[signature] 8/27/96

Andrew Mosholder, M.D.
Medical Officer, DNDP

NDA 20-243/SE5-006
HFD-120/Laughren/David/Dubitsky/Mosholder
HFD-710/Choudhury/Sahlroot

11-13-96

I agree that this supplement is approvable. See my memo to file for more detailed comments.

Thomas P. Laughren, MD
TL, PDP

TABLE 34.
Treatment Emergent Signs and Symptoms
Intent-to-Treat Safety Sample

(CONTINUED)

COSTART Body System and Preferred Term		TREATMENT			
		Fluvoxamine		Placebo	
		57		63	
		N	%	N	%
DIGESTIVE	APPETITE INC	0	0	2	3.17
	DIARRHEA	9	15.79	7	11.11
	DYSPEPSIA	8	14.04	4	6.35
	FLATUL	3	5.26	0	0
	NAUSEA	10	17.54	13	20.63
	NAUSEA VOMIT	0	0	1	1.59
	RECTAL DIS	0	0	1	1.59
	TOOTH CARIES	0	0	1	1.59
	TOOTH DIS	0	0	1	1.59
	VOMIT	5	8.77	5	7.94
	BODY SYSTEM TOTAL	24	42.11	24	38.10
HEMATIC AND LYMPH	ECCHYMOSIS	2	3.51	0	0
	EOSINOPHILIA	0	0	1	1.59
	BODY SYSTEM TOTAL	2	3.51	1	1.59
METABOLIC AND NUTRITIONAL	WEIGHT DEC	2	3.51	0	0
	WEIGHT INC	0	0	1	1.59
	BODY SYSTEM TOTAL	2	3.51	1	1.59
MUSCULOSKELETAL	ARTHRALGIA	1	1.75	0	0
	CRAMPS LEG	0	0	1	1.59
	MYALGIA	1	1.75	2	3.17
	MYASTHENIA	0	0	1	1.59
	BODY SYSTEM TOTAL	2	3.51	4	6.35
NERVOUS	AGITATION	7	12.28	2	3.17

TABLE 34.
Treatment Emergent Signs and Symptoms
Intent-to-Treat Safety Sample

(CONTINUED)

COSTART Body System and Preferred Term		TREATMENT			
		Fluvoxamine		Placebo	
		57		63	
		N	%	N	%
NERVOUS	AKATHISIA	0	0	1	1.59
	AMNESIA	1	1.75	0	0
	ANXIETY	1	1.75	1	1.59
	DEPRESSION	3	5.26	0	0
	DIZZINESS	5	8.77	5	7.94
	DREAM ABNORM	2	3.51	4	6.35
	DRY MOUTH	2	3.51	0	0
	EMOTION LABIL	2	3.51	1	1.59
	HOSTILITY	1	1.75	1	1.59
	HYPERKINESIA	7	12.28	2	3.17
	HYPERTONIA	1	1.75	0	0
	INSOMNIA	17	29.82	6	9.52
	MANIC REACT	2	3.51	0	0
	NERVOUSNESS	3	5.26	5	7.94
	PARESTHESIA	0	0	2	3.17
	PERSON DIS	1	1.75	0	0
	SLEEP DIS	0	0	1	1.59
	SOMNOLENCE	6	10.53	1	1.59
	SUICIDAL IDEATION	1	1.75	0	0
	THINKING ABNORM	2	3.51	0	0
	TREMOR	0	0	1	1.59
	VASODILAT	0	0	1	1.59
	BODY SYSTEM TOTAL	31	54.39	21	33.33
RESPIRATORY	BRONCHITIS	0	0	3	4.76
	COUGH INC	5	8.77	4	6.35

FEB 20 1997

REVIEW AND EVALUATION OF CLINICAL DATA

NDA 20-243

SPONSOR: Solvay Pharmaceuticals

DRUG: Fluvoxamine maleate (Luvox)

MATERIAL SUBMITTED: Supplement 6 for Pediatric Labeling/Response to Approvable Letter

DATE SUBMITTED: 12/13/96

Tab 78

DATE RECEIVED: 12/16/96

MEDICAL OFFICER: Andrew Mosholder, M.D.

REVIEW COMPLETED: 2/12/97

Background

This supplement provides for pediatric use labeling for fluvoxamine maleate (Luvox), based on the results of a randomized controlled trial, study 114.02.01. On 11/27/96 the Division sent Solvay an approvable letter for this supplement, and the present submission is Solvay's response. In the approvable letter, the Division proposed changes to the sponsor's draft labeling, and requested a Phase IV commitment for an efficacy study in adolescents. The latter request was made because of an age by treatment interaction noted in the results of study 114.02.01, in which there was little evidence for efficacy in the adolescent age group. Also requested was a safety update, a world literature update, a foreign regulatory update, and development of a 25 mg tablet strength. This submission contains the sponsor's response to all of these points.

Labeling

1. The sponsor has added the sources of starch, namely potato and corn, to the inactive ingredients listed in the Description section. I see no objection to this.

2. In the Clinical Trials section, the sponsor has made some editorial changes to the outcome classification tables, and has agreed to include language describing the age by treatment interaction. With respect to the latter, Solvay added some wording emphasizing the post hoc nature of this analysis. I find the sponsor's proposed changes acceptable.

3. Uunder Drug Interactions Solvay added the requested labeling regarding a putative interaction with sumaptriptan.

4. Under Precautions/Activation of mania/hypomania, the sponsor has added "n=2" to show that the 4% incidence of mania represented two patients. I see no objection to this but favor providing the complete numbers for both drug and placebo.

5. As requested, Solvay has removed from the Adverse Reactions section the table of treatment emergent adverse event incidences in the pediatric study (formerly Tabel 2A). In its place, they have simply listed the adverse events not already listed in the existing Table 2 for the adult studies, providing they occurred in at least two children and were more common with Luvox. Also listed are the adverse events more frequent in the placebo group, again providing that they occurred in at least two children, but I am not convinced this adds much of value. I have proposed some modifications to this section.

It is of interest that in the adult studies, the incidence of agitation was 2% and 1% for fluvoxamine and placebo, respectively, while for the pediatric study, the corresponding incidences were 12% and 3%. That is, the risk ratio for adults was 2 and for children was 4. It is possible that this reflects a real difference in adverse reactions between adults and children. There is an emerging literature pointing to behavioral reactions to SSRI drugs in children (for a review, see Devane et al., J Clin Psychiatry 1996;57:55-66). This is also reflected in Pfizer's recently submitted study of sertraline in the treatment of juvenile OCD. Here, the incidence of agitation was 13% in the sertraline treated children and 2.1% in the placebo treated children (p=.005). Comparable figures for the adult OCD studies with sertraline were 6% and 3%, respectively.

It may be that this is a reaction to SSRIs that is more prominent in children than adults; further data would help clarify this.

Safety Update

Solvay provided safety data on the open label extension phases for the original study. There was a one year open label extension which enrolled 99 patients, designated study 114.02.01E. Subsequently, 21 of these patients received further open label fluvoxamine treatment in an extension protocol, designated 114.02.01H. There were 12 premature discontinuations for adverse events and 4 serious adverse events during the first extension study 114/02.01E, and a single premature discontinuation for an adverse event from the following study 114.02.01H. These cases are summarized in the sponsor's table which is attached to this review. It will be seen that most of the reasons for discontinuation represent types of disinhibited behavior. One could speculate that fluvoxamine has a disinhibiting effect in children, and indeed there is some support for this from the controlled trial data about agitation, but absent a control group for comparison it is difficult to conclude anything from open label adverse event reports.

At our request, Solvay provided additional information on 2 patients who discontinued prematurely from open label treatment (fax 2/12/97, to be submitted to NDA). Both patients had a variety of ECG abnormalities as read by the computer program. For patient 65815, these abnormalities were deemed to be insignificantly changed from baseline, although I noted that the patient's QTc interval increased from a baseline of 454 msec to 492 msec on fluvoxamine. For patient 65848, the ECG findings suggested right ventricular hypertrophy, but an echocardiogram failed to confirm this. Thus neither patient appeared to have important treatment emergent cardiac toxicity, despite the ECG abnormalities.

Solvay also compiled all postmarketing reports through 12/2/96 involving fluvoxamine treatment of patients up to age 18 years. This yielded a total of 106 reports, including 39 serious adverse events and one death.

The death occurred in a 10 year old boy who had been receiving fluoxetine for OCD and had been switched to fluvoxamine treatment (100 mg/d) for one week. He died suddenly and unexpectedly; the autopsy revealed multifocal, probably viral myocarditis, and small coronary artery disease. While one could speculate that fluvoxamine treatment contributed in some way to this boy's death, there seems to have been sufficient cardiac pathology to account for death regardless of drug treatment.

Other notable adverse events included one case of toxic epidermal necrolysis in a 15 year old girl after 8 days of fluvoxamine therapy (case FLUV001930086), and a case of erythema multiforme in a 7 year old boy (case FLUV002950428). Toxic epidermal necrolysis and Stevens Johnson syndrome are both noted in the current fluvoxamine labeling under postmarketing reports.

There was one case (FLUV002950163) designated as serotonin syndrome, in a 13 year old girl, treated with fluvoxamine for 4 days at 50-100 mg/d. She developed tremor followed by seizures; other symptoms included dyspnea, fever, sweating and abnormal gait. EEG and clinical laboratories were normal. She was admitted to the hospital and treated with diphenhydramine. Serotonin syndrome is not noted in the current Luvox labeling.

In addition to the last case, there were 6 other case reports of convulsions.

One 16 year old anorexic girl developed pancytopenia and sepsis while receiving fluvoxamine; this case was confounded by severe anorexia, however, which can affect the status of the bone marrow (case FLUV001890637).

Another interesting case described treatment emergent Tourette's syndrome in a 14 year old boy (case FLUV001949196). Notably, the TS symptoms resolved after discontinuing fluvoxamine but emerged again when the patient was rechallenged. After the second course of fluvoxamine was discontinued the TS symptoms again resolved.

World Literature Update

Solvay conducted a world literature search through 11/21/96 for articles dealing with pediatric safety of fluvoxamine. Their review team, lead by Dr. Eric Phillips, the Director of Drug Safety and Surveillance, found no additional information that would affect the conclusion that fluvoxamine is safe and effective in pediatric patients. A bibliography and selected reprints were supplied with the submission. Several of the publications represented case reports which Solvay provided under postmarketing reports. Although only a selected number of reprints was available to me, I am inclined to agree that no hitherto unsuspected concerns about use of fluvoxamine in children are represented in the literature.

Miscellaneous

Solvay would like to meet with the Agency regarding the best way to study the age interaction. With respect to the 25 mg dosage strength, this has apparently been approved but Solvay has not yet marketed it. Finally, regarding foreign regulatory actions, Luvox is not indicated for pediatric use anywhere in the world.

Conclusions and Recommendations

In my opinion, this supplement may be approved with some minor revisions to the sponsor's proposed labeling.

Andrew Mosholder 2/12/97

Andrew Mosholder, M.D.
Medical Officer, DNDP

NDA 20-243
Div file
HFD-120/Laughren/David/Dubitsky/Mosholder

2-20-97

I agree that this supplement can now be approved. See more detailed response in memo to file.

T. Laughren

ATTACHMENT SPONSOR'S TABLE

SUMMARY TABLE OF PATIENT NARRATIVES
LUVOX® PEDIATRIC OCD EXTENSION STUDIES

PATIENT NUMBER	AGE[1] (YRS)	GENDER	RACE	INVESTIGATOR'S TERM	DOSE[2] (mg)	OUTCOME
PREMATURE WITHDRAWALS						
65130-E	11	F	Caucasian	Behavioral disinhibition, Midnight awakening	50	AE still present, no further treatment
65148-E	16	M	Caucasian	Hypomania	200	AE still present, no further treatment
65230-E	8	F	Caucasian	Hyperactivity, Tiredness, Dizziness	100	Recovered, no sequelae (hyperactivity), AE still present, no further treatment (tiredness, dizziness)
65231-E	11	M	Caucasian	Hyperactivity	200	AE still present, no further treatment
65253-E	10	M	Caucasian	Aggressive behavior	150	Recovered, without sequelae
65811-E[3]	10	M	Caucasian	Hyperactivity	150	AE still present, no further treatment
65815-E	15	M	Caucasian	Suicidal ideation, Suicidal gesture	100	Recovered, without sequelae
65818-E	12	M	Caucasian	Agitation	50	Recovered, without sequelae
65824-E	14	M	Caucasian	Difficulty falling asleep	150	AE still present, no further treatment
65848-E	10	M	Caucasian	Hyperactivity, oppositional behavior	50-75	AE still present, no further treatment
65853-E[3]	13	M	Caucasian	Dangerous (behavioral) events	200	Not recorded
65855-E	17	M	Caucasian	Gastrointestinal gas	25	AE still present, no further treatment
SERIOUS ADVERSE EVENTS						
65811-E[3]	10	M	Caucasian	Hospitalized for broken arm	150	Recovered, without sequelae
65816-E	11	F	Caucasian	Hospitalized for elective surgery to correct scoliosis	0	Recovered, without sequelae
65853-E[3]	13	M	Caucasian	Hospitalized for cracked ribs, fractured right elbow, amnesia	200	Recovered, without sequelae (ribs), AE still present, no further treatment (elbow), Not recorded (amnesia)
66052-E	15	F	Caucasian	Hospitalized for anxiety and suicidal ideation	200	Not recorded
HUMANITARIAN PREMATURE WITHDRAWALS						
65249-H	15	F	Caucasian	Panic attacks	150	AE still present, no further treatment

[1] age at start of Core Study
[2] dose at first occurrence of adverse event leading to withdrawal
[3] serious adverse event and separate adverse event leading to withdrawal

DEPARTMENT OF HEALTH & HUMAN SERVICES

Public Health Service
Food and Drug Administration
Rockville MD 20857

NDA 20-243/S-021

Tab 79

Solvay Pharmaceuticals
Attention: J. Greg Perkins, Ph.D.
Vice President Regulatory Science
901 Sawyer Road
Marietta, Georgia 30062

SEP 28 2000

Dear Dr. Perkins:

Please refer to your supplemental new drug application dated and received December 2, 1999, submitted under section 505(b) of the Federal Food, Drug, and Cosmetic Act for Luvox (fluvoxamine maleate) 25 mg, 50 mg, and 100 mg Tablets.

Additionally, we acknowledge receipt of your submissions dated May 31, and June 30, 2000.

Reference is also made to an Agency letter dated March 25, 1997, providing for the approval of supplemental application S-006 to use Luvox to treat obsessive compulsive disorder in the pediatric population. This letter also committed that Solvay explore further the effects of Luvox in obsessive compulsive disorder (OCD) patients between the ages of 12 – 17 years old as a Phase 4 commitment.

We additionally refer to a series of faxes dated September 21, 24, and 26, 2000 in which labeling for this supplemental application, S-021, was agreed upon by Solvay and the Agency.

This supplemental new drug application provides for revised labeling of Luvox based upon the results of a long-term, open-label safety study and a pharmacokinetic study in children and adolescents with OCD.

We have completed the review of this supplemental application, as amended, and have concluded that adequate information has been presented to demonstrate that the drug product is safe and effective for use as recommended in the agreed upon enclosed labeling text. Accordingly, this supplemental application is approved effective on the date of this letter.

Additionally, this data completely fulfills your Phase 4 commitment for S-006 as enumerated in our March 25, 1997, Agency letter.

The final printed labeling (FPL) must be identical to the enclosed labeling (text for the package insert).

Please submit 20 paper copies of the final printed labeling ten of which are individually mounted on heavy weight paper or similar material. Alternatively, you may submit the FPL electronically according to the guidance for industry titled *Providing Regulatory Submissions in Electronic Format - NDAs* (January 1999). For administrative purposes, this submission should be designated "FPL for approved supplement NDA 20-243/S-021". Approval of this submission by FDA is not required before the labeling is used.

ATTACHMENT
NDA 20-243/S-021

[Note: Below is the labeling for Luvox. This labeling was agreed upon by Solvay and the Agency in a series of faxes dated September 21, 24, and 26, 2000. The labeling is identical to your last approved labeling supplement, S-022, which was approved in an Agency letter dated August 9, 2000, except for the highlighted revisions. These revisions to labeling are based on the labeling changes proposed in your December 2, 1999 submission (S-021) as well as labeling revisions requested in an Agency letter dated June 1, 2000 (S-017). Double underline font denotes additions to the labeling, and strikeout font denotes deletions to the labeling.]

LUVOX®
(Fluvoxamine Maleate) Tablets
25 mg, 50 mg and 100 mg

DESCRIPTION
Fluvoxamine maleate is a selective serotonin (5-HT) reuptake inhibitor (SSRI) belonging to a new chemical series, the 2-aminoethyl oxime ethers of aralkylketones. It is chemically unrelated to other SSRIs and clomipramine. It is chemically designated as 5-methoxy-4'-(trifluoromethyl)valerophenone-(E)-O-(2-aminoethyl)oxime maleate (1:1) and has the empirical formula $C_{15}H_{21}O_2N_2F_3$ $C_4H_4O_4$. Its molecular weight is 434.4.

The structural formula is:

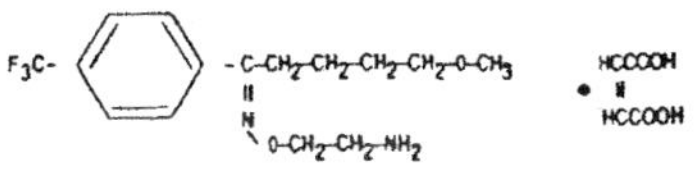

Fluvoxamine maleate is a white or off white, odorless, crystalline powder which is sparingly soluble in water, freely soluble in ethanol and chloroform and practically insoluble in diethyl ether.

LUVOX® (Fluvoxamine Maleate) Tablets are available in 25 mg, 50 mg and 100 mg strengths for oral administration. In addition to the active ingredient, fluvoxamine maleate, each tablet contains the following inactive ingredients: carnauba wax, hydroxypropyl methylcellulose, mannitol, polyethylene glycol, polysorbate 80, pregelatinized starch (potato), silicon dioxide, sodium stearyl fumarate, starch (corn), and titanium dioxide. The 50 mg and 100 mg tablets also contain synthetic iron oxides.

CLINICAL PHARMACOLOGY
Pharmacodynamics
The mechanism of action of fluvoxamine maleate in Obsessive Compulsive Disorder is presumed to be linked to its specific serotonin reuptake inhibition in brain neurons. In preclinical studies, it was found that fluvoxamine inhibited neuronal uptake of serotonin.

It is likely that this experience significantly underestimates the degree of accumulation that might occur with repeated diazepam administration. Moreover, as noted with alprazolam, the effect of fluvoxamine may even be more pronounced when it is administered at higher doses.

Accordingly, diazepam and fluvoxamine should not ordinarily be co-administered.

Theophylline: The effect of steady-state fluvoxamine (50 mg bid) on the pharmacokinetics of a single dose of theophylline (375 mg as 442 mg aminophylline) was evaluated in 12 healthy non-smoking, male volunteers. The clearance of theophylline was decreased approximately three-fold. Therefore, if theophylline is co-administered with fluvoxamine maleate, its dose should be reduced to one third of the usual daily maintenance dose and plasma concentrations of theophylline should be monitored. No dosage adjustment is required for LUVOX® Tablets.

Warfarin: When fluvoxamine maleate (50 mg tid) was administered concomitantly with warfarin for two weeks, warfarin plasma concentrations increased by 98% and prothrombin times were prolonged. Thus patients receiving oral anticoagulants and LUVOX® Tablets should have their prothrombin time monitored and their anticoagulant dose adjusted accordingly. No dosage adjustment is required for LUVOX® Tablets.

PRECAUTIONS

General

Activation of Mania/Hypomania: During premarketing studies involving primarily depressed patients, hypomania or mania occurred in approximately 1% of patients treated with fluvoxamine. In a ten week pediatric OCD study, 2 out of 57 patients (4%) treated with fluvoxamine experienced manic reactions, compared to none of 63 placebo patients. Activation of mania/hypomania has also been reported in a small proportion of patients with major affective disorder who were treated with other marketed antidepressants. As with all antidepressants, LUVOX® Tablets should be used cautiously in patients with a history of mania.

Seizures: During premarketing studies, seizures were reported in 0.2% of fluvoxamine-treated patients. LUVOX® Tablets should be used cautiously in patients with a history of seizures. It should be discontinued in any patient who develops seizures.

Suicide: The possibility of a suicide attempt is inherent in patients with depressive symptoms, whether these occur in primary depression or in association with another primary disorder such as OCD. Close supervision of high risk patients should accompany initial drug therapy. Prescriptions for LUVOX® Tablets should be written for the smallest quantity of tablets consistent with good patient management in order to reduce the risk of overdose.

Hyponatremia: Several cases of hyponatremia have been reported. In cases where the outcome was known, the hyponatremia appeared to be reversible when fluvoxamine was discontinued. The majority of these occurrences have been in elderly individuals, some in patients taking diuretics or with concomitant conditions that might cause hyponatremia. In patients receiving LUVOX® Tablets and suffering from Syndrome of Inappropriate Secretion of Antidiuretic Hormone (SIADH), displacement syndromes, edematous states, adrenal disease or conditions of

MEMORANDUM

Tab 80

DEPARTMENT OF HEALTH AND HUMAN SERVICES
PUBLIC HEALTH SERVICE
FOOD AND DRUG ADMINISTRATION
CENTER FOR DRUG EVALUATION AND RESEARCH

DATE: November 14, 1996

FROM: Thomas P. Laughren, M.D. Thomas P. Laughren
Team Leader, Psychiatric Drug Products
Division of Neuropharmacological Drug Products
HFD-120

SUBJECT: Recommendation for Approvable Action for Luvox (fluvoxamine) for Pediatric OCD

TO: File NDA 20-243/S-006
[**Note:** This overview should be filed with the 12-21-95 original submission.]

1.0 BACKGROUND

Luvox (fluvoxamine) is a selective serotonin reuptake inhibitor that was approved for the treatment of obsessive compulsive disorder (OCD) 12-5-94 (NDA 20-243). Supplement S-006 includes data from a single clinical trial supporting the use of fluvoxamine in the treatment of OCD in pediatric patients with this condition, in a dose range of 50-200 mg/day.

Since the proposal is to use the currently approved Luvox formulations for this expanded population, there was no need for chemistry, pharmacology, or biopharmaceutics reviews of this supplement. Consequently, the focus was on clinical data. The primary review of the efficacy and safety data was done by Andrew Mosholder, M.D. from the clinical group, and Japo Choudhury, Ph.D., from the Division of Biometrics also reviewed the efficacy data.

This study, RH.114.02.01, was conducted under IND 11,925. The original supplement for OCD (S-006) was submitted 12-21-95.

It should be noted that, at the current time, there are 5 drugs specifically approved for the treatment of obsessive compulsive disorder (OCD) in the US. The first of these to be approved was Anafranil, a tricyclic antidepressant, and this was followed by the 4 SSRIs, 3 of which were originally approved and marketed in the US for the treatment of depression (Prozac, Paxil, and Zoloft). Luvox is approved only for OCD. Of these 5 drugs, data were provided in support of the pediatric use in OCD only for Anafranil.

Anafranil does not have a separate indication for OCD in pediatric patients, but rather, it has a general indication for OCD, along with a description of the clinical trial conducted in the pediatric age group with OCD under Clinical Pharmacology. This approach to labeling is in fact consistent with current thinking about OCD, i.e., an illness that typically has its onset in childhood and very often continues on into adulthood. It is widely believed to be the same condition in both adults and children, both phenomenologically and regarding response to pharmacological treatment. This view supports both our approach to labeling and also the acceptablilty of basing an expansion of the claim into the pediatric age range on a single efficacy study.

We decided not to take this supplement to the Psychopharmacological Drugs Advisory Committee.

2.0 CHEMISTRY

Luvox is a marketed product, and there were no chemistry issues requiring review for this supplement. One possible concern, as noted by Dr. Mosholder, is the fact that the 50 mg tablet is currently the lowest available strength. While this tablet is scored, it would be necessary to break tablets to obtain 25 mg strengths to use during initial dosing and for upward titration. We may want to note this potential problem in the approvable letter.

3.0 PHARMACOLOGY

There were no pharmacology issues requiring review for this supplement.

4.0 BIOPHARMACEUTICS

There were no biopharmaceutics issues requiring review for this supplement.

5.0 CLINICAL DATA

5.1 Efficacy Data

5.1.1 Summary of Study RH.114.02.01

As noted, this supplement provided data for a single study.

This was a randomized, 20-center (all US), double-blind, parallel group, 10-week, flexible-dose study comparing fluvoxamine in a dose range of 50-200 mg/day vs placebo for the treatment of OCD in 120 pediatric outpatients, ranging in age from 8 - 17 and meeting DSMIIIR criteria for OCD. In addition to meeting diagnostic criteria, patients were required to (1) have at an NIMH-OC score of at least 7 and a C-YBOCS score of at least 15, at both screening and baseline visits, and (2) have a Children's Depression Rating Scale (CDRS) score of $\leq$ 40 at screening and baseline. In addition, they could not meet diagnostic criteria for Tourette's Disorder, other major Axis 1 disorders, or mental retardation.

The study began with a 1-2 week single-blind placebo phase, and was followed by the 10-week double-blind treatment phase. The initial dose was 25 mg in the evening, and dosage was subsequently titrated, in increments of 25 mg q 3-4 days, up to a maximum dose of 100 mg bid, presumably to maximize efficacy and tolerability. The minimum dose was to be 50 mg/day. Dosing was on a bid schedule. An open label extension followed the double-blind phase for responding patients, and nonresponding patients could enter this phase after 6 weeks.

Efficacy assessments included: (1) C-YBOCS; (2) NIMH-OC; (3) CGI severity and improvement ratings for OCD. Assessments were done at baseline and at the ends of weeks 1, 2, 3, 4, 6, 8, and 10.

We focused on 4 key efficacy variables: (1) change from baseline in the C-YBOCS total score, NIMH-OC score, CGI severity score, and (2) CGI improvement score.

Patients were approximately 47% female, predominantly white, and the mean age was 13. The age distribution was roughly 50:50 between the 8-11 and 12-17 age ranges. The treatment groups were comparable at baseline on the demographic and key efficacy variables.

There were 57 patients assigned to fluvoxamine and 63 to placebo. Of the placebo patients, 57% completed to 10 weeks, compared to 67% of fluvoxamine patients. There was a distinct dropoff at week 6, at which time nonresponding patients could enter the open label phase. The mean fluvoxamine dose for completers to week 10 was 156 mg/day.

The sponsor used a 2-way ANOVA as the primary analysis. Dr. Choudhury conducted alternative analyses for several of these variables.

The results of this study are summarized in tables on pages 10-11 of this memo, i.e., a summary of the significance of pairwise comparisons by week for LOCF and OC of the intent-to-treat sample on p. 10 and a summary of effect sizes for the 4 key variables, as measured by difference between drug and placebo in mean scores at week 10, on p. 11.

Fluvoxamine was superior to placebo on reduction of C-YBOCS score in the LOCF analyses and also the OC analyses up through week 6. The OC analyses were not significant at weeks 8 and 10. This outcome may have resulted from dropouts due to nonresponse from the placebo group at week six, since the protocol provided for such patients to enter the open extension at that point. In fact, more patients dropped from the placebo group for lack of effect than from the fluvoxamine group. In addition, an analysis of dropout cohorts by Dr. Choudhury suggested that, at the point of dropout, fluvoxamine patients were always doing at least as well as placebo patients, and generally better. Thus, this loss of significance in the OC analysis late in the trial is less troubling.

However, a more troubling finding for the C-YBOCS variable was an interaction based on an age grouping. The sample was divided into 2 groups, i.e., 8-11 (n=44) and 12-17 (n=76) for this analysis. For the 8-11 group, the outcome was still highly significant in favor of fluvoxamine. Indeed, for the LOCF analysis at week 10, the mean reduction from baseline for fluvoxamine was almost 10 units on the C-YBOCS compared to slightly less than 4 units for placebo. On the other hand, for the 12-17 group, the group having a larger n, there was no statistically significant difference between fluvoxamine and placebo. For the LOCF analysis at week 10, the mean change from baseline for fluvoxamine was only 4 units on the C-YBOCS compared to slightly less than 4 units for placebo. Thus, the placebo response was roughly the same in the two subgroups, but a treatment effect was apparent only in the 8-11 age group.

For the NIMH-OC variable, the outcome favored fluvoxamine over placebo on both the ANOVA and also on 2 nonparametric tests that may have been more valid, given the non-normal distribution of the data. Again, there was some loss of significance for the OC analysis late in the trial, likely due to the reasons given earlier.

For the CGI Improvement and Severity scores, fluvoxamine was also favored over placebo, for both LOCF and OC analyses, except late in treatment. The loss of significance for the OC analysis late in the trial was again likely due to the reasons given earlier.

Impression: Overall, I consider this a positive study, providing support for the effectiveness of fluvoxamine as a treatment for OCD in a pediatric population. The one troubling finding was the strong interaction on the basis of age, with a strong effect in the 8-11 age group and essentially no demonstrable effect in the 12-17 age group.

5.1.2 Comment on Other Important Clinical Issues Regarding the Efficacy of Luvox for Obsessive Compulsive Disorder in Pediatric Patients

Evidence Bearing on the Question of Dose/Response for Efficacy

There were no data specifically pertinent to the question of dose dependency for effectiveness in this supplement. While the mean dose for completers to 10 weeks was 156 mg/day in study 114, this finding is difficult to interpret, since the tendency in the somewhat artificial circumstances of a flexible dose clinical trial is to push patients to the highest tolerable dose. Thus, it seems reasonable to recommend 50 mg as the initial target dose for fluvoxamine in pediatric patients with OCD. However, it also seems reasonable to recommend 200 mg/day as the maximum recommended dose and suggest that, although not proven, some patients may benefit from doses above 50 mg/day.

Clinical Predictors of Response

The patients in this trial were almost all Caucasian, so a subgroup analysis on this variable was not possible.

A gender by treatment analysis revealed no statistically significant interaction, however, there was a tendency for male patients to do better than female patients early in the trial.

As noted earlier, there was a significant age by treatment interaction, revealing a highly significant drug effect in the 8-11 group and essentially no effect in the 12-17 group.

Size of Treatment Effect

Overall, there was a roughly 3 unit difference between fluvoxamine and placebo in reduction from baseline on the C-YBOCS, for LOCF at week 10. If one focuses on the 8-11 subgroup, where the drug effect was most prominent, the difference was 6 units. Changes of this magnitude are generally consistent with what has been seen with other drugs recently approved for OCD, and I believe that the Solvay has met the test of law in demonstrating that fluvoxamine has anti-OCD activity in this pediatric population. However, this is not a cure for this condition. As Dr. Mosholder pointed out in his review, a majority of patients at the end of the trial would still have been eligible for study entry based on their C-YBOCS scores, despite having experienced a significant reduction in their level of symptoms.

Duration of Treatment

No data were provided in this supplement to address the question of long-term effectiveness for OCD in this population. However, the sponsor has underway a relapse prevention trial in adults that is adequate by design to address this issue, and if that study is positive, I think it would be reasonable to extrapolate to the pediatric population. In the meantime, the labeling for Luvox acknowledges the absence of sufficient relapse prevention data generally, yet suggests that it would not be unreasonable to continue responding patients beyond the acute treatment phase.

5.1.3 Conclusions Regarding Efficacy Data

I believe that Solvay has provided evidence for the effectiveness of fluvoxamine in the treatment of OCD in pediatric patients with this disorder. Given the general view that OCD is essentially the same disorder in adults and children, I consider one study sufficient to support extrapolation of the claim into the pediatric age group. The one troubling and puzzling finding here is the strong age by treatment interaction observed in this study. This finding is puzzling since it would be unusual to see the kind of discontinuity in effect that this finding suggests. If fluvoxamine works in adults and in children aged 8-11, why should it fail to work in adolescents. I still believe that the study as a whole must be considered positive, since the hypothesis was that fluvoxamine has an anti-OCD effect in the age group studied, i.e., 8-17, and, overall, that hypothesis was supported. The apparent lack of an effect in the 12-17 age group is a post hoc finding that essentially generates an additional hypothesis, i.e., that fluvoxamine may not be equally effective in all age groups. As such, it needs to be addressed, certainly by further inquiry, and probably in labeling as well.

We will ask Solvay in the approvable letter to further explore this finding with the data available in this study. One possible explanation is lack of compliance in the adolescent population. Another possibiltiy is to look at the characteristics of the adolescents recruited to see if anything about them, e.g., associated psychiatric illnesses, would predict a poorer response. We will ask Solvay to examine whatever records are available from this study to try to assess compliance and any other predictors of poor response.

In the meantime, however, I think it would be reasonable to allow an extension of the claim by permitting this trial to be described in the Clinical Trials section of Clinical Pharmacology.

5.2 Safety Data

Since Luvox has been available in the US for the treatment of OCD in adults for approximately 2 years and elsewhere for the treatment of depression and OCD for much longer, our approach to the safety data was, in part, to compare the findings from the relatively small pediatric OCD database with the databases for depression and OCD. Dr. Mosholder concluded that Luvox is acceptably safe for use in the treatment of OCD in the pediatric age group, and I agree with that conclusion.

The safety data for this review were derived entirely from study 114 which, as described above, was a 10-week, placebo controlled flexible dose study involving 57 pediatric patients exposed to fluvoxamine in a dose range of 50-200 mg/day. The cutoff date for the study report for 114 was August, 1995. No analysis of postmarketing reports for Luvox related specifically to the treatment of pediatric patients with OCD was included in this supplement.

The mean age of patients in this study was 13, with roughly half in each of 2 age groups (8-11 and 12-17). Patients were also distributed roughly 50:50 by gender. The mean dose for fluvoxamine completers was 156 mg/day.

There were no deaths in this study, and no serious events in the short-term phase. None of the 4 serious events reported in fluvoxamine patients during the extension phase could be reasonably considered drug-related.

The overall pattern of dropouts was as expected, with about twice the rate of dropouts for lack of efficacy among placebo patients (35%) compared to fluvoxamine patients (16%). Three fluvoxamine patients (5%) discontinued for adverse events compared to 1 placebo patient (2%). One of the fluvoxamine dropouts was for a manic reaction and one for agitation, anxiety, impulsivity, and decreased attention span.

The common and drug-related adverse events overall from study 114 (incidence ≥ 5% and at least twice the placebo rate) included: agitation, anorexia, depression, dysmenorrhea, dyspepsia, flatulence, hyperkinesia, insomnia, rash, and somnolence. This list overlapped to some extent with the adverse events associated with Luvox in the adult depression and OCD databases.

Explorations of data from study 114 for laboratory, vital signs, and ECG variables, did not reveal any consistent findings for fluvoxamine.

In conclusion, the safety experience for Luvox in pediatric patients with OCD did not reveal any adverse findings that are unique for this population and none that would preclude its use in this population. Of note, there were 3 fluvoxamine patients who met criteria for potentially clinically significant weight loss compared to none for placebo. Also, as noted, there was one dropout for each of agitation and manic reaction among fluvoxamine exposed subjects.

We have requested a safety update in the approvable letter, including an update on spontaneous reports, particularly for adverse events pertinent to the use of Luvox in a pediatric population.

5.3 Clinical Sections of Labeling

We have made several changes in the clinical sections of the draft labeling that is included with the approvable letter. The explanations for the changes are provided in bracketed comments in the draft labeling. I will briefly note here several of the more critical issues needing modification:

-I modified the description of the clinical study in pediatric OCD, by noting the significant age interaction.

-Solvay had wanted a specific indication for pediatric OCD, however, given the general view that OCD is essentially the same disorder in adults and children, I don't see any justification for such a claim. Rather, it is more appropriate to support an expanded claim by permitting a description of the additional pediatric study in the Clinical Trials subsection, as has been done.

-I added a statement summarizing the findings pertinent to the induction of mania from the pediatric OCD study to the mania statement under Precautions.

-Under Pediatric Use in Precautions, I added a class statement recommending monitoring of weight and growth in children treated chronically with SSRIs, given the general finding of appetite suppression and weight loss with this class of drugs.

-Solvay had proposed the addition of a separate adverse events incidence table for study 114. However, I did not add that table, since the overall profile of adverse events for that study was similar to that seen in the adult studies, as labeling already acknowledges. I do not feel that this table contributes sufficient new information to justify its considerable length. Rather, I have asked them to prepare a brief subsection noting any important differences between tables 2 and 2A, similar to the subsection noting the differences between the OCD studies and the pooled OCD and depression studies in adults.

-Finally, I have added Solvay's proposed changes in the Dosage and Administration section to accomodate the expanded OCD claim, with essentially no modification.

6.0 WORLD LITERATURE

A literature review regarding the use of Luvox for the treatment of OCD in the pediatric population was not included as part of this supplement. We will ask for a literature review on this topic in the approvable letter.

7.0 FOREIGN REGULATORY ACTIONS

Luvox is marketed in a number of countries around the world for the treatment of depression and OCD, and in the US for the treatment of OCD. To my knowledge, it is not yet marketed anywhere for the treatment of OCD in the pediatric age group. We will ask for an update on the regulatory status of Luvox for OCD in the pediatric age group in the approvable letter.

8.0 PSYCHOPHARMACOLOGICAL DRUGS ADVISORY COMMITTEE (PDAC) MEETING

We decided not to take this supplement for the use of Luvox in the treatment obsessive compulsive disorder in the pediatric age group to the PDAC.

9.0 DSI INSPECTIONS

DSI's current policy is to not conduct routine inspections for supplemental indications, but rather, only if there is some specific concern that would justify an inspection. There were no such issues, consequently none of the study sites for the key trial supporting the extension of the OCD claim into the pediatric age group have been inspected.

10.0 LABELING AND APPROVABLE LETTER

10.1 Final Draft of Labeling Attached to Approvable Package

Our proposed draft of labeling is attached to the approvable letter. As noted, we have made several changes to the sponsor's draft dated 12-21-95.

10.2 Foreign Labeling

Luvox is not marketed anywhere at this time for the treatment of OCD in the pediatric age group.

10.3 Approvable Letter

The approvable letter includes draft labeling and requests for a safety update, a literature update, a regulatory status update, a commitment to further explore the age interaction observed in study 114, and a recommendation for a 25 mg strength.

11.0 CONCLUSIONS AND RECOMMENDATIONS

I believe that Solvay has submitted sufficient data to support the conclusion that Luvox is effective and acceptably safe in the treatment of OCD in the pediatric age group. The concern about the possibility of differential effectivenss on the basis of age in the pediatric population needs to be further explored, but I don't think that concern should preclude the extension of the claim into the pediatric population overall. I recommend that we issue the attached approvable letter with our labeling proposal and the above noted requests for updates and further explorations of the age interaction, in anticipation of final approval.

cc:
Orig NDA
HFD-120
HFD-120/TLaughren/PLeber/AMosholder/PDavid

DOC: MEMLVOCD.AE1

Summary of Significance Levels[1] (2-Sided) for Pairwise Comparisons (Fluvoxamine vs Placebo) in Study 114

Key Outcome Variables	Fluvoxamine vs Placebo						
	Week[2]						
	1	2	3	4	6	8	10
C-YBOCS[3]							
LOCF	*	*	*	*	*	-	*
OC	*	*	*	*	*	-	-
CGI Severity[3]							
LOCF	*	*	*	*	*	*	*
OC	*	*	*	*	*	-	-
CGI Improvement[3]							
LOCF	*	*	*	*	*	*	*
OC	*	*	*	*	*	-	-
NIMH-OC[4]							
LOCF	t	*	*	*	*	*	-
OC	t	*	*	*	t	-	-

1 * = $p \leq 0.05$
t = $p \leq 0.10$
- = $p > 0.10$

2 End of weeks 1, 2, 3, 4, 6, 8, and 10

3 p-values for this variable based on 2-way ANOVA

4 p-values for this variable based on Block-Wilcoxon Test

Size of Treatment Effect in Study 114			
CGI Improvement Score			
Group	Baseline[1]	Wk 10	Difference[2]
Placebo	-	3.8	
Fluvoxamine	-	3.1	0.7
C-YBOCS Score			
Group	Baseline[3]	BL - Wk 10[4]	Difference[5]
Placebo	24	- 3	
Fluvoxamine	24	- 6	3
NIMH-OC Score			
Group	Baseline[3]	BL - Wk 10[4]	Difference[5]
Placebo	9.4	- 1.1	
Fluvoxamine	9.5	- 2.0	0.9
CGI Severity Score			
Group	Baseline[3]	BL - Wk 10[4]	Difference[5]
Placebo	4.7	- 0.4	
Fluvoxamine	4.8	- 0.9	0.5

1 Baseline score not relevant for this variable
2 Difference between drug and placebo in mean CGI Improvement score at week 10
3 Mean score at baseline
4 Mean Change from baseline to week 10 (LOCF)
5 Difference in mean change from baseline to week 10 endpoint (LOCF) between fluvoxamine and placebo

REVIEW AND EVALUATION OF CLINICAL DATA

Tab 81

APPLICATION INFORMATION

NDA #	19-839, Supplement # 02 Safety Update
Sponsor:	Pfizer, Inc.

DRUG NAME

Generic Name:	Sertraline Hydrochloride
Trade Name:	Zoloft®

DRUG CHARACTERIZATION

Pharmacological Category:	Selective serotonin reuptake inhibitor
Proposed Indication:	Obsessive Compulsive Disorder
Dosage Forms, Strengths & Routes of Administration:	Marketed 50 and 100 mg Tablets

REVIEWER INFORMATION

Clinical Reviewer:	James F. Knudsen, Ph.D., M.D.
Review Completion Date:	March 28,1996

1.2 Related Reviews

NDA #19-839 Sertraline in the treatment of depression

NDA #19-839/S-002 Sertraline in the treatment of obsessive compulsive disorder (OCD)

2.0 Background

Supplement S-002 to NDA 19-839 for Zoloft® (sertraline) tablets in the treatment of OCD was submitted on May 14, 1992 and included data from 2 placebo-controlled studies 371/372 and 237/248 and one uncontrolled study #494. Data from a third placebo-controlled study (protocol 546) were submitted on January 13, 1994. The clinical review of the application was completed on March 1, 1995. An approvable letter was sent on August 1, 1995. The present submission is a safety update report and includes routine clinical data collected from the OCD NDA submitted on May 14, 1992 plus data from an additional group of OCD patients who participated in sertraline studies subsequent to the OCD NDA cut-off date of April 17, 1991 and up through June 30, 1995, the cut-off date for this safety update.

In addition, the sponsor has submitted a separate pediatric/adolescent section which includes safety data collected in completed pediatric/adolescent OCD studies as of the data cut-off of June 30, 1995. For both the adult and pediatric/adolescent studies, serious adverse experiences were in a database that included all completed as well as ongoing studies as of the cut-off date for the safety update of June 30, 1995.

2.1 Indication

Sertraline is a selective serotonin reuptake inhibitor (SSRI) marketed in the United States for the treatment of depression and more recently approved for the treatment of OCD in adults.

2.2 Related INDs and NDAs

Unchanged from those noted in the original OCD NDA submission.

2.3 Administrative History

The following is a brief history.

August 1, 1995 Correspondence stating application for sertraline in treatment of OCD was approvable.

August 10, 1995 Pfizer's letter of intent to file an amendment to S-002.

December 7, 1995 Amendment including safety update to S-002 submitted.

2.4 Proposed Direction for Use

The text from the Division's August 1, 1995 draft of labeling was included in section 1 (volume 1) of this safety update submission and is not repeated in the present review of safety data.

Percentage of Patients Dropping out In Adult OCD Placebo-Controlled Trials

	SERTRALINE (N=533)	PLACEBO (N=373)
Psychiatric Disorders		
Insomnia	2.6	0.8
Somnolence	1.9	0.3
Gastro-Intestinal Disorders		
Nausea	2.8	0.3
Diarrhea	2.1	0.8

Adapted from Sponsor's Table 32, Vol. 2, P. 341.
Pooled data from 237/248, 371/372 (weeks 1-12), 546, 495 and 336.

In both the original OCD NDA database and this safety update database, adverse events associated with dropouts in sertraline-treated patients were concentrated mainly in the psychiatric and gastrointestinal systems.

The table which follows displays those adverse events most frequently associated with dropouts (in the placebo-controlled OCD trials) in at least 1% of sertraline-treated patients and at least twice the placebo rate in the pediatric/adolescent OCD database.

Percentage of Patients Dropping Out From Pediatric/Adolescent OCD Placebo-Controlled Trials

	Sertraline (N=92)	Placebo (N=95)
Psychiatric Disorders		
Agitation	3.3	0.0
Insomnia	2.2	1.1
Concentration Impaired	2.2	0.0

Adapted from Sponsor's Table 61, Vol. 2, P. 473.
Data from placebo-controlled study number 498.

The adverse events most frequently associated with dropouts were grouped with psychiatric disorders.

The adverse events associated with discontinuations in the adult OCD database were most frequently reported to be gastrointestinal and psychiatric side effects, whereas, in the pediatric database the most frequently occurring adverse events were psychiatric in nature.

8.4 Other Specific Search Strategies

8.4.1 Serious Adverse Events

As of the OCD safety update cut-off date of June 30, 1995, 1,581 adult patients in completed and ongoing studies had received treatment with sertraline; 426 with placebo and 308 with active control drugs. There were 30 reports (2%) of adverse experiences reported as serious in sertraline-treated patients compared to 11 reports (3%) in the placebo treatment group and 8 (3%) patients in the active-control group and 8 patients on blinded therapy for which the blind had not been broken.

In the completed and ongoing studies of the pediatric/adolescent OCD program, serious adverse experiences were reported in 16 (7.3%) of 220 sertraline-treated patients and none of the 95 placebo-treated patients.

Narrative summaries of drop-outs due to medical events were reviewed for serious adverse events. No additional serious adverse events were located.

Serious adverse events possibly or probably related to sertraline will be discussed under specific subsections of this safety review. Events not related, in my opinion, to sertraline use are tabulated and appear in the table of serious events not considered drug-related (Appendix 8.7).

8.4.2 Search for Emergence of Suicidality

There were no reports of completed suicides in either the adult OCD database (N=1581) or the pediatric/adolescent database (N=220). The table which follows summarizes the incidence of serious adverse experiences associated with suicidality in the adult and pediatric/adolescent database.

Summary of Suicidality in All Adult and Pediatric/Adolescent OCD Studies (cut-off date June 30, 1995)

Protocols	Treatment Groups	N	Attempts	Gesture	Ideation	Total Suicidality (%)
Adult	Sertraline	1581	2	1	6	0.6%
	Placebo	426	0	0	1	0.2%
	Active Control	308	3	0	0	0.1%
Pediatric/Adolescent	Sertraline	220	1	2	3	3.0%
	Placebo	95	0	0	0	0.0%

When results are expressed as percent of patient per treatment group and as a function of exposure to treatment (incidence per patient exposure year) the incidence of suicidality was 0.035/PEY for the adult sertraline-treated group (PEY=225.7) compared to 0.25PEY for the pediatric/adolescent group (PEY=24.37). The final adult OCD database compares favorably with that of the original OCD NDA report of less than 1% incidence of suicidality in sertraline-treated patients. In the small pediatric/adolescent pooled population of OCD patients, the incidence of suicidality in sertraline-treated patients was five fold greater than the adult OCD sertraline-treated patients. A summary of the medical history of the 6 pediatric/adolescent cases is located in appendix 8.4.2.

Of the 6 cases, 3 occurred in protocol 525, 2 in protocol 536 and 1 in protocol 550. The one placebo reported case occurred in protocol 498. There were 3 males and 3 females. The mean age of the six patients was 14 years (range 8-17 years). Four of the 6 were reported to have a comorbid diagnosis of major depression. Four of the 6 patients had received a maximum dose of 200mg prior to the report of suicidality, which occurred over a wide range of days, (8 to 136 days of sertraline exposure). The one placebo-treated patient (protocol 498) of which there is limited data had a report of suicidal ideation classified as mild in intensity (data from table 60, p. 470 in volume #2).

Suicidal acts or emergence of suicidal thoughts in depressed patients treated with other SSRIs have been discussed and revealed no association with an increased risk (Beasley et al., BMJ 303:685,1991). Obsessive compulsive disorder has a substantial comorbidity with major depression and other anxiety disroders (Weissman et al. J Clin Psychiatry 55:3(Supp.),5:1994) and depression is an important risk factor for suicide. Before receiving sertraline, 4 of the 6 pediatric patients had a comorbid diagnosis of major depression and therefore may have been more suicidal at start of treatment. Similar cases of self-injurious ideation or behavior have been reported in fluoxetine-treated young OCB patients (10 to 17 years old). Four of the 6 had major risks for self-destructive behavior including depression (King et al. J. Am. Acad Child Adolesc Psychiatry 30:179,1991.)

8.5 Other Safety Findings

8.5.1 Adverse Events Incidence Table

Appendix Table 8.5.1.1 is the safety update table which displays the adverse events occurring at a rate of 1% or greater in the adult sertraline-treated OCD patients in the combined placebo-controlled clinical trials. The table is ordered from the system with the most frequently reported adverse experiences to the system with the fewest reports of experiences. Long-term data from the 40-week continuation phase of protocol 371/372 are not included in this table. The incidence of adverse experiences differed only slightly depending on whether the data included weeks 1-12 or weeks 1-52 from this protocol which was discussed in the original OCD NDA.

All adverse experiences whether observed or listed by the investigator or reported by the subject were recorded in CRFs. All adverse experiences were included in this section whether or not the investigator deemed them to be related to the study medication. The adverse experiences were auto encoded from the investigator's term to body system and preferred term using the WHO-AE dictionary. Each adverse experience was only counted once for a given subject, regardless of the number of times a given adverse experience was reported. For patients with more than one treatment-emergent adverse experience with the same preferred term, the events with greater severity or more probable relationship to the medication was chosen.

Common and Possible Sertraline-Related Adverse Experiences in Placebo-Controlled Pediatric/Adolescent OCD Studies (Protocol 498)

Adverse Experiences	Sertraline (N=92) %	Placebo (N=95) %
Psychiatric		
Insomnia	37	13
Nervousness	15	6
Agitation	13	2
Central and Peripheral Nervous Systems		
Dizziness	12	6
Hyperkinesia	9	4
Tremor	6	0
Gastro-Intestinal		
Nausea	17	7
Anorexia	13	5
Body As A Whole		
Fatigue	8	2
Skin and Appendages		
Rash	5	1

Commonly occurring adverse experiences in the sertraline pediatric/adolescent treatment group not reported at a comparable rate in the adult OCD group were: nervousness, agitation, hyperkinesia, fatigue and rash. Whereas, in the adult OCD's sertraline treatment group the commonly occurring adverse experiences not reported at a comparable rate in the pediatric/adolescent treatment group were: decreased libido, ejaculatory failure, diarrhea, dyspepsia, and increased sweating.

Evidence of Dose-Relatedness to Certain Adverse Experiences

The multi center outpatient study 371/372 was a fixed-dose study (50,100 or 200mg/day or placebo) and included a 12-week treatment phase followed by an additional 40 weeks of double-blind treatment for responders. These data were discussed in the original OCD NDA. To summarize, 4 adverse experiences showed a statistically significant dose-related increase in incidence. These were: ejaculation failure, tremor, dyspepsia and yawning. The adverse experience profile during the long-term treatment phase of this protocol (1-52 weeks) was similar to that of the 1-12 week exposure. In addition to the 4 adverse experiences (ejaculation failure, tremor, dyspepsia and yawning) which showed a statistically significant dose-related increase in incidence during weeks 1-12, two other adverse expeirences showed a dose-related increase during weeks 1-52, namely an increase in weight and sweating.

10.0 Conclusions

The safety profile of sertraline in the safety update compares favorably with the safety profile previously established in the OCD NDA for the daily dose range 50 to 200. The majority of side effects in clinical trials were psychiatric and gastrointestinal in nature, transitory and mild or moderate in severity.

The safety profile of sertraline in pediatric OCD patients was similar to the safety profile in the adult OCD patients with some exceptions. Adverse events associated with discontinuations in the pediatric database were most frequently psychiatric in nature and included agitation, insomnia, concentration impairment and nervousness. In the adult OCD database discontinuations were associated with, for the most part, different psychiatric adverse events than the pediatric patients (insomnia, somnolence and anxiety) and in addition, gastrointestinal side-effects (nausea, diarrhea). Dose reduction in these children may have ameliorated some of the behavioral side-effects.

The incidence of suicidality was higher in the pediatric/adolescent database than the adult OCD database and may be a result of psychiatric/neurologic comorbidity (major depression) in the former group. The incidence of seizures was higher in the pediatric/adolescent group than adult OCD group and with the data available does not appear causally related to the sertraline use. The incidences of clinically significant laboratory abnormalities (transaminase, cholesterol, uric acid analytes) were similar in the pediatric/adolescent and adult OCD groups and consistent with the current product labeling.

The overall incidence of clinically significant vital sign measurements was similar in the pediatric and adult databases. Although the incidence of vital sign abnormalities, particularly decreased diastolic blood pressure measurements, was higher in the pediatric database. There were no serious adverse experiences associated with the decreased blood pressure.

11. Recommendations

There are no safety issues that would preclude approval of this safety update.

James F. Knudsen

James F. Knudsen, M.D., Ph.D.

cc: Original NDA 19-839
Div. File HFD-120/
/CSO/PDavid/
/Tlaughren/
/JKnudsen/

4-2-96

I agree that we can now proceed with the approval of this supplement. However, there are some labeling issues that still need violations. See my memo to the file for my more detailed comments.

Thomas P. Laughren, MD

GL, PDP

PUBLIC HEALTH LINK

Tab 82

To: Directors of Public Health of PCTs to forward to:

- All GENERAL PRACTITIONERS - please ensure this message is seen by all practice nurses and non-principals working in your practice and retain a copy in your 'locum information pack'.
- Deputising services
- Community Paediatricians
- Project manager/Nurse lead in Walk in Centres
- Lead nurses in PCTs to forward to school nurses and young people's health services
- Leads at nurse-led PMS Pilots
- PCT Pharmaceutical Advisers to forward to community pharmacists
- PCT Prescribing Advisers

To: Medical Directors of NHS Trusts to forward to:
- Consultant psychiatrists
- Consultant paediatricians
- Nurse Executive Directors of NHS Trusts and Mental Health Trusts and NHS Trusts with Child and Adolescent Mental Health Services
- Trust Chief Pharmacists to forward to Medicines Information Pharmacists

Cc:
- Regional Directors of Public Health
- Directors of Public Health of Strategic Health Authorities to forward to: SHA pharmaceutical advisers and SHA lead nurses
- UK CMOs
- Chairmen of Professional Executive Committee

From: Professor Gordon Duff, Chairman – Committee on Safety of Medicines

Date: 10th December 2003
Reference: CEM/CMO/2003/20, Gateway ref: 2369
Category: **URGENT MESSAGE**
**PLEASE ACTIVATE THE CASCADE **

Dear Colleague

SELECTIVE SEROTONIN REUPTAKE INHIBITORS - USE IN CHILDREN AND ADOLESCENTS WITH MAJOR DEPRESSIVE DISORDER

I wrote to you in June and September to inform you that paroxetine and the related antidepressant, venlafaxine should not be used to treat depressive illness in children and adolescents under the age of 18 years. Since then the Expert Working Group of the Committee on Safety of Medicines (CSM) has completed its review of the safety and efficacy of the SSRI class in the treatment of paediatric major depressive disorder.

On the basis of this review of the available clinical trial data, CSM has advised that the balance of risks and benefits for the treatment of major depressive disorder (MDD) in under 18s is judged to be unfavourable for sertraline, citalopram and escitalopram and unassessable for fluvoxamine. Only fluoxetine (Prozac) has been shown in clinical trials to have a favourable balance of risks and benefits for the treatment of MDD in the under 18s.

In adults, on the basis of evidence to date, the benefits of treatment are considered to outweigh the risks for all SSRIs.

Like paroxetine and venlafaxine, none of these drugs has ever been licensed for use in depressive illness in under 18s but we know they are used in this age group outside their licensed indications. Sertraline and fluvoxamine are licensed for treatment of obsessive compulsive disorder (OCD). This new advice does not relate to use in OCD.

Summary of advice
In patients under 18 years old:
* Paroxetine, venlafaxine, sertraline, citalopram and escitalopram are now contraindicated in paediatric MDD in the under 18s.
* There are no data on the safety and efficacy of fluvoxamine in paediatric MDD. Safety and efficacy in adults cannot be extrapolated to those under 18 and therefore this product should not be used in this age group.
* The balance of risks and benefits of fluoxetine in the treatment of MDD in under 18s appears to be favourable.

General prescribing advice for paroxetine, venlafaxine, sertraline, citalopram escitalopram and fluvoxamine:

1. These products should not be prescribed as new therapy for patients under 18 years of age with depressive illness.

2. If your patient is being successfully treated with any of these products, then the normal completion of the planned treatment course should be considered as an option in the management of the illness.

3. If your patient is not doing well on any of these products, change of treatment should be considered.

4. A decision to prescribe any of these for paediatric MDD, for example if a patient is intolerant to fluoxetine, should only be made with specialist advice and after careful consideration of all available information.

Fluoxetine does not have a marketing authorisation for MDD in under 18 year olds. However the CSM has considered the clinical trial data and advised that the balance of risks and benefits is favourable. Again, a decision to prescribe fluoxetine for paediatric MDD in a patient under 18 should be made with specialist advice.

Stopping SSRIs

No SSRI should be stopped abruptly. Gradual decrease in dose may be required, particularly for venlafaxine and paroxetine. Information on what to expect when stopping individual products is already present in product information.

Further information

1. Attached is an overview of the regulatory status of these products and the advice of CSM. We fully appreciate the need for prescribers to have access to the data supporting the regulatory decisions and to this end we have published on the Medicines and Healthcare products Regulatory Agency (MHRA) website two further levels of detailed information. One contains a summary of the safety and efficacy data for each product in paediatric MDD and the other describes the individual trials reviewed by the CSM. This information is provided to enable

prescribers to make informed decisions on the management of their paediatric patients who may already be receiving treatment with SSRIs or who may need pharmacotherapy for MDD.

2. A leaflet for patients about SSRIs and depression is also attached.

3. Further information for prescribers and patients including questions and answers and the SSRI fact sheet issued together with Current Problems in Pharmacovigilance in September 2003 is available on the website of the MHRA (http://www.mhra.gov.uk).

Please report any suspected adverse reactions to SSRIs via the Yellow Card reporting scheme to the CSM/ MHRA.

Should you require any additional information, please telephone 020 7084 2000 at the MHRA.

Professor Gordon Duff
Chairman - Committee on Safety of Medicines

Level 1 – Overview of regulatory status and CSM advice relating to major depressive disorder in children and adolescents

	Fluoxetine	**Sertraline**	**Citalopram**	**Escitalopram**	**Fluvoxamine**	**Paroxetine**	**Venlafaxine**
Drug class	SSRI	SSRI	SSRI	SSRI (active constituent of citalopram)	SSRI	SSRI	Serotonin and noradrenaline reuptake inhibitor (SNRI)
Licensed indications children and adolescents	None	Obsessive compulsive disorder	None	None	Obsessive compulsive disorder	None	None
Efficacy in major depressive disorder (MDD) in children and adolescents	Demonstrated in controlled clinical trials	Not demonstrated in controlled clinical trials	Not consistently demonstrated in controlled clinical trials	No data from clinical trials	No data from clinical trials	Not demonstrated in controlled clinical trials	Not demonstrated in controlled clinical trials
Safety profile in MDD trials in children and adolescents	Mania and hypomania more frequently reported than in adults, perhaps as a result of differing inclusion criteria in clinical trials. No increased rate of self-harm and suicidal thoughts compared with placebo.	Rate of events including agitation, anorexia, insomnia and suicidal thoughts and self harm increased compared with placebo.	Increased rate of self-harm compared with placebo in 1 of 2 trials.	No data from clinical trials	No data from clinical trials	Increased rate of self-harm and suicidal thoughts compared with placebo.	Increased rate of self-harm and suicidal thoughts compared with placebo.
CSM advice in relation to MDD in children and adolescents	**Risk/benefit balance is favourable.**	**Risk/benefit balance is unfavourable.**	**Risk/benefit balance is unfavourable.**	**Risk/benefit balance is presumed unfavourable. (Extrapolation from citalopram.)**	**Risk/benefit balance is not assessable – safety and efficacy in adults cannot be extrapolated to under 18 year olds.**	**Risk/benefit balance is unfavourable.**	**Risk/benefit balance is unfavourable.**

Leaflet for patients

SELECTIVE SEROTONIN REUPTAKE INHIBITORS

USE IN CHILDREN AND TEENAGERS WITH DEPRESSION

Doctors have been told that some medicines used to treat depression in adults (SSRIs) are not suitable for use in children and teenagers under the age of 18 years to treat depression. This note is to explain what it's all about.

What are SSRIs?
SSRIs are medicines that are mostly used to treat depression. Some of them have other uses as well, for example to treat obsessive compulsive disorder. This note is just about the treatment of depression. It is nothing to do with obsessive compulsive disorder.
The following medicines are SSRIs:

- Sertraline (commonest brand Lustral)
- Citalopram (commonest brand Cipramil)
- Escitalopram (commonest brand Cipralex)
- Paroxetine (commonest brand Seroxat)
- Fluoxetine (commonest brand Prozac)
- Fluvoxamine (commonest brand Faverin)

Also there is a similar medicine called

- Venlafaxine (commonest brand Efexor ER)

So what's new?
For any medicine, a balance has to be made between any harmful effects of taking a medicine and whether it will make you better. This is known as the balance of the improvements against the side effects (or in other words, the good against the harm).

A group of experts, called the Committee on Safety of Medicines, advises the Government on the safe and effective use of medicines. It has looked at the results of research on these medicines in children and teenagers with depression. For sertraline, citalopram and escitalopram, the experts have decided that these medicines may do more harm than good in the treatment of depression in under 18s. (Previously the experts have also decided that paroxetine and venlafaxine may do more harm than good as well.) For fluvoxamine the experts could not make a decision as there is no proper research in children and teenagers with depression. Only one medicine, fluoxetine, seems to do more good than harm for the treatment of depression in the under 18s.

What does this mean?

Doctors have been told that, for children and teenagers with depression,

* Seroxat (paroxetine), Efexor (venlafaxine), Lustral (sertraline), Cipramil (citalopram) and Cipralex (escitalopram)
  - should not be used in children and teenagers.
* Faverin (fluvoxamine)
  - should not be used because there has been no proper research in this age group.
* Prozac (fluoxetine)
  - Can be used in children and teenagers.

What does this mean for me?

* If you are being treated with any of these medicines at the moment and you are doing well on the medicine then you can finish the tablets you've got, if you and your doctor think that this is a good idea.

* If you are being given any of these medicines at the moment and you are not doing well on the medicine, then you should talk to your doctor about a change of treatment.

* If you have recently become depressed and you need a medicine your doctor should avoid giving you Seroxat, Efexor, Lustral, Cipralam, Cipralex or Faverin, if he/she possibly can.

* If your doctor thinks that he needs to give you one of the medicines listed above, say if you don't feel well taking fluoxetine, he or she will only do this if they are a specialist or if a specialist has said it's OK.

Why is Prozac OK?

The group of experts has looked at the research with Prozac and decided that on balance it does more good than harm in most of the under 18s.

If you are depressed and under 18 your doctor will ask a specialist before he or she gives you Prozac and will only give it if the specialist has said that it's OK.

Stopping SSRI medicines

You should not suddenly stop taking these medicines. The dose needs to be lowered slowly especially if you are taking the ones called Efexor or Seroxat.

Further information

Further information on your medicine can be found in the patient information leaflet which accompanies the medicine.

Further explanations of the new advice can be found on the website of the MHRA at http://www.mhra.gov.uk/

Tab 83

Efficacy of Paroxetine in the Treatment of Adolescent Major Depression: A Randomized, Controlled Trial

MARTIN B. KELLER, M.D., NEAL D. RYAN, M.D., MICHAEL STROBER, PH.D., RACHEL G. KLEIN, PH.D., STAN P. KUTCHER, M.D., BORIS BIRMAHER, M.D., OWEN R. HAGINO, M.D., HAROLD KOPLEWICZ, M.D., GABRIELLE A. CARLSON, M.D., GREGORY N. CLARKE, PH.D., GRAHAM J. EMSLIE, M.D., DAVID FEINBERG, M.D., BARBARA GELLER, M.D., VIVEK KUSUMAKAR, M.D., GEORGE PAPATHEODOROU, M.D., WILLIAM H. SACK, M.D., MICHAEL SWEENEY, PH.D., KAREN DINEEN WAGNER, M.D., PH.D., ELIZABETH B. WELLER, M.D., NANCY C. WINTERS, M.D., ROSEMARY OAKES, M.S., AND JAMES P. McCAFFERTY, B.S.

ABSTRACT

Objective: To compare paroxetine with placebo and imipramine with placebo for the treatment of adolescent depression. **Method:** After a 7- to 14-day screening period, 275 adolescents with major depression began 8 weeks of double-blind paroxetine (20–40 mg), imipramine (gradual upward titration to 200–300 mg), or placebo. The two primary outcome measures were endpoint response (Hamilton Rating Scale for Depression [HAM-D] score ≤8 or ≥50% reduction in baseline HAM-D) and change from baseline HAM-D score. Other depression-related variables were (1) HAM-D depressed mood item; (2) depression item of the Schedule for Affective Disorders and Schizophrenia for Adolescents-Lifetime version (K-SADS-L); (3) Clinical Global Impression (CGI) improvement scores of 1 or 2; (4) nine-item depression subscale of K-SADS-L; and (5) mean CGI improvement scores. **Results:** Paroxetine demonstrated significantly greater improvement compared with placebo in HAM-D total score ≤8, HAM-D depressed mood item, K-SADS-L depressed mood item, and CGI score of 1 or 2. The response to imipramine was not significantly different from placebo for any measure. Neither paroxetine nor imipramine differed significantly from placebo on parent- or self-rating measures. Withdrawal rates for adverse effects were 9.7% and 6.9% for paroxetine and placebo, respectively. Of 31.5% of subjects stopping imipramine therapy because of adverse effects, nearly one third did so because of adverse cardiovascular effects. **Conclusions:** Paroxetine is generally well tolerated and effective for major depression in adolescents. *J. Am. Acad. Child Adolesc. Psychiatry,* 2001, 40(7):762–772. **Key Words:** paroxetine, imipramine, major depression, adolescent.

The treatment of depression in adolescents is an area of burgeoning interest. Unfortunately, few well-controlled, large-scale, randomized clinical trials have been conducted in this population. Data from the 1,769 adolescents and

Accepted February 15, 2001.

From the Department of Psychiatry and Human Behavior, Brown University, Providence, RI (Dr. Keller); Department of Psychiatry, University of Pittsburgh School of Medicine (Drs. Ryan, Birmaher); UCLA Medical Center (Drs. Strober, Feinberg); New York University Child Study Center (Drs. Klein, Koplewicz); Department of Psychiatry, Dalhousie University, Halifax, Nova Scotia (Dr. Kutcher); Department of Psychiatry, University of Pennsylvania, Philadelphia (Dr. Hagino); Department of Child and Adolescent Psychiatry, State University of New York at Stony Brook (Dr. Carlson); Center for Health Research, Portland, OR (Dr. Clarke); Department of Psychiatry, University of Texas Southwestern Medical Center, Dallas (Dr. Emslie); Department of Psychiatry, Washington University School of Medicine, St. Louis (Dr. Geller); Department of Psychiatry, Grace-1WK Hospital, Halifax, Nova Scotia (Dr. Kusumakar); Department of Psychiatry, Sunnybrook Health Science Centre, University of Toronto (Dr. Papatheodorou); Department of Psychiatry, Oregon Health Sciences University, Portland (Drs. Sack, Winters); New York State Psychiatric Institute, New York (Dr. Sweeney); Department of Psychiatry and Behavioral Sciences, University of Texas Medical Branch, Galveston (Dr. Wagner); Department of Psychiatry, Children's Hospital of Philadelphia (Dr. Weller); North America Medical Affairs, GlaxoSmithKline, Collegeville, PA (Ms. Oakes, Mr. McCafferty).

This study was supported by a grant from GlaxoSmithKline, Collegeville, PA. The authors acknowledge the contributions of the following individuals: Jill M. Abbott, Ellen Basian, Ph.D., Carolyn Boulos, M.D., Elyse Dubo, M.D., Mary A. Fristad, Ph.D., Joan Hebeler, M.D., Kevin Kelly, Ph.D., Sharon Reiter, M.D., and Ronald A. Weller, M.D. Editorial assistance was provided by Sally K. Laden, M.S.

Reprint requests to Dr. Keller, Department of Psychiatry and Human Behavior, Brown University School of Medicine, 345 Blackstone Blvd., Providence, RI 02906.

young adult participants in the National Comorbidity Survey (Kessler and Walters, 1998) indicate a lifetime prevalence rate of 15.3% for major depression, comparable with the 17% lifetime prevalence of depression in adults (Kessler et al., 1994). As with adults, the course of major depression in adolescents is often characterized by protracted episodes, frequent recurrence, and impairment in social and academic domains (Rao et al., 1995). Suicide is the third leading cause of death in adolescents, and depressive disorders are strongly correlated with suicide attempts (Eisenberg, 1984; Kovacs et al., 1993). Depressed adolescents grow up to be depressed adults and, compared with healthy controls, have higher rates of suicide, psychiatric and medical hospitalizations, and impairment in work, family, and social lives (Weissman et al., 1999).

The efficacy of tricyclic antidepressants has been investigated in at least 11 double-blind, randomized studies (Dulcan et al., 1998; Ryan and Varma, 1998), none demonstrating superiority of active treatment over placebo. However, methodological deficiencies in these studies, including very small sample sizes and diagnostic heterogeneity, limit statistical inference and generalizability of the findings. At the same time, cardiovascular effects and lethality in overdose associated with the tricyclic agents have greatly limited their use in clinical practice.

Since the selective serotonin reuptake inhibitors (SSRIs) became commercially available, the safety, tolerability, and efficacy of these agents in treating major depression in adolescents have been noted in several open-label reports (Ambrosini et al., 1999; Apter et al., 1994; Masi et al., 1997; McConville et al., 1996; Rey-Sanchez and Gutierrez-Casares, 1997; Rodriguez-Ramos et al., 1996; Simeon et al., 1998). Placebo-controlled trials, which remain the standard against which efficacy is determined, number only two, both with fluoxetine (Emslie et al., 1997; Simeon et al., 1990). A small study by Simeon and associates (1990) was negative. In contrast, a large-scale trial by Emslie and colleagues (1997) showed a 23% drug-placebo difference in overall clinical improvement. The findings of a third study, which used a historical case-control design (Strober et al., 1999), suggested greater efficacy of fluoxetine compared with imipramine in a severely ill, inpatient population of adolescents with major depression. We now report principal findings from the first double-blind, placebo-controlled comparison of an SSRI, paroxetine, and a placebo-controlled comparison with a tricyclic antidepressant, imipramine, in the treatment of adolescents with major depression.

METHOD

Study Design

This was an 8-week, multicenter, double-blind, randomized, parallel-design comparison of paroxetine with placebo and imipramine with placebo in adolescents with major depression. The trial was conducted at 10 centers in the United States and 2 in Canada. Four hundred twenty-five subjects were screened for eligibility, and 275 subjects were randomly assigned to experimental treatment. The trial was conducted in accordance with good clinical practices and the Helsinki Declaration. All subjects and their parent(s) provided written informed consent before entry into the study; the identity of all subjects is completely blinded in this report. Funding for this study was provided by GlaxoSmithKline; each author had access to data and signed off on the manuscript before it was submitted for publication.

Patient Eligibility

Male and female subjects, aged 12 through 18 years, fulfilling the *DSM-IV* (American Psychiatric Association, 1994) criteria for a current episode of major depression of at least 8 weeks in duration were enrolled. Major depression was diagnosed by a systematic clinical interview which used the juvenile version of the Schedule for Affective Disorders and Schizophrenia for Adolescents-Lifetime version (K-SADS-L) rating scale. The K-SADS-L was developed by one of the authors (R.G.K.) through modification of the adult SADS assessment technique (Endicott and Spitzer, 1978) by providing uniform anchors so that symptoms were specifically rated for clinical relevance and by adding items to generate *DSM-IV* diagnoses. The K-SADS-L uses separate patient and parent reports to assess lifetime presence of affective and schizophrenic disorders, as well as the full range of childhood and adolescent psychopathological conditions. In addition to fulfilling *DSM-IV* criteria for major depression, subjects were required to have a total score of at least 12 on the 17-item Hamilton Rating Scale for Depression (HAM-D), a score of less than 60 on the Children's Global Assessment Scale, and a score of at least 80 on the Peabody Picture Vocabulary Test. All subjects were medically healthy.

Potential subjects in the study were screened initially by telephone, and candidates who were considered likely to meet diagnostic criteria were evaluated at the study site. Adolescents and parents were interviewed separately. For those cases in which there existed a significant discrepancy between information provided by the adolescent and information provided by the parent, the clinician met with both to discuss the information obtained and then rendered a rating. Eligible subjects and their parent(s) were required to reach agreement with the site investigator that the subject had a disorder requiring treatment. In cases in which the diagnosis was not certain, audiotapes of the screening interview were to be reviewed and the diagnosis was to be verified further by an independent expert from another participating site prior to certifying study eligibility.

Subjects with a current or lifetime *DSM-IV* diagnosis of bipolar disorder, schizoaffective disorder, eating disorder, alcohol or substance use disorder, obsessive-compulsive disorder, autism/pervasive developmental disorder, or organic brain disorder were excluded from consideration. A diagnosis of posttraumatic stress disorder within 12 months of recruitment was also exclusionary, as was current suicidal ideation with intent or specific plan, a history of suicide attempts by drug overdose, any medical condition in which the use of an antidepressant was contraindicated, current psychotropic drug use, an adequate trial of antidepressant medication within 6 months of study entry, or exposure to investigational drug use either within 30 days of study entry or within five half-lives of the drug. Females who were pregnant or breastfeeding and those who were sexually active and not using reliable contraception were also excluded.

Blinding, Randomization, and Treatment

All subjects underwent a 7- to 14-day screening phase to determine persistence and severity of entry diagnostic and eligibility criteria and to obtain baseline global functioning scores, physical examination, and clinical laboratory studies. Placebo was not administered during the screening phase. By means of a computer-generated list, subjects who still met entry criteria were randomly assigned to an 8-week course of treatment with paroxetine, imipramine, or placebo in a 1:1:1 ratio. Tablets were overencapsulated in matching Supro B locking capsules to preserve medication blinding. Subjects assigned to paroxetine treatment received 20 mg/day in the morning for weeks 1 through 4. Optional dosage increases to 30 mg of paroxetine per day (divided dose) were allowed at week 5 and to 40 mg per day (divided dose) at weeks 6 through 8 if deemed necessary by the treating clinician. Imipramine treatment was initiated with a forced titration schedule in which subjects received daily doses of 50 mg during week 1, 100 mg during week 2, 150 mg during week 3, and 200 mg during week 4. Thereafter, optional dosage increases to 250 mg/day (during week 5) and to 300 mg/day (during weeks 6 through 8) were allowed if judged necessary by the research study clinician. Imipramine administration was divided between morning and evening for all daily doses of 100 mg or greater.

Subjects were instructed to take their medication twice daily, once in the morning and again in the evening. The number of active drug or matched placebo capsules administered per day was identical for each treatment group during forced titration. During weeks 1 and 2, subjects in the paroxetine or imipramine groups received one active drug capsule in the morning and one active drug or matched placebo capsule in the evening. Subjects in the placebo group received one capsule in the morning and one in the evening. During week 3, subjects received one active drug capsule in the morning and two active drug or matched placebo capsules in the evening. At week 4, subjects received one active drug capsule plus one matched placebo capsule in the morning and two active drug or matched placebo capsules in the evening. Beginning at week 5, subjects either remained at the week 4 dose level (i.e., four capsules per day) or were titrated upward to five or six capsules per day. Subjects who completed the study were offered the option of continuing blinded treatment at the same dose for 6 additional months. If subjects withdrew from the study prematurely for any reason, the dose of medication was gradually tapered over a 7- to 17-day period.

Supportive case management was provided to all subjects at each weekly clinic visit according to the method described by Fawcett et al. (1987). Such management was limited to psychosocial interaction that enabled observation of treatment effects. Interpersonal or cognitive-behavioral psychotherapeutic interventions were strictly prohibited.

Efficacy and Safety Evaluation

After randomization, subjects were seen at weekly intervals and evaluated with standardized instruments and global assessments for efficacy. The protocol described two primary outcome measures: (1) response, which was defined as a HAM-D score of ≤8 or a ≥50% reduction in baseline HAM-D score at the end of treatment; and (2) change from baseline in HAM-D total score. Five other depression-related variables were declared a priori: (1) change in the depressed mood item of the HAM-D; (2) change in the depression item of the K-SADS-L; (3) Clinical Global Impression (CGI) improvement scores of 1 (very much improved) or 2 (much improved); (4) change in the nine-item depression subscale of the K-SADS-L; and (5) mean CGI improvement scores.

Assessment of multiple domains of functioning, general health, and behavior consisted of (1) Autonomous Function Checklist, completed by the parent, which assessed the subject's autonomy in performing daily activities (Sigafoos et al., 1988); (2) Self-Perception Profile, completed by the subject to measure self-esteem (Harter, 1988); and (3) Sickness Impact Scale, completed by the subject, to measure present health and quality of life (Bergner et al., 1981).

Adverse events, heart rate, blood pressure, and body weight were determined at each weekly visit. Rhythm strip electrocardiograms (ECGs) were obtained at each visit, and 12-lead ECGs were obtained during the screening phase and at weeks 4 and 8. Routine clinical laboratory studies were conducted during the screening phase and at week 8, or upon study withdrawal.

If changes in cardiovascular parameters occurred, then dosage reductions were required. Doses were reduced by 10 mg for paroxetine doses of 30 mg or 40 mg; subjects receiving 20 mg of paroxetine were withdrawn from the study. Similarly, imipramine doses of 250 mg or 300 mg per day were reduced by 50 mg, and subjects receiving ≤200 mg of imipramine were withdrawn from the study. Cardiovascular parameters necessitating dosage reduction or study withdrawal were defined prospectively as heart rate ≥110 beats per minute (bpm) at two consecutive visits or heart rate ≥130 bpm at a single visit; systolic blood pressure >140 mm Hg or diastolic blood pressure >85 mm Hg; PR interval ≥0.21 seconds; QRS interval ≥0.12 seconds and ≥150% of baseline; or QT_C interval ≥0.48 seconds.

Blood samples were obtained from all patients at weeks 4 and 8 for determination of plasma concentrations of imipramine, desmethylimipramine (the major, pharmacologically active metabolite of imipramine), and paroxetine. Subjects were withdrawn from the study if the combined imipramine and desmethylimipramine concentration exceeded 500 ng/mL.

Statistical Methods

A sample size of 90 patients per arm was required to provide approximately 80% power to detect an effect size of 0.4 between an active regimen and placebo with an α level of 5% (two-tailed). The change from baseline in the HAM-D total score was used.

The efficacy analyses were performed on the population of patients who were randomized and had at least one postbaseline efficacy evaluation. Two datasets from this population were examined: (1) a last observation carried forward dataset in which the last observation on treatment was carried forward to estimate missing data for patients who withdrew prior to completing 8 weeks of treatment, and (2) a completer dataset that examined results in patients who received study medication for the full 8 weeks. Missing data were not estimated for the completer dataset.

Continuous variables, such as changes from baseline to endpoint in the HAM-D total score, CGI improvement scale, and K-SADS-L, were analyzed by a two-factor analysis of variance using the general linear model procedure of the Statistical Analysis System (SAS). The model included terms for treatment and investigator. Categorical variables, such as percentage of subjects responding to treatment, were analyzed with logistic analysis implemented in the categorical modeling procedure (CATMOD) of the SAS; the model included effects for investigator and treatment. Pairwise comparisons between each active treatment and placebo were two-tailed and performed at an α level of .05. Data are reported as least square means (±SD or SE).

RESULTS

Treatment groups were similar with regard to demographic characteristics and psychiatric profile (Table 1). Most subjects had a first-degree relative with major depression and were experiencing their first episode of major depression. The mean duration of the current depressive episode was more than 1 year, with a mean baseline HAM-D total score between 18 and 19. Features of melancholic or endogenous depression were exhibited by 35% to 40% of patients, and 20% had features of atypical depression. Despite exclusion criteria that limited many comorbid conditions, psychiatric comorbidity was common. Comorbid anxiety disorders, such as separation anxiety and social anxiety disorder, and externalizing disorders were present at the time of screening in 19% to 28% of subjects.

Premature Discontinuation

A total of 190 subjects (69% of 275) completed the 8-week study. Premature withdrawal rates were 24% for placebo, 28% for paroxetine ($p = .60$ versus placebo), and 40% for imipramine ($p = .02$ versus placebo). Premature study discontinuation due to adverse effects occurred at a rate of 6.9% in the placebo group. Study withdrawal due to adverse effects was the most common reason for discontinuation in the paroxetine (9.7%; $p = .50$ versus placebo) and imipramine (31.5%; $p < .01$ versus placebo) groups, respectively. Cardiac adverse effects consisting of tachycardia (8 patients), postural hypotension (2), prolonged QT intervals (2), arrhythmia (1), atrioventricular block (1), abnormal ECG (1), extrasystole (1), and hypertension (1) led to withdrawal among 14% of subjects in the imipramine group (13 subjects). Protocol violation, including lack of compliance, was the most common reason for withdrawal in the placebo group (8.0%).

Efficacy Results

Of the depression-related variables, paroxetine separated statistically from placebo at endpoint among four of the parameters: response (i.e., primary outcome measure), HAM-D depressed mood item, K-SADS-L depressed mood item, and CGI score of 1 (very much

TABLE 1
Demographic Characteristics and Mean Baseline Depression Scores for 275 Randomized Subjects

Parameter	Paroxetine ($n = 93$)	Imipramine ($n = 95$)	Placebo ($n = 87$)
Gender, M/F	35/58	39/56	30/57
Age, mean ± SD (yr)	14.8 ± 1.6	14.9 ± 1.6	15.1 ± 1.6
Race, no. (%)			
White	77 (82.8)	83 (87.4)	70 (80.5)
African American	5 (5.4)	3 (3.2)	6 (6.9)
Asian American	1 (1.1)	2 (2.1)	2 (2.3)
Other	10 (10.8)	7 (7.4)	9 (10.3)
CGAS, mean ± SD	42.7 ± 7.5	42.5 ± 7.4	42.8 ± 8.3
Duration of current depressive episode, mean ± SD (months)	14 ± 18	14 ± 18	13 ± 17
No. of prior depressive episodes (%)			
0	81	79	77
1	12	14	14
≥2	7	6	8
First-degree relative with major depression (%)	86	90	95
Age at onset of first episode, mean ± SD (yr)	13.1 ± 2.8	13.2 ± 2.7	13.5 ± 2.3
Mean baseline HAM-D total score	18.98 ± 0.43	18.11 ± 0.43	18.97 ± 0.44
Features of melancholic or endogenous depression	36	35	40
Features of atypical depression (%)	25	16	9
Current comorbid psychiatric diagnosis (%)			
Any diagnosis	41	50	45
Anxiety disorder[a]	19	26	28
Externalizing disorder[b]	25	26	20

Note: CGAS = Children's Global Assessment Scale; HAM-D = Hamilton Rating Scale for Depression.
[a] Includes separation anxiety, panic ± agoraphobia, agoraphobia, social anxiety disorder, generalized anxiety disorder.
[b] Includes conduct disorder, oppositional defiant disorder, and attention-deficit/hyperactivity disorder.

improved) or 2 (much improved) and trended toward statistical significance on two measures (K-SADS-L nine-item depression subscore and mean CGI score) (Table 2). The response to imipramine was not significantly different from that for placebo across any of the seven depression-related variables.

A total of 63.3% of paroxetine subjects (57/90; $p = .02$ versus placebo), 50% of imipramine subjects (47/94; $p = .57$ versus placebo), and 46% of placebo subjects (40/87) achieved a HAM-D total score of ≤8 at endpoint (Fig. 1). The time course of response in mean HAM-D total score is shown in Figure 2. Among patients who completed 8 weeks of treatment, 76.1% of paroxetine subjects (51/67; $p = .02$ versus placebo), 64.3% of imipramine subjects (36/56; $p = .44$ versus placebo), and 57.6% of placebo subjects (38/66) achieved a mean HAM-D total score of ≤8. In the paroxetine group, 65.6% of patients were considered very much or much improved on the CGI ($p = .02$ versus placebo); rates for the imipramine and placebo groups were 52.1% ($p = .64$ versus placebo) and 48.3%, respectively. Improvement in baseline depressed mood as measured by the HAM-D and the K-SADS-L depressed mood items was significantly greater than placebo in the paroxetine group, but not significantly greater than placebo in the imipramine group. Improvements in the K-SADS-L depression subscore ($p = .07$) and mean CGI score ($p = .09$) trended toward statistical significance in the paroxetine group, but not in the imipramine group ($p = .98$ and $p = .90$, respectively) (Table 2).

Although neither paroxetine nor imipramine separated statistically from placebo across the nonsymptom measures of functioning, health, and behavior, improvements over baseline were achieved for each active treatment group. Placebo-treated subjects also improved along the behavioral measures, but to a lesser extent than patients in the active treatment groups.

Dosage Titration

Nearly half of subjects in the paroxetine group remained at the initial starting dose of 20 mg/day (48%). Mean dose at study endpoint for paroxetine was 28.0 mg (SD ±8.54 mg) and for imipramine was 205.8 mg (SD

TABLE 2
Mean Scores of Depression-Related Variables in Adolescents With Major Depression[a]
Who Were Treated With Paroxetine, Imipramine, or Placebo

	Paroxetine				Imipramine				Placebo		
Variable	Mean	(SE)	*n*	p^b	Mean	(SE)	*n*	p^b	Mean	(SE)	*n*
HAM-D ≤8											
Week 8 endpoint	63.3%	(—)	90	.02	50.0%	(—)	94	.57	46.0%	(—)	87
HAM-D ≤8 or 50% reduction in baseline HAM-D											
Week 8 endpoint	66.7%	(—)	90	.11	58.5%	(—)	94	.61	55.2%	(—)	87
HAM-D depressed mood item											
Baseline	2.99	(0.08)	90		2.79	(0.08)	94		2.86	(0.08)	87
Week 8 endpoint	0.99	(0.14)	9	.001	1.17	(0.14)	94	.14	1.53	(0.14)	87
K-SADS-L depressed mood item											
Baseline	4.57	(0.09)	83		4.29	(0.09)	87		4.63	(0.09)	85
Week 8 endpoint	2.37	(0.18)	83	.05	2.52	(0.18)	87	.87	2.90	(0.18)	85
CGI score of 1 or 2[c]											
Week 8 endpoint	65.6%	(—)	90	.02	52.1%	(—)	94	.64	48.3%	(—)	87
K-SADS-L 9-item depression subscore											
Baseline	28.25	(0.52)	83		27.54	(0.51)	88		28.84	(0.52)	85
Week 8 endpoint	16.59	(0.84)	83	.07	17.99	(0.83)	88	.98	19.27	(0.83)	85
Mean CGI score											
Week 8 endpoint	2.37	(0.16)	90	.09	2.70	(0.15)	94	.90	2.73	(0.16)	87
HAM-D total score											
Baseline	18.98	(0.43)	90		18.11	(0.43)	94		18.97	(0.44)	87
Week 8 endpoint	8.24	(0.81)	90	.13	9.2	(0.81)	94	.87	9.88	(0.83)	87

Note: HAM-D = Hamilton Rating Scale for Depression; K-SADS-L = Schedule for Affective Disorders and Schizophrenia for Adolescents-Lifetime version; CGI = Clinical Global Impression.

[a] The last evaluation during treatment for subjects who did not complete the entire study (i.e., the last observation carried forward) is reported.

[b] The *p* values compare treatment difference in active versus placebo groups.

[c] CGI score of 1 = very much improved; CGI score of 2 = much improved.

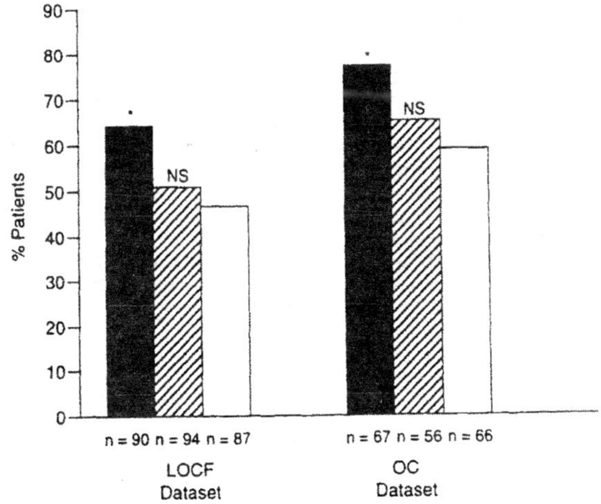

Fig. 1 Percentage of subjects treated with paroxetine (■), imipramine (▨), and placebo (□) who achieved a HAM-D total score ≤8 in the LOCF and completer (OC) subgroups at week 8. *p = .02; NS = $p \geq .44$. HAM-D = Hamilton Rating Scale for Depression; LOCF = last observation carried forward; OC = observed cases.

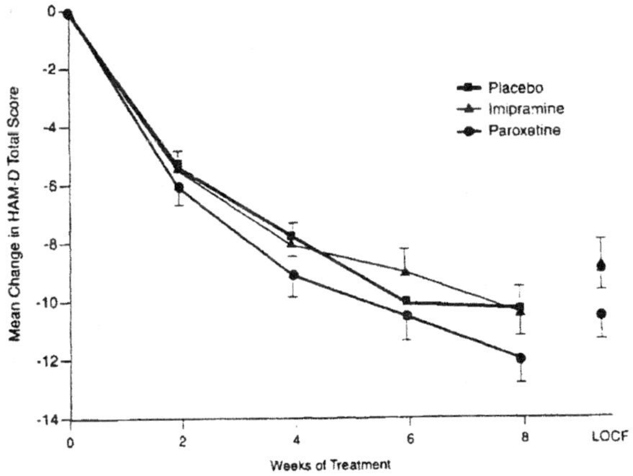

Fig. 2 Least square mean change HAM-D total score (±SEM) during an 8-week course of paroxetine (n = 90), imipramine (n = 94), and placebo (n = 87) administration in adolescents with major depression. HAM-D = Hamilton Rating Scale for Depression; LOCF = last observation carried forward.

±63.94 mg). The most common "doses" of placebo (administered as divided doses) were four capsules per day (31.0%) and six capsules per day (41.4%).

Adverse Effects

Paroxetine was generally well tolerated in this adolescent population, and most adverse effects were not serious. The most common adverse effects reported during paroxetine therapy were headache, nausea, dizziness, dry mouth, and somnolence (Table 3). These occurred at rates that were similar to rates in the placebo group with the exception of somnolence, which occurred at rates of 17.2% for paroxetine and 3.4% for placebo. Dizziness, dry mouth, headache, nausea, and tachycardia were most commonly reported during imipramine treatment. Tremor occurred in 10.8% of paroxetine-, 14.7% of imipramine-, and 2.3% of placebo-treated subjects.

Adverse effects in all treatment groups occurred most often during the first week of therapy. Dosage reductions were most often required for somnolence, insomnia, and restlessness among paroxetine-treated subjects. Dry mouth, constipation, and tremor were the most common adverse effects leading to imipramine dose reductions. Premature withdrawal from the study because of adverse effects occurred at rates of 9.7% for paroxetine, 31.5% for imipramine, and 6.9% for placebo. Clinically significant

TABLE 3
Adverse Effects Occurring in ≥5% of Subjects in the Paroxetine, Imipramine, and Placebo Groups

Adverse Effect	Paroxetine (n = 93)	Imipramine (n = 95)	Placebo (n = 87)
Cardiovascular system			
Tachycardia	2 (2.2)	18 (18.9)	1 (1.1)
Postural hypotension	1 (1.1)	13 (13.7)	1 (1.1)
Vasodilation	0 (0)	6 (6.3)	2 (2.3)
Chest pain	2 (2.2)	5 (5.3)	2 (2.3)
Digestive system			
Dry mouth	19 (20.4)	43 (45.3)	12 (13.8)
Nausea	22 (23.7)	23 (24.2)	17 (19.5)
Constipation	5 (5.4)	9 (9.5)	4 (4.6)
Decreased appetite	7 (7.5)	2 (2.1)	4 (4.6)
Diarrhea	7 (7.5)	3 (3.2)	7 (8.0)
Dyspepsia	6 (6.5)	9 (9.5)	4 (4.6)
Tooth disorder	5 (5.4)	2 (2.1)	2 (2.3)
Vomiting	3 (3.2)	8 (8.4)	6 (6.9)
Abdominal pain	10 (10.8)	7 (7.4)	10 (11.5)
Nervous system			
Dizziness	22 (23.7)	45 (47.4)	16 (18.4)
Emotional lability	6 (6.5)	3 (3.2)	1 (1.1)
Hostility	7 (7.5)	3 (3.2)	0 (0)
Insomnia	14 (15.1)	13 (13.7)	4 (4.6)
Nervousness	8 (8.6)	6 (6.3)	5 (5.7)
Somnolence	16 (17.2)	13 (13.7)	3 (3.4)
Tremor	10 (10.8)	14 (14.7)	2 (2.3)
Headache	32 (34.4)	38 (40.0)	34 (39.1)
Respiratory system			
Cough increased	5 (5.4)	3 (3.2)	6 (6.9)
Pharyngitis	5 (5.4)	12 (12.6)	8 (9.2)
Respiratory disorder	10 (10.8)	7 (7.4)	11 (12.6)
Rhinitis	7 (7.5)	3 (3.2)	5 (5.7)
Sinusitis	6 (6.5)	2 (2.1)	7 (8.0)
Other			
Sweating	1 (1.1)	6 (6.3)	1 (1.1)
Abnormal vision	1 (1.1)	7 (7.4)	2 (2.3)
Asthenia	10 (10.8)	7 (7.4)	10 (11.5)
Back pain	4 (4.3)	2 (2.1)	10 (11.5)
Infection	10 (10.8)	5 (5.3)	9 (10.3)
Trauma	2 (2.2)	3 (3.2)	6 (6.9)

Note: Values represent no. (%).

increases or decreases in body weight were not observed among any of the three treatment arms of this study.

Serious adverse effects occurred in 11 patients in the paroxetine group, 5 in the imipramine group, and 2 in the placebo group. An event was defined as serious if it resulted in hospitalization, was associated with suicidal gestures, or was described by the treating physician as serious. The serious adverse effects in the paroxetine group consisted of headache during discontinuation taper (1 patient) and various psychiatric events (10 patients): worsening depression (2); emotional lability (e.g., suicidal ideation/gestures [5]); conduct problems or hostility (e.g., aggressiveness, behavioral disturbance in school [2]); and euphoria/expansive mood (1). Seven patients were hospitalized: 2 with worsening depression, 2 with emotional lability, 2 with conduct problems, and 1 with euphoria. Of the 11 patients, only headache (1 patient) was considered by the treating investigator to be related to paroxetine treatment.

The 5 serious adverse effects in the imipramine group consisted of maculopapular rash (1 patient), dyspnea/chest pain (1), hostility (1), emotional lability (1), and visual hallucinations/abnormal dreams (1). Two of the adverse effects (i.e., hallucinations, rash) were considered related to imipramine. All 5 patients were withdrawn from the study, and the patients with hostility or emotional lability were hospitalized. In the placebo group, emotional lability (1 patient) and worsening depression (1) were considered serious. The placebo-treated patient with emotional lability, which was considered to be related to placebo, was withdrawn from the study.

Of subjects in the imipramine group who stopped therapy because of adverse effects, nearly one third (13.7%) did so because of cardiovascular effects, including tachycardia, postural hypotension, and prolonged QT interval. Mean standing heart rate increased by 17 bpm over baseline among subjects treated with imipramine. Neither paroxetine nor placebo was associated with changes in heart rate.

DISCUSSION

This is the first study to compare efficacy of an SSRI and a tricyclic antidepressant with placebo in the treatment of major depression in adolescents. Paroxetine was significantly more effective than placebo with regard to achievement of both HAM-D total score ≤8, CGI score of 1 (very much improved) or 2 (much improved), and improvements in the depressed mood items of the HAM-D and the K-SADS-L. Paroxetine did not separate statistically from placebo for K-SADS-L depression subscore, mean CGI score, or HAM-D total score.

The demonstration of efficacy for paroxetine in this study is in accordance with findings of open-label studies of SSRIs (Ambrosini et al., 1999; Apter et al., 1994; Masi et al., 1997; McConville et al., 1996; Rey-Sanchez and Gutierrez-Casares, 1997; Rodriguez-Ramos et al., 1996; Simeon et al., 1998) and results from placebo-controlled (Emslie et al., 1997) and historical case-control (Strober et al., 1999) studies. These findings of efficacy for paroxetine and other SSRIs are notable in that randomized, double-blind, placebo-controlled trials (Geller et al., 1990; Hughes et al., 1990; Kashani et al., 1984; Klein et al., 1998; Kramer and Feiguine, 1981; Kutcher et al., 1994; Kye et al., 1996; Petti and Law, 1982; Preskorn et al., 1987) and one meta-analysis (Hazell et al., 1995) have not shown efficacy for the tricyclic antidepressants in the treatment of adolescent depression. Because efficacy has not been demonstrated for the tricyclic antidepressants and because these agents are associated with an unacceptably high risk of cardiotoxicity, especially in children, further controlled studies are not likely to be conducted. As such, future research involving bupropion or noradrenergic antidepressants not yet clinically available will be required to address more fully the question of preferential efficacy of the SSRIs in this age group.

Our study used a flexible-dose design in which doses could be adjusted on the basis of clinical response and tolerability. Roughly half of subjects were maintained at the paroxetine starting dose of 20 mg. The mean daily dose of paroxetine in this study, 28 mg, is comparable with that reported in flexible-dose trials in adults (Claghorn, 1992; Cohn and Wilcox, 1992; Dunbar et al., 1991; Fabre, 1992; Feighner and Boyer, 1992; Shrivastava et al., 1992; Smith and Glaudin, 1992).

The adverse-effect profile of paroxetine in this adolescent population was concordant with that reported in studies of adult patients with depression (Claghorn, 1992; Cohn and Wilcox, 1992; Dunbar et al., 1991; Fabre, 1992; Feighner and Boyer, 1992; Shrivastava et al., 1992; Smith and Glaudin, 1992). Serious adverse effects were reported during treatment with paroxetine (11 patients), imipramine (5), and placebo (2). Because these serious adverse effects were judged by the investigator to be related to treatment in only 4 patients (paroxetine, 1; imipramine, 2; placebo, 1), causality cannot be determined conclusively. Adverse cardiovascular effects were not observed in subjects treated with paroxetine. In contrast, tachycardia, postural hypotension, and prolongation of QT intervals during imipramine therapy resulted in treatment discontinuation in one third of the 31.5% of subjects who stopped treatment prematurely with the tricyclic antidepressant.

Limitations

A high placebo response rate was observed in this study, which is not unusual for clinical trials of major depression in either pediatric or adult populations. In studies of pediatric patients with major depression, placebo response rates range from 20% to 80% (Birmaher et al., 1998; Emslie et al., 1997; Geller et al., 1992; Jensen et al., 1992; Kowatch et al., 1999). Placebo response also is high in adults with major depression as demonstrated by mean placebo response rates of approximately 30% to 40% in short-term studies (Brown, 1994; Schatzberg and Kraemer, 2000; Trivedi and Rush, 1994).

Several factors possibly contributed to the observed placebo response rate. A probable contributing factor was the weekly supportive case management sessions, which may have contributed to clinical improvement for patients in the placebo and active-treatment groups. In addition, the lack of a placebo run-in before randomization may have contributed to a higher placebo response. Inclusion of patients with externalizing disorders (e.g., conduct disorder, oppositional defiant disorder) also could be argued to have increased the placebo response rate. A post hoc analysis was conducted to assess this issue. However, the separate analysis of our database revealed that response rates to paroxetine, imipramine, and placebo among patients with attention-deficit/hyperactivity disorder (ADHD) were significantly lower than in patients without ADHD, regardless of treatment group assignment, including placebo (Birmaher et al., 2000).

The mean HAM-D total score from our sample at baseline in all three groups was 18 (±0.43), possibly accounting for the high placebo response. In fact, there appears to be an inverse relationship between placebo response in adults and clinical severity of depression. Adults with less severe depression exhibit greater placebo response rates than more seriously ill patients. Mild to moderate depression (i.e., HAM-D total score <19 in one study [Stewart et al., 1983], <13 in another [Paykel et al., 1988]) was associated with no drug–placebo difference in tricyclic antidepressant treatment studies of adult outpatients. Moreover, in contrast with our study, the mean baseline HAM-D total scores in short-term adult SSRI studies range from 23 to 28 (Cohn and Wilcox, 1985; Dunbar et al., 1991; Feighner and Overø, 1999; Reimherr et al., 1990; Stark and Hardison, 1985). It is important to emphasize, however, that comparisons in HAM-D scores between adults and adolescents may not be valid because of possible age-related variability in HAM-D.

Another methodological limitation must be acknowledged: the study was not designed to directly compare paroxetine with imipramine. The objective of the study was to determine the efficacy of two antidepressants with different mechanisms of action. To conduct a traditional three-arm comparative trial, this study would require testing at p values of .0167 rather than .05. To power a study at this level, it would have been necessary to enroll a greater number of patients, thus exposing more adolescents to the potential risks of clinical research.

Clinical Implications

Major depression in adolescents is an increasingly recognized clinical problem that is remarkably understudied. The majority of treatment studies involve the tricyclic antidepressants. Because these agents are associated with poor efficacy and cardiovascular adverse effects, their use is not recommended. In contrast, there are few large, well-controlled studies of SSRIs in adolescents. Our findings are therefore relevant to clinicians who are faced with treatment decisions for depressed adolescents and a relative paucity of data guiding therapeutic choice. Despite some methodological limitations, resulting in a high placebo response rate (outlined above), our study demonstrates that treatment with paroxetine results in clinically relevant improvement in depression scores. The SSRIs are the medications of choice for the treatment of major depression in adolescents because they are the only agents that have been shown to be efficacious in this population; they have a safer side-effect profile than other antidepressants, particularly in overdose; and they can be administered once daily. Clinicians should be aware that 8 weeks of treatment may not be sufficient to achieve a full clinical response, that some patients may benefit from higher doses, and that some as-yet unidentified groups of patients (e.g., more severely depressed; non-ADHD) may exhibit more robust responses to SSRI therapy.

Conclusion

The findings of this study provide evidence of the efficacy and safety of the SSRI, paroxetine, in the treatment of adolescent depression. Additional studies are called for to define the optimal length of therapy and dose of SSRIs in this population.

REFERENCES

Ambrosini PJ, Wagner KD, Biederman J et al. (1999), Multicenter open-label sertraline study in adolescent outpatients with major depression. *J Am Acad Child Adolesc Psychiatry* 38:566–572

American Psychiatric Association (1994), *Diagnostic and Statistical Manual of Mental Disorders, 4th edition (DSM-IV)*. Washington, DC: American Psychiatric Association

Apter A, Ratzoni G, King RA et al. (1994), Fluvoxamine open-label treatment of adolescent inpatients with obsessive-compulsive disorder or depression. *J Am Acad Child Adolesc Psychiatry* 33:342–348

Bergner M, Bobbitt RA, Carter WB, Gilson BS (1981), The Sickness Impact Profile: development and final revision of a health status measure. *Med Care* 19:787–805

Birmaher B, McCafferty JM, Bellew KM, Beebe KL (2000), Comorbid ADHD and other disruptive behavior disorders as predictors of response in adolescents treated for major depression. Abstract presented at American Psychiatric Association Annual Meeting, Chicago, May

Birmaher B, Waterman GS, Ryan ND et al. (1998), Randomized, controlled trial of amitriptyline versus placebo for adolescents with "treatment-resistant" major depression. *J Am Acad Child Adolesc Psychiatry* 37:527–535

Brown WA (1994), Placebo as a treatment for depression. *Neuropsychopharmacology* 10:265–269

Claghorn JL (1992), The safety and efficacy of paroxetine compared with placebo in a double-blind trial of depressed outpatients. *J Clin Psychiatry* 53(suppl):33–35

Cohn JB, Wilcox C (1985), A comparison of fluoxetine, imipramine, and placebo in patients with major depressive disorder. *J Clin Psychiatry* 46(suppl):26–31

Cohn JB, Wilcox CS (1992), Paroxetine in major depression: a double-blind trial with imipramine and placebo. *J Clin Psychiatry* 53(suppl):52–56

Dulcan MK, Bregman J, Weller EB, Weller R (1998), Treatment of childhood and adolescent disorders. In: *Textbook of Psychopharmacology*. 2nd ed. Schatzberg AF, Nemeroff CB, eds. Washington, DC: American Psychiatric Press, pp 803–850

Dunbar GC, Cohn JB, Fabre LF et al. (1991), A comparison of paroxetine, imipramine, and placebo in depressed outpatients. *Br J Psychiatry* 159:394–398

Eisenberg L (1984), The epidemiology of suicide in adolescents. *Pediatr Ann* 13:47 54

Emslie GJ, Rush AJ, Weinberg WA et al. (1997), A double-blind, randomized, placebo-controlled trial of fluoxetine in children and adolescents with depression. *Arch Gen Psychiatry* 54:1031–1037

Endicott J, Spitzer RL (1978), A diagnostic interview: the Schedule for Affective Disorders and Schizophrenia. *Arch Gen Psychiatry* 35:837–844

Fabre LF (1992), A 6-week, double-blind trial of paroxetine, imipramine, and placebo in depressed outpatients. *J Clin Psychiatry* 53:40–43

Fawcett J, Epstein P, Fiester SJ, Elkin I, Autry JH (1987), Clinical management: imipramine/placebo administration manual. *Psychopharmacol Bull* 23:309–324

Feighner JP, Boyer WF (1992), Paroxetine in the treatment of depression: a comparison with imipramine and placebo. *J Clin Psychiatry* 53(suppl):44–47

Feighner JP, Overø K (1999), Multicenter, placebo-controlled, fixed-dose study of citalopram in moderate-to-severe depression. *J Clin Psychiatry* 60:824–830

Geller B, Cooper TB, Graham DL, Fetner HH, Marsteller FA, Wells JM (1992), Pharmacokinetically designed double-blind placebo-controlled study of nortriptyline in 6- to 12-year-olds with major depressive disorder. *J Am Acad Child Adolesc Psychiatry* 31:34–44

Geller B, Cooper TB, Graham DL, Marsteller FA, Bryant DM (1990), Double-blind placebo-controlled study of nortriptyline in depressed adolescents using a "fixed plasma level" design. *Psychopharmacol Bull* 26:85–90

Harter S (1988), *Manual for the Self Perception Profile for Adolescents*. Denver: University of Denver

Hazell P, O'Connell D, Heathcote D, Robertson J, Henry D (1995), Efficacy of tricyclic drugs in treating child and adolescent depression: a meta-analysis. *BMJ* 310:897–901

Hughes CW, Preskorn SH, Weller E, Weller R, Hassanein R, Tucker S (1990), The effect of concomitant disorders in childhood depression on predicting treatment response. *Psychopharmacol Bull* 26:235–238

Jensen PS, Ryan ND, Prien R (1992), Psychopharmacology of child and adolescent major depression: present status and future directions. *J Child Adolesc Psychopharmacol* 2:31–45

Kashani JH, Shekim WO, Reid JC (1984), Amitriptyline in children with major depressive disorder: a double-blind crossover pilot study. *J Am Acad Child Psychiatry* 23:348–351

Kessler RC, McGonagle KA, Zhao S et al. (1994), Lifetime and 12-month prevalence of *DSM-III-R* psychiatric disorders in the United States: results from the National Comorbidity Survey. *Arch Gen Psychiatry* 51:8–19

Kessler RC, Walters EE (1998), Epidemiology of *DSM-III-R* major depression and minor depression among adolescents and young adults in the National Comorbidity Survey. *Depress Anxiety* 7:3–14

Klein RG, Mannuzza S, Koplewicz HS et al. (1998), Adolescent depression: controlled desipramine treatment and atypical features. *Depress Anxiety* 7:15–31

Kovacs M, Goldston D, Gatsonis C (1993), Suicidal behaviors and childhood-onset depressive disorders: a longitudinal investigation. *J Am Acad Child Adolesc Psychiatry* 32:8–20

Kowatch RA, Carmody TJ, Emslie GJ, Rintelmann JW, Hughes CW, Rush AJ (1999), Prediction of response to fluoxetine and placebo in children and adolescents with major depression: a hypothesis generating study. *J Affect Disord* 54:269–276

Kramer AD, Feiguine RJ (1981), Clinical effects of amitriptyline in adolescent depression: a pilot study. *J Am Acad Child Psychiatry* 20:636–644

Kutcher S, Boulos C, Ward B et al. (1994), Response to desipramine treatment in adolescent depression: a fixed-dose, placebo-controlled trial. *J Am Acad Child Adolesc Psychiatry* 33:686–694

Kye CH, Waterman GS, Ryan ND et al. (1996), A randomized, controlled trial of amitriptyline in the acute treatment of a major depression. *J Am Acad Child Adolesc Psychiatry* 35:1139–1144

Masi G, Marcheschi M, Pfanner P (1997), Paroxetine in depressed adolescents with intellectual disability: an open label study. *J Intellect Disabil Res* 41:268–272

McConville BJ, Minnery KL, Sorter MT, West SA, Friedman LM, Christian K (1996), An open study of the effects of sertraline on adolescent major depression. *J Child Adolesc Psychopharmacol* 6:41–51

Paykel ES, Hollyman JA, Freeling P, Sedgwick P (1988), Predictors of therapeutic benefit from amitriptyline in mild depression: a general practice placebo-controlled trial. *J Affect Disord* 14:83–95

Petti TA, Law WD III (1982), Imipramine treatment of depressed children: a double-blind pilot study. *J Clin Psychopharmacol* 2:107–110

Preskorn SH, Weller EB, Hughes CW, Weller RA, Bolte K (1987), Depression in prepubertal children: dexamethasone nonsuppression predicts differential response to imipramine vs placebo. *Psychopharmacol Bull* 23:128–133

Rao U, Ryan ND, Birmaher B et al. (1995), Unipolar depression in adolescents: clinical outcome in adulthood. *J Am Acad Child Adolesc Psychiatry* 34:566–578

Reimherr FW, Chouinard G, Cohn CK et al. (1990), Antidepressant efficacy of sertraline: a double-blind, placebo- and amitriptyline-controlled, multicenter comparison study in outpatients with major depression. *J Clin Psychiatry* 51(suppl B):18–27

Rey-Sanchez F, Gutierrez-Casares JR (1997), Paroxetine in children with major depressive disorder: an open trial. *J Am Acad Child Adolesc Psychiatry* 36:1443–1447

Rodriguez-Ramos P, de Dios-Vega JL, San Sebastian-Cabases J, Sordo-Sordo L, Mardomingo-Sanz MJ (1996), Effects of paroxetine in depressed adolescents. *Eur J Clin Res* 8:49–61

Ryan ND, Varma D (1998), Child and adolescent mood disorders: experience with serotonin-based therapies. *Biol Psychiatry* 44:336–340

Schatzberg AF, Kraemer HC (2000), Use of placebo control groups in evaluating efficacy of treatment of unipolar major depression. *Biol Psychiatry* 47:736–744

Shrivastava RK, Shrivastava SH, Overweg N, Blumhardt CL (1992), A double-blind comparison of paroxetine, imipramine, and placebo in major depression. *J Clin Psychiatry* 53(suppl):48–51

Sigafoos AD, Feinstein CB, Damond M, Reiss D (1988), The measurement of behavioral autonomy in adolescence: the autonomous functioning checklist. *Adolesc Psychiatry* 15:432–462
Simeon JG, Dinicola VF, Ferguson HB, Copping W (1990), Adolescent depression: a placebo-controlled fluoxetine treatment study and follow-up. *Prog Neuropsychopharmacol Biol Psychiatry* 4:791–795
Simeon JG, Nixon MK, Milin RP, Spenst W, Smith D (1998), Sertraline in adolescent depression and dysthymia: a six-month open trial. Presented at the 151st Annual Meeting of the American Psychiatric Association; May 30–June 4; Toronto
Smith WT, Glaudin V (1992), A placebo-controlled trial of paroxetine in the treatment of major depression. *J Clin Psychiatry* 53:36–39
Stark P, Hardison CD (1985), A review of multicenter controlled studies of fluoxetine vs. imipramine and placebo in outpatients with major depressive disorder. *J Clin Psychiatry* 46:53–58
Stewart JW, Quitkin FM, Liebowitz MR, McGrath PJ, Harrison WM, Klein DF (1983), Efficacy of desipramine in depressed outpatients: response according to research diagnosis criteria diagnoses and severity of illness. *Arch Gen Psychiatry* 40:202–207
Strober M, DeAntonio M, Schmidt-Lackner S et al. (1999), The pharmacotherapy of depressive illness in adolescents: an open-label comparison of fluoxetine with imipramine-treated historical controls. *J Clin Psychiatry* 60:164–169
Trivedi MH, Rush H (1994), Does a placebo run-in or a placebo treatment cell affect the efficacy of antidepressant medications? *Neuropsychopharmacology* 11:33–43
Weissman MM, Wolk S, Goldstein RB et al. (1999), Depressed adolescents grown up. *JAMA* 281:1707–1713

Tab 84

Wyeth®

August 22, 2003

Dear Health Care Professional,

Wyeth wishes to inform you about an update to the prescribing information for Effexor® (venlafaxine HCl) Tablets and Effexor® XR (venlafaxine HCl) Extended-Release Capsules to reflect important safety information on the use of venlafaxine in children and adolescents. In clinical studies in pediatric patients (ages 6 to 17), efficacy was not established for major depressive disorder (MDD) or generalized anxiety disorder (GAD), and there were increased reports among those patients on Effexor XR, vs. placebo, of hostility and suicide-related adverse events, such as suicidal ideation and self-harm. Effexor and Effexor XR have not been and are not now recommended for use in pediatric patients. We have updated the prescribing information for Effexor and Effexor XR with the following information shown here in italics:

PRECAUTIONS

Usage in Children/ Pediatric Use

Safety and effectiveness in pediatric patients (individuals below 18 years of age) have not been established.

In pediatric clinical trials, there were increased reports of hostility and, especially in Major Depressive Disorder, suicide-related adverse events such as suicidal ideation and self-harm.

The most common adverse events leading to discontinuation in at least 1% of children and adolescents treated with Effexor XR, and at a rate twice that of placebo, were as follows (percentages listed for Effexor XR and placebo, respectively): MDD studies, hostility (2%, <1%) and suicidal ideation (2%, 0%); GAD studies, abnormal/changed behavior (1%, 0%). In these clinical trials there were no suicides.

Venlafaxine is a serotonin and norepinephrine reuptake inhibitor. Effexor XR Extended-Release Capsules are indicated in adults for the treatment of MDD, GAD, and social anxiety disorder (SAD). Effexor Tablets are indicated in adults for the treatment of MDD.

In light of this important information, you should be alert to signs of suicidal ideation in children and adolescent patients prescribed Effexor or Effexor XR. You may need to reassess the benefit-risk balance when treating individual patients with Effexor or Effexor XR. If a decision is made to discontinue a patient from Effexor or Effexor XR, treatment should not be discontinued abruptly, due to risk of discontinuation symptoms. A gradual reduction in dose under medical supervision is recommended. Please see the prescribing information for additional information with regard to discontinuation.

Wyeth is committed to global surveillance of all its products and to providing you with current product information, and therefore is sending you this letter. Should you have any questions, or wish to report any adverse event associated with Effexor or Effexor XR, please call Wyeth at 1-800-934-5556. In addition, you can send adverse event information directly to Wyeth Global Safety Surveillance and Epidemiology (GSSE) by fax to 610-989-5544 or by mail to GSSE, 500 Arcola Road, Collegeville, PA 19426.

Adverse event information may also be reported to the FDA's MedWatch Reporting System by phone (1-800-FDA-1088), fax (1-800-FDA-0178), via the MedWatch Web site at www.fda.gov/medwatch, or by mail (using postage paid form) to MedWatch, HF-2, 5600 Fisher's Lane, Rockville, MD 20852-9787.

Enclosed is a copy of the revised labeling for Effexor and Effexor XR.

Sincerely,

Victoria Kusiak

Victoria Kusiak, M.D.
Vice President, Global Medical Affairs and
North American Medical Director for Wyeth Pharmaceuticals

Enclosures

Tab 85

Efficacy of Sertraline in the Treatment of Children and Adolescents With Major Depressive Disorder

Two Randomized Controlled Trials

Karen Dineen Wagner, MD, PhD
Paul Ambrosini, MD
Moira Rynn, MD
Christopher Wohlberg, MD, PhD
Ruoyong Yang, PhD
Michael S. Greenbaum, MD
Ann Childress, MD
Craig Donnelly, MD
Deborah Deas, MD
for the Sertraline Pediatric Depression Study Group

Context The efficacy, safety, and tolerability of selective serotonin reuptake inhibitors (SSRIs) in the treatment of adults with major depressive disorder (MDD) are well established. Comparatively few data are available on the effects of SSRIs in depressed children and adolescents.

Objective To evaluate the efficacy and safety of sertraline compared with placebo in treatment of pediatric patients with MDD.

Design and Setting Two multicenter randomized, double-blind, placebo-controlled trials were conducted at 53 hospital, general practice, and academic centers in the United States, India, Canada, Costa Rica, and Mexico between December 1999 and May 2001 and were pooled a priori.

Participants Three hundred seventy-six children and adolescents aged 6 to 17 years with *Diagnostic and Statistical Manual of Mental Disorders, Fourth Edition*–defined MDD of at least moderate severity.

Intervention Patients were randomly assigned to receive a flexible dosage (50-200 mg/d) of sertraline (n=189) or matching placebo tablets (n=187) for 10 weeks.

Main Outcome Measures Change from baseline in the Children's Depression Rating Scale–Revised (CDRS-R) Best Description of Child total score and reported adverse events.

Results Sertraline-treated patients experienced statistically significantly greater improvement than placebo patients on the CDRS-R total score (mean change at week 10, −30.24 vs −25.83, respectively; $P=.001$; overall mean change, −22.84 vs −20.19, respectively; $P=.007$). Based on a 40% decrease in the adjusted CDRS-R total score at study end point, 69% of sertraline-treated patients compared with 59% of placebo patients were considered responders ($P=.05$). Sertraline treatment was generally well tolerated. Seventeen sertraline-treated patients (9%) and 5 placebo patients (3%) prematurely discontinued the study because of adverse events. Adverse events that occurred in at least 5% of sertraline-treated patients and with an incidence of at least twice that in placebo patients included diarrhea, vomiting, anorexia, and agitation.

Conclusion The results of this pooled analysis demonstrate that sertraline is an effective and well-tolerated short-term treatment for children and adolescents with MDD.

JAMA. 2003;290:1033-1041 www.jama.com

Major depressive disorder (MDD) occurs not only in adults but also in children and adolescents.[1-11] Prevalence rates of up to 3% in children and 8% in adolescents have been reported,[3] and the lifetime prevalence rate for depression in youths aged 15 to 18 years has been estimated at 14% to 15%,[12] which is comparable with that in adults.[13] In general, the clinical course of the disease is similar in pediatric and adult patients, although there is some evidence that early-onset MDD may represent a more pernicious form of the disease.[4,14] Patients diagnosed as having MDD during childhood or adolescence face a 2- to 4-fold greater risk of developing depression as young adults than do children or adolescents without MDD.[14-16]

For editorial comment see p 1091.

The social and economic costs associated with pediatric MDD are high and may carry over into adulthood, including more frequent hospitalizations and lower educational and earning potential.[14,15,17] In addition, a quarter of adolescents with MDD develop substance

Author Affiliations, Financial Disclosures, and the Sertraline Pediatric Depression Study Group Investigators are listed at the end of this article.
Corresponding Author and Reprints: Karen Dineen Wagner, MD, PhD, University of Texas Medical Branch, Department of Psychiatry and Behavioral Sciences, Division of Child and Adolescent Psychiatry, 301 University Blvd, Galveston, TX 77555-0188 (e-mail: kwagner@utmb.edu).

abuse disorders[3] and approximately half attempt suicide at some time during their lives. Among children with MDD, there is a 4- to 5-fold higher lifetime risk of suicide attempt than in healthy controls.[14,15,18]

Despite the costs and prevalence of the disorder, MDD is frequently underdiagnosed and inadequately treated.[19] For pediatric patients, this problem has been compounded by the discouraging results of early psychopharmacological studies, in which tricyclic antidepressants were consistently found to be no more effective than placebo in treating depressed youths.[20] On the basis of their good safety profile and established efficacy in treatment of adults with MDD, selective serotonin reuptake inhibitors (SSRIs) are routinely cited as the best available treatment option for depressed children and adolescents.[21,22] Empirical evidence of the effectiveness of SSRIs in this patient population has been limited, however. Several small uncontrolled trials of SSRIs[23-28] and a single-center (N=96) placebo-controlled trial of fluoxetine[29] have suggested efficacy. Published reports of 2 large multicenter, placebo-controlled studies of fluoxetine[30] and paroxetine[31] also reported favorable results, but statistical significance was not achieved for their primary end points.

Encouraging results have been reported in 3 small, open-label studies of sertraline in adolescents with MDD[32-34] and in a retrospective chart review of pediatric patients.[35] Herein, we report the pooled results of 2 identically designed, concurrently conducted 10-week international, multicenter, randomized, double-blind, placebo-controlled, parallel-group trials of sertraline vs placebo in children and adolescents with MDD.

METHODS

Study Participants

Participants were outpatients aged 6 to 17 years who met the diagnostic criteria for MDD, as defined in the *Diagnostic and Statistical Manual of Mental Disorders, Fourth Edition* (*DSM-IV*)[1] and as determined by the Kiddie Schedule for Affective Disorders and Schizophrenia for School-Age Children–Present and Lifetime Version (K-SADS-PL).[36] For study entry eligibility, these diagnostic criteria had to be met at the first and third visits during a 2-week screening period and the current episode of major depression had to be of at least 6 weeks' duration. At all 3 visits during the screening period, patients were required to have a Children's Depression Rating Scale–Revised (CDRS-R) score of at least 45[37,38] and a Clinical Global Impression of Severity of Illness (CGI-S) rating of at least 4,[39] indicating at least moderate severity of illness. Exclusion criteria included current, primary, *DSM-IV*–defined diagnosis of attention-deficit/hyperactivity disorder, conduct disorder, obsessive-compulsive disorder, or panic disorder; history of bipolar disorder; any current psychotic features; and history of psychotic disorders or autistic spectrum disorders. Patients who had previously attempted suicide or who were judged to pose a significant suicidal or homicidal risk were also excluded. Patients were also excluded if screening electrocardiographic or laboratory test results, vital signs, or body weight were clinically significantly outside the normal range. Other exclusion criteria included a positive serum β-human chorionic gonadotropin pregnancy test (among girls aged 12-17 years) at the second screening visit, previous enrollment in a sertraline study, medical contraindications to treatment with SSRIs, and history of failure to respond to a clinically adequate dosing regimen of an SSRI. Patients were required to be free of psychotropic medication (with the exception of diphenhydramine or chloral hydrate as sleep aids) for at least 2 weeks (at least 4 weeks for fluoxetine) prior to initiation of double-blind study drug treatment.

Study Design

The 2 trials, developed in response to a US Food and Drug Administration (FDA) written request, were identically designed and were conducted at 53 hospital, general practice, and academic centers in the United States, India, Canada, Costa Rica, and Mexico. Participation in the study was based on inspection of the study site by 1 of the authors (C.W.) or a designate. Criteria for investigator participation included but was not limited to previous experience with multicenter research trials, expertise in pediatric psychiatry, and a clear understanding of Good Clinical Practices, as outlined in the US Code of Federal Regulations. Additionally, study conduct was reviewed at investigators' meetings, and all investigators who conducted interviews using the CDRS-R were required to first pass a certification test. During the study, all sites were regularly monitored. When necessary, additional training regarding completion of study documents, retention of source documents, and conduct of ratings was provided on a personal level. All data collected were reviewed for errors in formatting and for inconsistency.

Enrollment began in December 1999 and follow-up ended in May 2001. Both trials were approved by institutional review boards or ethics committees for each study center. Informed assent or written permission of the child or adolescent and written informed consent of at least 1 parent or legal guardian were obtained.

The trials began with the 2-week pretreatment screening period. During these screening visits, diagnosis of MDD was confirmed using the K-SADS-PL and clinical history and symptom severity was assessed using the CDRS-R and CGI-S. Physical and laboratory evaluations were performed at the second screening visit. At the third screening visit (baseline), patients who remained eligible for study entry were randomly assigned to double-blind receipt of either sertraline or matching placebo for 10 weeks in a 1:1 ratio using a computer-generated randomization code. To ensure that each treatment group included similar numbers of younger and older children, patients were stratified into 2 age groups: children (aged 6-11 years) and adolescents (aged 12-17 years). Study drug was packaged in identical blister packs containing 25-mg and/or 50-mg sertraline tablets or matching placebo. For all patients, treatment was initiated at a dosage of 25 mg/d for the first 3 days and was continued at a dosage of 50 mg/d through the end of the second week. Thereafter, in the absence of dose-limiting adverse events, the dosage could be flexibly titrated upward in increments of 50 mg/d every 2 weeks to a maximum of 200 mg/d until a satisfactory clinical response was achieved. Both patients and clinicians were blinded to group assignment.

With the exception of diphenhydramine and chloral hydrate, which could be used intermittently as sleep aids, concomitant treatment with a psychotropic drug was not permitted. Patients were not permitted to receive cognitive behavioral therapy during the study. Other types of psychotherapy were permitted, provided that they did not specifically address issues of depression and had been under way for at least 2 months prior to the initial screening visit. Patients could be discontinued from the study at an investigator's discretion for reasons such as adverse events and failure to improve despite increases in the study drug dosage.

Outcome Measures, Schedule of Assessments, and Sample Size

The primary efficacy rating scale was the CDRS-R, a validated 17-item, clinician-rated instrument that measures the severity of a patient's depressive symptoms, with total possible scores ranging from 17 to 113. Fourteen of the 17 items are rated on a scale from 1 to 7, with an item score of 3 suggestive of mild, 4 or 5 moderate, and 6 or 7 severe symptoms. The other 3 items are rated on a scale from 1 to 5. Both children and their parents provide input into the first 14 items of the scale. A child's nonverbal behavior is rated by the observer for items 15 through 17. The prospectively defined primary efficacy outcome measure was the CDRS-R Best Description of the Child total score, which is based on the highest (most severe) rating provided for each item by a valid, reliable source, in the judgment of the investigator; sources included the child, parent or legal guardian, and other available sources.[37,38] Secondary efficacy measures included the proportion of CDRS-R responders, defined a priori as patients who had at least a 40% decrease in the adjusted CDRS-R total score (CDRS-R total minus 17, the minimum possible total score); scores on the CGI-S and the Clinical Global Impression of Improvement (CGI-I) scales, clinician-rated instruments that assess a patient's severity of illness and global improvement, respectively[39]; and the proportion of CGI-I responders, defined as patients with a CGI-I score of 2 or lower ("very much" or "much" improved). The CDRS-R and CGI-S measurements were collected at all 3 screening visits and, along with the CGI-I, at the end of weeks 1, 2, 3, 4, 6, 8, and 10 of double-blind treatment (or at the time of early discontinuation).

Patient-rated secondary efficacy measures included the Multidimensional Anxiety Scale for Children (MASC), which is used to assess symptoms of anxiety[40]; the Children's Global Assessment Scale (CGAS), which measures a patient's social functioning[41]; and the total score on the 15-item Pediatric Quality of Life Enjoyment and Satisfaction Questionnaire (PQ-LES-Q), a measure of a patient's quality of life (Jean Endicott, PhD, unpublished data, 2002). This scale was adapted from the Q-LES-Q, a validated instrument that assesses quality of life in adults and that has been shown to be sensitive to drug-placebo differences in mood and anxiety.[42] These assessments were made at baseline and at the end of week 10 of double-blind treatment (or at the time of early discontinuation).

Safety data were collected from the first day of double-blind study drug receipt through 7 days after the last dose of double-blind study drug was taken and included vital signs (blood pressure and pulse), body weight, and all adverse events reported by patients or observed by investigators. A serious adverse event was defined, according to established criteria, as any event that resulted in death or was life-threatening or that resulted in inpatient hospitalization or prolongation of a hospital stay, persistent or significant disability/incapacity, or a congenital anomaly/birth defect. Blood samples for routine hematologic and serum chemistry studies and urine samples for routine urinalysis and drug testing were obtained at screening and the end of weeks 4 and 10 (or at the time of early discontinuation). Thyroid function was tested at screening and the pregnancy test was repeated at the end of weeks 4 and 10. A 12-lead electrocardiogram was obtained and a physical examination was performed at screening and the end of week 10 (or at the time of early discontinuation).

Based on the single-center study reported by Emslie et al,[29] a sample size for each trial of 160 patients, with 80 patients per treatment group, was calculated to provide 88% power for a 2-sided test at an α level of .05 to detect differences between treatment groups. The studies were not powered to detect differences between treatment groups within age groups.

Statistical Analyses

Data from both studies were pooled in a prospectively defined combined analysis. Using a repeated-measures mixed-model analysis, the mean changes from baseline to each postbaseline visit in the CDRS-R total and the CGI-S score were compared between treatment groups. For each measure, the mean changes from baseline to each postbaseline visit week were then averaged to give a mean overall change from baseline, and the mean overall changes from baseline were compared between treatment groups. The model included the baseline effect as covariate, the random subject effect, and the fixed effects of site, treatment, age group, week, and week-by-treatment interaction. The same mixed model (without the baseline

Figure 1. Flow of Patients Through the 2 Trials

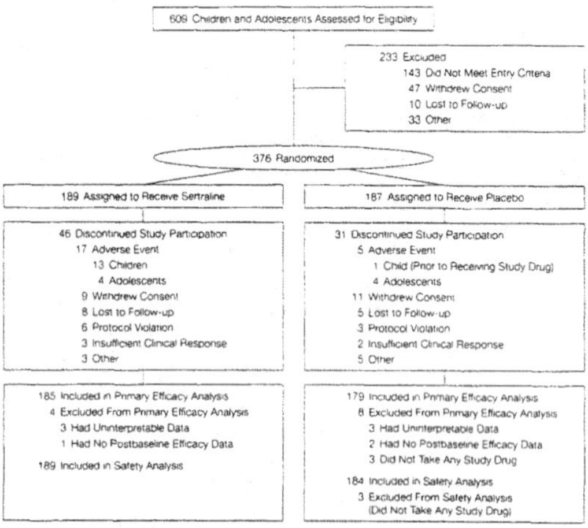

effect) was used to compare the CGI-I scores at each postbaseline visit as well as the mean overall CGI-I score in each treatment group. Categorical variables (proportions of CDRS-R responders and CGI-I responders at study end point) were compared between treatment groups using Cochran-Mantel-Haenszel methods with centers as strata. Changes from baseline to study end point in the MASC, CGAS, and PQ-LES-Q total scores (using the last-observation-carried-forward method) were compared between treatment groups using an analysis of covariance model that contained study treatment group, age group, and baseline effects. As described in the statistical analysis plan, centers with fewer than 4 patients were combined to form 1 pooled center within each trial, and an additional pooled center was generated from centers with exactly 4 patients. This "sort and pool" procedure was chosen as the most objective and conservative way to pool because selective factors such as location and language/culture were not used. For all statistical tests, a 2-sided $P \leq .05$ was considered significant. Assumptions regarding the linearity of data were made in the analysis plan and were tested following database release. No gross violation of linear model assumptions was detected; therefore, nonparametric analyses were not performed. Descriptive statistics were used to summarize safety results. SAS version 8.2 (SAS Institute Inc, Cary, NC) was used for the efficacy analysis and SAS version 6.12 was used for safety data.

RESULTS

Patient Disposition

As shown in FIGURE 1, 376 patients were randomly assigned to double-blind treatment with either sertraline (n=189) or placebo (n=187). All 189 patients randomized to sertraline and 184 of the patients randomized to placebo received at least 1 dose of double-blind study drug and were included in the safety evaluation. Patients were randomized by the following countries: United States, 297; India, 44; Costa Rica, 16; Canada, 14; and Mexico, 5. The intention-to-treat population was modified as follows: 1 sertraline-treated and 2 placebo patients were excluded from the efficacy analysis because no postrandomization efficacy data were collected, and 3 sertraline-treated and 3 placebo patients, all from 1 US site, were excluded because of problems with data collection. Thus, 185 sertraline-treated patients (98%) and 179 placebo patients (97%) were included in the efficacy analysis. Forty-six sertraline-treated patients (24%) and 31 placebo patients (17%) discontinued the study early. Among patients treated with sertraline, the most common reasons for discontinuation were adverse events (n=17; 9%), withdrawal of consent (n=9; 5%), and loss to follow-up (n=8; 4%). Similar proportions of placebo patients discontinued from the study because they withdrew consent (n=11; 6%) or were lost to follow-up (n=5; 3%); fewer placebo patients (n=5, 1 of whom had not received study drug; 3%) discontinued because of adverse events. This difference was more apparent in children, among whom 13 sertraline-treated patients but no placebo patients discontinued because of adverse events.

Demographic and Background Characteristics

The 2 treatment groups were evenly balanced with respect to race, weight, clinical characteristics, and psychosocial stressors at baseline (TABLE 1). There was a statistically significant between-group difference in sex (57% of sertraline-treated and 45% of placebo patients were female; $P=.02$) but no significant interaction by age group for the primary and secondary efficacy variables. The majority of patients in both treatment groups (≥86%) were in their first lifetime MDD episode, whereas the others (<14%) were having a recurrent episode. In both subsets of patients, onset of illness occurred at approximately 10 years of age. There were no statistically significant differences in mean baseline CDRS-R or CGI-S scores between treatment groups. Nearly 40% of patients had at least 1 comorbid psychiatric disorder, with the most common (occurring in ≥5% of patients) being oppositional defiant disorder, anxiety, adjustment reaction, and phobic disorders. More than half of patients had a family history of MDD. The most common stressors included parental divorce or separation and death of a relative or friend. Only about half of patients were living with their biological father.

Efficacy

As can be seen in FIGURE 2 and TABLE 2, sertraline-treated patients exhibited significantly greater improvement over the course of the study than those receiving placebo on the CDRS-R (mean change in scores of −22.84 vs −20.19, respectively; $P = .007$), as well as on the CGI-S and CGI-I. Similar outcomes favoring sertraline were observed among patients who completed all 10 weeks of double-blind treatment (mean changes in the CDRS-R total score of −30.24 vs −25.83, respectively, $P = .001$; and in the CGI-S of −1.99 vs −1.58, respectively, $P = .001$; and mean CGI-I scores of 2.02 and 2.30, respectively, $P = .009$). Week-by-week analyses showed that significant differences in favor of sertraline were apparent as early as week 1 on the CGI-I and week 3 on the CDRS-R and the CGI-S ($P < .05$).

Table 1. Baseline Demographic, Clinical, and Psychosocial Characteristics of Patients by Treatment Group*

Characteristics	Sertraline (n = 189)	Placebo (n = 187)
Demographic characteristics		
Sex		
Male	81 (42.9)	103 (55.1)
Female	108 (57.1)	84 (44.9)
Age group, y		
6-11 (Children)	86 (45.5)	91 (48.7)
12-17 (Adolescents)	103 (54.5)	96 (51.3)
Race		
White	135 (71.4)	130 (69.5)
Asian	26 (13.8)	23 (12.3)
Hispanic	15 (7.9)	19 (10.2)
Black	7 (3.7)	9 (4.8)
Other	6 (3.2)	6 (3.2)
Clinical characteristics		
Patients with single-episode MDD, mean (range)†		
Age at onset of illness, y	10.0 (1.3-16.8)	10.1 (1.2-16.9)
Duration of illness, mo	22.1 (1.5-107.6)	19.1 (1.1-119.3)
Patients with recurrent MDD, mean (range)†		
Age at onset of illness, y	9.6 (3.0-15.8)	10.3 (4.0-14.5)
Duration of illness, mo	43.7 (3.0-132.0)	39.8 (6.0-108.0)
CDRS-R score, mean (SD)‡	64.3 (11.0)	64.6 (11.0)
CGI-S score, mean (SD)§	4.6 (0.6)	4.5 (0.7)
Psychosocial characteristics		
≥1 Other psychiatric disorder	73 (38.6)	71 (38.0)
Family history of MDD	97 (51.3)	104 (55.6)
Parents were divorced or separated	80 (42.3)	86 (45.9)
Experienced death of close family member/friend	73 (38.6)	64 (34.2)
Biological mother living in same household	164 (86.7)	168 (89.8)
Biological father living in same household	92 (48.6)	98 (52.4)

Abbreviations: CDRS-R, Children's Depression Rating Scale–Revised Best Description of Child total score; CGI-S, Clinical Global Impression of Severity of Illness scale; MDD, major depressive disorder.
*Data are expressed as No. (%) unless otherwise indicated.
†For sertraline, n = 171 with single episodes and n = 18 with recurrent episodes; for placebo, n = 161 with single episodes and n = 26 with recurrent episodes.
‡For sertraline, n = 185 and for placebo, n = 179 patients in efficacy analysis.
§For sertraline, n = 185 and for placebo, n = 178 patients in efficacy analysis.

The adjusted mean change from baseline to study end was assessed for the individual items of the CDRS-R. Statistically significantly greater improvement was noted with sertraline treatment for 5 of the 17 items, including irritability ($P < .001$), low self-esteem ($P = .02$), excessive weeping ($P = .003$), listless speech ($P = .005$), and hypoactivity ($P = .03$). The change in depressed feelings was of borderline significance ($P = .05$), as was difficulty having fun ($P = .09$). No statistically significant difference was noted between treatment groups for suicidal ideation ($P = .78$), and the mean change was of similar magnitude between sertraline (−0.58) and placebo (−0.60).

Although the study was not powered to detect differences between age groups, a slightly greater difference in the CDRS-R mean change between treatment groups was noted in adolescents (sertraline, −21.55 vs placebo, −18.20; $P = .01$) than in children (sertraline, −24.05 vs placebo, −22.20; $P = .19$). Following 10 weeks of treatment, the difference in CDRS-R scores was of borderline significance in children (sertraline, −31.44 vs placebo, −27.56; $P = .05$) and remained significant in adolescents (sertraline, −28.95 vs placebo, −24.11; $P = .01$).

At study end point, using the last observations carried forward and the Cochran-Mantel-Haenszel method of analysis between treatment groups, 69% of sertraline-treated patients and 59% of placebo patients met the CDRS-R responder criteria ($P = .05$), and 63% of sertraline-treated patients compared with 53% of placebo patients met the CGI-I responder criteria ($P = .05$). In addition, significantly more sertraline-treated patients than placebo patients met the CDRS-R responder criteria at the end of weeks 1, 3, and 10 and the CGI-I responder criteria at the end of weeks 1, 2, 3, 4, and 10 ($P < .05$). With a 10% difference in responder rates for both the CDRS-R and CGI-I, the number needed to treat to expect a difference in response between sertraline and placebo would be 10 using either criterion. Patients treated with sertraline also had numerically better scores at study end point compared with placebo patients on the MASC,

PQ-LES-Q, and CGAS (Table 2). However, the differences between treatment groups did not reach statistical significance.

Tolerability

The mean dosage of study drug administered to patients who completed 10 weeks of double-blind treatment was 131 mg/d of sertraline and 144 mg/d of placebo equivalent, and the median duration of exposure to study drug was the same in both treatment groups (68 days). Sertraline in the dosage range of 50 to 200 mg/d was generally well tolerated. In the majority (>90%) of patients, adverse events were mild or moderate in intensity. There were 4 adverse events that occurred in at least 5% of sertraline-treated patients and with an incidence of at least twice that in placebo patients: diarrhea, vomiting, anorexia, and agitation (TABLE 3). Seventeen sertraline-treated patients (9%) discontinued the study because of adverse events; 13 of these patients were children. Seven sertraline-treated patients and 6 placebo patients had adverse events that met the established criteria for a "serious" adverse event, including suicide attempt (2 sertraline and 2 placebo), suicidal ideation (3 sertraline), and aggressive reaction (1 sertraline), as well as medical hospitalizations (1 sertraline and 4 placebo). There were no clinically important differences between the 2 treatment groups with respect to laboratory test, vital sign, physical examination, or electrocardiographic findings. The mean change in body weight from baseline to the final visit was −0.38 kg among patients treated with sertraline and +0.78 kg among placebo patients ($P = .001$).

Figure 2. Weekly and Overall Adjusted Mean CDRS-R Scores

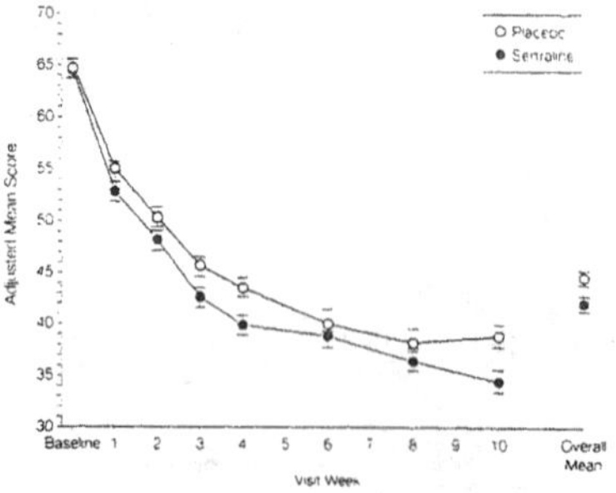

CDRS-R indicates Children's Depression Rating Scale–Revised Best Description of Child total score. Data are least square means at each visit week, with mean scores averaged to give the overall mean, from a repeated-measures mixed-model analysis with age category, site, treatment, week, and week-by-treatment interaction used as fixed effects, subject as a random effect, and baseline effect as a covariate. Error bars indicate SE of the adjusted means, derived from the repeated-measures mixed-model procedure. P values are as follows: week 1, $P = .09$; week 2, $P = .08$; week 3, $P = .01$; week 4, $P = .008$; week 6, $P = .37$; week 8, $P = .18$; week 10, $P = .001$; and mean response, $P = .007$.

COMMENT

In the trials reported here, sertraline was found to be more effective than placebo for treatment of pediatric MDD, with statistically greater improvement occurring as early as week 3. Of the 3 randomized, double-blind, placebo-controlled trials of an SSRI in pediatric MDD that have been published to date,[29-31] only 1, the study by Emslie et al[29] of fluoxetine, reported statistically significantly better results for the prospectively defined primary end point, and this was a comparatively small (n=96) single-center trial. Thus, our trials describe the largest positive psychopharmacological study of pediatric MDD, using an international multicenter study design.

The significance of the results is clinically as well as statistically relevant.

Table 2. Secondary End Point Measures

Measures	Baseline Score, Mean (SD)		Adjusted Overall Score, Mean (SE)*		Adjusted Change in Score From Baseline, Mean (SE)*		P Value†
	Sertraline	Placebo	Sertraline	Placebo	Sertraline	Placebo	
CGI-I	NA	NA	2.56 (0.06)	2.75 (0.06)	NA	NA	009
CGI-S	4.57 (0.64)	4.54 (0.66)	3.33 (0.05)	3.55 (0.05)	−1.22 (0.05)	−1.01 (0.05)	.005
CGAS	50.21 (7.07)	49.71 (7.17)	66.00 (1.04)	64.69 (1.04)	16.04 (1.04)	14.74 (1.04)	.38
MASC	51.06 (19.0)	51.85 (20.09)	45.90 (1.17)	48.35 (1.16)	−5.56 (1.17)	−3.11 (1.16)	.14
PQ-LES-Q	49.43 (10.82)	48.92 (10.94)	55.63 (0.68)	53.85 (0.68)	6.46 (0.68)	4.68 (0.68)	.07

Abbreviations: CGAS, Children's Global Assessment Scale; CGI-I, Clinical Global Impression of Improvement scale; CGI-S, Clinical Global Impression of Severity of Illness scale; MASC, Multidimensional Anxiety Scale for Children; NA, not applicable; PQ-LES-Q, Pediatric Quality of Life Enjoyment and Satisfaction Questionnaire.

*For the CGI-I and CGI-S, least square means and SEs are provided from a repeated-measures, mixed-model analysis with age category, site, treatment, week, and week-by-treatment interaction used as fixed effects in the model and subject used as a random effect. Baseline CGI-S score was used as a covariate for the analysis of CGI-S. Change from baseline of CGI-S and observed value of CGI-I were analyzed. For the CGAS, MASC, and PQ-LES-Q, last-observation-carried-forward least square means and SEs are provided from analysis of covariance, including protocol number, treatment, age, and baseline effects. Repeated-measures analysis was not used for these end points because values were collected only at baseline and study end.

†P values were derived from t tests and are the same for both adjusted overall scores and adjusted changes in scores.

Variability of response is typical in pediatric trials and was clearly evident in our study, as demonstrated by the high placebo response rates.[43] Larger variation in response is expected with greater numbers of participating sites because random errors from subject and measurement variation (particularly with subjective measurements) increase with a larger number of investigators with different degrees of experience.[44,45] We used a large number of sites (53) compared with a relatively small number of sites in the fluoxetine studies (15 and 1).[29,30] Additionally, the multinational nature of this study possibly contributed to the variability seen. While no statistically significant treatment-by-center, study, sex, or age interactions were noted, this does not entirely preclude an effect of variability, as long as the effect size from center to center was similar. The fact that no placebo-controlled study of tricyclic antidepressants in children has ever shown significant difference from placebo[20] suggests that even though the differences observed in this study were numerically small, they are nonetheless important.

Mean baseline levels of symptom severity were moderate to severe, as judged by the CDRS-R total scores, and these levels were mild following 10 weeks of treatment. Additionally, the degree of drug-placebo difference was similar to that observed with fluoxetine,[30] which was recently approved by the FDA for treatment of pediatric MDD. In fact, the magnitude of response was greater for sertraline (the mean change from baseline to study end point in CDRS-R total score was −22.0 for fluoxetine vs −14.9 for placebo; mean change from baseline to study end point in CDRS-R total score was −27.31 for sertraline vs −23.89 for placebo). A larger-than-expected percentage of patients in the fluoxetine study had self-rated depression scores that were in the lower range of severity, and approximately one third of those patients had comorbid attention-deficit/hyperactivity disorder, while less than 10% (36/376) of our patients did. It is unknown, however, whether these differences account for the differential treatment responses observed between the fluoxetine study results and ours.

The treatment effect size observed in these studies was modest in comparison with that typically observed in adult studies.[46] In part, this appears to be related to the relatively high rate of response to placebo in our patient sample (53%, CGI-I response rate). High placebo response rates have been a consistent feature of psychopharmacological studies of depressed adults,[46] and although studies of depressed youths are comparatively small in number, the data suggest that the placebo response rate is at least as high in this age population.[20,21,29-31] In our study, the exact nature of the high placebo response rate is unclear, but possible factors include frequent follow-up visits, the relatively large number of centers involved (increased variability), and language/cultural factors. Increased visit frequency and the attention associated with these visits may have an intrinsic component of therapy and is different than a "waiting period" control, in which there is no interaction. Furthermore, 8 placebo patients (4.3%) were receiving some form of psychotherapy during the course of the study and 29 (15.7%) had received psychotherapy prior to enrollment, potentially providing these patients with access to previously learned exercises. Thus, randomization to receipt of placebo does not imply complete lack of treatment.

Suicidality is an important concern in depressed patients. [Recently, regulators in the United States and the United Kingdom have issued advisories about the use of paroxetine, another SSRI, in the treatment of children and adolescents with MDD. The FDA is currently reviewing these data and a final determination regarding paroxetine and suicide risk has not yet been reached.] In our sertraline study, the number of suicide attempts was the same in each treatment group (2 for sertraline and 2 for placebo). Our trials showed a lack of significant difference in suicidal ideation between sertraline-treated and placebo patients, as measured by the CDRS-R. In patients who continued into the 24-week open-label extension study, only 1 episode of suicidal ideation was reported, and the investigator attributed this event to teasing by classmates. Additionally, the Best Pharmaceuticals for Children Act requires a review of adverse events for a period of 1 year after a drug is granted pediatric exclusivity. This review of sertraline's safety data was recently conducted by the FDA. The agency concluded: "These reports do not provide any safety signals that indicate that the Agency needs to do anything except continue to actively assess the evolving benefit-risk profile of these products [sertraline]."[47] Regardless, it is important to carefully supervise and assess the potential for suicidality in all patients with MDD, and larger studies on this issue should be conducted.

Table 3. Treatment-Emergent Adverse Events in Patients Analyzed for Safety*

Adverse Events	Sertraline	Placebo
Children†		
Insomnia	17 (19.8)	7 (8.0)
Diarrhea	13 (15.1)	4 (4.5)
Anorexia	9 (10.5)	2 (2.3)
Vomiting	8 (9.3)	4 (4.5)
Agitation	7 (8.1)	2 (2.3)
Urinary incontinence	6 (7.0)	0
Purpura	5 (5.8)	1 (1.1)
Adolescents‡		
Vomiting	8 (7.8)	3 (3.1)
Diarrhea	7 (6.8)	3 (3.1)

*Data are expressed as No. (%) for events occurring in at least 5% of sertraline-treated patients and with an incidence of at least 2 times that seen in placebo patients.
†For sertraline, n = 86 and for placebo, n = 88.
‡For sertraline, n = 103 and for placebo, n = 96.

Although our trials were not powered to detect differences by age group, there was some suggestion that sertraline may be more effective in adolescents. Further studies may be helpful to determine whether both age groups respond equally well to drug therapy.

Sertraline appears to be generally well tolerated, although these trials were powered only for efficacy. Patients treated with sertraline more frequently experienced agitation, anorexia, diarrhea, nausea, purpura, urinary incontinence, and vomiting. Although the incidence of discontinuations due to adverse events was similar between treatment groups in adolescents, a higher proportion of sertraline-treated children discontinued because of adverse events. The nature of this difference is unclear, although identical dosing regimens were used for both age groups and it is possible that the higher serum levels of sertraline in children[48] resulted in the greater incidence of adverse events. This may suggest a need for reduced initial doses or slower titration of sertraline in children compared with adolescents in an effort to improve tolerability. Regardless of age, careful symptomatic monitoring is warranted in all patients with MDD.

Discontinuation of sertraline was not associated with withdrawal symptoms in either the 10-week double-blind trials or the 24-week open-label extension study. All patients entering the extension study began open-label treatment with 50 mg/d of sertraline, regardless of their dosage in the double-blind study, and no significant untoward reactions were noted as a result of this dosage change.

The clinical importance of the weight difference noted in the 10-week trials is unclear, but in a subset of patients (n=226) who continued into the 24-week open-label extension study, this pattern was reversed and patients previously treated with sertraline displayed a mean weight gain (+2.98 kg) that was greater than in patients previously randomized to placebo (+1.22 kg).[49] Because appetite and weight changes are common in MDD, it is advisable for practitioners to monitor weight patterns in all patients with depression.

Acute studies such as reported here are limited by several factors, including the subjective nature of rating scales and the relatively short duration of treatment exposure. The applicability of these scales to younger patients with less developed insight and ability to form abstract thought is unclear. In addition, most patients were treated with doses of study drug lower than the maximum allowed by the protocol, and it is possible that in a longer-term study, investigators would have titrated the dosage to higher levels. Although no dose-response relationship for sertraline has been demonstrated, patients who do not respond initially to lower dosages may respond to dosage escalation, up to a maximum of 200 mg/d.

Major depressive disorder is a serious public health problem that is frequently underdiagnosed and inadequately treated.[10] Given the paucity of empirical data available to guide physicians in the psychopharmacological treatment of pediatric MDD, further research is needed. Whether lower initial dosages in children would improve tolerability or long-term sertraline treatment in children and adolescents would result in maintenance of effect and an improvement of quality of life deserves study. Nonetheless, the results reported here support the conclusion that sertraline is an effective, safe, and well-tolerated short-term treatment for children and adolescents with MDD.

Author Affiliations: University of Texas Medical Branch, Galveston (Dr Wagner); Drexel University College of Medicine (Dr Ambrosini) and University of Pennsylvania (Dr Rynn), Philadelphia; Pfizer Inc, New York, NY (Drs Wohlberg and Yang); Ingenium Clinical Research, Libertyville, Ill (Dr Greenbaum); Nevada Behavioral Health Inc, Las Vegas (Dr Childress); Dartmouth Medical School, Lebanon, NH (Dr Donnelly); and the Medical University of South Carolina, Charleston (Dr Deas).

Financial Disclosures: Dr Wagner has received research support from Abbott, Bristol-Myers Squibb, Eli Lilly, Forest Laboratories, GlaxoSmithKline, Organon, Pfizer, and Wyeth-Ayerst; has served as a National Institute of Mental Health consultant to Abbott, Bristol-Myers Squibb, Cyberonics, Eli Lilly, Forest Laboratories, GlaxoSmithKline, Novartis, Otsuka, Janssen, Pfizer, and UCB Pharma; and has participated in speaker's bureaus for Abbott, Eli Lilly, GlaxoSmithKline, Forest Laboratories, Pfizer, and Novartis. Dr Ambrosini has received honoraria and funds for clinical trials from Pfizer. Dr Rynn has been a consultant to Pfizer, PharmaStar, and Eli Lilly. Drs Wohlberg and Yang, as employees of Pfizer, hold stock options in the company. Dr Donnelly has been a consultant and speaker for Pfizer and has participated in speaker's bureaus for Eli Lilly and GlaxoSmithKline.

Author Contributions: Dr Wagner, as principal author of this article, and Dr Yang, as principal statistician for the analyses, had full access to all study data and take responsibility for the integrity of the data and the accuracy of the data analyses. All coauthors also had access to the data.

Study concept and design: Wagner, Ambrosini, Wohlberg

Acquisition of data: Wagner, Ambrosini, Rynn, Wohlberg, Greenbaum, Childress, Donnelly, Deas.

Analysis and interpretation of data: Wagner, Ambrosini, Wohlberg, Yang.

Drafting of the manuscript: Wagner, Wohlberg, Yang, Donnelly

Critical revision of the manuscript for important intellectual content: Wagner, Ambrosini, Rynn, Wohlberg, Greenbaum, Childress, Donnelly

Statistical expertise: Yang

Obtained funding: Wohlberg

Administrative, technical, or material support: Ambrosini, Wohlberg, Donnelly

Study supervision: Wohlberg

Sertraline Pediatric Depression Study Group Investigators: United States: M. Bangs, L. Beckett, C. Borchardt, R. Brown, J. Danziger, S. Dubovsky, C. Foley, D. Geenens, R. Hendren, H. Johnston, S. Kronmal, E. Lee, M. Levin, M. Liebowitz, P. Londborg, J. March, C. Merideth, M. Minto, W. Murphy, J. Oldroyd, H. Quintana, M. Rapaport, R. Ricardi, M. Rieser, D. Robbins, W. Rosenfeld, B. Sangal, K. Saylor, V. Sharma, R. Steingard, J. Walkup, K. Toups, K. Weihs, D. Weisbrot; Canada: A. Duffy, S. Fisman, W. Fleisher, J. Garland, T. Wilkes; Costa Rica: Y. Jaramillo-Borges; Mexico: A. Ontiveros, Brazil: S. Ines Ruschel; India: S. Derasari, P. Satya Venkata Narsimha Sharma, S. Parkar, K. Kumar Ayyappan, T. John, S. Srinath, D. Mohan, G. Devi Mandadi, N. Brahmavar Pai.

Funding/Support: Funding for these trials was provided by Pfizer Inc.

Role of the Sponsor: Pfizer Inc participated in the completion of the study protocol based on input from study investigators, monitored the study, produced the statistical output, and assisted in the generation of the manuscript. Final approval of the manuscript content was provided by the principal author and was not under the control of the sponsor.

REFERENCES

1. American Psychiatric Association. *Diagnostic and Statistical Manual of Mental Disorders. Fourth Edition.* Washington, DC: American Psychiatric Association; 1994.
2. Emslie GJ, Kennard BD, Kowatch RA. Affective disorders in children: diagnosis and management. *J Child Neurol.* 1995;10(suppl):42-49.
3. Birmaher B, Ryan ND, Williamson DE, et al. Childhood and adolescent depression: a review of the past 10 years, part 1. *J Am Acad Child Adolesc Psychiatry.* 1996;35:1427-1439.
4. Kovacs M. Presentation and course of major depressive disorder during childhood and later years of the life span. *J Am Acad Child Adolesc Psychiatry.* 1996;35:705-715.
5. McCauley E, Myers K, Mitchell J, Calderon R, Schloredt K, Treder R. Depression in young people: initial presentation and clinical course. *J Am Acad Child Adolesc Psychiatry.* 1993;32:714-722.
6. Birmaher B, Brent DA, Benson RS. Summary of the practice parameters for the assessment and treatment of children and adolescents with depressive disorders. *J Am Acad Child Adolesc Psychiatry.* 1998;37:1234-1238.
7. Kovacs M, Feinberg TL, Crouse-Novak M, Paulauskas SL, Pollock M, Finkelstein R. Depressive disorders in childhood, I: a longitudinal prospective study of characteristics and recovery. *Arch Gen Psychiatry.* 1984;41:229-237.
8. Lewinsohn PM, Clarke GN, Seeley JR, Rohde P. Major depression in community adolescents: age at onset, episode duration, and time to recurrence. *J Am Acad Child Adolesc Psychiatry.* 1994;33:809-818.
9. Kovacs M, Feinberg TL, Crouse-Novak M, Paulauskas SL, Pollack M, Finkelstein R. Depressive disorders in childhood, II: a longitudinal study of the risk for a subsequent major depression. *Arch Gen Psychiatry.* 1984;41:643-649.
10. Klerman GL, Weissman MM. Increasing rates of depression. *JAMA.* 1989;261:2229-2235.
11. Gershon ES, Hamovit JH, Guroff JJ, Nurnberger JI. Birth-cohort changes in manic and depressive disorders in relatives of bipolar and schioaffective patients. *Arch Gen Psychiatry.* 1987;44:314-319.

12. Kessler RC, Walters EE. Epidemiology of *DSM-III-R* major depression and minor depression among adolescents and young adults in the National Comorbidity Survey. *Depress Anxiety*. 1998;7:3-14.

13. Blazer DG, Kessler RC, McGonagle KA, Swartz MS. The prevalence and distribution of major depression in a national comorbidity sample: the National Comorbidity Survey. *Am J Psychiatry*. 1994;151:979-986.

14. Weissman MM, Wolk S, Wickramaratne P, et al. Children with prepubertal-onset major depressive disorder and anxiety grown up. *Arch Gen Psychiatry*. 1999;56:794-801.

15. Weissman MM, Wolk S, Goldstein RB, et al. Depressed adolescents grown up. *JAMA*. 1999;281:1707-1713.

16. Pine DS, Cohen P, Gurley D, Brook J, Ma Y. The risk for early-adulthood anxiety and depressive disorders in adolescents with anxiety and depressive disorders. *Arch Gen Psychiatry*. 1998;55:56-64.

17. Berndt ER, Koran LM, Finkelstein SN, et al. Lost human capital from early-onset chronic depression. *Am J Psychiatry*. 2000;157:940-947.

18. Rao U, Weissman MM, Martin JA, Hammond RW. Childhood depression and risk of suicide: a preliminary report of a longitudinal study. *J Am Acad Child Adolesc Psychiatry*. 1993;32:21-27.

19. Ornstein S, Stuart G, Jenkins R. Depression diagnoses and antidepressant use in primary care practices: a study from the Practice Partner Research Network (PRPNet). *J Fam Pract*. 2000;49:68-72.

20. Hazell P, O'Connell D, Heathcote D, Robertson J, Henry D. Efficacy of tricyclic drugs in treating child and adolescent depression: a meta-analysis. *BMJ*. 1995;310:897-901.

21. Ambrosini PJ. A review of pharmacotherapy of major depression in children and adolescents. *Psychiatr Serv*. 2000;51:627-633.

22. Kastelic EA, Labellarte MJ, Riddle MA. Selective serotonin reuptake inhibitors for children and adolescents. *Curr Psychiatry Rep*. 2000;2:117-123.

23. Boulos C, Kutcher S, Gardner D, Young E. An open naturalistic trial of fluoxetine in adolescents and young adults with treatment-resistant major depression. *J Child Adolesc Psychopharmacol*. 1992;2:103-111.

24. Colle LM, Belair J-F, DiFeo M. Extended open-label treatment of adolescents with major depression. *J Child Adolesc Psychopharmacol*. 1994;4:225-232.

25. Ghaziuddin N, Naylor MW, King CA. Fluoxetine in tricyclic refractory depression in adolescents. *Depression*. 1995;2:287-291.

26. Findling R, Fiala S, Myers C. Putative determinants of paroxetine response in pediatric patients with major depression [abstract]. *Psychopharmacol Bull*. 1996;32:446.

27. Rey-Sanchez F, Gutierrez-Casares JR. Paroxetine in children with major depressive disorder: an open trial. *J Am Acad Child Adolesc Psychiatry*. 1997;36:1443-1447.

28. Apter A, Ratzoni G, King RA, et al. Fluvoxamine open-label treatment of adolescent inpatients with obsessive-compulsive disorder or depression. *J Am Acad Child Adolesc Psychiatry*. 1994;33:342-348.

29. Emslie GJ, Rush J, Weinberg WA, et al. A double-blind, randomized, placebo-controlled trial of fluoxetine in children and adolescents with depression. *Arch Gen Psychiatry*. 1997;54:1031-1037.

30. Emslie GJ, Heiligenstein JH, Wagner KD, et al. Fluoxetine for acute treatment of depression in children and adolescents: a placebo-controlled, randomized clinical trial. *J Am Acad Child Adolesc Psychiatry*. 2002;41:1205-1215.

31. Keller MB, Ryan ND, Strober M, et al. Efficacy of paroxetine in the treatment of adolescent major depression: a randomized, controlled trial. *J Am Acad Child Adolesc Psychiatry*. 2001;40:762-772.

32. McConville BJ, Minnery KL, Sorter MT, West SA, Friedman LM, Christian K. An open study of the effects of sertraline on adolescent depression. *J Child Adolesc Psychopharmacol*. 1996;6:41-51.

33. Ambrosini PJ, Wagner KD, Biederman J, et al. Multicenter open-label sertraline study in adolescent outpatients with major depression. *J Am Acad Child Adolesc Psychiatry*. 1999;38:566-572.

34. Nixon MK, Milin R, Simeon JG, Cloutier P, Spenst W. Sertraline effects in adolescent major depression and dysthymia: a six-month open trial. *J Child Adolesc Psychopharmacol*. 2001;11:131-142.

35. Tierney E, Joshi PT, Llinas JF, Rosenberg LA, Riddle MA. Sertraline for major depression in children and adolescents: preliminary clinical experience. *J Child Adolesc Psychopharmacol*. 1995;5:13-27.

36. Kaufman J, Birmaher B, Brent D, et al. Schedule for affective disorders and schizophrenia for school-age children—present and lifetime version (K-SADS-PL): initial reliability and validity data. *J Am Acad Child Adolesc Psychiatry*. 1997;36:980-988.

37. Poznanski EO, Freeman LN, Mokros HB. Children's Depression Rating Scale—Revised (September 1984). *Psychopharmacol Bull*. 1985;21:979-989.

38. Poznanski EO, Mokros HB. *Children's Depression Rating Scale, Revised (CDRS-R) Manual*. Los Angeles, Calif: Western Psychological Services; 1995.

39. Guy W. *ECDEU Assessment Manual for Psychopharmacology*. Rockville, Md: National Institute of Mental Health; 1976.

40. March JS, Parker JD, Sullivan K, Stallings P, Conners CK. The multidimensional anxiety scale for children (MASC): factor structure, reliability, and validity. *J Am Acad Child Adolesc Psychiatry*. 1997;36:554-565.

41. Schaffer D, Gould MS, Brasic J, et al. A Children's Global Assessment Scale (CGAS). *Arch Gen Psychiatry*. 1983;40:1228-1231.

42. Endicott J, Nee J, Harrison W, Blumenthal R. Quality of Life Enjoyment and Satisfaction Questionnaire: a new measure. *Psychopharmacol Bull*. 1993;29:321-326.

43. Findling R, Reed M, Blumer J. Pharmacological treatment of depression in children and adolescents. *Paediatr Drugs*. 1999;1:161-182.

44. Amsterdam J, Brunswick D. Site variability in treatment outcome in antidepressant trials. *Prog Neuropsychopharmacol Biol Psychiatry*. 2002;26:989-993.

45. Small G, Schneider, L, Hamilton S, et al. Site variability in a multisite geriatric depression trial. *Int J Geriatr Psychiatry*. 1996;11:1089-1095.

46. Walsh BT, Seidman SN, Sysko R, Gould M. Placebo response in studies of major depression. *JAMA*. 2002;287:1840-1847.

47. *FDA Discusses Pediatric Drug Safety With its Advisory Subcommittee Under Best Pharmaceuticals for Children Act*. Washington, DC: US Food and Drug Administration; 2003. FDA Talk Paper T03-41.

48. Alderman J, Wolkow R, Chung M, Johnston HF. Sertraline treatment of children and adolescents with obsessive-compulsive disorder or depression: pharmacokinetics, tolerability, and efficacy. *J Am Acad Child Adolesc Psychiatry*. 1998;37:386-394.

49. Rynn M, Wagner KD, Donnelly C, Ambrosini PJ, Landau P, Wohlberg C. Long-term safety and tolerability of sertraline in children and adolescents with MDD. Paper presented at: 156th Annual Meeting of the American Psychiatric Association; May 17-22, 2003; San Francisco, Calif.

Psychopharmacological Treatment of Major Depressive Disorder in Children and Adolescents

Christopher K. Varley, MD

THE REPORT BY WAGNER AND COLLEAGUES[1] IN THIS ISsue of THE JOURNAL, a pooled analysis of 2 multicenter, double-blind, randomized placebo-controlled trials evaluating the effect of the selective serotonin reuptake inhibitor (SSRI) sertraline on children and adolescents aged 6 to 17 years with major depressive disorder (MDD), constitutes the largest positive psychopharmacological study of MDD in this age group reported to date. The primary outcome was change from baseline in the Children's Depression Rating Scale–Revised (CDRS-R), with a prospectively determined primary efficacy measure of the CDRS-R Best Description of Child total score; secondary efficacy measures included the proportion of CDRS-R responders, defined as patients who had at least a 40% decrease in the adjusted CDRS-R total score. The results indicate a statistically significant improvement for patients receiving active drug vs those receiving placebo.

An increasing body of knowledge confirms that depression is a common and serious illness in youth, affecting 3% to 8% of children and adolescents.[2] Moreover, rates of depression increase dramatically as children move into adolescence.[3] An estimated 20% of adolescents have had at least 1 episode of MDD by age 18 years, while 65% report transient, less severe depressive symptoms.[4,5] Depression compromises the developmental process; feelings of worthlessness, low self-esteem, and thoughts of suicide are common, as are difficulties with concentration and motivation.[6] As many as 20% of adolescents each year have suicide ideation and 5% to 8% attempt suicide.[7] While the majority of attempts are not lethal, suicide is a leading cause of death in adolescents and is a major health care concern. One of the major risk factors associated with suicide is depression.

Depressive disorders in children and adolescents can be chronic and recurrent. The mean length of a major depressive episode in youth aged 6 to 17 years is 7 to 9 months, with remittance commonly occurring over a 1½- to 2-year period.[8] Longitudinal studies suggest a strong potential for recurrence; 48% to 60% of this age group have recurrence of major depression after an initial MDD episode within 5 years.[6,8]

See also p 1033.

Although depression in youth is now recognized as a significant health concern, identification of safe and effective treatment has been challenging. The study by Wagner et al in this issue of THE JOURNAL is the fourth published double-blind, placebo-controlled study demonstrating efficacy in the treatment of MDD in children and adolescents; all studies included SSRIs. In 1997, Emslie et al[9] reported the first randomized controlled trial examining the efficacy of an antidepressant (fluoxetine) in the treatment of MDD. In 2001, Keller et al[10] reported a trial showing the efficacy of paroxetine. In 2002, Emslie et al[11] reported another positive study with fluoxetine. In 2001, Wagner et al[12] presented data from a positive double-blind, placebo-controlled trial of citalopram, but to date, the results have not been published in a peer-reviewed journal.

A number of psychotropic medications established as safe and effective in the treatment of MDD in adults have been investigated in youth but may not be effective, including tricyclic antidepressants, monoamine oxidase inhibitors, and venlafaxine.[13,14] There are also safety concerns regarding the use of tricyclic antidepressants in children and adolescents, including lethality in overdose and cardiac conduction delays (and possibly increased risk of sudden death) in therapeutic dosages.[15]

On the basis of the 2 positive studies,[9,11] fluoxetine has received US Food and Drug Administration (FDA) labeling as safe and effective for the treatment of MDD in children and adolescents. However, the SSRI findings are not without controversy. The beneficial effects in both fluoxetine studies were modest,[9,11] and in the second, larger multicenter study,[11] not all of the prospectively identified primary outcome measures were significantly different than with placebo.

Similarly, in the study by Keller et al,[10] the response rate for patients receiving paroxetine was 63% compared with 50% for imipramine and 46% for placebo. Only 1 of 2 prospectively identified primary outcome measures achieved statistical significance. Two other large placebo-controlled trials of paroxetine in MDD were negative (written com-

Author Affiliation: Division of Child and Adolescent Psychiatry, Department of Psychiatry and Behavioral Sciences, University of Washington School of Medicine, Seattle.
Corresponding Author and Reprints: Christopher K. Varley, MD, Division of Child and Adolescent Psychiatry, Department of Psychiatry and Behavioral Sciences, University of Washington School of Medicine, Box 359300/CL-08, Seattle, WA 98195 (e-mail: cvarley@u.washington.edu).

nunication, Philip Perera, MD, Medical Information Department, GlaxoSmithKline, July 9, 2003).[16]

In the current study by Wagner et al, 69% of the patients receiving sertraline were considered responders compared with 59% of those receiving placebo, a difference of only 10%.[1] These findings suggest that children may be more responsive than adults to nonspecific measures of support that are included in the placebo response, possibly because children and adolescents are in a more dependent and reactive developmental state.

Despite this limited evidence base, prescription of psychotropic medications for the treatment of depression in children and adolescents has increased dramatically.[17] In a study of almost 900000 youths enrolled in 3 large health care systems, antidepressant medication prevalence increased in the period 1987-1996 by a factor of 3.6 at one site, 6.2 at a second, and 10.4 at a third.[17]

One attractive feature of the SSRIs has been their relative safety profile. Previous concerns regarding a possible association with suicidal ideation and attempts in adults led to scientific review, as well as congressional hearings, ultimately revealing no causal link.[18]

Recent reports by regulatory agencies have expressed concern regarding the use of paroxetine in children and adolescents. On June 10, 2003, Gordon Duff, chairman of the Committee on Safety in Medicines in Great Britain, wrote that paroxetine was now contraindicated and "should not be used in children and adolescents under the age of 18 years to treat depressive illness."[19] This message came 2 weeks after new data from clinical trials sponsored by the manufacturer of paroxetine were received by the Medicines and Health Care Products Regulatory Agency (MHRA). These trials of paroxetine included more than 1000 patients aged 7 to 17 years (written communication, Philip Perera, MD, Medical Information Department, GlaxoSmithKline, July 9, 2003). There were no deaths due to suicide, although the rates of suicidal thinking and suicide attempt were higher among those receiving paroxetine compared with placebo. An expert working group reviewed the data and concluded that paroxetine did not demonstrate efficacy in depressive illness in this age group. In addition, the risk of harmful outcomes, including episodes of self-harm and potentially suicidal behavior, was estimated to be between 1.5 and 3.2 times higher with paroxetine than with placebo. The balance of risks and benefits with paroxetine was assessed to be "unfavourable when used to treat depressive illness in this age group."[19]

On June 19, 2003, the FDA posted a talk paper indicating that the possible increased risk of suicidal thinking and suicide attempts in youth younger than 18 years who were treated with paroxetine for MDD was being reviewed.[20] The FDA recommended that paroxetine not be used in children and adolescents with MDD while this issue was under review. Both the FDA and the MHRA suggest that there is no evidence that paroxetine is effective in children or adolescents with MDD,[19,20] even though the study by Keller et al[10] reported some benefit.

In addition, in the study by Keller et al,[10] serious adverse events were defined as those that resulted in hospitalization, were associated with suicidal gestures, or were described by the treating physician as serious. Serious adverse events occurred in 11 patients treated with paroxetine, 5 with imipramine, and 2 with placebo. The serious adverse events in the paroxetine group included 10 patients with various psychiatric events, including worsening of depression (n=2), emotional lability, which included suicidal ideation and gestures (n=5), conduct problems or hostility, including aggressiveness (n=2), and euphoric mood or expansiveness (n=1). Seven patients in the paroxetine group were hospitalized because of worsening depression (n=2), emotional lability (n=2), conduct problems (n=1), or euphoria (n=1). In the placebo group, 1 patient had emotional lability and 1 patient had worsening depression; both were considered serious adverse events.

In the study by Wagner and colleagues, sertraline was reported as generally well tolerated, although more patients receiving the active drug (9%) than receiving placebo (3%) discontinued medication because of adverse events, most commonly reported as abdominal pain, diarrhea, and nausea.[1] Serious adverse events included suicide attempts in 2 patients in the sertraline group and 2 patients in the placebo group; 3 patients receiving sertraline had suicidal ideation and 1 receiving sertraline had an aggressive reaction.

In contrast, the fluoxetine studies do not report higher rates of adverse events, including mood symptoms or suicidal ideation, with active drug compared with placebo.[9,11]

Depression is an illness associated with agitation, despair, self-loathing, and suicide. Suicide attempts may occur as depression is lifting and an individual is energized enough to act on thoughts of self-harm. Since suicide is rare in children and adolescents, ascertaining whether there is a meaningful increased risk of suicidal ideation, suicide attempts, or suicide completion associated with any medication used to treat depression will require review of large numbers of patients.

Until this issue is resolved, prudent practice in the treatment of depressive illnesses in children and adolescents must include careful attention to the decision to treat a child or adolescent with medication for MDD; clinical expertise with mental health assessment, consideration of varied treatment modes including cognitive behavioral or interpersonal psychotherapy, partnership with patients and their parents, and careful attention to symptom course, particularly emotional lability and the assessment of suicidal ideation in youth who are treated with antidepressant medications (specifically, SSRIs, and more particularly, paroxetine). Current evidence continues to support the use of SSRIs, particularly fluoxetine and sertraline, in the treatment of MDD in children and adolescents. Caution is indicated at this time regarding the use of paroxetine in children and adolescents with MDD, and a clinician would be ill-advised to begin treatment with paroxetine for a patient younger than 18 years with MDD. In patients who have been identified as having a robust response to paroxetine, it does not appear prudent to switch to another SSRI based on current data.

REFERENCES

1. Wagner KD, Ambrosini P, Rynn M, et al. Efficacy of sertraline in the treatment of children and adolescents with major depressive disorder: two randomized controlled trials. *JAMA*. 2003;290:1033-1041.
2. Birmaher B, Ryan ND, Williamson DE, et al. Childhood and adolescent depression: a review of the past 10 years: part 1. *J Am Acad Child Adolesc Psychiatry*. 1996;35:1427-1439.
3. Compass BE, Connor JK, Hinden BR. *New Perspectives on Depression During Adolescence: New Perspectives on Adolescent Risk Behavior*. Cambridge, England: Cambridge University Press; 1998:319-362.
4. Lewinsohn PM, Hops H, Roberts RE, Seeley JR, Andrews JA. Adolescent psychopathology, I: prevalence and incidence of depression and other *DSM-III-R* disorders in high school students. *J Abnorm Psychol*. 1993;102:133-144.
5. American Academy of Child and Adolescent Psychiatry (1998) practice parameters for the assessment and treatment of children and adolescents with depressive disorders. *J Am Acad Child Adolesc Psychiatry*. 1998;37(suppl):63S-83S.
6. McCauley E, Myers K. Longitudinal course of depressive disorders in young people. *Child Adolesc Psychiatr Clin N Am*. 1992;1:183-196.
7. Grunbaum JA, Kann L, Kinchen SA, et al. Youth risk behavior surveillance—United States, 2001. *MMWR CDC Surveill Summ*. 2002;51(SS-4):1-62.
8. McCauley E, Myers K, Mitchell J, Calderon R, Schloredt K, Treder R. Depression in young people: initial presentation and clinical course. *J Am Acad Child Adolesc Psychiatry*. 1993;32:714-722.
9. Emslie GJ, Rush AJ, Weinberg WA, et al. A double-blind, randomized, placebo-controlled trial of fluoxetine in children and adolescents with depression. *Arch Gen Psychiatry*. 1997;54:1031-1037.
10. Keller MB, Ryan ND, Strober M, et al. Efficacy of paroxetine in the treatment of adolescent major depressive disorder: a randomized, controlled trial. *J Am Acad Child Adolesc Psychiatry*. 2001;40:762-772.
11. Emslie GJ, Heiligenstein JH, Wagner KD, et al. Fluoxetine for acute treatment of depression in children and adolescents: a placebo-controlled, randomized clinical trial. *J Am Acad Child Adolesc Psychiatry*. 2002;41:1205-1215.
12. Wagner KD, Robb AS, Findling R, Tiseo PJ. Citalopram is effective in the treatment of major depressive disorder in children and adolescents: results of a placebo-controlled trial. Paper presented at: 40th Annual Meeting of the American College of Neuropsychopharmacology; December 9-12, 2001; Waikoloa, Hawaii.
13. Dulcan MK, Bregman J, Weller EB, Weller R. Treatment of childhood and adolescent disorders. In: Schatzberg AF, Nemeroff CB, eds. *Textbook of Psychopharmacology*. 2nd ed. Washington, DC: American Psychiatry Press; 1998:803-850.
14. Mandoki MW, Tapia MR, Tapia MA, Sumner GS, Parker JL. Venlafaxine in the treatment of children and adolescents with major depression. *Psychopharmacol Bull*. 1997;33:149-154.
15. Varley CK. Sudden death related to selected tricyclic antidepressants in children. *Paediatr Drugs*. 2001;3:613-627.
16. Milin RP, Simeon J, Spenst WP. Poster presented at: 46th Annual American Academy of Child and Adolescent Psychiatry Meeting; October 19-21, 1999; Chicago, Ill. Abstract NR67.
17. Zito JM, Safer DJ, DosReis S, et al. Rising prevalence of antidepressant treatment for US children and adolescents. *Pediatrics*. 2000;109:721-727.
18. Khan A, Khan S, Kolts R, Brown WA. Suicide rates in clinical trials of SSRIs, other antidepressants, and placebo: analysis of FDA reports. *Am J Psychiatry*. 2003;160:790-792.
19. Duff G. Safety of Seroxat (paroxetine) in children and adolescents under 18 years, contraindication in the treatment of depressive illness. United Kingdom's Department of Health's Chairman of Committee of Safety of Medicine's message on paroxetine. Available at: http://www.mca.gov.uk. Accessibility verified August 6, 2003.
20. US Food and Drug Administration. FDA statement regarding the antidepressant Paxil for pediatric depression. FDA Talk Paper. June 19, 2003. Available at: http://www.fda.gov/bbs/topics/ANSWERS/2003/ANS01230.html. Accessibility verified August 8, 2003.

Tab 86

Pediatric Program Summary Statistics

Since the pediatric exclusivity program began, 283 Written Requests have been issued and 88 drugs have been granted exclusivity. Among these, only fluoxetine has been approved for the treatment of major depressive disorder in pediatric patients; the labeling changes for pediatric major depressive disorder that were made following these studies are summarized as follows:

- Effectiveness established in patients 8-17 years of age for MDD
- Decreased weight gain has been observed in association with the use of fluoxetine, as with other SSRIs. In one 19-week clinical trial pediatric subjects treated with fluoxetine gained an average of 1.1cm less in height (p=0.004) and 1.1 kg less in weight (p=0.008) than those treated with placebo. Therefore, height and weight should be monitored periodically in pediatric patients treated with fluoxetine.
- Mania/hypomania led to discontinuation of 1.8% of fluoxetine treated patients vs. 0% of placebo controlled patients in the three placebo-controlled trials combined. Regular monitoring for the occurrence of mania/hypomania is recommended
- Higher average steady state fluoxetine and norfluoxetine concentrations were observed in children than in adolescents. These differences were almost entirely explained by differences in weight.
- Separate dosing recommendations in lower weight children

The Division of Neuropharmacologic Drug Products has developed a template for pediatric written requests for the study of antidepressants, which is provided here.

****

Sample Written Request for Antidepressants

This is a sample Written Request outlining the pediatric studies the Agency believes will provide a meaningful health benefit to the pediatric population for antidepressants. An actual Written Request may differ from this sample depending upon the nature of the specific drug product and any other indications for which it is used. To receive a formal Written Request for pediatric studies under section 505A of the Federal Food, Drug, and Cosmetic Act for a particular antidepressant agent, please submit a proposed pediatric study request to the Division of Neuropharmacologic Drug Products. The proposed pediatric study request should incorporate the material in this sample and include descriptions of any other studies necessary to provide a meaningful health benefit to pediatric populations. Please refer to the outline in the "Guidance For Industry - Qualifying for Pediatric Exclusivity Under Section 505A of the Federal Food, Drug, and Cosmetic Act," for additional information.

NDA XX-XXX
Sponsor
Attention: Contact
Address

Three Years From the
Date of the Original WR__________

Dear Contact:

Reference is made to your Proposed Pediatric Study Request submitted on [Insert date] to your New Drug Application for [Insert Drug].

To obtain needed pediatric information on [Insert drug], the Food and Drug Administration (FDA) is hereby making a formal Written Request, pursuant to Section 505A of the Federal Food, Drug, and Cosmetic Act (the Act), that you submit information from the trials in pediatric patients with depression described below.

PEDIATRIC DEPRESSION

Background Comments on Pediatric Depression

Under current regulations [21 CFR 201.57(f)(9)(iv)], a new claim in a pediatric population could be established by extrapolating the effectiveness results of adequate and well controlled studies in adults for the same entity if it were believed that depression was essentially the same disease in adults and children. Under FDAMA (1997), a claim might be based on a single study in pediatric patients along with confirmatory evidence from another source, perhaps adult data for that disorder, an approach considered in the draft guidance document entitled "Guidance for Industry - Providing Clinical Evidence of Effectiveness for Human Drug and Biological Products". This approach too requires some degree of belief that the course of the disease and the effects of the drug are sufficiently similar in the pediatric and adult populations to make data from the adult efficacy studies pertinent to pediatric patients. Unfortunately, in our view there is little reason to assume continuity between adult and pediatric depression and our concern about the extrapolability of adult depression data to pediatric depression is more than theoretical. While we, of course, acknowledge the one published positive report of fluoxetine in pediatric depression (Emslie, et al, 1997), we are concerned about the preponderance of negative studies of antidepressants in pediatric populations. We recognize that all of these negative studies utilized tricyclic antidepressants, and that, in addition, there are other possible explanations for the negative outcomes, e.g., sample size, entry criteria, outcome measures, etc. Nevertheless, these negative trials (at least 12 in number) lead to a substantial concern about the ability to extrapolate positive antidepressant findings from adult to pediatric patients. Consequently, we believe that a pediatric depression claim for any antidepressant already approved in adult depression would need to be supported by two independent, adequate and well controlled clinical trials in pediatric depression. In addition, a pediatric depression program would need to include pharmacokinetic information and safety information in the relevant pediatric age groups. For pediatric depression, we consider the relevant age groups to include children (ages 7 through 11) and adolescents (ages 12 through 17).

Specific Study Requirements for Development Program in Pediatric Depression

Types of Studies:

Pediatric Efficacy and Safety Studies
Pediatric Pharmacokinetic Study
Pediatric Safety Study

Objective/Rationale:

The overall goal of the development program is to establish the safety and efficacy of the study drug in the treatment of pediatric depression, and to develop other information, e.g., pharmacokinetic, pertinent to using the drug in the pediatric population.

Study Design:

Pediatric Efficacy and Safety Studies

For the controlled efficacy studies, conduct two randomized, double-blind, parallel group, placebo-controlled acute treatment trials, with a recommended duration of at least 6 to 8 weeks. We recommend that at least one of the two studies should be a fixed dose study including two or more fixed doses of the study drug. You may consider dosing patients on the basis of patient weight. Randomization must be stratified by the two age groups studied. Ideally, a relapse prevention trial would follow from the acute treatment trials, involving the randomization of responders from the acute treatment trials to continuation on either study drug or placebo, with follow-up observation for relapse for a period of 6 months or more. Please note that a relapse prevention trial is not required under this written request.

Pediatric Pharmacokinetic Study

A pharmacokinetic study to provide information pertinent to dosing of the study drug in the relevant pediatric population. These data could come from traditional pharmacokinetic studies, or alternatively, from population kinetic approaches applied to controlled efficacy trials or to other safety trials. You should be aware that a guidance document on population pharmacokinetic studies is available under [www.fda.gov/cder/guidance/1852fnl.pdf].

Pediatric Safety Study

Safety data should be collected in the controlled efficacy trials. Longer-term safety data should be generated in longer-term open extensions from these trials and/or in separate longer-term open safety studies.

Age Group in Which Study(ies) will be Performed - All Studies:

Both children (ages 7 to 11) and adolescents (ages 12 to 17) should be equally represented in the samples, and there should be a reasonable distribution of both sexes in these strata.

Number of Patients to be Studied or Power of Study to be Achieved:

Pediatric Efficacy and Safety Studies
While it is difficult to specify the sample size needed to show a difference between drug and placebo in this population, it should be noted that, in the only published positive antidepressant trial in pediatric depression (Emslie, et al, 1997), there were 48 patients in each of the two treatment arms.
Pediatric Pharmacokinetic Study
A sufficient number of subjects to adequately characterize the pharmacokinetics in the above age groups.
Pediatric Safety Study
A sufficient number of pediatric patients to adequately characterize the safety of [Insert drug] at clinically effective doses for a sufficient duration.
Entry Criteria:
The protocols should include a valid and reliable diagnostic method for recruiting children and adolescents with major depressive disorder.
Study Endpoints:
Pediatric Efficacy and Safety Studies
It is essential to identify a single primary outcome for the controlled efficacy trials, and ordinarily this should be change from baseline to endpoint on whatever symptom rating scale you have chosen for your trials.
Pediatric Pharmacokinetic Study
Pharmacokinetic measurements as appropriate.
Pediatric Safety Study
Appropriately frequent standard measures of safety (clinical - including signs and symptoms and laboratory).
Statistical Information:
Pediatric Efficacy and Safety Studies
These trials should have a detailed statistical plan. Ordinarily these trials should be designed with at least 80% statistical power to detect a treatment effect of conventional (p=0.05) statistical significance.
Pediatric Pharmacokinetic Study
Descriptive analysis of the pharmacokinetic parameters.
Pediatric Safety Study
Descriptive analysis of the safety data.
Study Evaluations:
Pediatric Efficacy and Safety Studies
A scale specific to pediatric depression and sensitive to the effects of drug treatment of pediatric depression, e.g., the Children's Depression Rating Scale-Revised, and a global measure, e.g., the Clinical Global Impression (CGI).
Pediatric Pharmacokinetic Study
The pharmacokinetic assessments should be made with respect to the study drug and any metabolites that make substantial contributions to its efficacy and/or toxicity. For the parent and each metabolite followed, the data collected should provide estimates of the pharmacokinetic parameters including AUC, half-life, C_{max}, t_{max}, and apparent oral clearance in pediatric subjects in the relevant age range. You should be aware that a draft guidance document on pediatric pharmacokinetic studies is available under [www.fda.gov/cder/guidance/index.htm, under Clinical/Pharmacological (Draft)].
Pediatric Safety Study
Routine safety assessments should include vital signs, weight, clinical laboratory, ECGs, and monitoring for adverse events. Although not a part of this Written Request, we remind you that it may be important to determine the effect of the study drug on the growth and development of pediatric patients, and we encourage you to consider longer-term studies of a year or more to address this question if the acute studies demonstrate antidepressant activity.
Drug Information:
Use age appropriate formulations in the studies described above. Since the pediatric patient population consists of both children (ages 7 to 11) and adolescents (ages 12 to 17), your marketed dosage formulation should be adequate for these studies.
Drug Concerns:
Specific concerns, if any, related to administration of drug to pediatric patients is to be conveyed in this paragraph.
Labeling that may result from the studies:
The pediatric depression efficacy, safety, and pharmacokinetic studies described in this request could result

in the addition to labeling of information pertinent to these studies.

Format of reports to be submitted:

Full study reports or analyses, not previously submitted to the Agency, addressing the issues outlined in this request, with full analysis, assessment, and interpretation. In addition, the reports are to include information on the representation of pediatric patients of ethnic and racial minorities. Include other information as appropriate

Timeframe for submitting reports of the Study(ies):

Reports of the above studies must be submitted to the Agency within 3 years from the date of this letter to be eligible to qualify for pediatric exclusivity extension under Section 505A of the Act. Please remember that pediatric exclusivity attaches only to existing patent protection or exclusivity that has not expired at the time you submit your reports of studies in response to this Written Request.

Response to Written Request:

As per the Best Pharmaceuticals for Children Act, section 4(A), within 180 days of receipt of this Written Request you must notify the Agency as to your intention to act on the Written Request. If you agree to the request then you must indicate when the pediatric studies will be initiated.

Please submit protocols for the above studies to an investigational new drug application (IND) and clearly mark your submission "**PEDIATRIC PROTOCOL SUBMITTED FOR PEDIATRIC EXCLUSIVITY STUDY**" in large font, bolded type at the beginning of the cover letter of the submission. Please notify us as soon as possible if you wish to enter into a written agreement by submitting a proposed written agreement. Clearly mark your submission "**PROPOSED WRITTEN AGREEMENT FOR PEDIATRIC STUDIES**" in large font, bolded type at the beginning of the cover letter of the submission.

Reports of the studies should be submitted as a supplement to your approved NDA with the proposed labeling changes you believe would be warranted based on the data derived from these studies. When submitting the reports, please clearly mark your submission "**SUBMISSION OF PEDIATRIC STUDY REPORTS - PEDIATRIC EXCLUSIVITY DETERMINATION REQUESTED**" in large font, bolded type at the beginning of the cover letter of the submission and include a copy of this letter. Please also send a copy of the cover letter of your submission, via fax (301-594-0183) or messenger to the Director, Office of Generic Drugs, HFD-600, Metro Park North II, 7500 Standish Place, Rockville, MD 20855-2773.

If you wish to discuss any amendments to this Written Request, please submit proposed changes and the reasons for the proposed changes to your application. Submissions of proposed changes to this request should be clearly marked "**PROPOSED CHANGES IN WRITTEN REQUEST FOR PEDIATRIC STUDIES**" in large font, bolded type at the beginning of the cover letter of the submission. You will be notified in writing if any changes to this Written Request are agreed upon by the Agency.

We hope you will fulfill this pediatric study request. We look forward to working with you on this matter in order to develop additional pediatric information that may produce health benefits to the pediatric population.

If you have any questions, contact [Insert Name], Regulatory Project Manager, at [Insert telephone number].

Sincerely yours,

[Office Directors Name]
Director
Office of Drug Evaluation I
Center for Drug Evaluation and Research

Drug Utilization for Selected Antidepressants Among Children & Adolescents in the U.S.

Tab 87

Gianna C. Rigoni, Pharm.D., M.S.
Epidemiologist
Division of Surveillance, Research & Communication Support
Office of Drug Safety, CDER, FDA

February 2, 2004

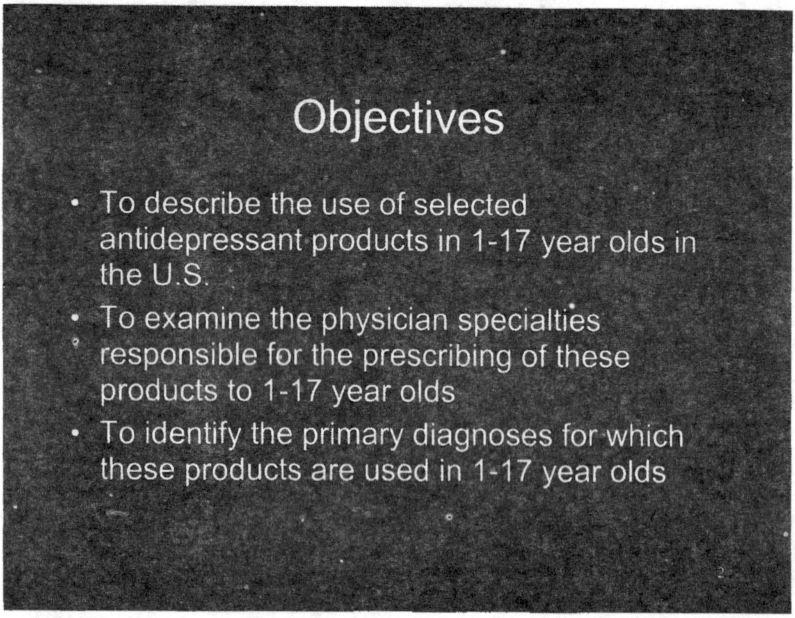
Objectives
To describe the use of selected antidepressant products in 1-17 year olds in the U.S.
To examine the physician specialties responsible for the prescribing of these products to 1-17 year olds
To identify the primary diagnoses for which these products are used in 1-17 year olds

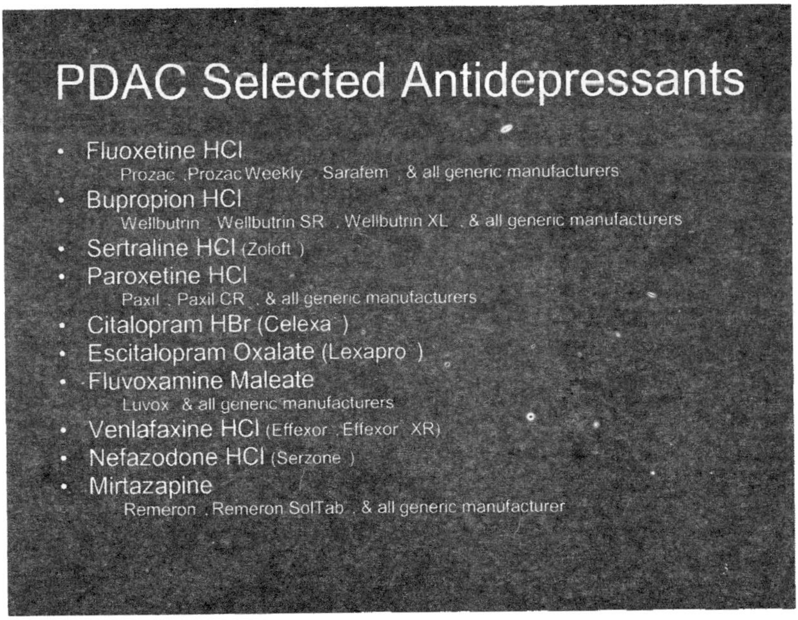
PDAC Selected Antidepressants
• Fluoxetine HCl
Prozac, Prozac Weekly, Sarafem, & all generic manufacturers
• Bupropion HCl
Wellbutrin, Wellbutrin SR, Wellbutrin XL, & all generic manufacturers
• Sertraline HCl (Zoloft)
• Paroxetine HCl
Paxil, Paxil CR, & all generic manufacturers
• Citalopram HBr (Celexa)
• Escitalopram Oxalate (Lexapro)
• Fluvoxamine Maleate
Luvox & all generic manufacturers
• Venlafaxine HCl (Effexor, Effexor XR)
• Nefazodone HCl (Serzone)
• Mirtazapine
Remeron, Remeron SolTab, & all generic manufacturer

FDA Labeled Indications for Antidepressant Use in Pediatrics

- Pediatric major depressive disorder (MDD)
  - Fluoxetine
- Pediatric obsessive-compulsive disorder (OCD)
  - Fluoxetine
  - Sertraline
  - Fluvoxamine

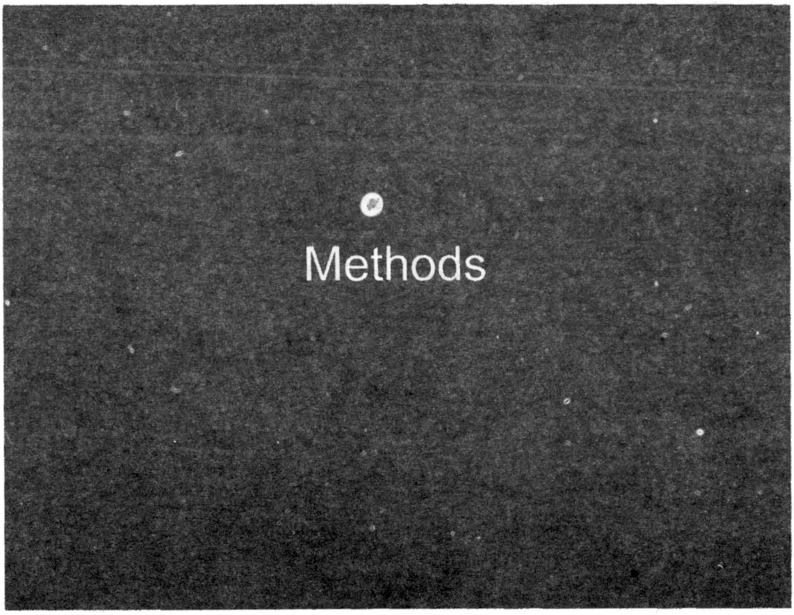
Methods

Methods

- Data analyzed from January 1988 – December 2002
- Outpatient Drug Utilization Data Sources
  - IMS Health, National Prescription Audit *Plus* (NPA *Plus*)
  - IMS Health, National Disease and Therapeutic Index (NDTI)

National Prescription Audit *Plus* (NPA *Plus*)

- Measures the "retail outflow" of prescriptions from pharmacies to consumers
  - Includes: chain, independent, mass merchandisers, food stores with pharmacies, mail-order, and long-term care pharmacies
- Number of dispensed prescriptions is obtained from a sample of approximately 22,000 pharmacies in the U.S.
  - Projected nationally

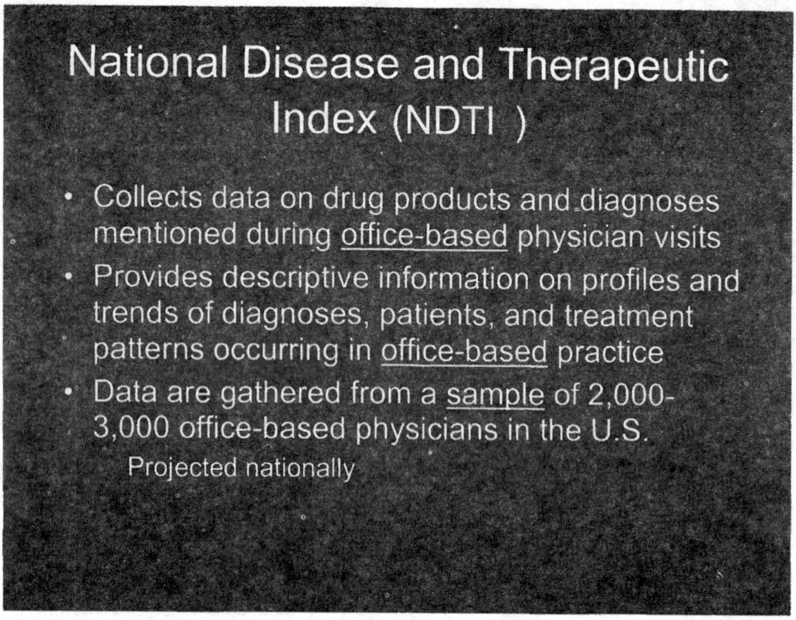
National Disease and Therapeutic Index (NDTI)
• Collects data on drug products and diagnoses mentioned during office-based physician visits
• Provides descriptive information on profiles and trends of diagnoses, patients, and treatment patterns occurring in office-based practice
• Data are gathered from a sample of 2,000-3,000 office-based physicians in the U.S.
Projected nationally

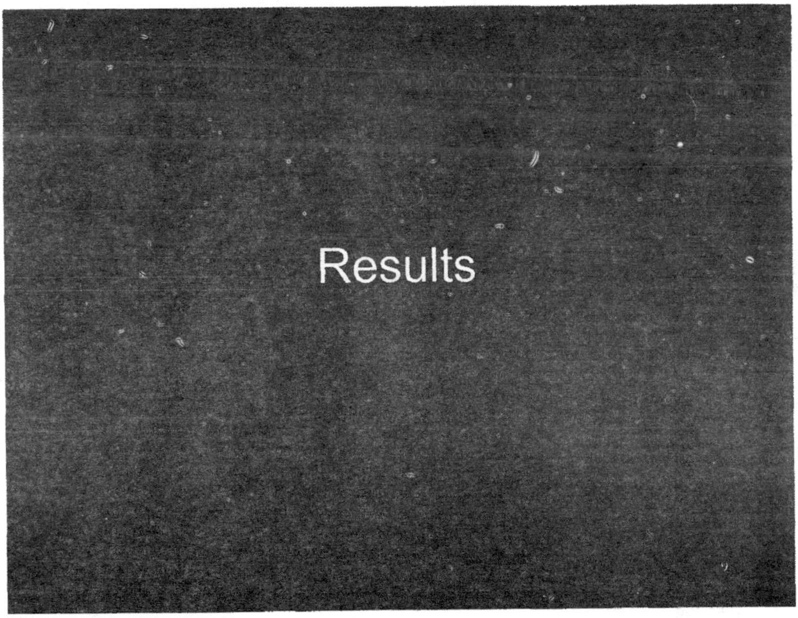
Results

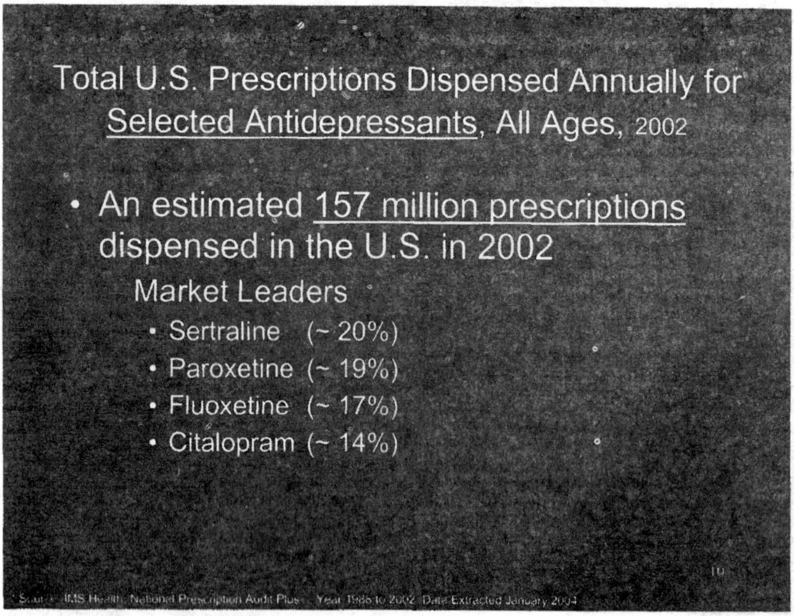
Total U.S. Prescriptions Dispensed Annually for Selected Antidepressants, All Ages, 2002
• An estimated 157 million prescriptions dispensed in the U.S. in 2002
Market Leaders
• Sertraline (~ 20%)
• Paroxetine (~ 19%)
• Fluoxetine (~ 17%)
• Citalopram (~ 14%)
10
Source: IMS Health, National Prescription Audit Plus, Year 1986 to 2002, Data Extracted January 2004

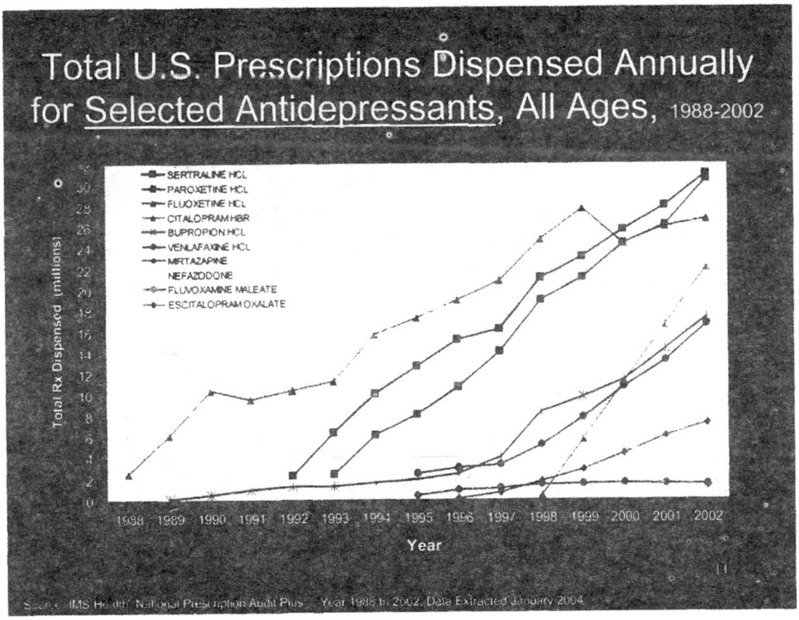
Total U.S. Prescriptions Dispensed Annually
for Selected Antidepressants, All Ages, 1988-2002
SERTRALINE HCL
PAROXETINE HCL
FLUOXETINE HCL
CITALOPRAM HBR
BUPROPION HCL
VENLAFAXINE HCL
MIRTAZAPINE
NEFAZODONE
FLUVOXAMINE MALEATE
ESCITALOPRAM OXALATE
Total Rx Dispensed (millions)
1988 1989 1990 1991 1992 1993 1994 1995 1996 1997 1998 1999 2000 2001 2002
Year
IMS Health, National Prescription Audit Plus Year 1988 to 2002, Data Extracted January 2004

Method for Estimating Use in 1-17 Year Olds from NPA *Plus*

- IMS Health NDTI™ data
  - Proportion of office-based physician visits that involved the mention of one of the selected antidepressants to 1-17 year olds
- IMS Health NPA *Plus*™ data
  - Applied NDTI proportion to the total number of prescriptions dispensed in the U.S. for that year

Source: IMS Health, National Prescription Audit Plus, National Disease and Therapeutic Index, Years 1998 to 2002, Data Extracted January, 2004

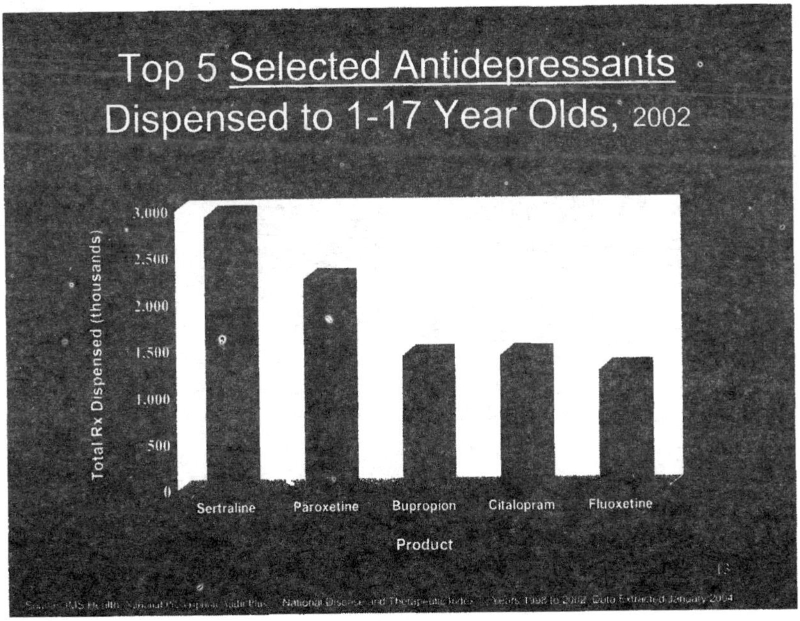
Top 5 Selected Antidepressants
Dispensed to 1-17 Year Olds, 2002
Total Rx Dispensed (thousands)
3,000
2,500
2,000
1,500
1,000
500
0
Sertraline
Paroxetine
Bupropion
Citalopram
Fluoxetine
Product
13

Total U.S. Prescriptions Dispensed Annually for Selected Antidepressants, Ages 1-17 Years, 2002

- Younger pediatric population (1-11 years)
  In 2002, an estimated 2.7 million prescriptions (~ 2% of total) dispensed
  - Sertraline (31%), paroxetine (18%), fluoxetine (16%)
- Adolescent population (12-17 years)
  In 2002, an estimated 8.1 million prescriptions (~ 5% of total) dispensed
  - Sertraline (26%), paroxetine (22%), bupropion (13%)

14

[illegible] National Disease and Therapeutic Index, Years 1998 to 2002. Data Extracted January 2004

Top Office-Based Prescriber Specialties Mentioning Selected Antidepressants, Ages 1-17 Years, 1998-2002

- Younger pediatric population (1-11 years)
  - Top ranked physician specialties have shifted slightly and relative proportions have also changed
    - **1998** Psychiatry (66%); Family Practice (10%); and Pediatrics (8%)
    - **2002** Psychiatry (64%); Pediatrics (17%); and Neurology (8%)
- Adolescent population (12-17 years)
  - Top ranked physician specialties have remained constant, but relative proportions have changed
    - **1998** Psychiatry (67%); Pediatrics (10%); and Family Practice (9%)
    - **2002** Psychiatry (65%); Pediatrics (17%); and Family Practice (9%)

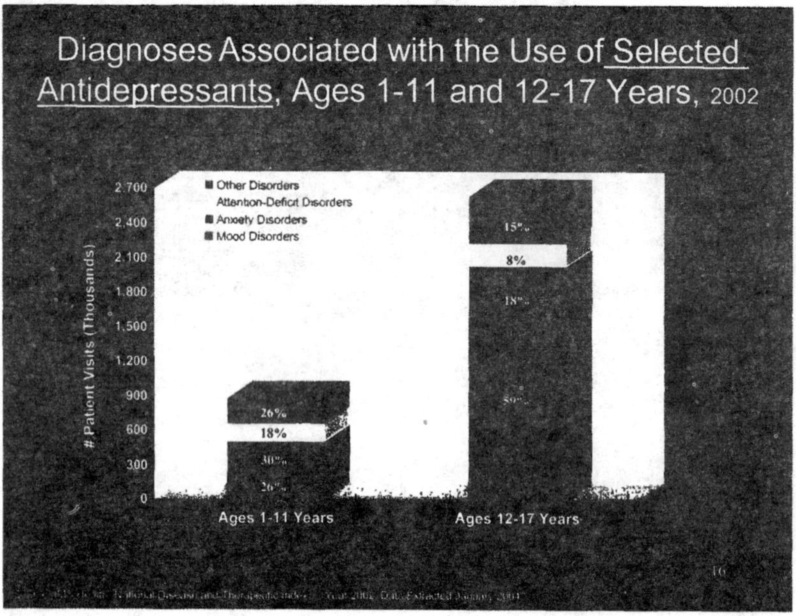
Diagnoses Associated with the Use of Selected Antidepressants, Ages 1-11 and 12-17 Years, 2002
Other Disorders
Attention-Deficit Disorders
Anxiety Disorders
Mood Disorders
Patient Visits (Thousands)
2,700
2,400
2,100
1,800
1,500
1,200
900
600
300
0
26%
18%
30%
26%
15%
8%
18%
Ages 1-11 Years
Ages 12-17 Years

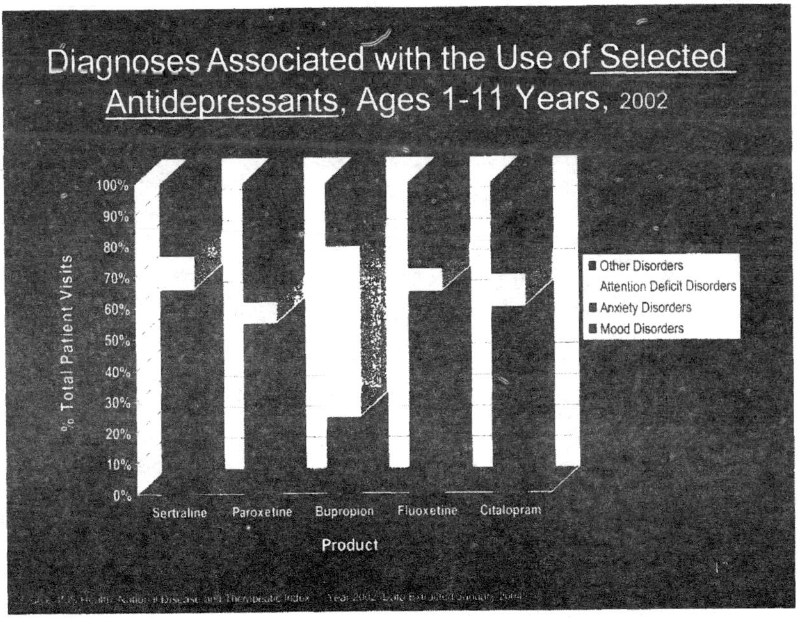
Diagnoses Associated with the Use of Selected Antidepressants, Ages 1-11 Years, 2002
100%
90%
80%
70%
60%
50%
40%
30%
20%
10%
0%
% Total Patient Visits
Sertraline
Paroxetine
Bupropion
Fluoxetine
Citalopram
Product
Other Disorders
Attention Deficit Disorders
Anxiety Disorders
Mood Disorders

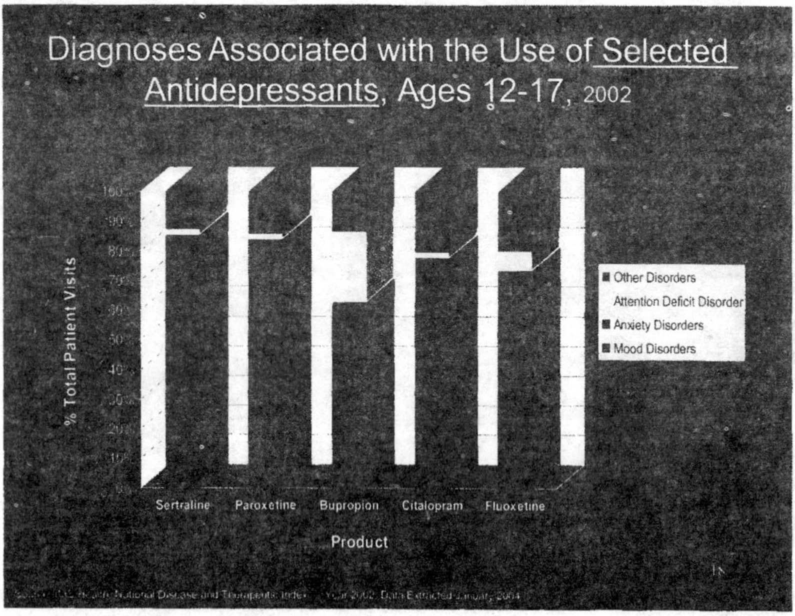
Diagnoses Associated with the Use of Selected Antidepressants, Ages 12-17, 2002
% Total Patient Visits
Other Disorders
Attention Deficit Disorder
Anxiety Disorders
Mood Disorders
Sertraline
Paroxetine
Bupropion
Citalopram
Fluoxetine
Product

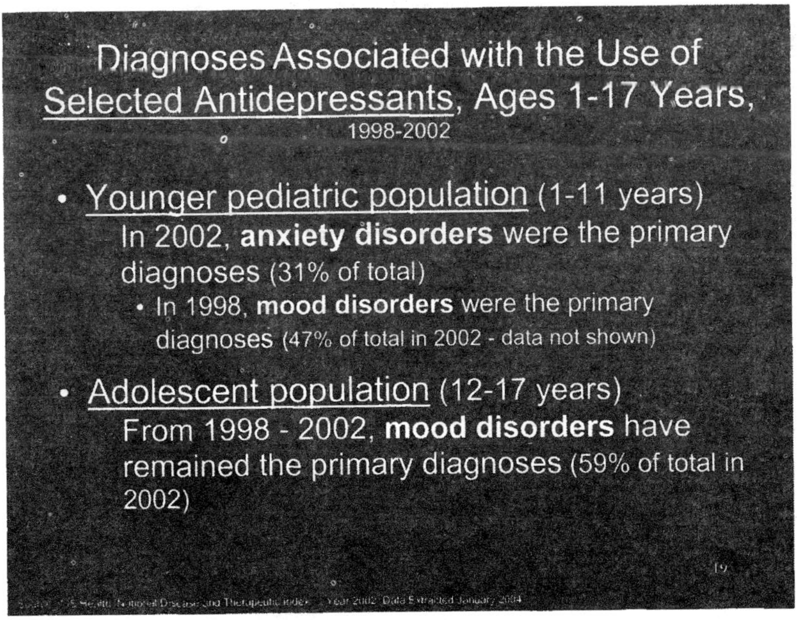
Diagnoses Associated with the Use of Selected Antidepressants, Ages 1-17 Years,
1998-2002
• Younger pediatric population (1-11 years)
In 2002, anxiety disorders were the primary diagnoses (31% of total)
• In 1998, mood disorders were the primary diagnoses (47% of total in 2002 - data not shown)
• Adolescent population (12-17 years)
From 1998 - 2002, mood disorders have remained the primary diagnoses (59% of total in 2002)

Limitations

- Outpatient Drug Use Data
  - Data on dispensed prescriptions include prescriptions filled in the outpatient pharmacy setting only
  - Prescriptions dispensed for ages 1-17 years extrapolated from physician office visit data
  - Data on prescriber specialties and indications
    - Taken from a sample of 2,000-3,000 office-based physicians
    - A mention of a product during a office visit may not result in a patient actually filling the prescription in a pharmacy

Conclusions

- Antidepressant use among children & adolescents appears to be widespread
  - Increasing annually since 1988
- Psychiatrists, pediatricians, and primary care providers continue to be the primary prescribers
- Diagnoses for the outpatient use of selected antidepressants
  - Ages 1-11 Years
    - Anxiety disorders (31%), mood disorders (27%), attention-deficit disorder (17%)
  - Ages 12-17 Years
    - Mood disorders (59%), anxiety disorders (18%), attention-deficit disorder (8%)

ONE HUNDRED EIGHTH CONGRESS

U.S. House of Representatives
Committee on Energy and Commerce
Washington, DC 20515–6115

JOE BARTON, TEXAS
CHAIRMAN

September 14, 2004

Tab 88

Janet Woodcock, M.D.
Deputy Commissioner for Operations
Food and Drug Administration
5600 Fishers Lane
Rockville, Maryland 20857

Dear Dr. Woodcock:

On September 9, 2004, you testified before the Subcommittee on Oversight and Investigations in a hearing entitled "Publication and Disclosure Issues in Anti-Depressant Pediatric Clinical Trials." We now ask for your responses to several additional questions (attached).

Because we wish to include the questions and responses in the printed record of this hearing, please respond no later than Tuesday, September 21, 2004. Please fax and e-mail the responses. The faxed response should be directed to Billy Harvard, Committee on Energy and Commerce, Majority staff, at 202-226-2447, and Voncille Hines, Committee on Energy and Commerce, Minority staff, at 202-225-5288. The e-mail copy of the response should be directed to (Billy.Harvard@mail.house.gov) and Voncille Hines (Voncille.Hines@mail.house.gov). Due to the uncertainties of postal deliveries on Capitol Hill, we ask that your responses not be sent through the postal service.

If you have any questions, please have your staff contact David Nelson, Minority Investigator/Economist, Committee on Energy and Commerce, at 202-226-3400.

Sincerely,

JOHN D. DINGELL
RANKING MEMBER

Attachment

Dr. Janet Woodcock
Page 2

cc: The Honorable Joe Barton, Chairman
Committee on Energy and Commerce

The Honorable Greg Walden, Vice Chairman
Subcommittee on Oversight and Investigations

The Honorable Peter Deutsch, Ranking Member
Subcommittee on Oversight and Investigations

Questions for Janet Woodcock, M.D.
Deputy Commissioner for Operations
Food and Drug Administration
from the Honorable John D. Dingell
Committee on Energy and Commerce
regarding the September 9, 2004, Subcommittee on Oversight and Investigations
Hearing entitled
"Publication and Disclosure Issues in Anti-Depressant Pediatric Clinical Trials"

1. Why did Organon not receive pediatric exclusivity for their drug Remeron?

2. How does the Agency react to a question, raised by at least one drug firm, of whether it is ethical to perform a long-term safety study if a clinical trial shows no efficacy in children?

3. Does the FDA have sufficient authority, under the Best Pharmaceuticals for Children Act, to require that drugs be studied to its satisfaction?

4. You testified that the FDA actively works to post summaries of pediatric trials in a timely manner. We know you did not in all but one of the drugs explored at this hearing. What other studies, which also have failed to show efficacy, has the FDA not yet released? Please provide a list of drugs that have failed to show efficacy in clinical trials in pediatric populations, as well as the dates the FDA received the study results.

5. I understand that the FDA has possession of studies that show that at least some of the anti-depressants, under discussion in this hearing, are not effective in some of the trials of adults with Major Depressive Disorder (MDD). Please tell us which of these drugs, that were not shown to be effective in pediatric studies, were also submitted with one or more failed trials to FDA for adult populations suffering from MDD.

6. You testified that the FDA asked manufacturers to change the labels of ten drugs to include stronger cautions and warnings about the need to monitor patients for worsening of depression and the emergence of suicidal behavior and ideation? You further state that the new warning language has now been added to the labels for seven of these products and that sponsors of the other three drugs have also agreed to adopt the language. Which three drugs have yet to make the appropriate changes to their labels? Why have they not changed their labels? Do they have a time limit for making these changes?

7. Please identify each official in the Office of Drug Safety, in the review division referred to as Neuropharm, or anywhere else in the Center for Drug Evaluation and Research, that reviewed, recommended (or failed to recommend), approved, concurred in the approval, or otherwise participated in the decision to request that Wyeth Laboratories moderate its labeled warning, or proposed labeled warning, regarding the dangers of Effexor in children and adolescents.

8. Please identify each official in the Office of Drug Safety, in the review division referred to as Neuropharm, or anywhere else in the Center for Drug Evaluation and Research, that reviewed, recommended (or failed to recommend), and/or approved the decision not to require GlaxoSmithKline to label their drug, Paxil, as having failed to show efficacy in at least one pediatric trial.

9. Please identify each official in the Office of Drug Safety, in the review division referred to as Neuropharm, or anywhere else in the Center for Drug Evaluation and Research, that reviewed, recommended (or failed to recommend), and/or approved the decision not to require Forest Laboratories to label their drug, Celexa, as having failed to show efficacy in a pediatric trial.

10. Please identify each official in the Office of Drug Safety, in the review division referred to as Neuropharm, or anywhere else in the Center for Drug Evaluation and Research, that reviewed, recommended (or failed to recommend), and/or approved the decision not to require Bristol-Myers Squibb, to label their drug, Serzone, as having failed to show efficacy in at least one pediatric trial.

11. Please identify each official in the Office of Drug Safety, in the review division referred to as Neuropharm, or anywhere else in the Center for Drug Evaluation and Research, that reviewed, recommended (or failed to recommend), and/or approved the decision not to require Organon to label their drug, Remeron, as having failed to show efficacy in at least one pediatric trial.

12. Please identify each official in the Office of Drug Safety, in the review division referred to as Neuropharm, or anywhere else in the Center for Drug Evaluation and Research, that reviewed, recommended (or failed to recommend), and/or approved the decision not to require Pfizer to label their drug, Zoloft, as having failed to show efficacy in at least one pediatric trial.

13. Please identify each official in the Office of Drug Safety, in the review division referred to as Neuropharm, or anywhere else in the Center for Drug Evaluation and Research, that reviewed, recommended (or failed to recommend), and/or approved the decision not to require Wyeth to label their drug, Effexor, as having failed to show efficacy in at least one pediatric trial.

**Questions for Janet Woodcock, M.D., Deputy Commissioner for Operations
Food and Drug Administration from
the Honorable Bart Stupak
Committee on Energy and Commerce regarding the September 9, 2004
Subcommittee on Oversight and Investigations Hearing entitled
"Publication and Disclosure Issues in Anti-Depressant Pediatric Clinical Trials"**

1. In the 9/9/2004 hearing and at this year's Advisory Committee hearings, FDA officials have said repeatedly that the data sets they have in which to determine the safety and efficacy of antidepressants to treat depression in children are too small. What changes need to be made to the Written Requests for pediatric trials in order for FDA officials to better determine efficacy and safety? What has FDA learned from its review of antidepressants about how this system should be changed? What changes have you implemented or will you implement? Does legislation need to be enacted to make the changes necessary?

2. Please provide the Committee with the number of spontaneous adverse events classified as suicide, suicidal behavior and ideation reported to the FDA through MedWatch for each year since the drugs Wellbutrin, Celexa, Prozac, Luvox, Serzone, Paxil, Remeron, Zoloft, and Effexor have been approved for use in adults. Please classify adverse events by age group (adult, adolescents, and children). Please also explain how the FDA has followed up on these reports and classified these events.

3. In Dr. Dianne Murphy's testimony before the Advisory Committee on September 13, 2004, she stated that over 293 Written Requests for products to be studied in children have been made by FDA since 1994, and that studies have been submitted on over 110 products. Please account for the 183 products that have had Written Requests issued, but have not had studies submitted. How many of those 293 Written Requests were unanswered? How many products have studies underway that have not been submitted to the FDA?

4. Dr. Murphy testified that 76 label changes have been made. Why have only 76 labels been changed? What is the status of the other 24 label changes? Why has the FDA only posted 41 product summaries on its Web site when over 110 products have studies completed and 76 products have label changes?

5. Dr. Dianne Murphy testified before the Advisory Committee on September 13, 2004, that "Under FDA's general disclosure provisions for approved applications, the summary for Prozac is available" on the FDA Web site. Why has the FDA not used those same disclosure provisions to publish the summaries of pediatric trials of other drugs?

June 16, 2004

VIA FACSIMILE & USPS (202) 690-8168

The Honorable Tommy G. Thompson
Secretary
Department of Health and Human Services
200 Independence Avenue, SW
Washington, DC 20201

Tab 89

Dr. Lester M. Crawford, D.V.M., Ph.D.
Acting Commissioner
U.S. Food and Drug Administration
5600 Fishers Lane
Rockville, MD 20857

Dear Secretary Thompson and Dr. Crawford:

Last March, I instructed my staff to review whether or not Dr. Andrew Mosholder, who works in the Office of Drug Safety (ODS), was precluded from delivering his analysis of clinical data relating to children, anti-depressants, and suicidal events to a Food and Drug Administration (FDA) Advisory Committee Meeting (ACM) on February 2, 2004. My concerns at the time centered around the public's right to know the possible effects of certain anti-depressants on children and reflected my deep and unbridled concern for the thousands of children across America who are faithfully taking potentially life-threatening medication, which have been found to be no better than placebo in the treatment of depression in children. In addition, I expressed concern to you regarding the investigation that was launched into the "leak" of Dr. Mosholder's analysis.

Let me begin by saying that Dr. Mosholder appears to be a man of great integrity, placing his findings and recommendations above all else, despite FDA efforts to limit and strategically manipulate information to be provided to the public. This country needs more civil servants with Dr. Mosholder's devotion to doing what is right in the face of adversity.

Interviews conducted during the course of this investigation have provided the Committee with a trove of information to consider. To begin with, it is necessary to address the ODS, both its function and mission. The ODS has a very specific mission: it "evaluates drug risks and promotes the safe use of drugs by the American people." In essence, ODS maintains a system of "postmarketing surveillance" to identify adverse effects that did not appear during the drug development process. This mission makes perfect sense. Clinical studies conducted, prior to a drug entering the U.S. market, involve a limited number of highly selected individuals and a similarly limited number of trials. In other words, the laboratory in which the drug is being tested for its usefulness is understandably small and controlled. As a result, the full range of possible adverse effects of a new drug does not always surface. Indeed, the real laboratory for new drugs occurs once the drug is dispensed across large numbers of people after marketing begins.

The ODS learns about adverse events through reporting by companies and through voluntary reports submitted to FDA's MedWatch program; a program for health professionals and consumers to report adverse events to FDA. Staff in ODS, like Dr. Mosholder, use this information to identify drug safety concerns and recommend actions to improve product safety and protect public health. Unfortunately, interviews with FDA employees suggest that a disconnect exists within the ODS, between its mission and its current operations.

According to staff interviews, Dr. Mosholder is a child psychiatrist who, prior to joining ODS, served for almost 10 years in the Division of Neuropharmacologic and Psychiatric Drugs (Neuropharm) within the Center for Drug Evaluation and Research (CDER) of FDA. Neuropharm, located within CDER's Office of New Drugs (OND), is responsible for approving drugs for entry into the marketplace. During his decade in Neuropharm, Dr. Mosholder was responsible for reviewing safety and effectiveness studies on anti-depressants and children. As a result of his unique knowledge and experience, Dr. Mosholder is the de facto expert at FDA for the efficacy of anti-depressants in children, and accordingly was sought out by Dr. Katz, the Director of Neuropharm, to do a "rush consult" to evaluate the clinical studies involving children, anti-depressants and suicide. This "rush consult" was sparked by several factors, including the availability of new data analyses indicating an increase in suicidal thoughts and behaviors in children treated with some of these drug agents. As a result of this consult, Dr. Mosholder was protected from all other assignments so that he could complete this important analysis quickly (the Mosholder Analysis).

Dr. Mosholder conducted his review of the clinical data, prepared his analysis, and provided that analysis, without recommendations, to his peers and superiors including, Drs. Mary Willy, Mark Avigan, and Anne Trontell in September 2003. Overall, the Mosholder Analysis was widely disseminated. Moreover, Dr. Mosholder's findings were and remain that there is a link between anti-depressant use by children and suicidal and self-injurious thoughts and behaviors. His report was well received. In fact, his immediate supervisor Dr. Willy noted a job well done, while Drs. Avigan and Tronell, both of whom would later write dissenting opinions to Dr. Mosholder's analysis, advised Dr. Mosholder that he had done a "great job" and "good job," respectively.

Over the course of the next several months, Dr. Mosholder said that he continued to refine his analysis, but his findings never changed, i.e., the link between children, anti-depressants and suicide was unmistakable. As a result of these and other events, a decision was made by Neuropharm and OND that Dr. Mosholder would present his analysis and findings at the February 2, 2004 Psychopharmacologic Drugs Advisory Committee Meeting (ACM), as noted in the Federal Register on October 31, 2003.

On December 10, 2003, the United Kingdom's Medicines and Healthcare Products Regulatory Agency (MHRA) issued a statement regarding children, anti-depressants and suicide. The MHRA noted that only Prozac should be given to children with depression and that the use of all other selective serotonin reuptake inhibitors (SSRI anti-depressants) was contraindicated. The FDA was well aware of this determination.

In anticipation of the February 2, 2004 ACM, a planning meeting took place in December 2003. During the course of that planning meeting, Dr. Mosholder distributed to all the attendees an outline of his talking points, which noted that a child taking an anti-depressant, other than Prozac, was twice as likely to have a suicidal event as a child taking a placebo. This was a significant finding and was consistent with the MHRA findings and the Lancet study.

Dr. Laughren, the Deputy Director of Neuropharm and formerly Dr. Mosholder's team leader during his tenure in Neuropharm, objected unexpectedly to Dr. Mosholder's methods at a December meeting. This was the case despite the fact that he had received a copy of the analysis and had an opportunity to review it several months earlier. It is my understanding that Dr. Laughren wanted to get further analysis of the data done by Columbia University before reaching a conclusion.

On January 6, 2004, Dr. Mosholder was contacted by Dr Katz. During a 20 minute conversation, Dr Katz informed Dr. Mosholder that he would no longer be presenting at the ACM because Dr. Mosholder: 1) reached a different conclusion than OND; and 2) utilized incomplete data. This decision was neither embraced by Dr. Mosholder, nor by his superiors in the ODS, but it appears that little could be done to ameliorate the situation.

During the course of this investigation, it has become increasingly more apparent that the ODS and the OND exist in a relationship that is best described as "separate but unequal." According to staff interviews, the ODS serves a subservient role to the OND. Indeed, the ODS was described by one employee as the "unwanted stepchild" at FDA, rather than a watchdog for the public at large. This observation merits further in-depth review because of the seriousness of the impact of any organizational weakness at the FDA upon public safety.

Subsequent to the decision to remove Mosholder from the agenda of the ACM, the FDA engaged in a series of other activities that are also very troubling. In anticipation of the fact that parties interested in the Mosholder analysis were expected to attend the ACM, including family members of children harmed by one or more anti-depressants, it appears the FDA: 1) prepared scripted answers for Dr. Mosholder to read if questioned at the ACM; 2) attempted to have Mosholder present data known to be unreliable and deceptively misleading; and 3) engaged in behavior that overall is unexpected from an organization charged with ensuring and protecting the safety of American consumers taking prescription medications.

To begin, Dr. Mosholder was advised at one point that if he were willing to modify his recommendations, perhaps he could present his analysis at the ACM. Indeed, new recommendations were drafted for his consideration. However, Dr. Mosholder refused to accept new, alternative language, stating that the alternative language misconstrued his recommendations.

In addition, Dr. Mosholder was told that he was not sitting at the meeting table during the ACM, despite the fact that he was providing information on another topic. This decision was made by the OND. Dr. Mosholder was advised that in the event he was asked any questions regarding his anti-depressant analysis, he was not allowed to speak about his analysis, he could only speak from the "prepared" answers. This seems like a peculiar way to treat the "established" expert in the area of SSRIs and children.

Perhaps most troubling, however, was the fact that OND attempted to have Dr. Mosholder present "reporting rates" of suicidal thoughts, rather than the available clinical trials data on anti-depressants and children, which formed the foundation of his analysis. This is bothersome for several reasons. "Reporting rates" are considered marginally reliable and clinical trials data have long been regarded by FDA as the most reliable type of data based upon the experts interviewed. As one interviewee stated, "clinical data trumps reporting data any time." These rates are derived from dividing the number of cases reported to the FDA by pharmacists, physicians and others and stored in the computerized Adverse Event Reporting System (AERS). AERS is a voluntary reporting system intended, among other things, to monitor the safety effects of drugs once they are approved by the FDA for marketing. In order to determine the reporting rate you simply take the AERS data for a particular drug and divide it by the number of prescriptions filled for that particular drug. This provides the "reporting rate" for that drug.

In the instant situation, the OND wanted Dr. Mosholder to present "reporting rates" of suicidal thoughts and behavior for anti-depressants in children at the ACM. However, Dr. Mosholder refused to do so because most serious adverse drug effects are never reported to FDA. Consequently, any "reporting rate" would be extremely low, not because the SSRI anti-depressants do not promote suicidal thoughts and behaviors in children, but because voluntary reporting is so poor and infrequent. The use of "reporting rates" at the ACM would be deceptively false and misleading and would provide a "false sense of security" to the public. Staff interviews suggest that had these reporting rates been presented at the ACM, the public, the media and the Congress probably would have concluded that anti-depressants are all extremely safe for children.

On one hand, it can be said that the public should be grateful that Dr. Mosholder held his ground and refused to present "reporting rates" at the ACM; yet, on the other hand, the fact that a high-level official at the OND/FDA would consider such an alternative is alarming. In fact, it begs the question: in how many other instances were reporting rates provided when more reliable data was available? In how many other instances has the OND manipulated its advisory committee meetings to withhold from the public and misrepresent safety information about marketed drugs of critical importance to patient safety?

It appears from this investigation to date, the turning point for removing the Mosholder Analysis from the ACM was not the fact that Columbia University was going to further analyze the data or that Dr. Mosholder's superiors had not "cleared" the consult, as reported in the press. After all, it was repeatedly reported to us that consults/analyses that had not been "cleared" were regularly presented to the ACM. The lynchpin for removal of the Mosholder consult from the ACM was the insertion of "recommendations." Specifically, Dr. Mosholder recommended that "a risk management strategy directed at discouraging off-label pediatric use of anti-depressant drugs, particularly the use of drugs other than fluoxetine (Prozac), in the treatment of pediatric MDD (major depressive disorder)."

During the course of discussions regarding the removal of the Mosholder Analysis from the ACM agenda, another matter of interest came to light. Specifically, staff interviews suggest that inserting recommendations into drug consults are neither encouraged nor wanted by the OND. In fact, one employee at the ODS stated, that he was "hazy" on whether or not recommendations should ever be written. Another employee stated that consult recommendations are outright discouraged because they force the hand of the OND to "do something" and that the OND preferred that ODS consults remain "sterile."

The fact that ODS employees believe that they should not insert recommendations in their consults appears to be in direct contravention of ODS claims. Specifically, the ODS's website states that ODS is to "identify drug safety concerns and recommend actions to improve product safety and protect the public health." It would seem that OND's decision to discourage scientists at ODS from recommending action intended to serve the public interest is inconsistent with its stated mission. More importantly, it is contrary to the basic fundamental principle upon which our government is built: that is; having independent and objective reviewers of fact to protect the American public in a timely and effective manner, particularly when it comes to the issues of public health.

A review of the facts surrounding the removal of the Mosholder Analysis from the ACM, coupled with efforts to have "reporting data" presented as opposed to clinical data at the ACM and attempts to modify Mosholder's recommendations, in return for a seat at the ACM table, lend themselves to a number of concerns. First, the relationship between the ODS and the OND does not appear to be in the best interest of the consumer. Indeed, some staff interviews noted that ODS is simply there to "serve" OND. Still others stated that perhaps ODS should consider re-naming itself to the "Office of Drug Safety Consultants" or the "Office of Dumb Simpletons."

In addition, I continue to be extremely interested in the investigation that was launched into the "leak" of information to the press and to Congress regarding the findings of the Mosholder Analysis. Although I am continuing my review of that matter, there is one point that must be made. My letter, dated March 25, 2004, asked: "What was the purpose of this alleged investigation?" In response, I was advised that: "This investigation was initiated to determine if there was an inappropriate disclosure of sensitive information." This response appears to be 1) not true; 2) an insult to the process in which I am engaged; and 3) at best, a misleading response to my inquiries.

It was well-established among ODS employees that the "leak" investigation was intended to ferret out the name or names of the individuals who contacted the press with Dr. Mosholder's findings. The investigation was a catalyst for fear and was, according to those interviewed to date, intended to target the "leak." In fact, none of the individuals interviewed had any recollection of the "leak" investigation being driven by a concern about the disclosure of sensitive information; rather they believed that FDA was after the "leaker," and if found, that individual(s) would likely suffer severe negative consequences. Accordingly, in the future, I would greatly appreciate that my inquiries be taken with the seriousness in which they are asked; I expect no less.

Thank you for your continued cooperation.

Sincerely,

Charles E. Grassley
Chairman

Tab 90

Review and Evaluation of Clinical Data

Drugs, NDAs, sponsors, and date of submissions:

1. Wellbutrin (Bupropion), NDA 18-644, GlaxoSmithKline, submissions dated 11/04/03, 4/15/04, 5/18/04
2. Remeron (mirtazapine), NDA 20-415, Organon, submissions dated 11/10/03 & 4/15/04
3. Luvox (fluvoxamine), NDA 21-519, Solvay, submissions dated 11/10/03 & 4/13/04
4. Effexor and Effexor XR (venlafaxine), NDAs 20-151 and 20-699, Wyeth, submissions dated 11/19/03 & 5/14/04
5. Zoloft (sertraline), NDA 19-839, Pfizer, submissions dated 11/21/03 & 4/15/04
6. Celexa (citalopram), NDA 20-822, Forest, submissions dated 11/21/03 & 4/15/04
7. Paxil (paroxetine), NDA 20-031, GlaxoSmithKline, submissions dated 11/24/03, 4/15/04, & 5/17/04
8. Prozac (fluoxetine), NDA 18-936, Lilly, submissions dated 12/4/03 & 4/20/04
9. Serzone (nefazodone), NDA 20-152, Bristol Myers Squibb, submissions dated 1/14/04 & 4/20/04

Subject: Relationship between psychotropic drugs and pediatric suicidality
Reviewer: Tarek A. Hammad, M.D., Ph.D., M.Sc., M.S.
Date Review Completed: 8/16/04

This document analyzes and evaluates data submitted by sponsors of several psychotropic drugs in response to FDA requests regarding data pertinent to pediatric suicidality.

Several hyperlinks (seen underlined in blue color) were put in place to facilitate navigating through the document.

Table of Contents

1 Background

On May 22, 2003, GlaxoSmithKline submitted an analysis of suicide-related[1] adverse events in pediatric trials of paroxetine. This analysis showed a statistically significant increase in such behavior with paroxetine treatment, compared to placebo. In order to provide a meaningful comparison to the paroxetine findings, the Division of Neuropharmacological Drug Products (DNDP) requested that the sponsors of eight other psychotropic drugs tested in children and adolescents conduct searches of their databases similar to the search performed by GlaxoSmithKline. The initial letters requesting these searches were issued on 7/22/03. Follow up requests to obtain additional information were issued on 11/24/03 & 12/9/03 (Appendix I). The latter requests were issued in part to cast an even broader net for events, since there was concern that event-finding by sponsors may not have been complete.[2]

Based on our initial assessments of the responses to our 7/22/03 letters, we decided that it may be useful to obtain patient-level datasets to permit an exploration for covariates to assess for possible imbalances among treatment groups. Requests for these data sets were issued on 10/3/03 & 10/28/03 (Appendix II).

Because of a very wide diversity in the events the sponsors had subsumed under the broad category of "possibly suicide-related," concerns were raised within the Division that not all captured events could be considered to reasonably represent suicidal thinking and behavior. At a joint meeting of the Psychopharmacological Drug Products Advisory Committee and Pediatric Subcommittee of the Infectious Diseases Advisory Committee held on February 2, 2004[3], the Division presented these concerns publicly, and proposed a plan for outsourcing a blinded review of the adverse events of interest to an expert group of suicidologists. Subsequently, all adverse events (AEs) identified by the sponsors as being suicide-related, as well as all serious AEs, all accidental injuries, and all accidental overdoses were independently blindly adjudicated by a group of ten suicidology experts assembled by Columbia University. The adjudication process was applied to the additional AEs mentioned above to provide reassurance that all suicide-related AEs had been identified.

On 3/17/04, while the AEs were being classified, DNDP requested additional data (Appendix III) on treatment-emergent suicidality among study patients as measured by the suicidality item(s) in various depression questionnaires (the questionnaires are provided in Appendix IV).

The purpose of this document is to evaluate and to analyze the suicide-related adverse

---

[1] The sponsor used an algorithm based on selected preferred terms to identify "suicide-related" adverse events.

[2] See Dr. Thomas P. Laughren memo to the PDAC meeting held on February 2, 2004. The memo was dated December 30, 2003.

[3] http://www.fda.gov/cder/drug/antidepressants/default.htm
http://cdernet.cder.fda.gov/ACS/Flash%20Minutes/Psychopharmacologic/psycho-Minutes_Quick_feb2.pdf

events identified by the blinded adjudication process described above in order to investigate the relationship between pediatric suicidality and psychotropic drugs.

2 Objectives

1- To investigate the relationship between psychotropic drugs and pediatric suicidality reported as AEs (AEs included in the analysis were the ones blindly classified by a group of suicidology experts assembled by Columbia University).

2- To investigate the relationship between psychotropic drugs and pediatric suicidality as suggested by scores on the suicidality item(s) reported in pertinent depression questionnaires.

3- To understand the sources of inconsistency - in any of the above outcomes - between trials and/or between drugs by investigating possible sources of variation or imbalance in the data e.g. trial design, duration of exposure, patient population, and other potential confounders.

3 Sources of data

In total, eight sponsors of nine psychotropic drugs provided datasets to DNDP culled from all the randomized controlled trials of their respective drug products conducted in the pediatric population as electronic files (in SAS transport file format). The variables included in these data provided detailed information about the individual patients. The variables are listed in the data requests in Appendix II and Appendix III.

The studied drugs included fluoxetine (Prozac), sertraline (Zoloft), paroxetine (Paxil), fluvoxamine (Luvox), citalopram (Celexa), bupropion (Wellbutrin), venlafaxine (Effexor), nefazodone (Serzone), and mirtazapine (Remeron).

A total of 25 pediatric trials from all drugs were submitted. The trials were conducted over a nearly 20 year period from 1983 to 2001; trial duration ranged from 4 to 16 weeks. The indications included Major Depressive Disorder [15 trials], Anxiety Disorders (Obsessive Compulsive Disorder [five trials], Generalized Anxiety Disorder [two trials], and Social Anxiety Disorder/Social Phobia [one trial]), and Attention Deficit Hyperactivity Disorder (two trials). Descriptive information for all trials included in this review is provided in Appendix V.

Only 23 of the trials were evaluable. Wellbutrin trial number "41" was excluded from the analysis because it was uncontrolled. Paxil trial number "453" was also excluded because its randomized withdrawal design did not allow direct comparison to the other 23 parallel arm trials[4].

[4] Trial 453 included two phases, an open-label phase (Phase I) in which patients received paroxetine for 16 weeks, and a 16 week double-blind placebo-controlled phase (Phase II) in which responders were eligible to participate. Although only data from the 16-week double-blind phase was included in the submitted

4 Operational Definitions

4.1 Outcome variables

4.1.1 Outcome variables under "objective 1"

AEs were captured on Case Report Forms (CRFs) during the course of these trials. Information in these CRFs (and possibly from other sources, e.g., hospital records) was used by the sponsor to write narratives for AEs that led to discontinuation from the trial or were categorized as "serious" by the regulatory definition[5]. As described above, narratives for AEs that were identified by the algorithm for suicide-related events, all serious AEs, all accidental injury AEs, and all accidental overdoses underwent blinded classification by an independent group of experts in suicidology assembled by Columbia University. The coordinating team at Columbia University, led by Dr. Kelly Posner, conducted a training session with the expert panel prior to their application of the coding scheme. The following listing shows the coding scheme used by the expert panel and the number of events that were classified to each type.

1: suicide attempt (n=27)
2: preparatory actions towards imminent suicidal behavior (n=6)
3: self-injurious behavior, intent unknown (n=24)
4: self-injurious behavior, no intent, primarily to affect circumstance (n=2)
5: self-injurious behavior, no intent, primarily to affect internal state (n=5)
6: suicidal ideation (n=45)
7: other: accident*
8: other: psychiatric*
9: other: medical*
10: not enough information (n=7)
11: self-injurious behavior, no suicidal intent (unspecified type, i.e. rater not sure if it is 4 or 5 [n=4])
12: "other" (some combination of 7, 8, and 9) *

* The total of codes 7, 8, 9, & 12 is 261 events.

For the purpose of investigating the data to fulfill objective number 1, codes of AEs were grouped into five outcomes as listed in the following table:

---

dataset, there was a concern that patients in this trial might not be comparable to patients in other trials because only patients who were already shown to tolerate and respond to the drug were randomized.

[5] An adverse event is categorized as "serious" if it results in any of the following outcomes: death, a life-threatening adverse drug experience, inpatient hospitalization or prolongation of existing hospitalization, persistent or significant disability/ incapacity, or a congenital anomaly/birth defect. Also other important medical events requiring interventions to prevent one of the outcomes listed above [21 CFR Ch. 1, 314.80].

Table 1: Outcomes investigated under objective number 1.

Outcomes	Description	Columbia codes
Outcome 1 (n=33)	Definitive suicidal behavior	1, 2
Outcome 2 (n=45)	Suicidal ideation (without behavior)	6
The primary outcome (outcome 3) (n=78)	Definitive suicidal behavior/ideation	1, 2, 6
Outcome 4 (n=109)	Possible suicidal behavior/ideation	1, 2, 3, 6, 10
Outcome 5 (n=11)	Self-injurious behavior, non-suicidal	4, 5, 11

The primary focus of the analysis was outcome 3. For the purpose of "casting the broadest net" to identify potentially suicide-related events, "serious" adverse events were included among the AEs sent for adjudication. Beyond that, the "serious" status of AEs was not utilized in this review because it is a regulatory definition that has no impact on the characterization of an event as suicidal or not (i.e., suicidal ideation or suicide attempt would not qualify as a serious adverse event if it did not meet the regulatory definition mentioned above in footnote. Instead, we relied on the classification resulting from the blinded adjudication process.

4.1.1.1 PHASE DEFINITIONS

Based on the timing of these events, they were grouped in six "phases" as defined in the table below:

Table 2: Definition of "phases" based on the timing of events.

Phases	Description
Phase 1	Event occurred in double-blind acute treatment phase or within one day of the end of this phase[6]. The end of trials with a tapering period was set to be at the beginning of the tapering period.
Phase 2	Event occurred during a taper phase following the end of the double-blind period
Phase 3	Event occurred during the discontinuation phase--this phase was defined as 2 to 8 days after the cessation of medication for all drugs except Prozac where it was 2 to 31 days after the cessation of medication because it has a long half life and active metabolites. For an event to be classified in this phase, the patient must not have been taking drug at the time of the event
Phase 4	Event occurred between 2 and 8 days (2 and 31 days for Prozac) after the cessation of double-blind acute phase study medication *and* the patient had continued in an extension phase or started on a prescription anti-depressant
Phase 5	Event occurred between 9 and 31 days after the cessation of double-blind acute phase study medication *and* the patient had continued in an extension phase or started on a prescription anti-depressant (this category would not apply to Prozac patients)

---

[6] One day was added onto the end of the exposure because if a patient took the last dose of study drug at night, the drug exposure would continue into the next day.

risk of suicidality. Assuming an incidence of 5% in the placebo group, trials with 100 patients in each arm had 80% power to detect about a 4 fold increase or more in the risk of suicidality.

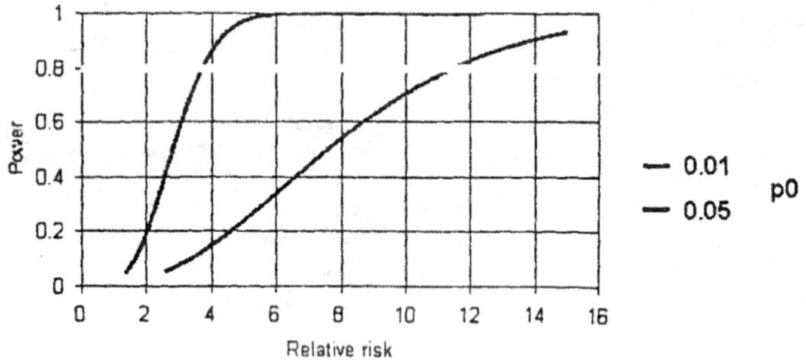

p0 = incidence of events in the placebo group.

6 Limitations of the current investigation

- It is worth noting that what is reported in this review represents a post-hoc analysis with multiple outcomes involved. This is complicated by the lack of statistical significance for many of the sub-analyses, which increase the level of uncertainty. Therefore, caution is warranted in the interpretation of the findings.

- Given the size of the individual trials and the background rates of suicide behavior/ideation, the conducted trials were capable of detecting an increase in the risk of suicidality of 4-12 fold. Therefore, none of the individual trials showed statistically significant results. Clearly, these trials were designed for efficacy and were not powered for safety purposes.

- The current analyses used short term data (4-16 weeks). Therefore we could possibly miss suicidality effects that require a cumulative exposure or long latency period that exceeds the trial duration

- Some of the covariates requested by the FDA to investigate their potential confounding effects on the risk estimates were missing from the submitted data. However, a reassuring finding is that in trials with complete data there were no significant imbalances detected between the drug and the placebo groups.

- Pooling data across drugs within a class assumes that the rate of suicidality is similar across that class of drugs, i.e. that there is a "class effect". In the current investigation, some of the drugs have smaller databases than others. Consequently, the smaller opportunity to observe suicidality may have resulted in none or fewer cases being observed for that drug. There is also the potential role for the immeasurable and uncontrollable differences in the level of ascertainment of events and completeness of narratives between various trials and various sponsors. Thus, observed differences in the risk between drugs may have several possible explanations, including a true difference between drugs, inadequate power for studies of some of the drugs, or because of differences between trials in ascertainment and reporting of adverse events.

- Observed rates of suicidality might not reflect actual rates among patients in the general population because patients participating in randomized clinical trials might be a selected subgroup of patients due to what is known as "volunteer's bias". Therefore, it might not be easy to generalize the findings of these analyses.

- Most trials were conducted with a flexible dosing scheme, which made investigating the dose effect difficult. The only information available for each patient is the maximal modal dose with no specification of which dose was associated with the event and the timing of event as it relates to changes in dose.

- The patterns and causes of premature discontinuation across these trials may be an important finding, but they are difficult to explore. Ignoring these patterns assumes that there is no informative censoring; however, it needs to be acknowledged that this is an important assumption, given the fact that discontinuations were as high as 50% in some trials.

- Adolescents are known to take their medications erratically, and medication compliance may have influenced the occurrence of events of interest. However, the extent of noncompliance was assessed differently across drug development programs.

7 Reviewer's Conclusions

- The involved search of adverse events in various drug development programs and the blinded classification process identified many events not previously identified and also eliminated a number of events that were not appropriately classified, thus reducing misclassification and providing more accurate risk estimates.

- It should be noted that, among the events considered representative of suicidality in these 25 pediatric antidepressant trials, there were no completed suicides.

- No individual trial showed a statistically significant signal for suicidality. However, many had a RR of 2 or more and some of the overall estimates, across various trial groupings, were statistically significant.

- The strength of the suicidality signal, although it varies from drug to drug, is comparable to previous findings for most drugs.

- The sensitivity analyses did not yield a meaningful difference in the magnitude of the estimated risks.

- The differences in the risk estimates between trials within the same drug in the same indication might be partially explained by some of the trials' design attributes.

- Most of the events occurred in trials with the highest proportion of patients with a history of suicide attempt or ideation at baseline.

- Notwithstanding the missing data on covariates, no meaningful effect modification or confounding was detected for any trial.

- The time to event analysis showed that the hazard may not be constant over time, and may not always be proportional between the drug and the placebo groups.

- Drug treatment is associated with symptoms of hostility or agitation. However, it was not possible to explore a possible link between the occurrence of these symptoms and suicidality due to limitations in the available data

18 APPENDIX XI: RRs and 95% CI for various outcomes overall and by indication

18.1 The primary outcome (outcome 3), all trials, all indications

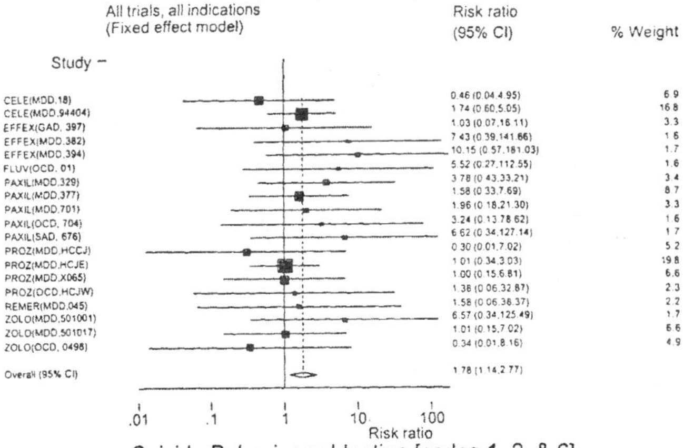

Suicide Behavior or Ideation [codes 1, 2, & 6]

18.2 Outcome 4, all trials, all indications

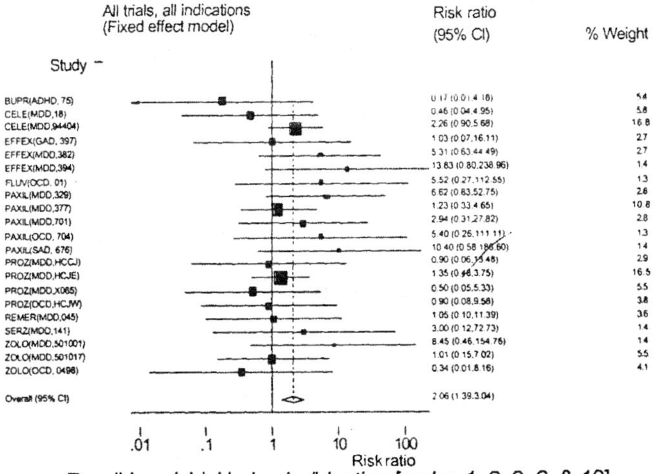

Possible suicidal behavior/Ideation [codes 1, 2, 3, 6, & 10]

18.5 Original sponsor's suicide-related events, all trials, all indications

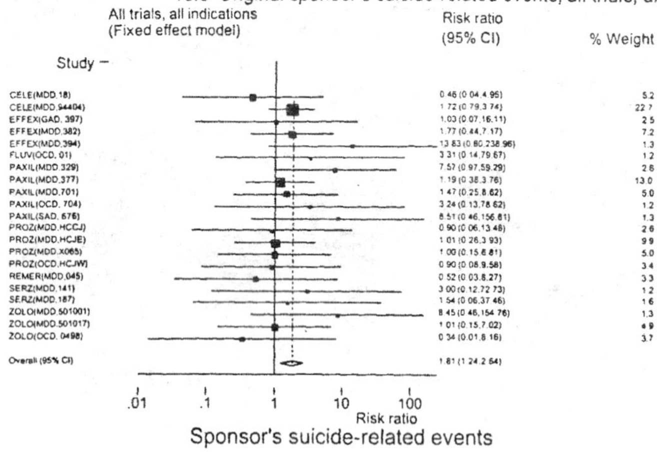

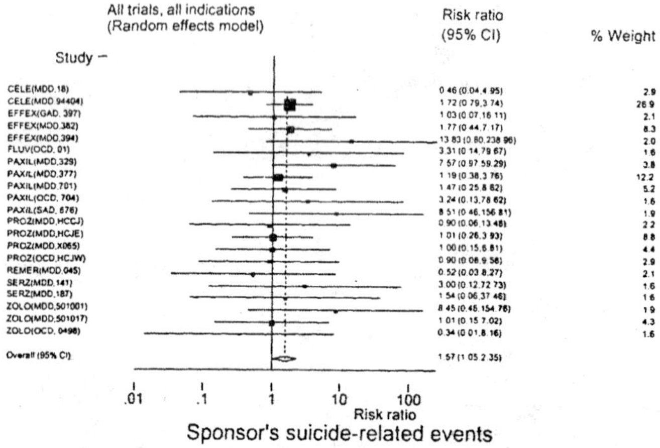

18.6 Original sponsor's suicide-related events, by indication

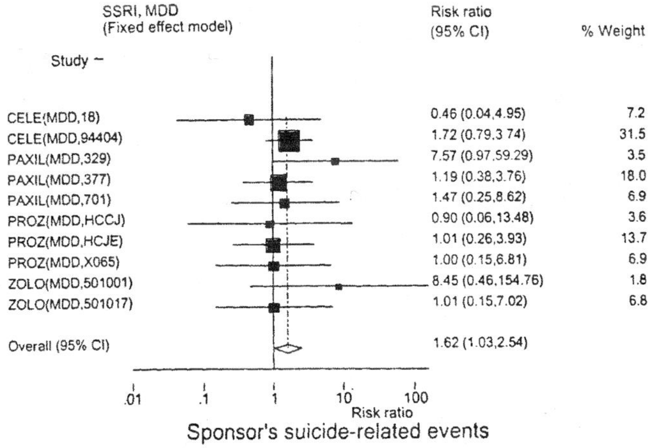

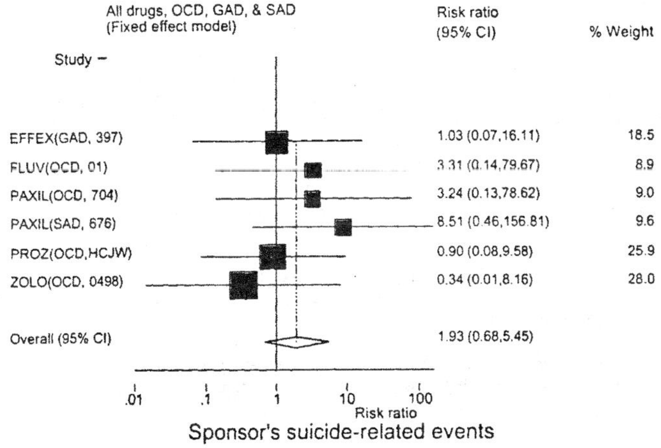

The New York Times

Tab 91

September 14, 2004

F.D.A. Links Drugs to Being Suicidal

By GARDINER HARRIS

BETHESDA, Md., Sept. 13 - Top officials of the Food and Drug Administration acknowledged for the first time on Monday that antidepressants appeared to lead some children and teenagers to become suicidal.

Dr. Robert Temple, director of the F.D.A.'s office of medical policy, said after an emotional public hearing here that analyses of 15 clinical trials, some of which were hidden for years from the public by the drug companies that sponsored them, showed a consistent link with suicidal behavior.

"I think that we now all believe that there is an increase in suicidal thinking and action that is consistent across all the drugs," Dr. Temple said, summarizing the agency's presentation to a special advisory committee. "This looks like it's a true bill."

The acknowledgement, made after the hearing, comes a year after the agency suppressed the conclusions of its own drug-safety analyst, Dr. Andrew Mosholder, who first found a link between the drugs and suicide in teenagers and children. Agency officials wrote in internal memorandums that Dr. Mosholder's analysis was unreliable, and they hired researchers at Columbia University to re-analyze the same data. That study recently reached conclusions nearly identical to Dr. Mosholder's.

The testimony came before an advisory committee of 31 independent experts that the F.D.A. has charged with making a recommendation about the labeling and use of antidepressants in children and teenagers.

Family members of suicide victims at the hearing angrily denounced agency officials for the delay in admitting the risk of antidepressants in children. The British health authorities decided in December to ban the use of most antidepressants in children and teenagers.

Mathy Milling Downing of Laytonsville, Md., whose 12-year-old daughter hanged herself in January, said: "Candace's death was entirely avoidable had we been given the appropriate warnings. "The blood of these children is on your hands."

Agency officials said that they had no regrets about the months of study. "I don't think the data were at that time reliable," Dr. Temple said. "Scaring people needlessly" or overdoing a warning is worrisome, he added.

The most popular pills are Zoloft, made by Pfizer; Paxil, made by GlaxoSmithKline; and Prozac, made by Eli Lilly & Company. In 2002, nearly 11 million children and teenagers were prescribed antidepressants.

The risk of suicide among patients given the pills is very small. If 100 children and teenagers are given antidepressants, 2 or 3 will become suicidal who otherwise would not have had they been given placebos, agency officials said. None of the children in the trials committed suicide, but some thought about or attempted suicide, researchers found.

In March, the agency required antidepressant manufacturers to include on labels a warning that therapy with antidepressants could lead some patients, both adults and children, to become suicidal. The committee must decide whether this warning is strong enough or whether the drugs should be banned for children. The advisory committee is expected to make a decision on Tuesday. The F.D.A. normally follows recommendations of its advisory committees.

It is a complex task. Most studies of the drugs have failed to show that they have any effect on depression in children and teenagers. But the drugs have proven effective in adults, and studies suggest that teenage suicide rates have dropped in countries where use of antidepressants is widespread. A large study of depressed teenagers conducted by the National Institute of Mental Health recently found that Prozac was far more effective in treating depression in children and teenagers than was talk therapy.

Several speakers noted that clinicians would have almost nothing to offer depressed teenagers and children if antidepressants were banned. Suicide is the third leading cause of death among teenagers, trailing only homicide and accidents. Without treatment, many more teenagers will die, several experts said. If the committee suggests an even stronger warning, some patients will resist therapy and could perhaps die, some speakers said.

The issue has roiled the agency and is likely to transform the way the drug industry markets its products. Committees in both the House and Senate have begun investigations following disclosures that Dr. Mosholder's analysis had been suppressed.

The New York State attorney general Eliot Spitzer, filed suit against GlaxoSmithKline, charging the drug maker with fraud for failing to disclose the results of clinical trials of Paxil that found no benefit while promoting the drug to physicians. The company settled the suit this summer by promising to disclose the results of all of its clinical trials of its marketed products dating back to 2000.

Editors of the nation's top medical journals have said they will not to accept for publication trials that have not been publicly registered, and legislation is expected to be offered in both the House and the Senate requiring the disclosure of the results of all major drug tests on humans.

For some bereaved parents, Monday's hearing was a chance to take drug makers and the F.D.A. to task.

Mark and Cheryl Miller of Overland Park, Kan.,, told the committee that their 13-year-old son, Matthew, had committed suicide seven months ago while taking Zoloft.

"Why haven't parents like Cheryl and myself and countless others been told the truth?" Mr. Miller asked.

But others said that antidepressants had helped millions. Dr. Suzanne Vogel-Sibilia of Beaver, Pa., said that she had brought her 15-year-old son, Tony, to the hearing to represent what she said were the vast majority of patients who had been helped by the drugs.

"Please help me preserve my future," Tony told the committee. "Don't take away my medication."

Claims that antidepressants cause patients to become acutely suicidal have been made since 1991, just

Tab 92

WSJ.com THE WALL STREET JOURNAL. ONLINE

September 13, 2004 2:56 p.m. EDT

FDA: Antidepressants Appear To Raise Juvenile Suicide Risk

By JENNIFER CORBETT DOOREN
September 13, 2004 2:56 p.m.

Of DOW JONES NEWSWIRES

WASHINGTON -- U.S. Food and Drug Administration medical experts said Monday there appeared to be an increased risk of suicidal behavior in adolescents taking antidepressants, but said there needed to be additional studies to determine the extent of the increase.

The FDA has convened a panel of outside physicians to discuss reports of suicide and antidepressants and to recommend what the agency should do about it. That panel is currently meeting and is expected to make its decision late Tuesday.

Data from small clinical trials in children taking antidepressants suggests that people under age 18 taking most antidepressants have almost twice the risk of suicidal behaviors as those taking placebos, or sugar pills, but that the drugs - with the exception of Eli Lilly & Co.'s (LLY) Prozac - don't work in kids. None of the data show a link between antidepressant use and an actual suicide. Prozac is the only FDA approved drug approved to treat major depression in children. Pfizer's (PFE) Zoloft is approved to treat obsessive compulsive disorder in people younger than age 18.

During the meeting FDA officials presented several analysis from the clinical trials, most of which have already been made public. But a new analysis adding the most recent data from a Prozac study that was published last month in the Journal of the American Medical Association suggests that all of the drugs increase the risk of suicidal behaviors, which are defined as suicidal thoughts, tendencies such as self-harm and violence.

The data showed about 78 serious judicial adverse events out of about 2,000 children, Dr. Robert Temple, head of the FDA's drug evaluation office told Dow Jones Newswires.

The increase in suicidal tendencies in kids on Prozac was extremely small and should probably be considered as not statistically significant, Temple and other FDA officials said.

"What's interesting and persuasive is that they all lean the same way," Temple said of the data on antidepressants.

During Monday's meeting, Dr. Andrew Mosholder, an FDA epidemiologist, was allowed to present his findings on antidepressants. Mosholder was banned in February from presenting his findings because his superiors said results were too preliminary.

Mosholder was given a round of applause from many of the 70 families who are testifying late Monday about their experiences with antidepressants. Several will tell stories about their children who committed suicide after taking antidepressants.

Mosholder said his analysis "indicates an association of adverse suicidal events with antidepressant drug treatment in short-term, placebo controlled pediatric trials." In a memo, he recommended the agency specifically discourage off-label use of antidepressants in children with the exception of Prozac, which is what British regulatory officials have done.

Earlier this year the FDA asked a panel of outside experts from Columbia University to look at the same data Mosholder did. Columbia's analysis, released last month, was similar to Mosholder's.

The FDA has been sharply criticized by Congress for its handling of the Mosholder matter and for being slow to release information.

Temple said he does not regret the decision to delay Mosholder's presentation until now, saying it was important for the FDA to get it right. He said it's difficult to interpret data on antidepressants and suicidal behavior because having depression alone increases those risks.

Dr. Wayne Goodman, the chairman of the psychiatry department at the University of Florida College of Medicine, and a member of the panel, said they must balance the risks and benefits of treating depression with drugs.

"Nothing in my experience is more tragic than the suicide of a young person," Goodman said. "To think that I prescribed an agent that might have contributed is unbearable. Equally unbearable is to think that I didn't do enough. That's the dilemma before us."

In March, the FDA suggested antidepressant manufacturers strengthen warning labels urging physicians to carefully monitor patients for worsening depression and suicidal thoughts.

The only FDA approved drug for treating kids with depression is Prozac, and most studies show it works. Various other antidepressants, however, are also routinely prescribed to people under age 18. Until recently, many physicians assumed they worked in kids because the drugs are proven effective in adults.

The FDA has struggled with how to handle the matter since it was alerted last year by GlaxoSmithKline (GSK) about clinical trial data that showed a statistically significant increase in so-called suicide-related adverse events in those taking the company's drug Paxil.

Last year, the FDA advised doctors not to prescribe Paxil to anyone younger than age 18.

In March, the FDA suggested antidepressant manufacturers strengthen warning labels urging physicians to carefully monitor patients for worsening depression and suicidal thoughts.

During a congressional hearing last week, officials from Wyeth (WYE), which makes Effexor, and Pfizer, which makes Zoloft, said they tried to strengthen warnings on their drug labels after studies of their drugs in children suggested they didn't work, but said the FDA suggested a more cautious approach.

In 2002, more than 10 million prescriptions were written for antidepressants for use by children,